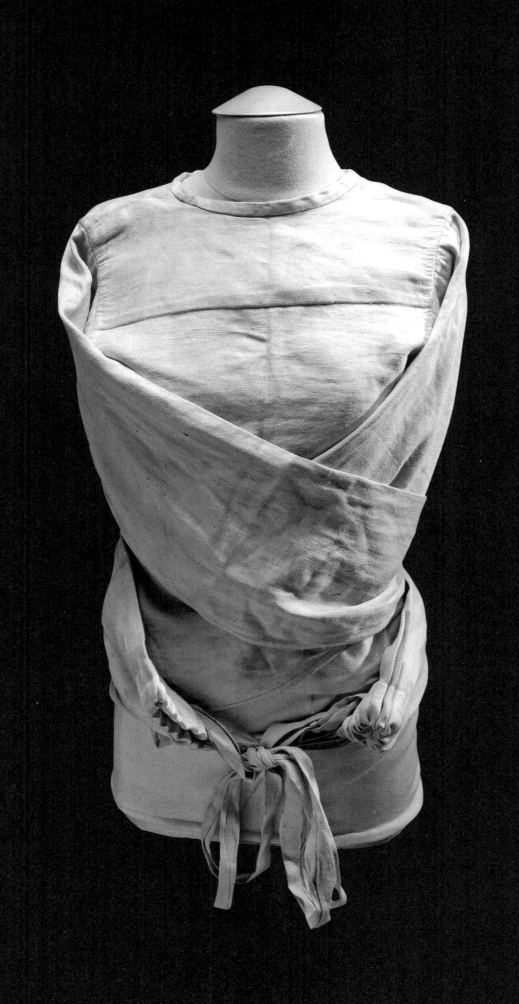

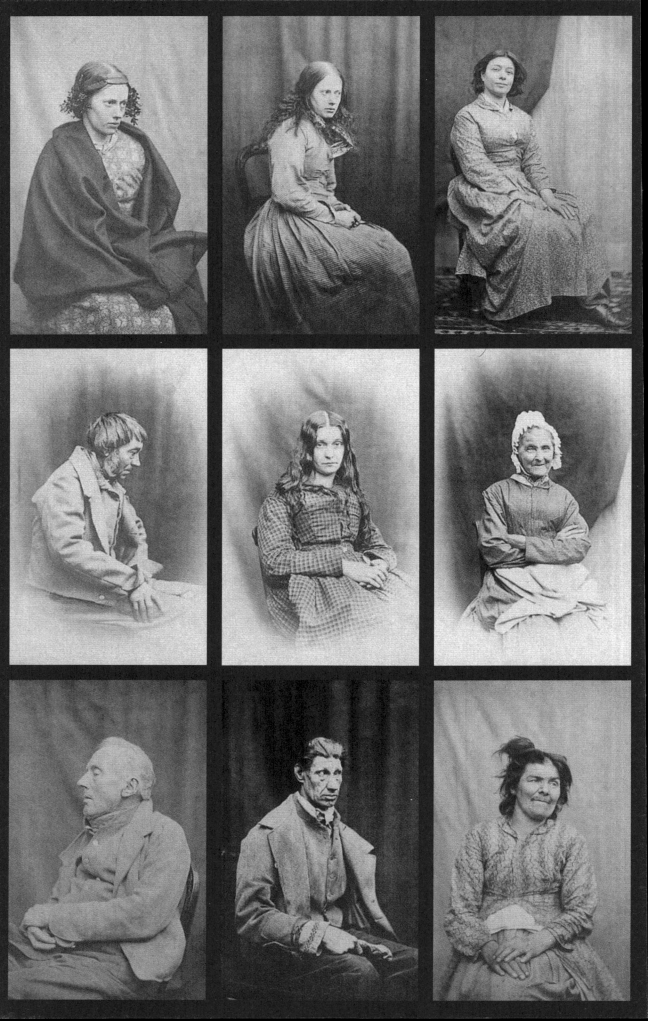

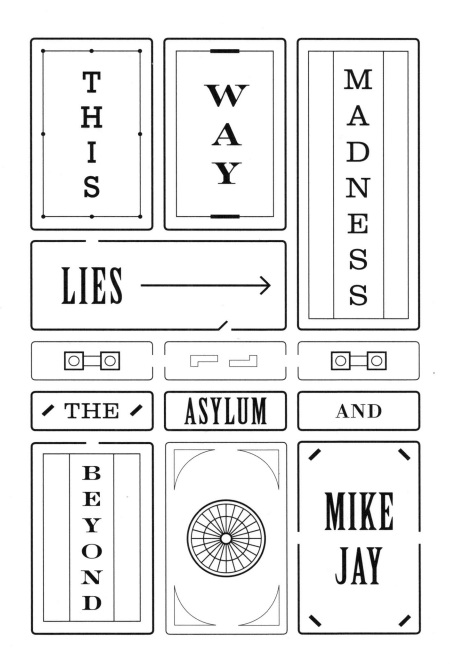

THIS WAY MADNESS LIES THE ASYLUM AND BEYOND

MIKE JAY

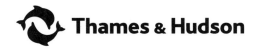
Thames & Hudson

wellcome collection

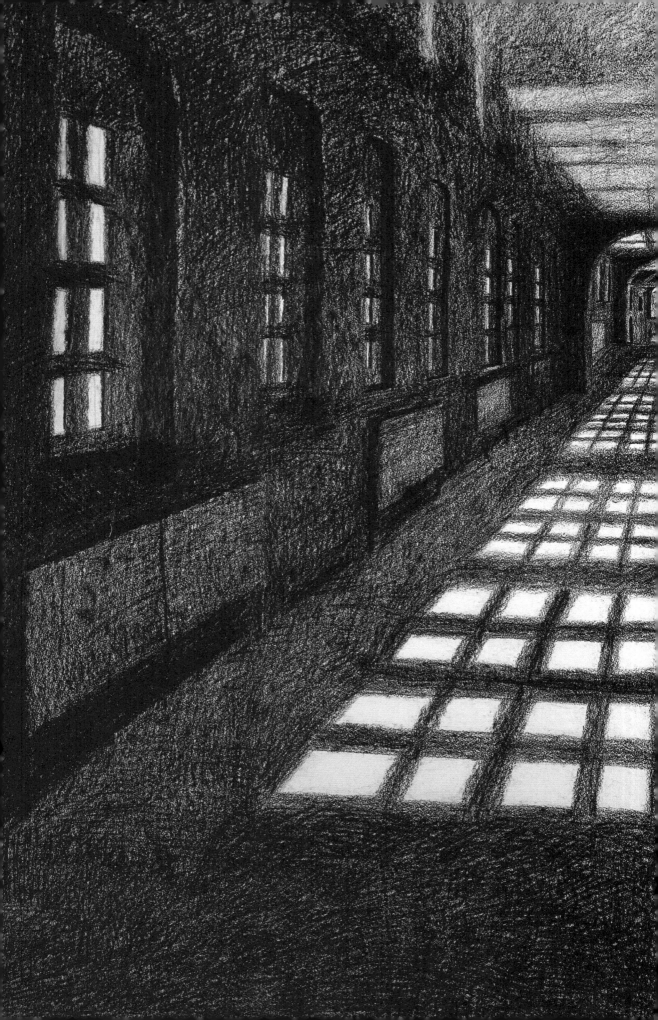

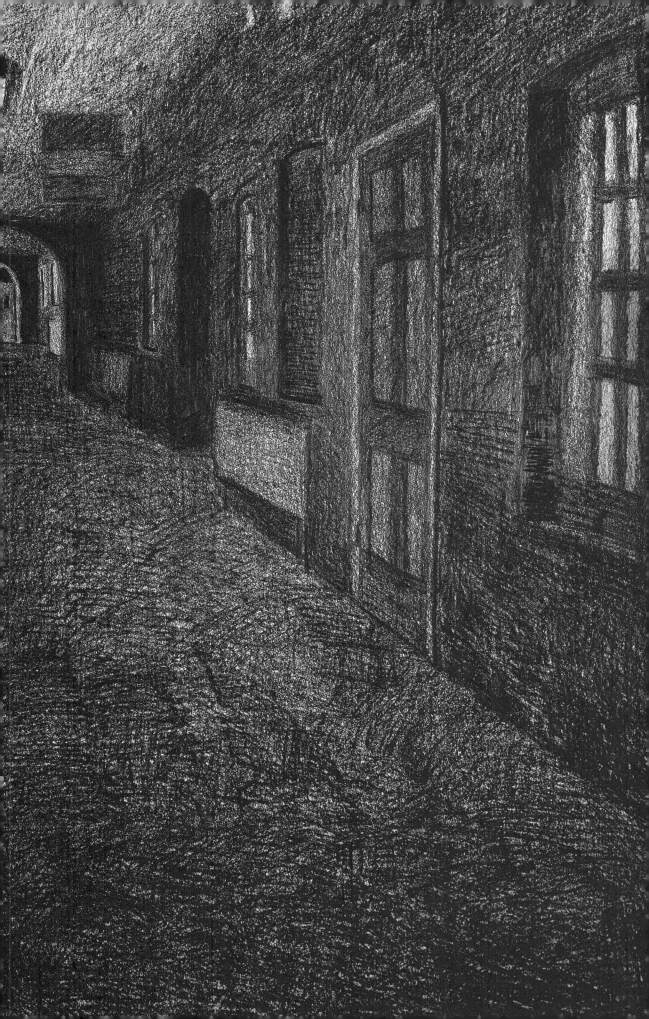

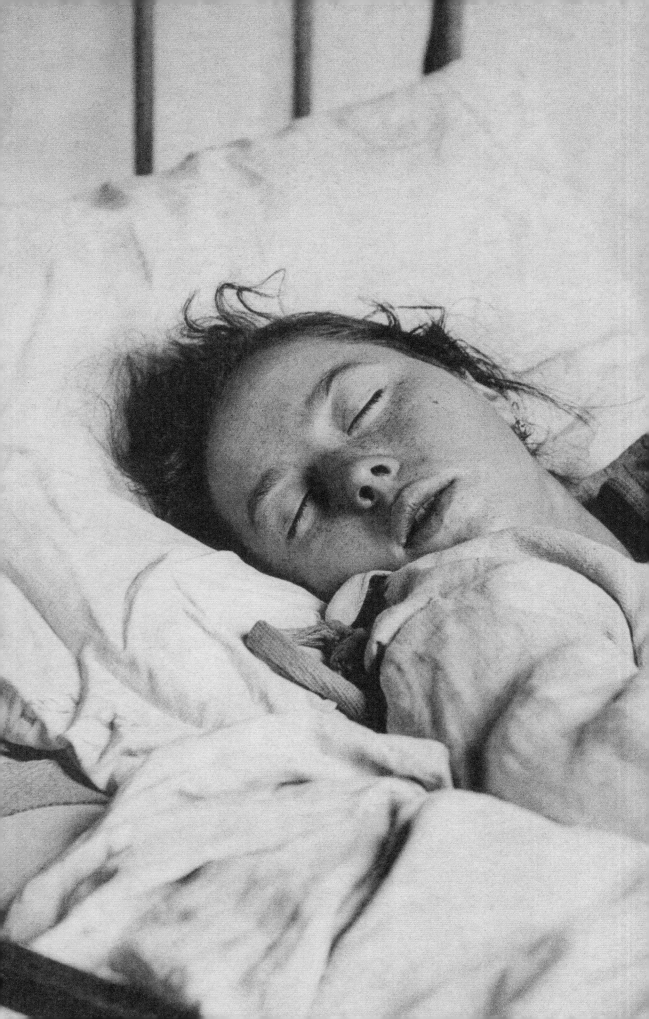

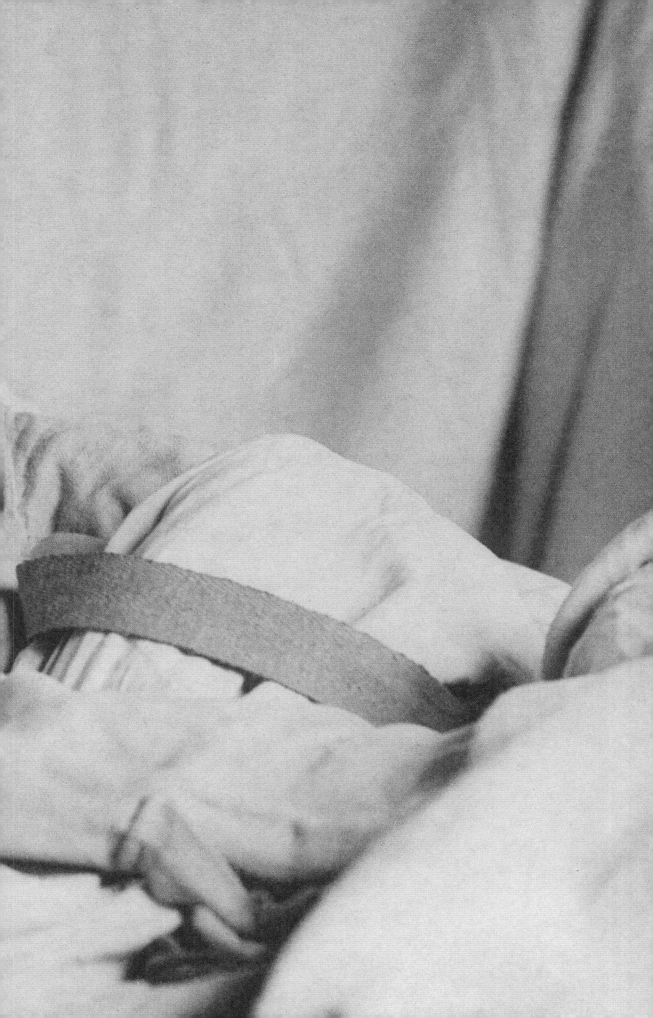

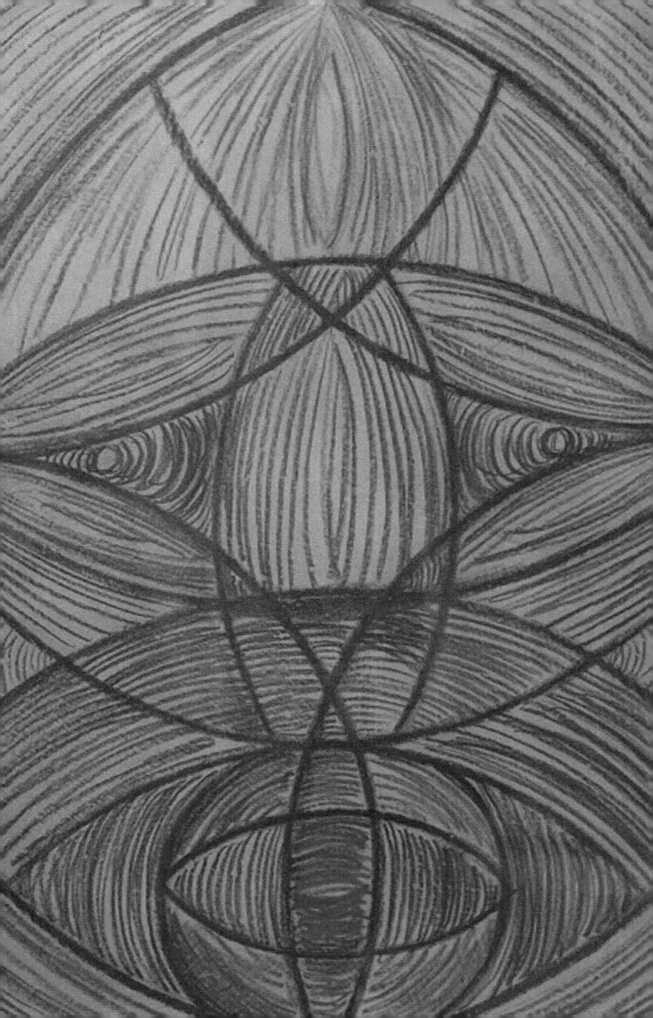

CONTENTS

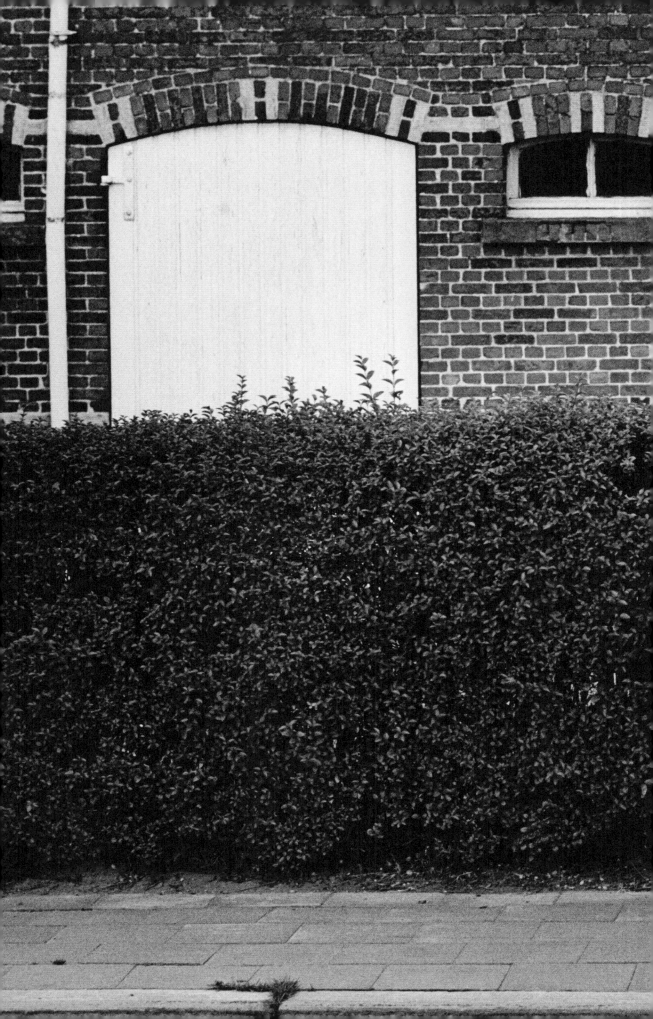

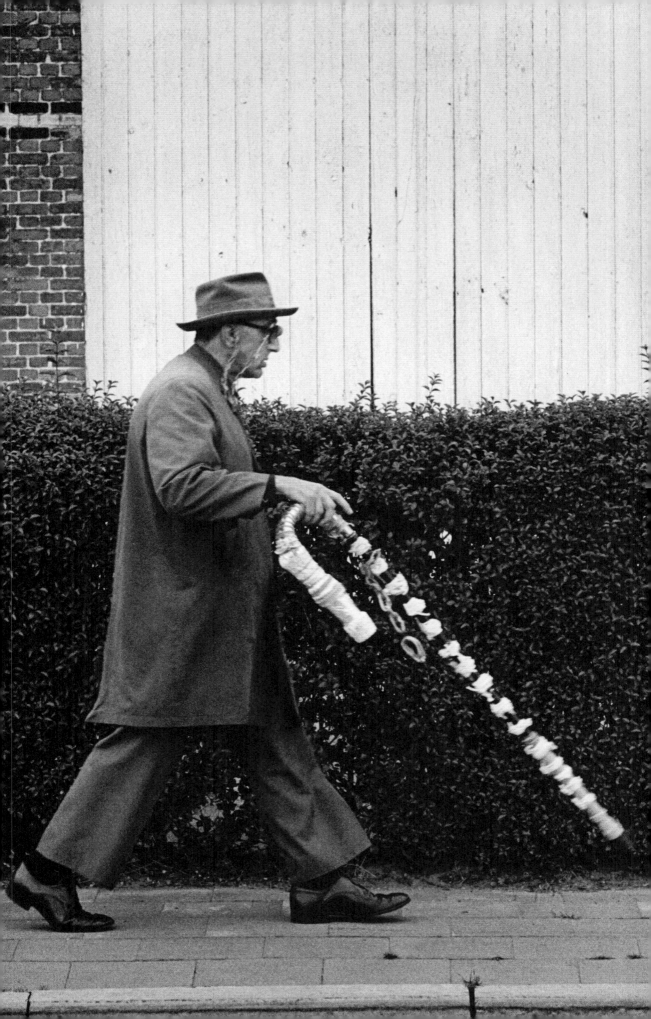

FOREWORD
—· WELLCOME COLLECTION ·—

The two words that recur frequently throughout this book, madness and asylum, carry with them powerful associations and the capacity to evoke vivid images. Published to accompany the Wellcome Collection exhibition "Bedlam: the asylum and beyond", the book traces the history and evolution of both words and their resonance today. Studying the lives and work of patients, artists, doctors and mental health campaigners across the centuries, both book and exhibition look at how we have sought to define and treat mental illness, how it is experienced and how we might come to terms with it in the future. The archival material and images included reflect an emphasis on lived experience and personal perspectives, with the work of artists often bridging artistic and therapeutic practice.

In recent times, one of the most important challenges facing mental health charities has been to raise awareness of just how many of us are affected by mental distress. The charity MIND, for example, estimates that one in four people in the United Kingdom will experience a mental health problem each year (MIND, 2016). Such statistics, as well as a growing concern about the low level of mental health care available to young people, and the rising numbers of older people suffering from dementia, have given renewed urgency to the questions of how, where and by whom affordable support and treatment are best provided. These questions are as old as the concept of 'madness' itself – likewise the tensions that they raise: between protection and restraint, between medical and psychosocial approaches to therapy, and whether to prioritize the creation of safe havens or to concentrate instead on integration into the wider world.

Mike Jay, co-curator of the exhibition and author of this book, examines these issues through the prism of 'Bedlam', the mythical domain of the mad, but also the bricks and mortar institution from which its name derives. The first three sections of the book follow the story of Bethlem Royal Hospital through its three incarnations: the 18th-century 'madhouse', the 19th-century asylum and the 20th-century mental hospital. Through analysis of these emblematic buildings, Jay considers the changing ideas of 'madness' that each generated. The closing section brings the story up to date, acknowledging that while the asylum as an institution is now largely consigned to the past, many of the questions it struggled so hard to address still persist.

Jay points out that in most areas of the history of medical care new knowledge brought new cures. The history of mental health care, however, seems to have been more cyclical. His descriptions of the cycles of abandonment, reform, forgetfulness, neglect and further reform demonstrate the perseverance required of 19th-century pioneers such as Samuel Tuke, a member of the Quaker family that opened the York Retreat, and the French physician Philippe Pinel. The lessons learned from their bold and often compassionate initiatives were all too often ignored in favour of short-term expediency, requiring the next generation to revisit them afresh. These swings

Page 01. Canvas straitjacket for adults, London, 1930–1960.
Page 02. Photographs by Hugh Welch Diamond of patients in Surrey Lunatic Asylum, 1850s.
Page 04–05. Pencil drawing (2004) by Paul Digby. A corridor in High Royds Hospital, Menston, Ilkley, Yorkshire, built in 1888.

JAMES PETO
HEAD OF PUBLIC PROGRAMMES

BÁRBARA RODRÍGUEZ MUÑOZ
CURATOR

of the pendulum reflect how mental illness has been defined and treated throughout history. Understanding the patterns of the past should help us to reassess our current attitudes towards the care of people with mental health issues.

In the popular imagination, 'Bedlam' may have been associated with restraint and isolation, but it originated in the 13th century as a place of refuge. Today, Bethlem Royal is a landscaped, open hospital providing targeted models of care and integration. Parallel to the story of Bethlem, Jay describes the evolution of Geel, Belgium's 'colony of the mad', whose model of providing care not through seclusion but through integration into the daily life of both home and work, can also be traced as far back as the 13th century. Having eventually been absorbed successfully into the Belgian State mental hospital system, Geel has consistently been held up as a beacon of good practice in the field of community care. The evolution and eventual waning of the asylum's dominance was, of course, heavily influenced in more recent times by new therapies emerging from bio-medicine and from the relatively young discipline of psychiatry. Drawing on examples from both northern and southern Europe and the United States, the later pages of the book look at some of the radical initiatives that accompanied these new therapies, as well as the resistance movements led by those who saw them as repressive or counterproductive, such as the Psichiatria Democratica organization, led by Italian psychiatrist Franco Basaglia from the 1960s.

One of the clearest messages to emerge from these international examples of different programmes and ideologies across the centuries is that providing genuine 'asylum' has always been hard work. At both the personal and the institutional level, it demands vigilance, dedication and imagination. This remains the case today in the post-asylum world, where prescription medications coexist with community projects, networked environments, creative therapies and spiritual approaches drawn from around the world. The internet, too, provides the opportunity for social interaction, peer support and treatment through online forums and the possibility of accessing advice and therapies. With that offer, however, comes the danger of an overloaded, confusing and sometimes expensive marketplace, and the risk of missing out on the kinds of direct relationships and personal support that can prove so valuable. In such a complicated environment, how do we ensure that the capacity for support available from family, community and institution is not exhausted?

The Wellcome Collection exhibition closes with a visionary collaborative project led by the artist the vacuum cleaner. Emerging from a series of workshops conducted in mental health settings, 'Madlove' aims to reimagine the original concept of the asylum as 'a safe place to go mad'. This section points to ways in which the notion of the asylum can be re-evaluated – if not as a place, at least as a state of safety, sanctuary and care. We hope that it also provides a context that can help us to negotiate more successfully the crowded landscape of different therapies available today and the continuing arguments about their respective values.

Page 06–07. Female patient diagnosed with 'hysteria-induced narcolepsy'; plate XLV from *Nouvelle iconographie de la Salpêtrière* published by Salpêtrière Hospital, Société de neurologie de Paris, 1889.

Page 08. *The Mask* (*c.* 1919) by Vaslav Nijinsky, pastel on paper (see p.133).

Page 10–11. Photograph from the series *Een gelaat van Geel* (*Faces of Geel*) by Hugo Minnen (1980–1981).

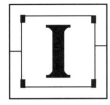**I**t may seem that mental illness has been with us forever, but it took root only around two hundred years ago and is a product of the Western world. Madness, by contrast, has been a part of every culture across the globe since the dawn of humanity. What we now call 'mental illness' encompasses a vast spectrum of conditions and experiences, and it has been obvious since ancient times that some of them have a physical component. At different times and places, this has been understood as possession by demons, an imbalance of humours in the body or a chemical deficit in the brain. However, in other cases there is no obvious physical cause, and the conditions manifest more as social problems than as medical ones: a personality spun out of control, an inability to interact with other people or a struggle to cope with the circumstances of life. Unlike physical diseases, mental illnesses can rarely be diagnosed simply by blood tests or brain scans. The symptoms of modern diagnoses, such as schizophrenia or depression, are all too real, but the biological mechanisms that underlie them are still unclear.

In the majority of fields of modern medicine, the source of an illness can be identified clearly via pathogens or genetic markers; more often than not, these point the way to a pharmaceutical or surgical remedy. Once this level of understanding has been achieved, medical history can be dismissed as little more than a curiosity: infection before antibiotics or surgery before anaesthesia may be rich in drama and period

In *Ship of Fools* (c. 1500) by Hieronymus Bosch, the passengers – indulging their passions – drift towards sin and loss of reason.

detail, but they have little direct relevance to the experience of patients or doctors today. By contrast, mental illness – or madness, as it has been known for most of its long lifetime – remains intimately connected to its past.

The story of psychiatry has had its medical breakthroughs, but it is also defined by repeated pendulum swings and unresolved questions. In recent years, far more attention has been paid to the social factors that are implicated in mental illness: schizophrenia, for example, remains frustratingly elusive in brain scans and gene sequences but has been shown to correlate significantly with childhood abuse, lack of family support, stress and cultural dislocation. Research of this kind is presented as a corrective to the tight biomedical focus that has dominated the field since the 1990s – designated by the US National Institute of Mental Health as the 'decade of the brain' – when it was expected that schizophrenia would soon be tracked back to a neurochemical root cause. This biomedical focus, in turn, emerged as a pushback against the sweeping claims of the mid-century's psychosocial theories, in which schizophrenia was held to be a consequence of rigid cultural norms and emotionally distanced parenting. And these psychosocial theories were a reaction against the biological ideas of heredity and drastic physical treatments espoused by the previous generation: the first generation to call themselves 'psychiatrists', for whom the science of their day offered the only hope of rescuing the legions of 'incurables' that were languishing in Victorian asylums.

INTRODUCTION

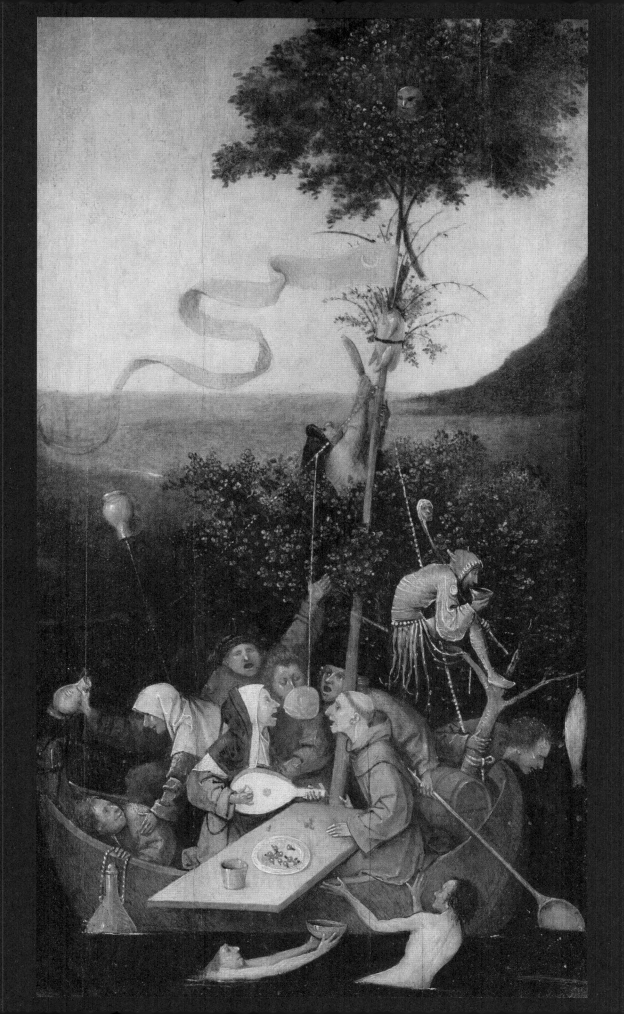

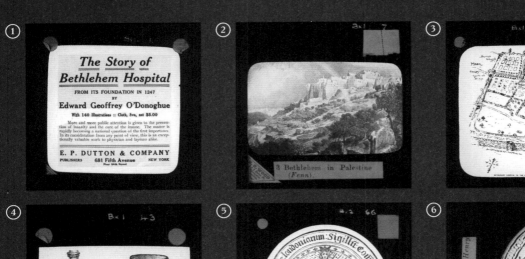
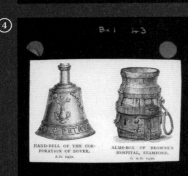
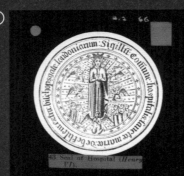
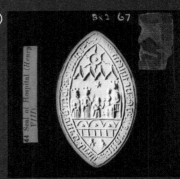
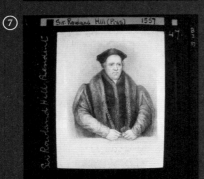
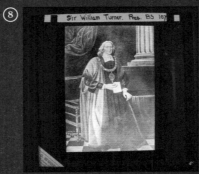
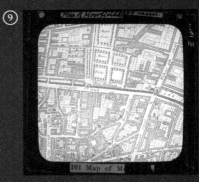
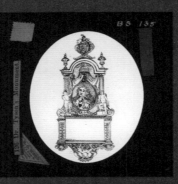
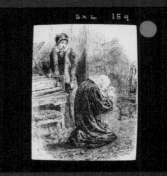
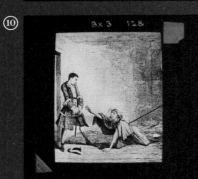
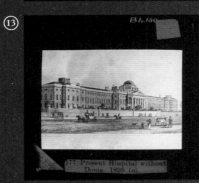
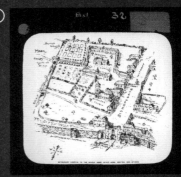
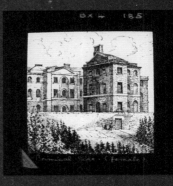
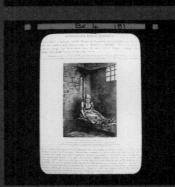

1.
The Story of Bethlehem Hospital
FROM ITS FOUNDATION IN 1247
BY
Edward Geoffrey O'Donoghue
With 140 Illustrations :: Cloth, 8vo, net $5.00

More and more public attention is given to the prevention of insanity and the care of the insane. The matter is rapidly becoming a national question of the first importance. In its consideration from any point of view, this is an exceptionally valuable work to physician and layman alike.

E. P. DUTTON & COMPANY
PUBLISHERS   681 Fifth Avenue   NEW YORK

2. 3 Bethlehem in Palestine (Fenn).

4. Bx1 43
HAND-BELL OF THE COR-PORATION OF DOVER. A.D. 1491.
ALMS-BOX OF BROWNE'S HOSPITAL, STAMFORD. c. A.D. 1470.

5. 43 Seal of Hospital (Henry I).

6. 44 Seal of Hospital (Henry VIII).

7. Sir Rowland Hill (Pres.) 1557

8. Sir William Turner. Pres. B.S. 107

9. 101 Map of M

10. Bx3 128

11. Dr. Tyson's Monument.

12. Bx1 159

13. 177 Present Hospital without Dome. 1825 (a)

14. Bx 4 181

15. Bx 4 185

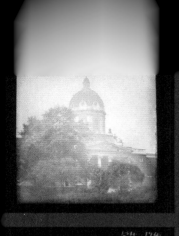

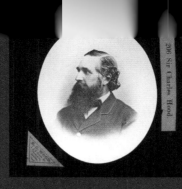

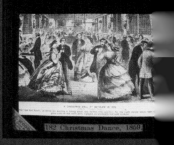

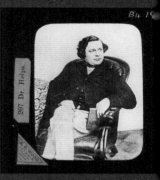

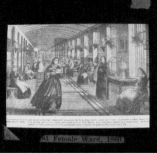

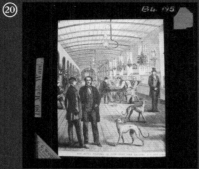

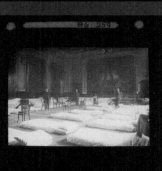

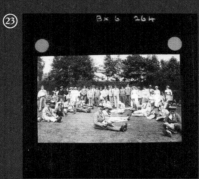

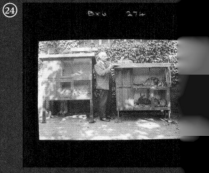

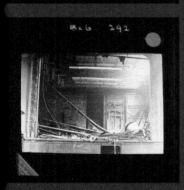

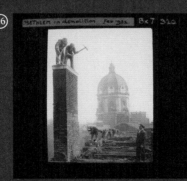

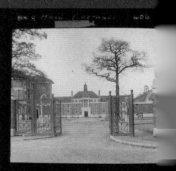

...cenes from the story of Bethlem hospital.

- Lantern slides assembled by Bethlem's chaplain in 1905
- Church of St Mary at Bethlehem
- Bethlem's first site at Bishopsgate
- Hand bell and alms box, 1491
- Bethlem's seal, reign of Henry VII
- Warden's seal, reign of Henry VIII
- Rowland Hill, Bethlem's president, 1557
- William Turner, president, 1669–1693
- Moorfields, London, 17th century

10. Highwayman Jack Sheppard visits his mother in Bethlem
11. Memorial to Edward Tyson, Bethlem physician, 1684–1708
12. George III kneeling at prayer
13. Bethlem at St George's Fields, Southwark
14. James Norris in chains, 1814
15. Female criminal lunatic wing, Southwark
16. Dome of Bethlem at Southwark
17. Charles Hood, superintendent, 1852–1862

18. Patient's dance at Bethlem, 1859
19. Female ward at Southwark, 1860
20. Male ward at Southwark, 1860
21. William Helps, physician, 1862–1865
22. Temporary dormitory after bombing, 1917
23. Wounded Soldiers' Day, Bethlem, 191[6]
24. Raising rabbits in captivity for food during World War 1
25. Fire-damaged recreation room, 1924
26. Demolishing Bethlem at Southwark, 1932
27. Bethlem at Beckenham, 1930

The Hospital of Bethlem at Moorfields, with visitors promenading in the grounds. Engraving after Robert Hooke, 1676.

These pendulum swings in medical opinion only lead us back into the shallow waters of history. Doctors have always had a place in the debates about madness, but it is only recently that we have come to view mental illness primarily in medical terms. Psychiatry was accepted as a proper branch of medicine only after a long struggle, both with the rest of the medical establishment and with society at large. The profession that defined mental illness originally was not medicine but the law, in which for centuries questions of guilt and mitigation have turned on concepts such as *compos mentis* (of sound mind), *mens rea* (guilty mind) and diminished responsibility. The legal term coined for it – 'insanity' – remains in common use today.

Yet the fundamental questions about madness predate both modern medicine and the law. Is it at root an illness of the body, or a disturbance of the mind? Or, to use the language of the deeper past, a sickness of the soul? Can it be treated in isolation like physical diseases, or does genuine healing need to involve the whole person? Should sufferers be encouraged to focus inwards and explore the roots of their distress, or outwards to distract them from it and allow them to forge a new life? Should they be kept secluded from society, which so often seems to be the cause of the illness, or is the solution to be found by integrating them more fully into it?

This last question has been the most crucial in shaping our modern story. It gave rise to the asylum, the institution that came to define madness and its treatment in the Western world. In its earliest form, the asylum promised sanctuary from the 'madding crowd' and religious consolation for the troubled soul. As modern ideas of therapy emerged and the state expanded its responsibilities, proponents of the asylum promised to turn it into a place of healing and cure. Gradually, the medical profession, with its promise that mental disorders were treatable diseases of the brain, assumed this role.

Each of these promises recreated the asylum in a new form that reflected the changing world around it. However, all of them remained unfulfilled, and by the time each had run its course

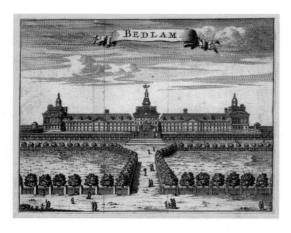

madness seemed to be more intractable than before. Every incarnation of the asylum followed the same trajectory: founded in an optimistic spirit of humanitarian reform and finally abandoned as a shaming reminder of a bygone era. In each case, the reason was the same: the confident promises on which the asylums were founded failed to materialize. None of them discovered a cure for madness, but we can recognize with hindsight that each contributed at least a grain of therapeutic truth. Their ideals and insights, as well as the inspiring and revolutionary figures who embodied them, formed the landscape of mental health today.

The arc of this story can be traced through a single institution: the Bethlem Royal Hospital in London, popularly known as 'Bedlam'. For centuries, Bedlam has been ingrained in the English language as the proverbial domain of the mad, but it is also a real hospital that still offers residential mental health care today. Over the centuries, it has occupied a succession of buildings that encapsulate the three ages of the asylum, and the views of madness that each represented.

During the 18th century, Bethlem was the archetypal madhouse: one of London's most famous landmarks and the subject of dozens of poems, plays, ballads and artworks in which it became the mythical home of madness itself. During the 19th century, it relocated to a new building: an archetypal Victorian asylum looming over the slums and factories on the south bank of the Thames. By then it was one among hundreds of asylums across Europe and the United States, the flowering of a humane and progressive movement that gradually gave way to despair as it struggled to cope with a rising tide of insanity. During the early 20th century, Bethlem moved to a modern site: a typical mental hospital, one among

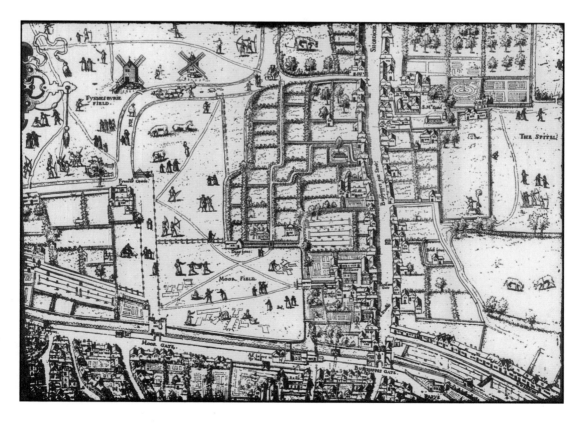

thousands across the globe, this time hidden away in London's leafy suburbs and dedicated to treating madness as a disease of the mind, utilizing the latest discoveries in medical science.

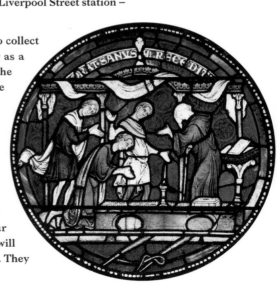

By the time of Bethlem's final incarnation, 'Bedlam' had become shorthand for all the cruelties – whips, chains, dungeons and straitjackets – that had been visited on the unfortunates of previous eras. However, the optimistic new therapies of the early 20th century, such as unmodified electroconvulsive therapy and lobotomy, have now been added to the list of past barbarities. When we recall scenes from Bedlam, it is usually to conjure the darkness of the past and to contrast it implicitly with our own enlightened modernity. But it would be rash to assume that the bleakest scenes of the 21st century – service users reduced by medication to obese zombies, or pushing abandoned shopping trolleys through blighted urban landscapes – will look any better to future generations. The dark mirror of Bedlam still reflects our world.

The true history of Bethlem hospital is another story. It begins in the 13th century, when it was founded by a London alderman named Simon FitzMary. The legend goes that while fighting in the Crusades he became detached from his party and found himself wandering alone in the desert at night, lost behind Saracen lines. Casting around helplessly in the darkness of the Holy Land, he saw a fixed point: a bright star over Bethlehem, which he followed to safety. On his return to London, he gave thanks for his salvation by founding a priory on his land at St Botolph without Bishopsgate – more or less the area now occupied by Liverpool Street station – dedicated to St Mary of Bethlehem.

The main function of the priory was to collect alms, but by 1400 it was also serving as a hospital, in the medieval sense of the word preserved in 'hospitality': a refuge for strangers in need, with no medical care implied. It housed a small number of charitable cases, including the old and infirm, but gradually began to specialize in those referred to as 'distracted', 'madde' or 'lunaticke'. These terms are difficult to translate, as our modern diagnoses probably will be for historians of the future. They were applied to those who were violent or delusional, or who had lost their reason, memory or speech; these included some whom we would now consider to be suffering from physical disorders, such as epilepsy or brain injury.

Madness could be interpreted in various ways. Some believed that its sufferers were tormented by demons; others saw them as victims of circumstance who had temporarily lost their reason through hardship or tragedy, or as sinners who had succumbed to pride and indulged their passions to self-destruction. It is hard to recover a clear sense of how they saw themselves. The best-documented case is that of Margery Kempe, who lived in Norfolk and between 1436 and 1438 dictated to a priest the first female autobiography. Many commentators have found in it evidence for what we would now diagnose as mental illness. After the birth of her first child she became deeply disturbed: hearing voices and falling into visions, attacking those around her and harming herself until she was physically restrained. Yet Kempe saw her experience in spiritual terms, as a punishment for her pride and vanity and a series of temptations by the Devil. She did penance and prayed, attracted followers, went on pilgrimage to the Holy Land and Rome, and is today venerated by the Church of England. If she suffered from post-natal depression or psychosis, she seems to have succeeded in turning it into a gift from God.

The stained glass in the Trinity Chapel of Canterbury Cathedral depicts the suffering of 'Mad Matilda of Cologne'.

Those deemed 'mad' were many and various, and they were only loosely distinguished from a wider cohort that included vagrants, beggars, petty criminals and the physically handicapped: those on the fringes of society, without family or resources to support themselves. It was in the courts of law that madness gradually took on a specific meaning. Under Britain's Anglo-Saxon laws, everyone had been straightforwardly liable for their actions, but the canon law introduced by the Normans included the idea of moral guilt, which considered the intentions and mental state of the perpetrator. The 13th-century jurist Henry de Bracton, who formalized the growing body of British law, stressed the importance of intention and formalized the concept of *mens rea*. From this it followed, in Bracton's words, that 'a madman is not liable'.[1] Madness, from this point onwards, was a legal concept that excused responsibility in some contexts but limited basic rights in others. The law was refined to make a distinction between 'natural fools' – those with congenital learning difficulties – and those suffering from madness, which might be periodic or temporary. The property of a madman, for example, was held in trust until such time as he might recover, whereas that of a fool

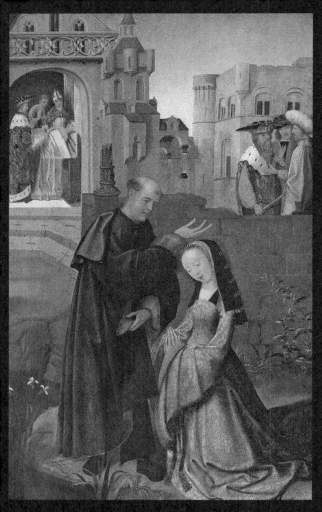

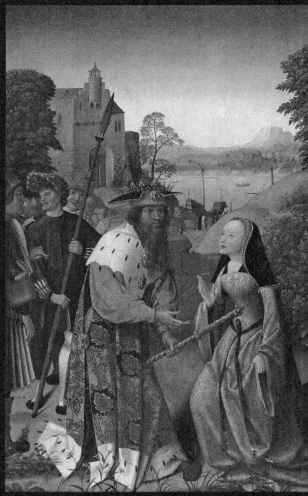

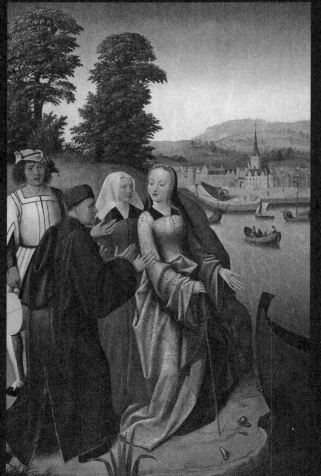

The legend of St Dymphna's martyrdom is depicted in Goswijn van der Weyden's series of panels, painted in Antwerp in 1505 and originally hung in the Abbey of Tongerlo near Geel.

The first of the *Seven Scenes from the Life and Veneration of St Dymphna* depicts her baptism by Gerebernus.

Dymphna's father, Damon the king of Oriel, tells his daughter of his misguided intention to wed her.

Accompanied by her retinue, Dymphna embarks on a journey to Belgium, where she hides in the town of Geel.

After it is discovered that Dymphna has fled the castle, the king's soldiers are sent out in search of her.

A faithful emissary reports to the king that his daughter has been discovered living in Geel in Flanders.

In a rage, the king kills the priest and his daughter. The residents collect their remains and return them to the town.

The body of fifteen-year-old Dymphna is laid to rest in Geel, where a church is later built in her memory.

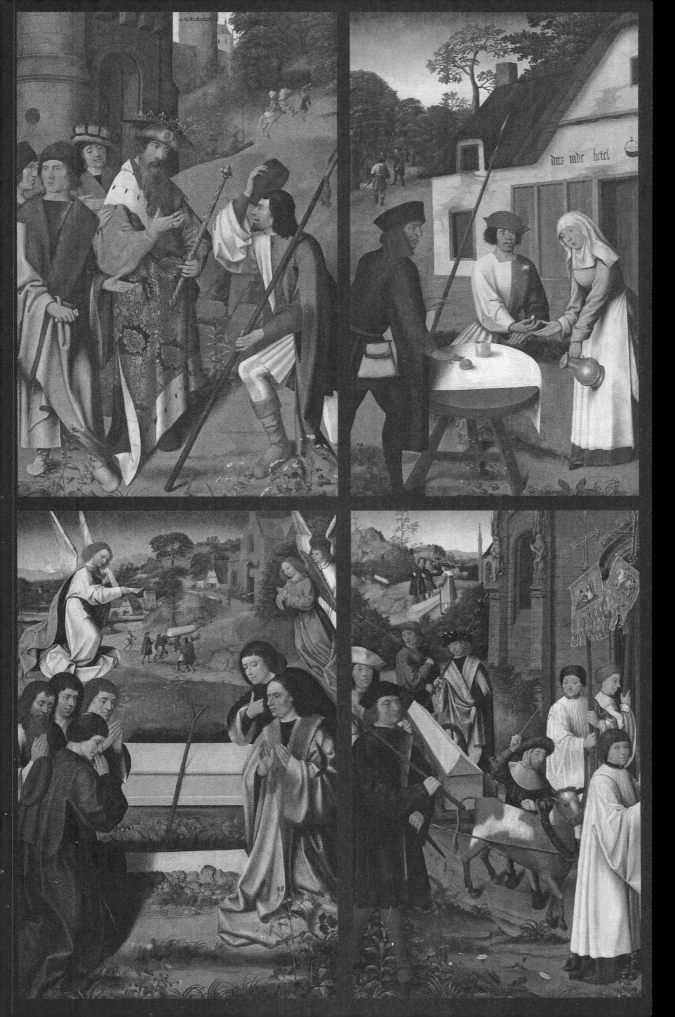

Dancers in Molenbeek (1592) by Pieter van Breughel. Those suffering from dancing mania were often led on curative pilgrimages.

became the property of the Crown. The term 'insanity' is first recorded in a legal source: 'madfolkes and lunaticke persons,' writes the ecclesiastical lawyer Henry Swinburne in 1590, 'during the time of their furor or insanitie of mind, cannot make a testament.'[2] It was only at this point that the modern concept of sanity emerged as the opposite of madness. Prior to this, sanity had referred to general health, but insanity gave it a more specific meaning, matching the legal term *compos mentis*. In this sense, it was the mad who defined the sane, not vice versa.

Bethlem was one of a handful of refuges that emerged across medieval Europe. Another that has endured is the town of Geel in Flanders, whose story begins, like that of Bethlem, in the 13th century and whose origin is similarly preserved in legend, in this case that of St Dymphna. Dymphna was a 7th-century Irish princess, whose father went mad with grief after the death of his wife and attempted to claim his daughter in marriage. In order to escape his incestuous passion, Dymphna fled to Europe and hid in the marshy flatlands of Flanders. Her father finally tracked her down in Geel and, when she refused him once more, beheaded her.

Over time, Dymphna became revered as a saint with powers of intercession for the mentally afflicted, and her shrine attracted tales of miraculous cures. Geel became a place of pilgrimage where, as at Bethlem, families could bring their distracted relatives for shelter and religious consolation. However, while Bethlem became an asylum, Geel took the opposite path. Those for whom the pilgrimage to St Dymphna brought no relief were often abandoned

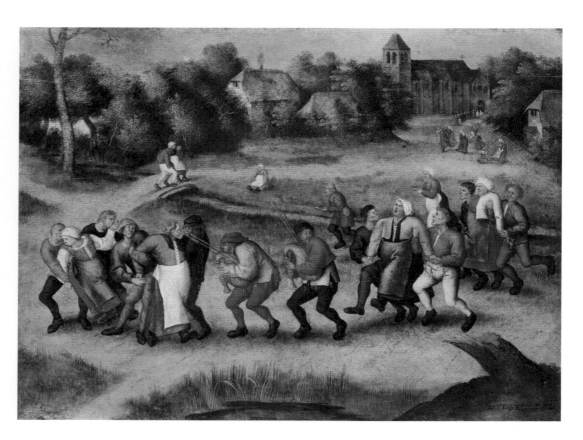

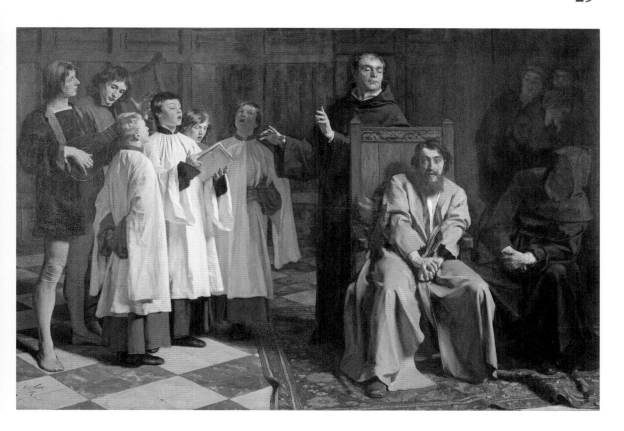

in her church. In 1480 a cloister was added to accommodate them, but it soon overflowed and local farmers began to take in the pilgrims, offering them board and lodging in their homes and putting them to work alongside their families. Over the centuries, Geel became widely known as a 'colony of the mad': an alternative to the asylum, where the mentally distracted were integrated into normal life rather than secluded from it. Geel, like Bethlem, still fulfils its ancient role today, and their stories illustrate how their contrasting approaches have fared over the centuries.

«GEEL BECAME KNOWN AS A 'COLONY OF THE MAD'»

By the time of Shakespeare, Bethlem was no longer a peaceful cloister. Its precincts had filled up with cell blocks, keepers' residences and rented accommodation; it was crowded and noisy, and a well-known landmark in what had become a teeming slum neighbourhood. Its mad folk had long been a familiar presence for Londoners, particularly through the tradition of plaintive 'Bedlam ballads' sung by itinerant musicians. However, it was the theatre that immortalized the asylum in popular culture. In the revenge tragedies and raucous satires of Jacobean drama, we witness Bethlem assuming its archetypal status: any madhouse could now be referred to as 'a Bedlam'. However, it also acquired a more expansive play of meanings, which extended beyond the madhouse.

The Madness of Hugo van der Goes (1872) by Emile Wauters. The Flemish artist entered a monastery to save his soul from damnation.

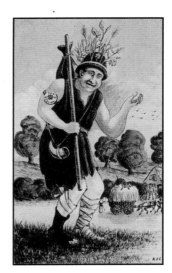

In the very early 17th century, 'Bedlam scenes' made a rapid transit from novelty to cliché. Characters visit Bedlam in Thomas Dekker and Thomas Middleton's *The Honest Whore, Part 1* (1604), and also in Dekker and John Webster's *Northward Ho* (1607). Webster parades the denizens of a madhouse in *The Duchess of Malfi* (1613/14), and in Thomas Middleton and William Rowley's *The Changeling* (1622) two characters impersonate madmen in an attempt to seduce a madhouse keeper's wife. Bedlam scenes were presented frequently as masques, dream-like pageants in which the inmates illustrated the variety of forms that madness could take. They were scenes in which extravagant lunacy was performed for entertainment, but also looking-glass worlds in which the rules of reality were suspended and the madness of modern society reflected.

Bedlam took on a mythic life of its own, bearing ever less resemblance to the real hospital on which it was based but reflecting an era in which madness was a source of popular fascination. A vocabulary had evolved, both in physicians' writings and in common speech, to distinguish between its varied forms. The minority in whom the condition was violent were often referred to as 'stark Bedlam mad': they were possessed by a fury or mania that made them commit acts that usually would be regarded as criminal, but in their case were senseless and self-destructive. These were the people who were most likely to be locked up for their own safety and for the public good. Then there were those who were 'distracted' or 'light-headed', who talked nonsensically or were gripped by some religious vision: this condition was regarded more often as a form of physical disease, analogous to the delusional babbling of a fever. And there were also the 'mopish', who were withdrawn and unable to engage with those around them: they were seen as troubled or 'not well in their wits'.

The condition that resonated most with the spirit of the age, however, was melancholy. This was a complex and troubling illness, believed to be physical in origin (an excess of black bile) but at the same time a malaise of the soul. The modern world seemed designed to incubate it – or, perhaps, the fashion for it allowed old forms of mental distress to be acted out in new and dramatic ways. In astrological terms, the melancholic were saturnine, under the influence of Saturn; in politics, they might become that dangerous type, the malcontent. Melancholy's symptoms overlapped to some extent with what today would be diagnosed as depression but also included violent fits and delusions: obsessions, hauntings, paranoid fantasies and visions of Satan. In its

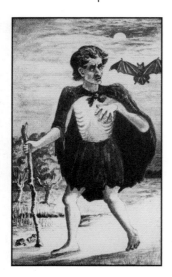

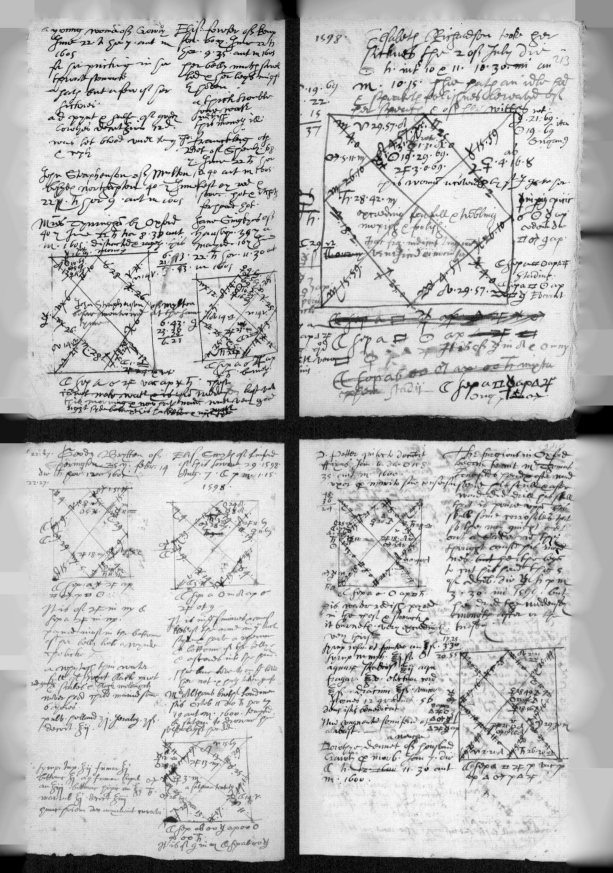

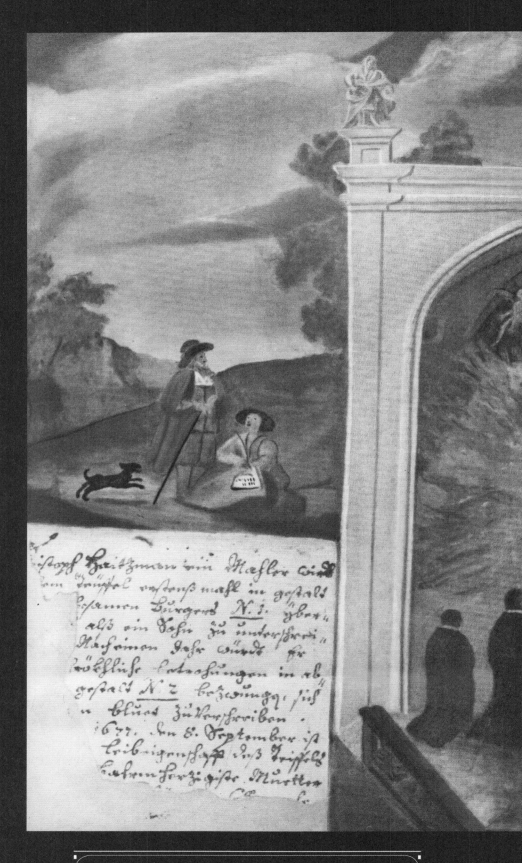

In 1677 Austrian painter Christoph Haizmann depicted his demonic possession in a series of tableaux. His case was studied by Sigmund Freud and has been identified by some psychiatrists as schizophrenia.

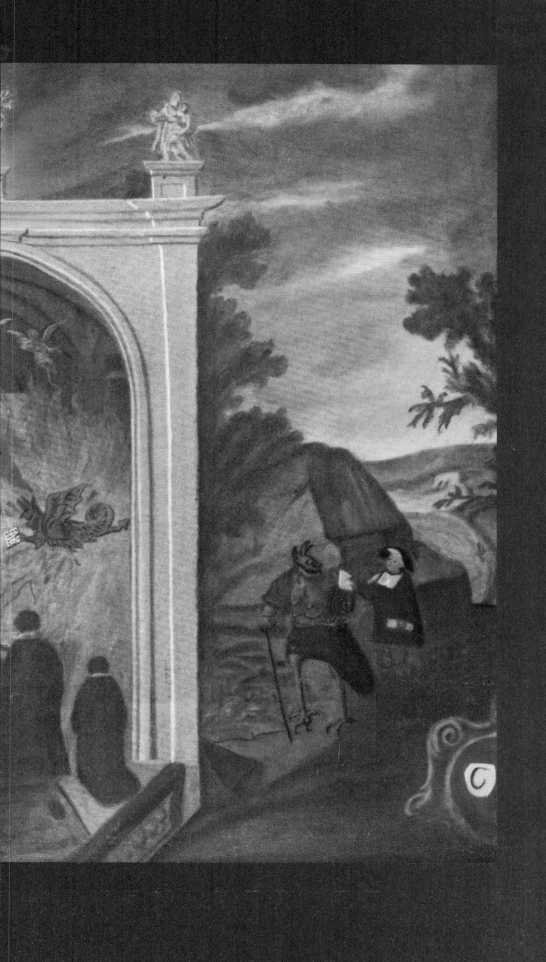

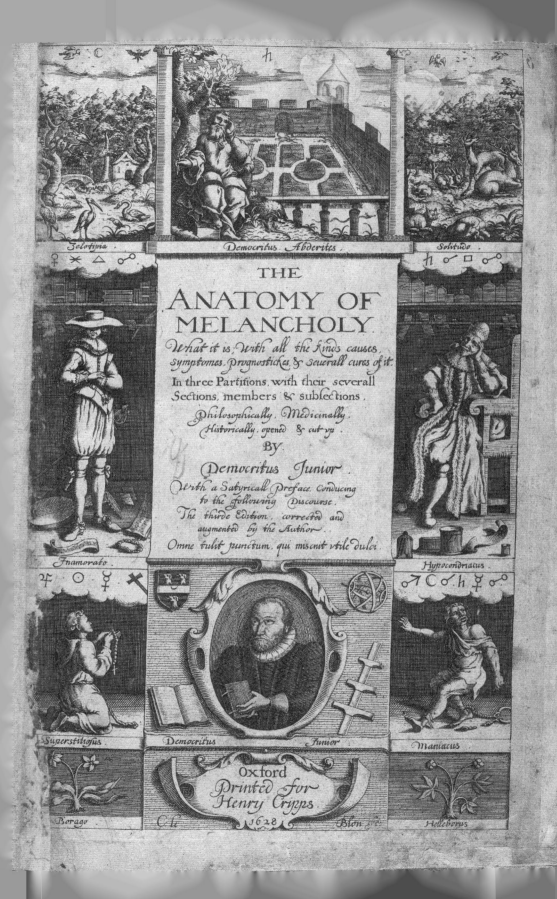

Zelotypia.

Democritus Abderites.

Solitudo.

Enamorato.

THE
ANATOMY OF
MELANCHOLY.

What it is. With all the kinds causes,
symptomes, Prognostickes, & seuerall cures of it.

In three Partitions, with their seuerall
Sections, members & subsections.

Philosophically, Medicinally,
Historically, opened & cut vp.

BY.

Democritus Junior.

With a Satyricall Preface, conducing
to the following Discourse.

The thirde Edition, corrected and
augmented by the Author.

Omne tulit punctum, qui miscuit vtile dulci.

Hypocondriacus.

Superstitiosus.

Democritus   Junior.

Maniacus.

Oxford
Printed for
Henry Cripps.
1628.

Borago.

Helleborus.

milder forms, it was a fashionable condition for brooding intellectuals, an existential alienation from mundane life, or a sign of seriousness and depth of character. But it was foolish to toy with it: the line between emotional sensitivity and madness was easy to cross.

The classic literary treatment of the subject is *The Anatomy of Melancholy*, the life's work of vicar Robert Burton, first published in 1621. It was a vast compendium of everything that had been said, from classical antiquity to the present, on the subject of melancholy's causes, symptoms and remedies. 'All the world is melancholy,' Burton wrote, 'I write of melancholy, by being busy to avoid melancholy.' He considered its source to be a humoral (today we would say chemical) imbalance, which produced symptoms that spanned the mental, psychological and spiritual. Melancholy might have physical causes, such as disease or heredity, but it was often provoked by the stresses of life – love, overwork, childbirth – or the corrosive effect of passions such as envy and pride. It was more than an illness: Burton saw melancholy as intimately linked to artistic and intellectual genius, and an inescapable part of life.

Madness also became a sign of the times because of changes in the law. The Poor Relief Act of 1601 consigned able-bodied paupers to workhouses, but obliged parishes to care for lunatics. As a result, some beggars took to feigning madness: ragged Tom o' Bedlams or Abraham-men, as they were known, were a familiar sight, and Bethlem was obliged to issue disclaimers that begging was not authorized by the hospital. Madness became a performance characterized by a stereotyped repertoire of puns, riddles, ditties and insults, elaborated by the stage fools and identity-swap plots of the theatre, recycled by wits and beggars on the street, and adopted in theatrical form by the mad folk themselves. The question of how to tell the real lunatic from the fake fed into broader themes of the age: the proliferation of spies and double agents, the need to dissemble in times of shifting religious loyalties, and the delicate line between the public and the private self.

Many of the great dramas of the age turned on questions of madness, including all of Shakespeare's major tragedies. In *Othello* it is the fruit of jealousy, in *Macbeth* the ruthless pursuit of power, and in *King Lear* its arrogant exercise. Hamlet pointedly satirizes the fashion for madness and explores the paradoxes opened up by attempting to distinguish its performance from its reality. In his opening soliloquy, Hamlet announces his deception to the audience: he will

Frontispiece to a 1638 edition of Robert Burton's *The Anatomy of Melancholy*: the classic compendium of causes, symptoms and remedies.

Etching by J. D. Nessenthaler, c. 1750. The mythological figures around the scholar represent the melancholy temperament.

«MADNESS BECAME A SIGN OF THE TIMES.»

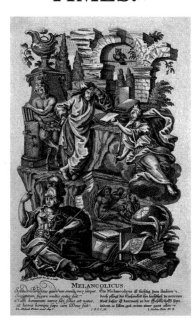

MELANCOLICUS.

'put an antic disposition on'. He proceeds to convince others of his lunacy, and by the end himself, too: before his climactic duel with Laertes, he makes the seemingly heartfelt confession that 'his madness is poor Hamlet's enemy'. Has it all been an act, or has he been deceiving himself that he is sane? Is Polonius right to suspect that 'though this be madness, yet there is method in't?'

Madness was the perfect subject for exposing the tricks that the mind plays on itself: as Sigmund Freud would acknowledge, 'The poets and philosophers before me discovered the unconscious.'[3] In *Don Quixote*, Miguel de Cervantes presents us with an accidental fake: someone who converts play-acting into full-blown madness without realizing he has done so. Quixote is, in conventional moral terms, undone by the sin of pride: his indulgence in the fantasies of chivalry and his obsession with bringing it back to life lead him into a delusional world, a hall of mirrors in which his vanity is reflected endlessly. He becomes grandiose and paranoid, creating a comedy of errors as he misreads situations and sees glory or persecution everywhere. Yet the way in which he banishes his doubts and pursues his dream is noble, even heroic, and his final repentance and return to sanity are tragic – a disenchantment of the world.

These ambivalent and ironic dramas caught the spirit of a rapidly modernizing age that was trying to define madness more tightly but finding the line that separated it from sanity impossible to fix. Plays, songs and riddles undermined the brittle certainties of lawyers and physicians; the theatre and the novel created alternate worlds in which the mad and the sane stepped casually into one another's shoes. The world had become, in a phrase that echoed through popular tracts and poems of the 17th century, 'a great Bedlam'. According to the title of Middleton's anarchic comedy of London life, first performed in 1605, this was *A Mad World, My Masters*; anyone who wishes to succeed in it, argues a character in John Ford's play *The Lover's Melancholy* (1628), 'must learn to be a madman or a fool'. As for those who were confined in Bedlam, who was to say whether they were truly mad or merely pretending – or, perhaps, saner than the rest of us? As Vindice, the revenger in disguise, asks in Middleton's *The Revenger's Tragedy* (1606):

'Surely we're all mad people, and they,
Whom we think are, are not.'

Thus, the stage was set for a new kind of institution, in which the drama of madness and the modern world would be performed in three acts.

The Cure of Folly (Extraction of the Stone of Madness, 1475–1480), a satire on medieval quack cures, by Hieronymus Bosch.

Frontispieces and illustrations from original editions of Cervantes's *The History of Don-Quixote*, volume 1 and volume 2.

Next page: 'Doctor Panurgus', by Martin Droeshout, *c.* 1620. Fantasies are distilled from the brain with chemical medicines.

---

1   Henry de Bracton, Thorne edition (Harvard, 1968–77), Volume 2, p. 424
2   Henry Swinburne, *A Treatise of Testaments and Last Wills*, Part 2 (Dublin: 1793)
3   Lionel Trilling, 'Freud and Literature' in *The Liberal Imagination* (1950) p. 34

VIDA Y HECHOS
Del Ingenioso Cavallero
DON QUIXOTE
DE LA MANCHA,
COMPUESTA
Por Miguel de Cervantes Saavedra.
PARTE PRIMERA.

Nueva Edicion, corregida y ilustrada con differentes Estampas muy donosas y apropriadas à la materia.

EN BRUSELAS,
De la Empresa de Juan Mommarte, Impresor jurado. Año 1662.
Con Licencia y Privilegio.

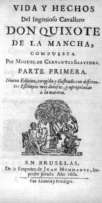
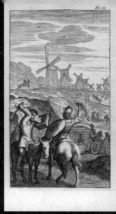
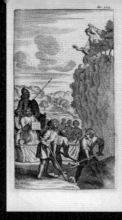
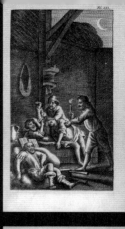

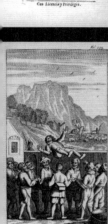
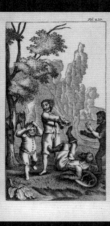
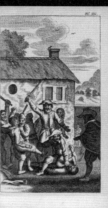
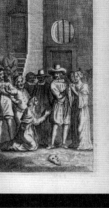

VIDA Y HECHOS
Del Ingenioso Cavallero
DON QUIXOTE
DE LA MANCHA,
COMPUESTA
Por Miguel de Cervantes Saavedra,
PARTE SEGUNDA.

Nueva Edicion, corregida y ilustrada con differentes Estampas muy donosas; y apropriadas à la materia.

EN BRUSELAS,
De la Empresa de Juan Mommarte, Impresor jurado. Año 1662.
Con Licencia y Privilegio.

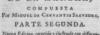
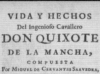

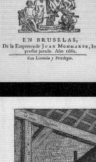
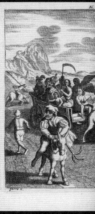
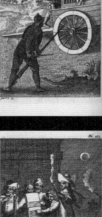
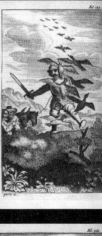

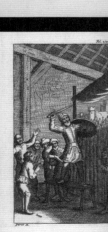
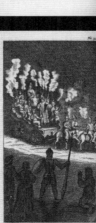
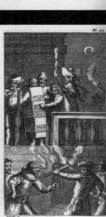
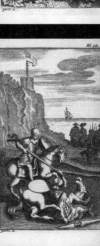

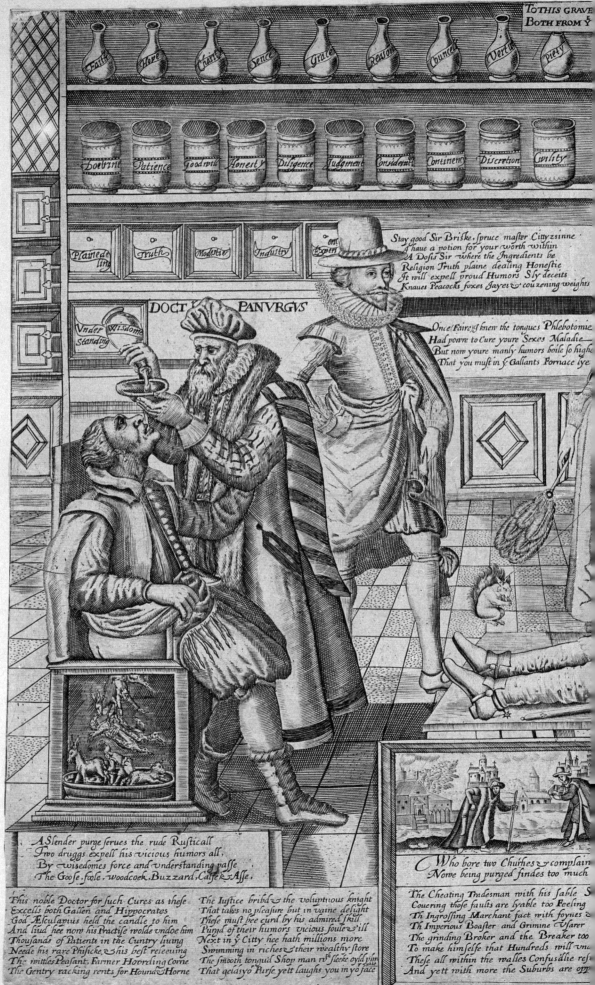

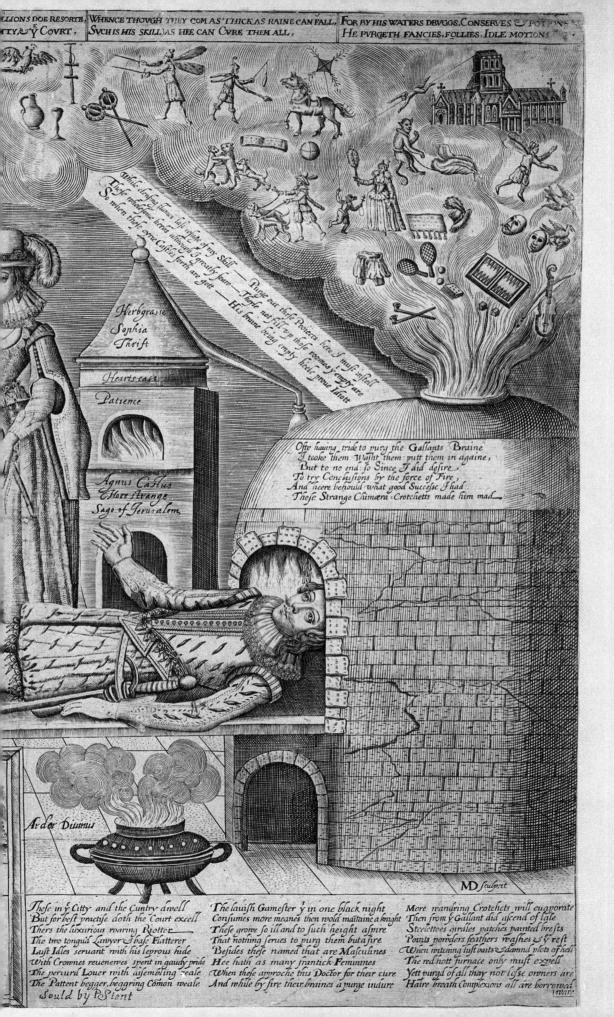

While dreffing thinges laft spake of my skill
Thefe wholefome herbs although I greatly feare
So when thefe evill Caftes forth are gott —
Purge out thefe Proiers here I muft myfelf
Thefe not fill up thofe roomes y empty are
His braine being empty heele proue Ifott

Herbgrasse
Sophia
Thrift

Hearts ease
Patience

Agnus Castus
Hore strange
Sage of Ierusalem

Ofte hauing tride to purg the Gallants Braine
I tooke them Washt them putt them in againe,
But to no end: so Since I did desire
To try Conclusions by the force of Fire,
And heere behould what good Succese I had
Thefe Strange Chimæra Crotchetts made him mad

Ardor Diurnus

MD sculpsit

Thefe in y Citty and the Cuntry dwell
But for beft practife doth the Court excell
Thers the luxurious roaring Riotter
The two tongud Lawyer & base Flatterer
Luft Idles seruant with his leprous hide
With Crownes reuenewes spent in gaudy pride
The periurd Louer with difsembling zeale
The Pattent begger, begging Comon weale
Sould by P Stent

The lauifh Gamefter y in one black night
Consumes more meanes then wold maintaine a knight
Thefe growe so ill and to such height aspire
That nothing serues to purg them but a fire
Besides thefe named that are Masculines
Hee hath as many frantick Feminines
When thefe approche this Doctor for their cure
And while by fire their braines a punge indure

More wandring Crotchets will euaporate
Then from y Gallant did ascend of late
Steelettoes girdles patches painted brefts
Points powders feathers wafhes & y reft
When witning luft baits & damnd plots of hell
The red hott furnace only muft expell
Yett purgd of all thay not lesse owners are
Haire breath Complexions all are borrowed
ware

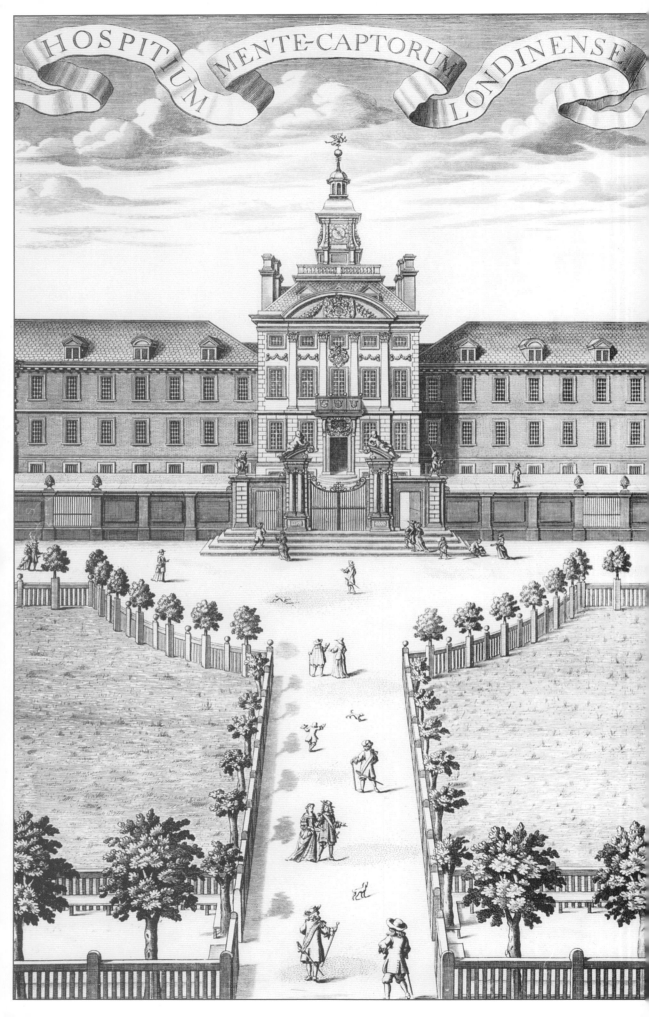

HOSPITIUM MENTE-CAPTORUM LONDINENSE.

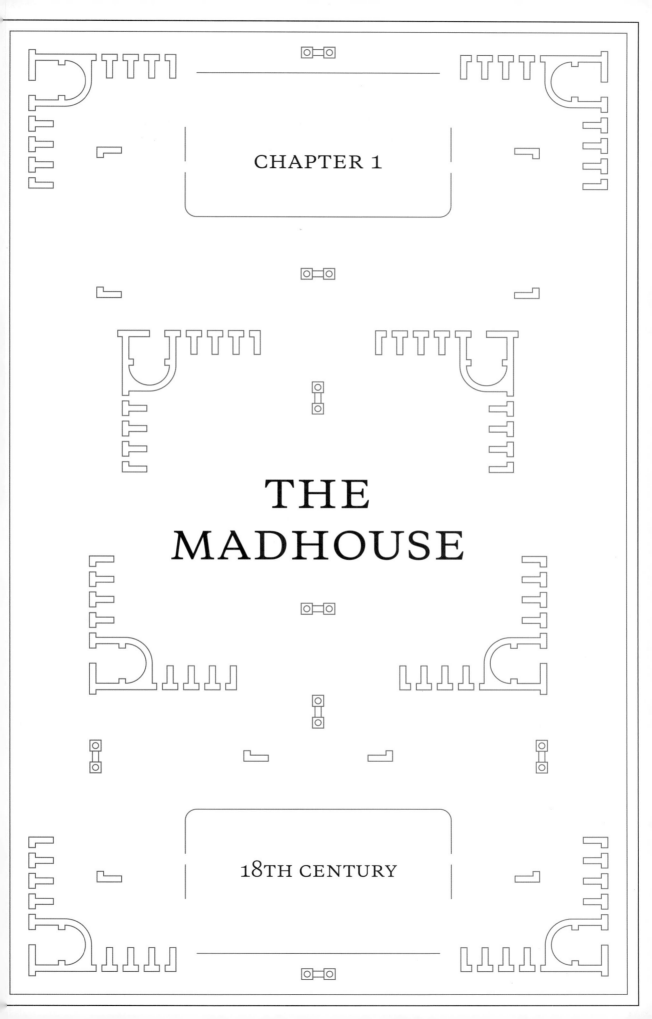

CHAPTER 1

THE MADHOUSE

18TH CENTURY

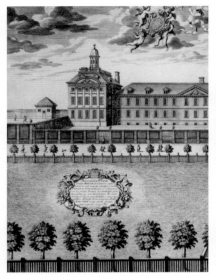
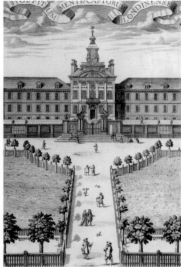
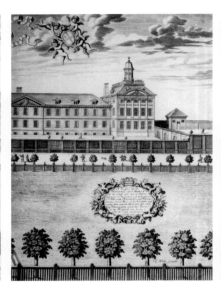

**THE SYMBOLISM WAS IMPOSSIBLE TO IGNORE:
A FACADE OF CARE CONCEALING A BLACK HOLE OF NEGLECT.**

above
Hospitium
Mente-
Captorium
Londinense
(c. 1690).
Engraving by
Robert White,
depicting the
new Bethlem.

The new Bethlem that arose in 1676 from the ashes of the Great Fire of London was hailed as one of the great ornaments of a city reinventing itself as the wonder of the age. London's medieval warrens of wattle and timber were replaced with a theatre of the modern world: the fashionable residences and entertainments of the West End; the financial hub of the City, where commodities were traded across the globe; and a raffish Grub Street and coffeehouse scene, where gossip and subversive ideas circulated and the follies of the powerful were satirized.

The old Bethlem priory was not destroyed in the Great Fire but many of the governors' residences were, and the staff used the hospital as temporary accommodation. A few winter nights demonstrated a fact that must have been obvious to Bethlem's residents for centuries: with stone floors, no fireplaces and no windows, it was barely fit for human habitation. A new site was chosen at Moorfields, on the edge of the city, and the brilliant polymath Robert Hooke – stalwart of the Royal Society, rival of Isaac Newton and assistant to Christopher Wren – was commissioned to design a public hospital that was fitting for the new city.

The result looked like no hospital in history. Its stone gates opened onto formal gardens with tree-lined, free-stone promenades, behind which rose an ornate facade modelled on Louis XIV's Tuileries Palace in Paris, with Corinthian columns, royal arms carved in stone and swagged with garlands, and a central balustrade leading up to an octagonal turret crowned with a shining cupola. It was a spectacular gesture of reinvention, not only of London but also of madness itself. Bethlem had stood for so long as the only public institution for the mad that its gloomy, draughty cells had become synonymous with the misery of the condition. But the new building was the envy of the city. In the words of *Bethlehems Beauty, Londons Charity, and the Cities Glory* (1676), the first of many poetic effusions published after its opening, it 'makes one Half-Madd to be a Lodger there'.

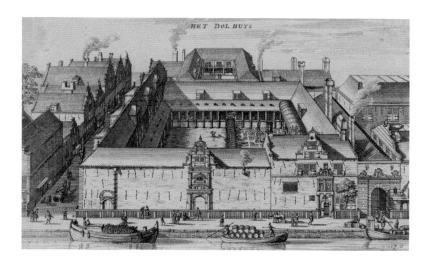

left
The
Amsterdam
dolhuis ,or
madhouse,
after the
completion of
its renovation
and extension
in 1617.

However, the face that the new Bethlem presented to the world was little more than a stage set. The building had no foundations: it had been erected on the waste ground beside the old Roman city wall, and six inches below ground its brick gave way to rubble. The weight of the facade bowed the flimsy structure behind it; the walls developed gaping cracks and ran with water whenever it rained. Before long, the chorus of praise for its grandeur was shadowed by jibes at its pretensions and paradoxes. 'The outside is a perfect mockery to the inside,' satirist Thomas Brown observed in 1699, making one wonder 'whether the persons that ordered the building of it, or those that inhabit it, were the maddest'.[1]

Moreover, the symbolism was impossible to ignore: a facade of care concealing a black hole of neglect. It was a cruel but accurate reflection of the mixed motives that had led to Bethlem's reinvention. The first examples of large-scale public madhouses had appeared earlier in the 17th century in the Dutch republics as expressions of civic pride in clean and orderly urban living. Known as *dolhuizen*, they were funded by public subscription, along with houses of correction for the idle and socially disruptive. In these buildings, work and discipline were the rule, and the mad were disruptive to the routine. The *dolhuizen* were humane and democratic in that they provided a place for those who would otherwise be abandoned on the street,

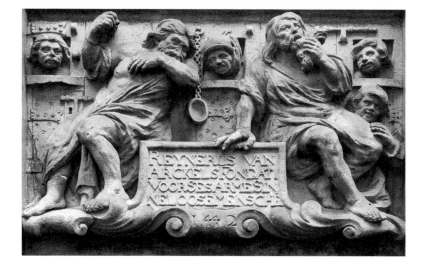

left
Relief depicting
the *dolhuis* in
's-Hertogenbosch,
by Pieter van
Coeverden (1686)

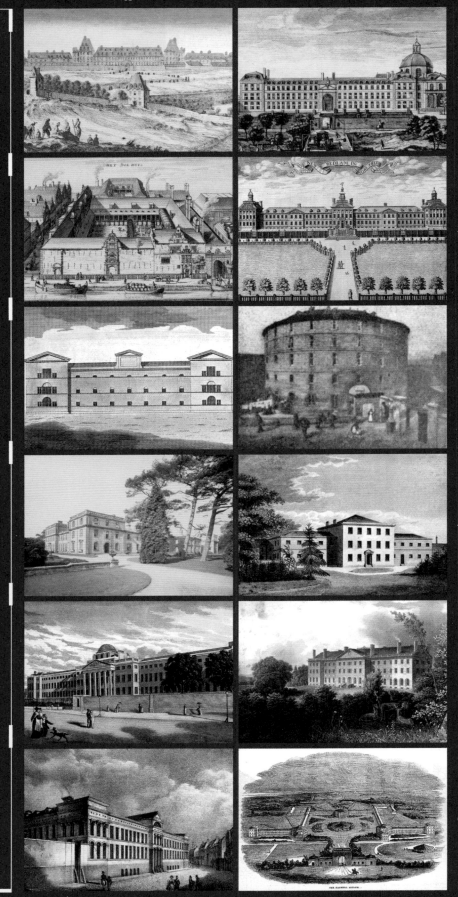

A

B

A1. Bicêtre Asylum, Paris, France, 1642

B1. Hopital Royal de la Salpêtrière, Paris, France, 1656

A2. Dolhuis, Amsterdam, Holland, 1663

B2. Bethlem, Moorfields, London, 1676

A3. St Luke's Lunatic Asylum, UK, 1751

B3. Der Narrenturm, Vienna, Austria, 1784

A4. Ticehurst House Hospital, UK, 1787

B4. York Retreat, UK, 1796

A5. New Bethlem, St George's Fields, London, 1815

B5. Bloomingdale Insane Asylum, New York, 1821

A6. Lunatic Asylum, Brussels, Belgium, 1825

B6. Hanwell Asylum, UK, 1831

C
D

1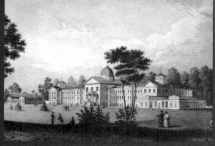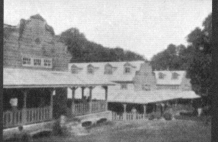

2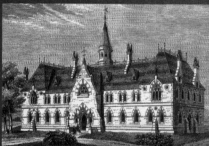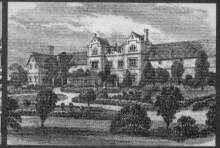

3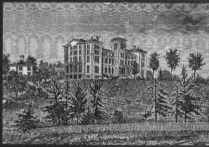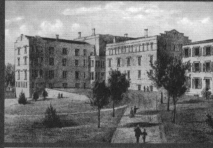

4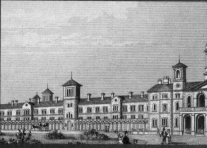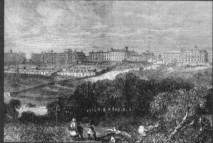

5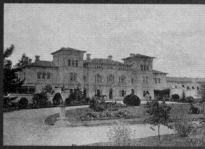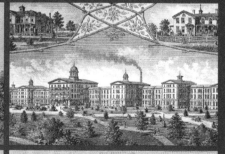

6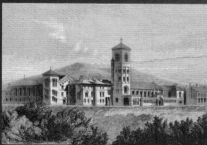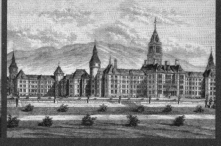

C1. Hospital for the Insane, Philadelphia, USA, 1841

D1. Kissy Asylum, Sierra Leone, 1844

C2. Colney Hatch Lunatic Asylum, Southgate, UK, 1851

D2. Lunatic Asylum, Adelaide, Australia, 1852

C3. New York State Asylum for Idiots, Syracuse, USA, 1855

D3. Juvenile Asylum, New York, USA, 1856

C4. Finlay Asylum, Quebec, Canada, 1860

D4. Asylum for Criminal Lunatics, Broadmoor, UK, 1864

C5. Insane Asylum, Beechworth, Victoria, Australia, 1867

D5. Northern Hospital for the Insane, Illinois, USA, 1872

C6. Lawrence Asylum, India, 1873

D6. Branch Insane Asylum, Napa, California, USA, 1873

below (left and right) **Engravings of the statues of *Raving* and *Melancholy Madness*, each reclining on one half of a pediment.**

but they also reflected a new intolerance for civil disorder. People wished for the mad to be treated humanely, but at the same time they believed that the less contact they had with others the better.

The madhouse stood in clear contrast to the system that emerged under the French monarchy: in 1656 Louis XIV founded a state system of institutions known as *hôpitals généraux*, where the mad were confined alongside beggars, criminals, prostitutes and vagabonds. In Paris the new prisons included the Bicêtre and the Salpêtrière, which would eventually become the city's two great

magnificent frontage was invisible to those inside it, who were confined in two gloomy and crumbling galleries, for male and female inmates. The exterior advertised its charitable largesse to the new city, but also served to distract from the conditions in which its charges were locked away.

The building's signature, crowning the main gates, was a pair of statues by renowned Danish sculptor Caius Gabriel Cibber titled *Raving* and *Melancholy Madness* (1676). These hulking figures would remain a London landmark for generations, the faces of madness frozen in stone. Their expressions

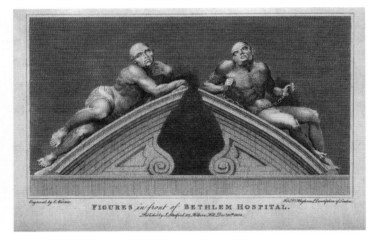

FIGURES *in front of* BETHLEM HOSPITAL.

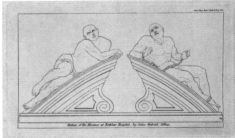

asylums for men and women, respectively. Their purpose was simply to remove beggars and other public nuisances from the streets, which they did in numbers that eventually rose to around six thousand. A letter from the king was enough to confine anyone for life without right of appeal.

Bethlem embodied the progressive sentiment that the mad were not to blame for their condition and should not be treated like criminals, but at the same time it was a pragmatic response to the disruption they caused in prisons and workhouses. Its

and poses could be read in many ways: as cautionary examples, as objects of pity, as medical illustrations. The contrast between them illustrated a classical idea of madness and its physical roots: on the left the torpor caused by black bile, and on the right the frenzy produced by excess of blood. At the same time, they characterized the types who were most likely to find themselves confined in Bethlem: those whose behaviour was chaotic and violent, and those who were too withdrawn to engage with the world around them. From another viewpoint,

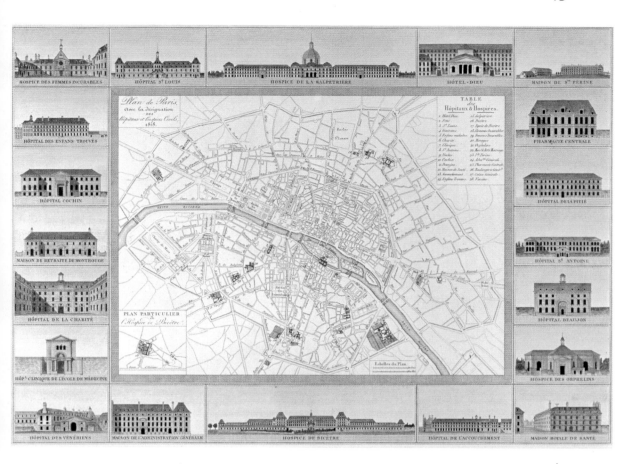

UNTIL THIS POINT THERE HAD ONLY BEEN TWO OPTIONS FOR THE MAD: LIVING WITH THEIR FAMILIES IF THEY WERE LUCKY, OR ROUGH ON THE ROADS IF THEY WERE NOT.

they epitomized the two problems that the madhouse had been built to address: the disruptive elements that needed to be isolated from civil society, and the demented or 'mopish' who were unable to contribute to the new economic order.

Bethlem's grandeur was also a response to the growth in private madhouses, a business sector that would become known in the 18th century as the 'trade in lunacy'. The old hospital had held a virtual monopoly on the care of the mad, but now it was competing with fashionable and well-funded rivals. Up to this point, besides Bethlem, there had been only two alternatives for those afflicted with madness: living with their families if they were lucky, or rough on the roads if they were not. The growing middle class now had a third option within their means: boarding their distressed or unmanageable relatives in specialist houses where they could be cared for with others of their kind.

Private madhouses tended to cluster together to share cleaners, nurses and medical staff; in London they were grouped in Chelsea to the west and Hackney to the east. They offered care that was beyond the reach of many families, especially the growing number obliged to choose between looking after their difficult relatives and earning money. The booming commercial worlds of trade, transport and craft guilds involved long hours of labour, travel and shift work, which loosened the ties of traditional family life. Bethlem's magnificence was a statement of intent for London's ambitions, but also an attempt to vault to the peak of this expanding market. In this it was relatively successful: the new hospital accepted fee-paying patients, who soon made up around one-third of the intake.

There are a few fragments of poetry written by Bethlem's early inmates, but the voices of the mad in this era mostly issue

above
Engraving by Etienne-Jules Thierry, 1818, published in 1820. The plan of Paris indicates the locations of civil hospitals and homes.

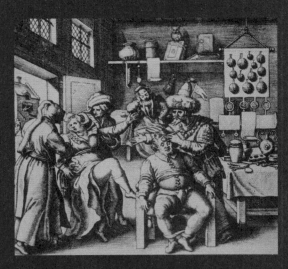
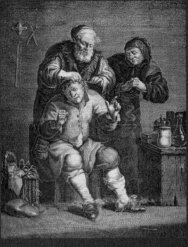

In these satirical works, quack doctors and itinerant surgeons operate on the mythical 'stone of folly'. They are depicted extracting the stones from the heads of grimacing patients, symbolizing the expulsion of 'folly' (insanity).

above (left) Photogravure, 1926
above (right) Engraving, 17th century.
below Mezzotint, David Teniers.

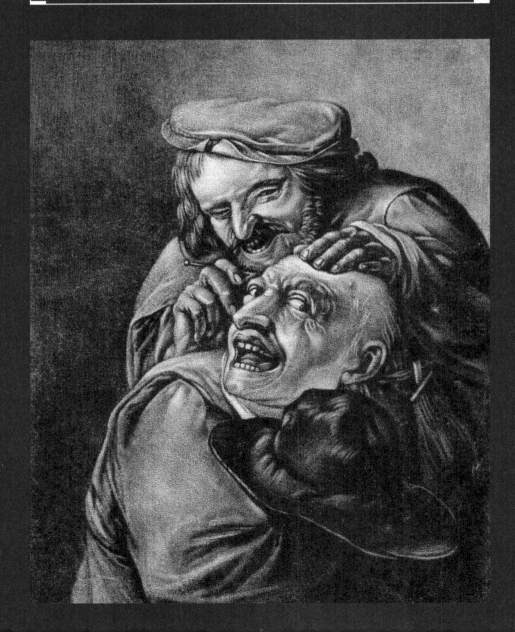

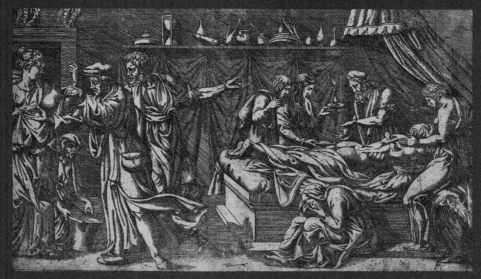

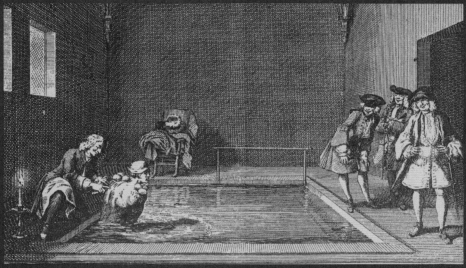

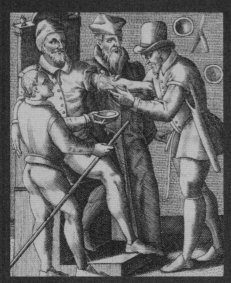

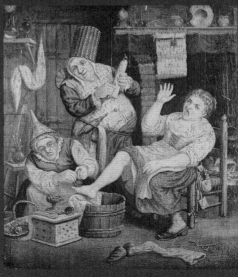

FROM THE BEGINNING, BETHLEM'S CARE
OF ITS INMATES WAS STRETCHED THIN.

from private madhouses, and particularly in the form of protests by those who were forced into them against their will. The Vagrancy Acts of 1714 and 1744 made a formal distinction between lunatics and other undesirables: the mad were protected from the public whipping to which other classes were subject, but they could be locked up if two Justices of the Peace agreed that they were a public danger. The Acts said little, however, about their rights to be released, and the complaints of those detained maliciously, for revenge or financial gain, became a staple of the scandal sheets. The best remembered is by Alexander Cruden, a devout Presbyterian bookseller, subject to wild romantic infatuations, who was locked up several times in order to restrain him from pursuing his love objects. His pamphlet of 1739, *The London Citizen Exceedingly Injured*, details his various imprisonments and daring escapes, as well as his terror that he would

end up in Bedlam, 'the sorest evil that could befall him, and which he dreaded more than death'. After his release, Cruden continued to publish pamphlets under the nom de plume 'Alexander the Corrector', in which he condemned the immorality of public life and pointed out grammatical errors in street signs. He also wrote *A Complete Concordance to the Holy Scriptures* (1737), which has never been out of print since it was published.

From the beginning, Bethlem's care of its inmates was stretched thin. The galleries were staffed by attendants, uniformed in the blue coats of charity workers, who fed their charges on porridge, bread and cheese, with meat three times a week. The inmates were cleaned and dressed, shaved and bathed, and occasionally ministered to by a surgeon. They received no special therapy for their mental conditions but were given general treatment aimed at restoring a healthy balance to the constitution. Its

right
The Hospital for Lunatics (1789) by Thomas Rowlandson, in which the incurable patients are represented by political figures.

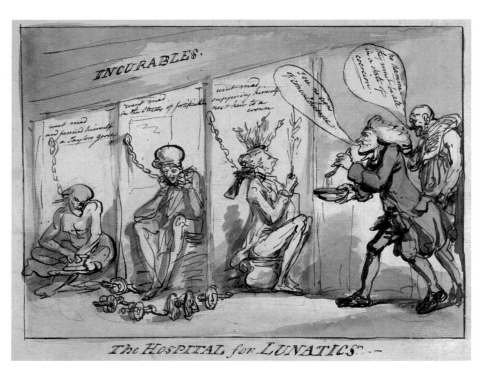

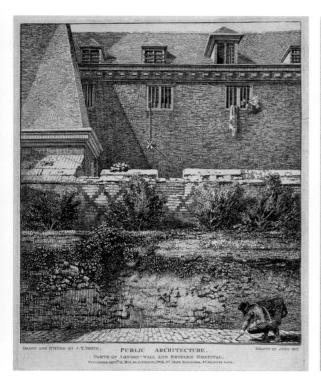

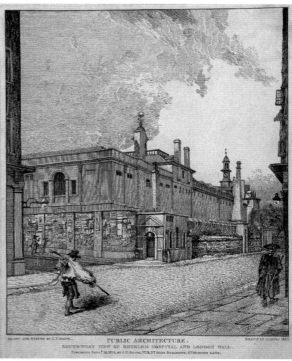

main features included bleeding – a seasonal practice, concentrated at the beginning and end of summer – purging with emetics and douching with cold showers.

The rationale for these treatments drew on the prevailing doctrine of humours, according to which violent behaviour could be calmed by drawing blood and black moods relieved by vomiting up substances that were blocking the digestion. However, they could also be deployed for the benefit of the keepers, whose jobs were demanding and unrewarding. They were entrusted with a steadily growing population of troubled and troublesome inmates, most of whom had ended up in Bethlem because everyone else had found them to be unmanageable. These inmates suffered from a variety of untreatable disorders and had nothing to occupy them. The priority of the staff was to maintain order, and the medical regime was deployed to serve this purpose. Bleeding weakened the inmates and made them more tractable; like purging and cold baths, it could be withheld from well-behaved patients and threatened to keep disruptive ones in check. They were 'treatment' in the sense of punishment as much as cure.

Pressure on resources led Bethlem to institute the policy that defines it in the public imagination to this day. With the charity of London's great and good spread among ever more worthy causes, and income from paying guests limited by the grim reputation that had so terrified Cruden, the governors decided to install donation boxes at the entrance of the new building and to open it for public visits. Londoners thronged to the new attraction: it joined a tourist trail that included the Tower, the royal palaces, the zoo, the theatres of Covent Garden and the promenade of the Strand. Visiting crowds attracted the same camp followers as elsewhere: street sellers, pickpockets and sex workers. The spectacular facade and grounds were an attraction in their own right, as well as the perfect proscenium for the continuous drama that played inside.

Many people left written descriptions of their visits and they often appear to have witnessed quite different scenes. There were certainly some visitors of the calibre that the governors had hoped for: 'persons of quality' attending in the spirit of charity and donating to the poor boxes, which accrued several hundred pounds a year. Samuel Pepys sent his out-of-town family to visit on their tour of the capital, and James Boswell noted his visit in his journal. Some visitors recorded pity and compassion for the inmates, whereas others took the experience as a moral lesson, 'there but for the grace of God go I'. For the serious-minded, a visit to Bethlem was an educative experience. Young

above (left and right) Etchings by John Thomas Smith, published in 1814. Two views of Bethlem hospital from the south and south-west, with part of the London Wall.

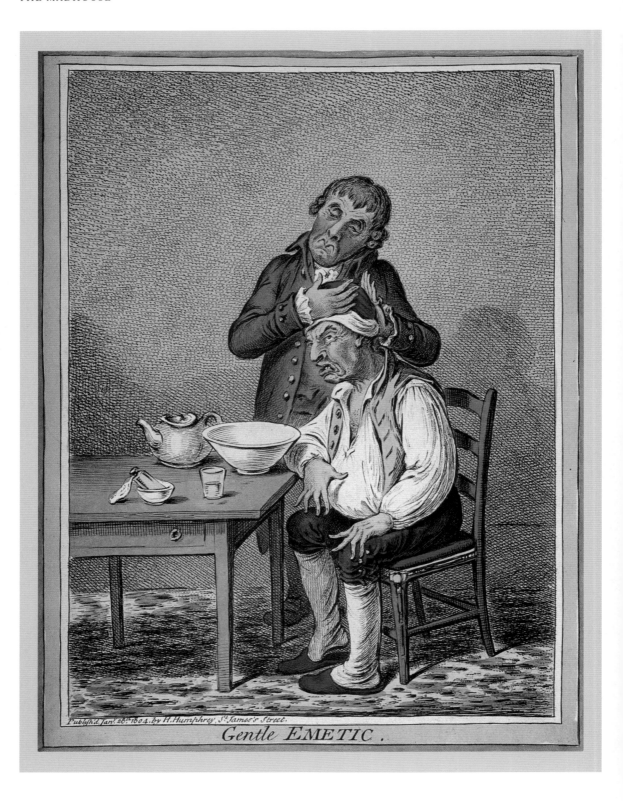

Gentle EMETIC.

above 'Gentle emetic', coloured print by
J. Sneyd, 1804, after an etching by James Gillray.
From a series by Gillray, satirizing bloodletting
and purging.

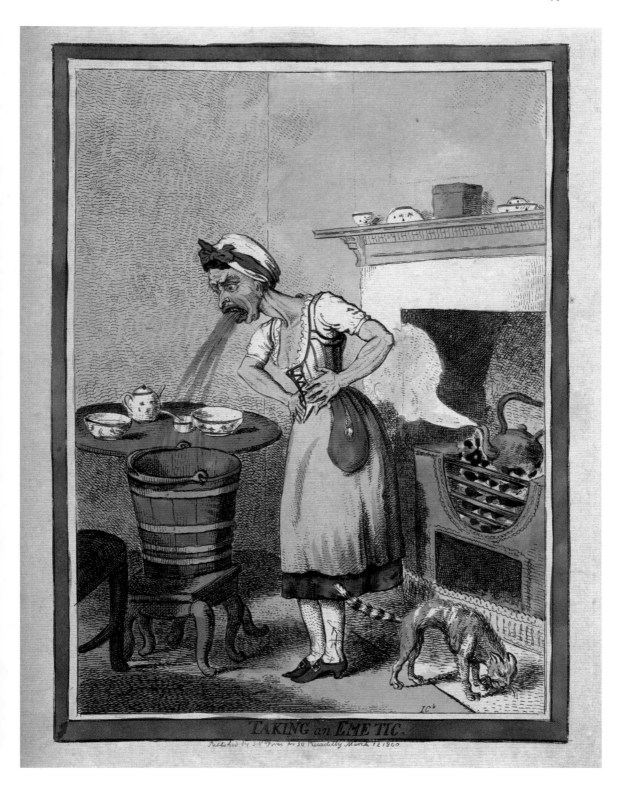

TAKING an EMETIC.

Published by S. W. Fores, No 50 Piccadilly March 12 1800

above Coloured etching by Isaac Cruikshank,
1800. A woman holds her stomach and vomits
violently into a bucket after self-administering
an emetic.

**VISITORS TO BETHLEM OFTEN APPEAR TO HAVE
WITNESSED QUITE DIFFERENT SCENES.**

---

people in particular should be shown what madness looked like, and the fate of those who suffered from it, as a warning against the dangers of pride, self-love and indulging the passions at the expense of reason.

Many visitors were relatives of the inmates, bringing them food and keeping them company. But plenty more came out of frank curiosity or for raucous entertainment. Particularly on Sundays and holidays, the scene in the galleries could be boisterous and rowdy. Like a ghost train or a freak show – or indeed the surgery and autopsy demonstrations that were also on offer to the London public at the time – it offered an extreme but safely contained experience, and a stage on which high-spirited visitors could perform acts of daring or display their wit. Some members of the public mocked and imitated the inmates, or pestered them with questions about why they were locked up. Many inmates gave as good as they got,

performing their madness in return, singing ditties or drawing sketches, and earning pennies or drink in reward.

The high-minded health campaigner Thomas Tryon was one of many visitors who disapproved of these spectacles, which in his view degraded everyone concerned. He firmly believed Bethlem to be 'one of the prime ornaments of the city, and a noble monument of charity'.[2] Public visits undermined the hospital's mission and encouraged the worst instincts in the visitors. The behaviour of young and drunken men and women, laughing and hooting, reduced them to the same level as those on the other side of the bars: each was performing for the other, indulging their pride and passions at the expense of their shared humanity. Tryon found the hospital's regime of bleeding and purging equally cruel and misguided, because in his view madness was not an imbalance of bodily humours

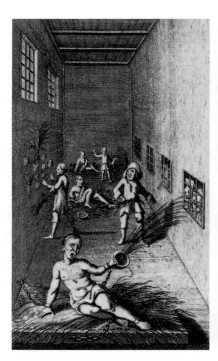

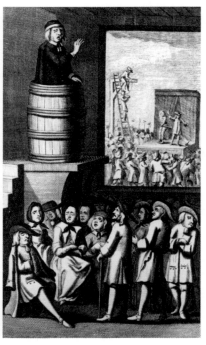

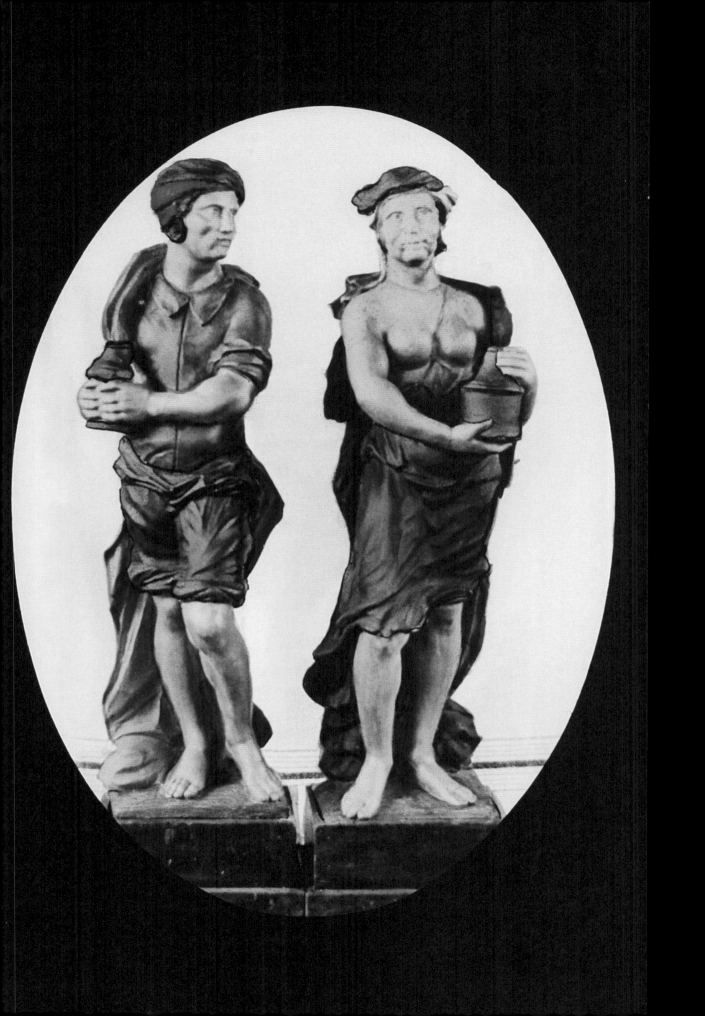

right
The Rake in Bedlam (1734), the final scene in William Hogarth's *The Rake's Progess*: the final degradation.

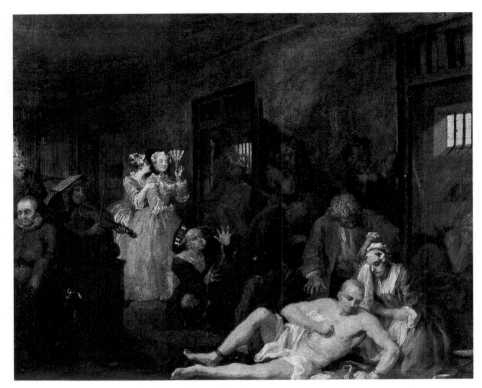

but an affliction of the soul. 'The world,' he concluded, 'has become a great Bedlam, where those who are more mad lock up those who are less.'[3]

The old Jacobean conceit that the sane were mad and the mad sane was frequently recalled and embellished. In 1703 Grub Street author Ned Ward included a lurid description of Bethlem in his salacious guide to London's low life, *The London Spy*, and then returned to the subject the following year with a lengthy broadside in verse titled *All Men Mad, or England a Great Bedlam*, in which he itemized the follies of the church and nobility, courtiers and politicians. In the same year, Jonathan Swift published *A Tale of a Tub*, in which he proposed that Bethlem's inmates might perform valuable service to the nation in these mad times. Surely the ranks of generals would be best supplied by one who is 'tearing his straw in piecemeal, swearing and blaspheming, foaming at the mouth and emptying his piss-pot in the spectators' faces'. Similarly, there must be

plenty of suitable lawyers, businessmen, poets and politicians among Bedlam's sorry and neglected ranks.

However, the satire that would do the most to fix the image of Bethlem, or rather Bedlam, in the public mind was the final painting of William Hogarth's sequence *The Rake's Progress*, completed in 1734. It was one of Hogarth's trademark 'modern moral subjects', following a wealthy and dissolute young man through a series of follies and indulgences – parties, expensive tailors, brothels, gambling dens – to debtors' prison and finally, violent and insane, to the gallery of Bedlam. The artist's tableau of demented and deluded lunatics, mocked by society visitors from behind their fluttering fans, conjured the nightmare scene described by observers such as Ward as a 'drumming of doors, ranting, holloaing, singing and rattling', which provoked in him lurid visions 'of the damn'd broke loose'.[4] In the age of Enlightenment, when the terrors of hell were waning,

Right page Plates 1 to 8 of William Hogarth's *The Rake's Progress*. Etchings and engravings, published in 1735. In Hogarth's most celebrated sequence of paintings, the young Tom Rakewell inherits a fortune and squanders it on fine clothes and high society. He marries for more money, gambles away his second fortune and is confined in debtor's prison; finally, insane and destitute, he finds himself in Bedlam – the lowest level to which a person can sink – much to the amusement of the visitors around him.

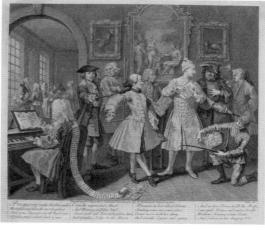

1

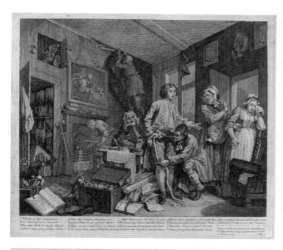

2

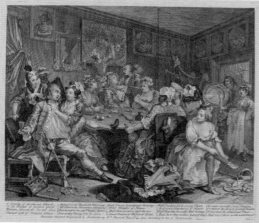

3

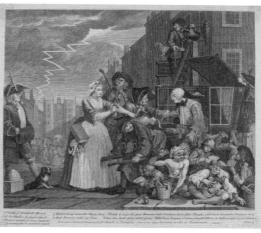

4

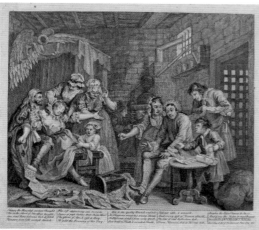

5

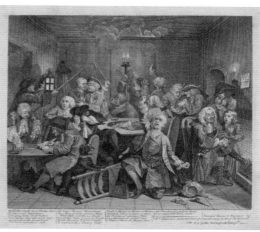

6

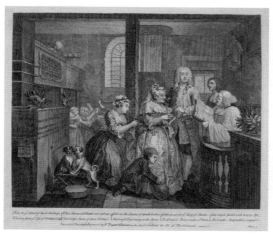

7

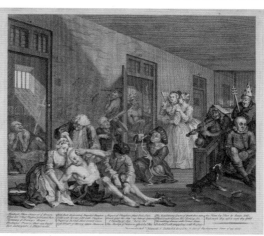

8

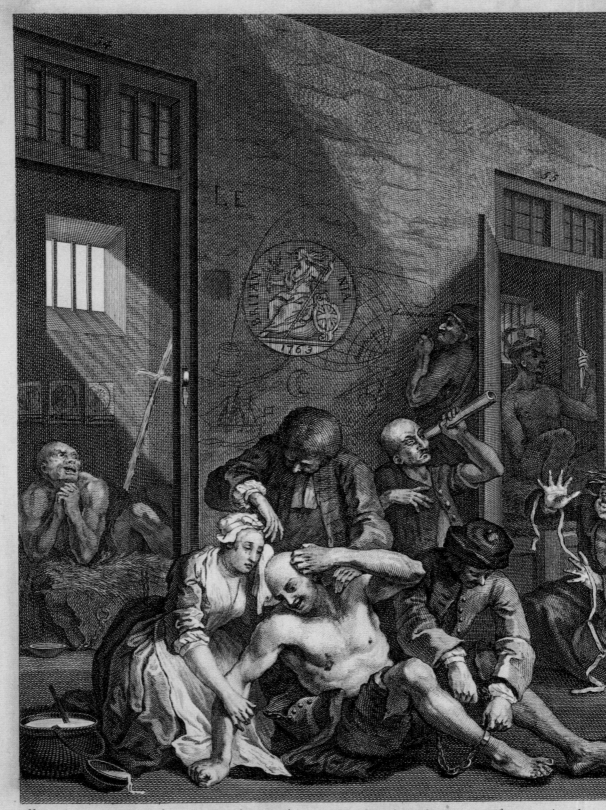

Madness, Thou Chaos of ȳ Brain,
What art? That Pleasure giv'st, and Pain?
Tyranny of Fancy's Reign!
Mechanic Fancy; that can build
Vast Labarynths, & Mazes wild,

With Rule disjointed, Shapeless Measure
Fill'd with Horror, fill'd with Pleasure!
Shapes of Horror, that wou'd even
Cast Doubt of Mercy upon Heaven.

Shapes of Pleasure, that but Seen
Wou'd split the Shaking Sides of Spleen
O Vanity of Age! here See
The Stamp of Heaven efac'd by Thee.

Invented &c. by Wᵐ Hoga

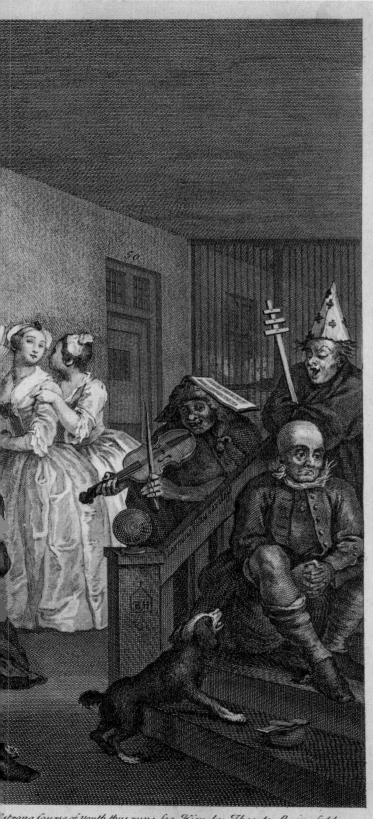

trong Course of Youth thus run, See Him by Thee to Ruin Sold,
fort from this darling Son! And curse thy self, & curse thy Gold.
g Chains with Terror hear,
eath grappling with Despair;

Retouch'd by the Author 1763

blish'd according to Act of Parliament June y.ᵉ 25. 1735.

right
*St Luke's
Hospital*
by Thomas
Rowlandson,
published
in 1809. The
cleanliness of
the women's
ward contrasts
with images
of Bethlem.

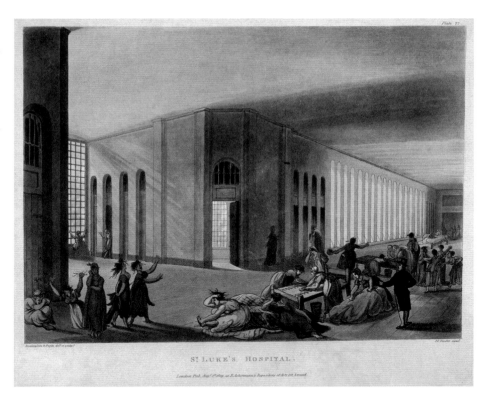

ST. LUKE'S HOSPITAL.

Bedlam was their secular equivalent: the lowest level to which a person could fall.

Like many before him, Hogarth had his eye not only on Bethlem but also on the world outside its walls. In a subsequent engraving of his painting in 1763, he made the link explicit by adding a new detail on the back wall: a circular emblem of Britannia, the coin of the realm. The grotesque spectacle being presented to us is not the madhouse but the nation. The mad bishop chanting to himself is a distorted reflection of the Church; the naked king clutching his orb and sceptre is the monarchy; the obsessive figure squinting through his telescope is the man of science; and the frenzied scribbler on the back wall, presumably, is the artist himself.

Along with satire and reflections on the moral state of the nation, the public visibility of madness prompted medical interest in the question of what it really was: what caused it and could it be cured? In 1751 a leading London physician and one of the governors of Bethlem, William Battie, established a rival hospital nearby, St Luke's Hospital for Lunatics, in which his new theories could be put to the test. Public visits were forbidden, and blistering, purging and bloodletting were replaced by a new therapeutic plan. In 1758 he published the groundbreaking *A Treatise on Madness*, in which he considered

the subject from a medical perspective and outlined the type of institution that would be most effective in treating it.

Battie distinguished between what he called 'original' madness, which was congenital, and 'consequential' madness, which was brought on by events. Original madness had no discernible cause and was incurable, but consequential madness could be traced to its source – perhaps a physical weakness or traumatic event – and in theory corrected. Various medicines were used at St Luke's – mercury for venereal diseases, opium for pain, cinchona bark for fever – but only for symptomatic relief. Battie entertained the hope that 'the antidote of madness is reserved in Nature's store, and will be brought to light in its appointed time';[5] until such time, however, most cases could at best be contained and managed. It was unjust for sufferers to be 'shut up in loathsome prisons as criminals or nuisances to the society', and remarkable results could be achieved in cases of consequential madness when the proper environment was created. A skilled practitioner, observing each individual case closely, could deduce and even orchestrate the circumstances in which the 'deluded imagination' might be restored to reason.

St Luke's was a teaching hospital, the first in which specialist techniques for what

> WHEN VISITING
> CAME TO AN END,
> BETHLEM RECEDED
> FROM PUBLIC VIEW,
> BUT ITS ERA OF
> NOTORIETY WAS
> NOT YET OVER.

was known as 'mad-doctoring' were passed on formally. It was also the foundation of a profitable business model, and Battie became extremely wealthy by passing trainees and patients on to the private madhouses that he ran in tandem with it.

As a cadre of specialist mad-doctors took shape, Bethlem's time-honoured regime was called into question and its resident physician, John Monro, replied to Battie's *Treatise* with a short and defensive pamphlet. Monro professed to be puzzled by Battie's confident classification of madness into 'original' and 'consequential', maintaining that it was 'a distemper of such a nature, that very little of real use can be said concerning it'.[6] Although the two men agreed on many points, this difference of opinion has the distinction of being the first public dispute in the history of what would later become psychiatry. But it hardly suggested that rapid progress was afoot. It was an argument between one doctor who believed a cure for madness might emerge in the distant future and another who thought it unlikely.

Public visits to Bethlem were ended in 1770 and they were replaced by a system of tickets authorized by the governors. This decision was not only a consequence of the notoriety of the visits, but also of changing public tastes, which were relegating cruel public spectacles, such as bear-baiting, to the lower orders of society. In addition, it reflected Battie's criticisms and the enlightened example he set at St Luke's. However, it was also because the hospital, thanks perhaps to its raised public profile, was now receiving more charitable donations and becoming self-sufficient.

The governors congratulated themselves that the end of visits had improved conditions, but the opinions of the inmates were not canvassed. A few examples of their poems and sketches have survived from the days of public visits, and it seems that there were some among them who enjoyed the attention of visitors. For others, no doubt, the experience was excruciating. When visiting came to an end, Bethlem receded from public view, but its era of notoriety was not yet over. Public visits would not be the last or the worst of its scandals.

In 1788 the debate over the nature of madness was revitalized by the best-known case of the 18th century, perhaps of all time. George III's indisposition began in his stomach as a bilious attack, but soon affected his mind. He rambled, then raved, and eventually foamed at the mouth, all the while refusing to accept medical attention or even to have his pulse checked. In public, his physicians announced that he was suffering from a fever; in private (and in Latin, for extra

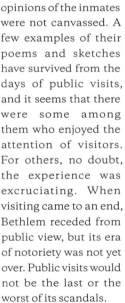

left (top to bottom)
This engraving by J. Peltro shows the facades of St Luke's, Hospital, Bethlem Hospital and St Paul's School.

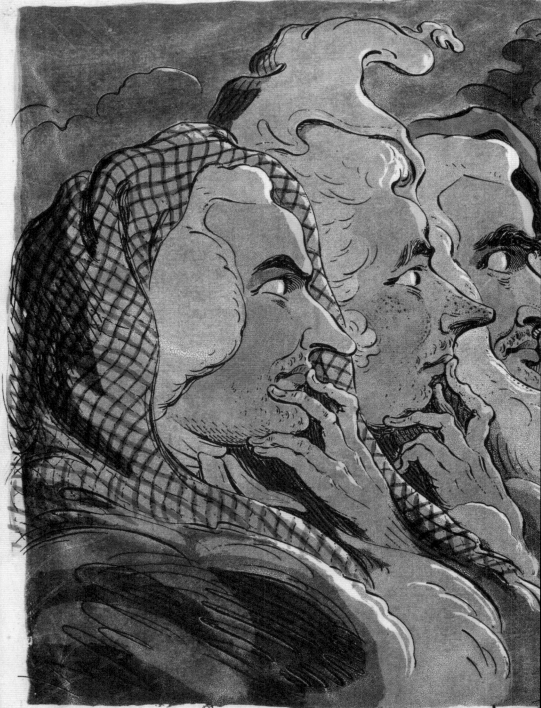

To H:Fuzelli Esq.ʳ this attempt in the

WIERD-SISTERS; MINISTER'S of
"They should be Women!— and yet th

Pub. Dec. 23. 1791.
by H.Humphrey N.º 18. Old Bond Street

...RKNESS: MINIONS of the MOON." 23 Dec. 1791.
...rds forbid us to interpret, — that they are so"

MADNESS HAD OVERTHROWN ROYAL PRIVILEGE; THE KING HAD BECOME THE MAD-DOCTOR'S SUBJECT.

---

discretion), they admitted he had become insane. He was removed from Windsor to his house at Kew, where his treatment could proceed with greater privacy.

There were competing opinions on the cause of the king's illness. For some, particularly his political opponents, it was a character weakness found out: absolute power had led to overweening pride and had corrupted his reason. Equally popular was the view that he was suffering from having eaten too many pears. His court physicians were of the opinion that it was a physical illness: a bad humour, perhaps, that had forced itself from his stomach into his brain. They were hopeful that he would recover spontaneously, but they had no idea how to assist the process. Other physicians offered advice, by letter and in the press. Some had deduced that it was a physical infection or fever, others that it was a sickness of spirit brought on by his royal responsibilities. They prescribed, variously, bleeding and blistering, music and fresh air, prayer and devotion.

As political pressure built and finding a cure became paramount, the court abandoned protocol and summoned a clergyman, from a provincial private madhouse, with a formidable reputation for achieving what Bethlem's physician believed to be impossible. The Reverend Dr Francis Willis had, it was reported in the House of Commons, 'cured nine out of ten'[7] of those in his care. Willis took what we would now call a psychological approach. At his madhouse in Lincolnshire, he put his patients to work in the fields, dressing them neatly to encourage self-respect and mending their spirits through exercise and good cheer. With the king, he deployed a mixture of morale boosting and strict discipline, and frequently used 'the eye', a fearsome stare with which he claimed he could subdue the most violent lunatic. When George disobeyed him, he forced him to wear a straitjacket. Previously, the court physicians had hardly dared to make any physical examination of the royal person, but Willis treated him, as he put it, just as he would one of Kew's gardeners. Madness had overthrown royal privilege; the king had become the mad-doctor's subject.

After eleven exhausting weeks, George's insanity abated and he was declared cured. Willis was rewarded with a pension of £1,000

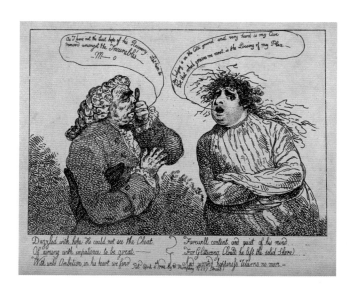

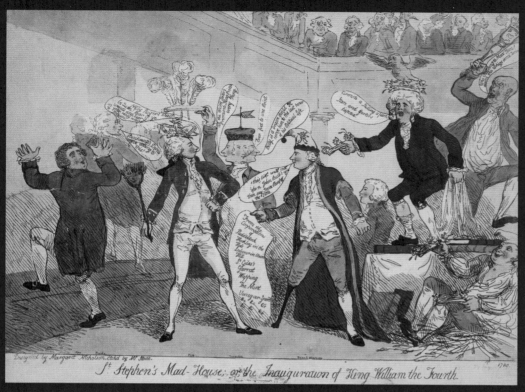

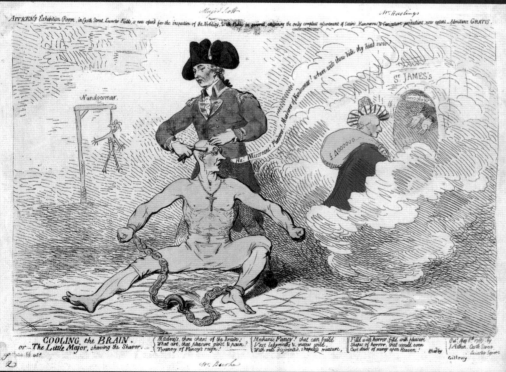

top In the satirical print *St Stephen's Mad-house* (1789), the House of Commons is depicted as Bedlam, with Prime Minister William Pitt holding a sweeping brush as a sceptre.

above In *Cooling the Brain. Or – the Little Major, Shaving the Shaver* (1789), British statesman Edmund Burke is portrayed as a violent lunatic chained up in Bedlam.

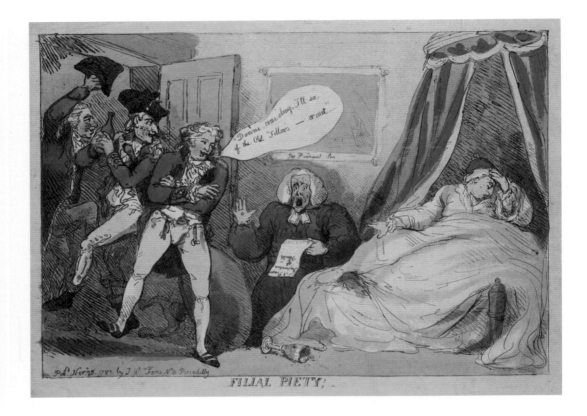

FILIAL PIETY!

a year and the demand for his services was such that he opened a second madhouse. However, it was also noted that the king's physical symptoms disappeared at exactly the same time as his mental ones. Today, it is widely believed that he was suffering from a physical illness, porphyria, which produces mental disturbances. This retrospective diagnosis has been called into question recently, but if it is correct the bewigged court physicians were broadly right and the royal patient would have recovered with or without Willis's unsparing treatment. Yet an important and highly visible precedent had been set. The authority of a mad-doctor had won the day, determining the course not only of the monarch's treatment but also of the nation's government.

Ten years later, George III was at the centre of another case that extended the reach of the mad-doctors into affairs of state. On 15 May 1800, as he was blowing a kiss to his subjects from the royal box at Drury Lane theatre, a pistol shot missed his head by inches. The would-be assassin was James Hadfield (see p.82), a soldier who had sustained sabre

wounds to the head while fighting in the British army against the French in 1794. He had subsequently become mentally unbalanced, fallen under the influence of a Pentecostal preacher and become convinced that the end of the world was at hand. It was revealed to him that he was God's instrument, and by killing the king he would initiate the Second Coming of the Messiah.

Hadfield was charged with high treason and defended in court by Thomas Erskine, a leading Whig politician and future Lord Chancellor, who accepted the facts of the case but denied the charge of treason. Hadfield had been acting 'for the benefit of mankind',[8] but under an insane delusion that made his act not a crime but a moral duty. Erskine called on the expert testimony of a physician to confirm that Hadfield was *non compos mentis* due to a physical injury, sustained in the service of his nation. It would be barbarous to convict him of treason, for which he might be hanged, drawn and quartered. Erskine's argument persuaded the Lord Chief Justice to halt the trial and announce that the defendant must be acquitted. There was no option but to free

RATIONAL EXPLANATIONS OF HOW THE MIND WORKED WERE GRADUALLY TRANSFORMING THEORIES OF MADNESS.

Hadfield immediately, which prompted a public outcry and forced Parliament to rush through a new law, the Criminal Lunatics Act, to close the loophole. It gave state madhouses the role of confining 'criminal lunatics', a new class who were excused guilt for their crimes but nevertheless imprisoned for the public good.

The philosophies of the Enlightenment had less impact on medicine than on the sciences, but rational explanations of how the mind worked were gradually transforming theories of madness and its meaning. In the influential *An Essay Concerning Human Understanding* (1689), John Locke had argued that a process of association creates thoughts and ideas; as a consequence, each person's understanding differs slightly from the next, and we all find each other eccentric to some degree. Some people, however, create connections between ideas that are wildly mistaken and lead to serious errors and delusions: this is the root

of much that we call madness. According to this view, the mad were not an inferior species of human who lacked reason, but those whom reason had led astray and could, in theory, correct.

These ideas found their moment in France after 1789, when the courtly physicians of the *ancien régime* were swept aside. Their figurehead was Philippe Pinel, who before the revolution had been a struggling provincial doctor with an interest in mental afflictions that developed after one of his friends suffered a breakdown. Pinel joined the republican administration and in 1793 was assigned to the Bicêtre hospital, which had been established by Louis XIV on the southern outskirts of Paris and was notorious as an indiscriminate dumping ground for undesirables, criminals, beggars, the physically disabled, the incurably sick and the mad. In order to assess the state of those in the lunatic wards, he took a step that few of his predecessors had

below
The King's Life Attempted, 15 May 1800, engraving published by Thomas Kelly in 1820. James Hadfield is seen firing a pistol at George III.

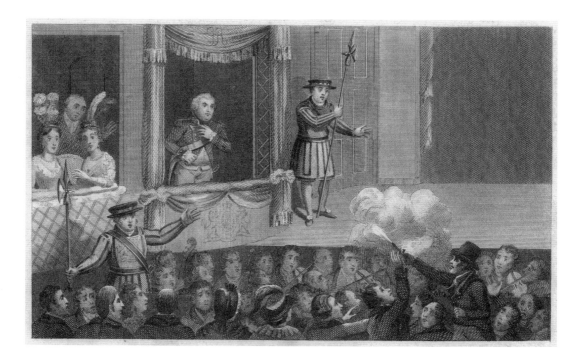

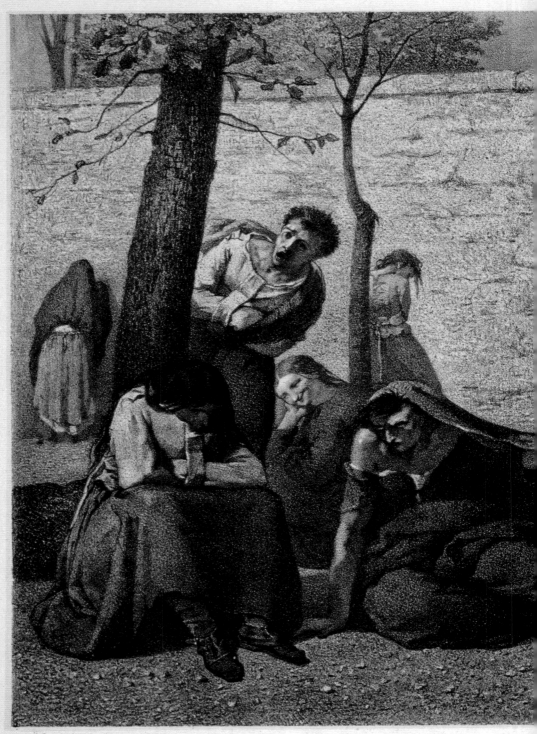

Amand Gautier, pinx et lith.

above Lithograph by A. Gautier, 1857. In the gardens of Salpêtrière hospital, women represent the conditions of dementia, megalomania, acute mania, melancholia, idiocy, hallucination, erotic mania and paralysis.

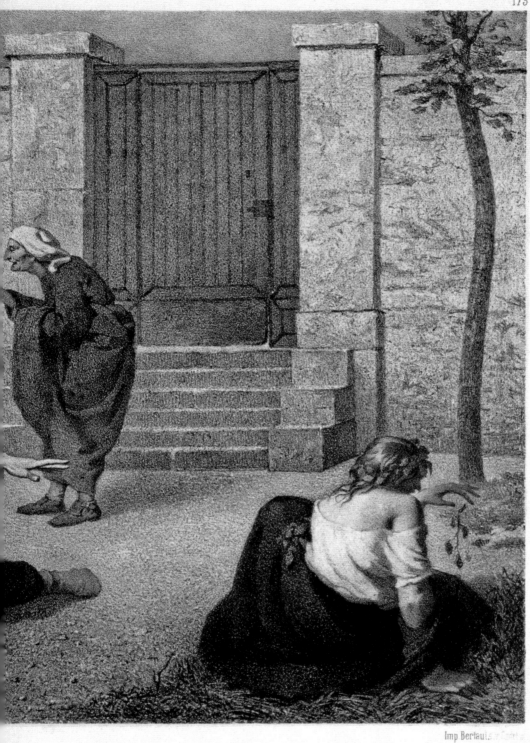

Imp Bertauts

THE MADHOUSE

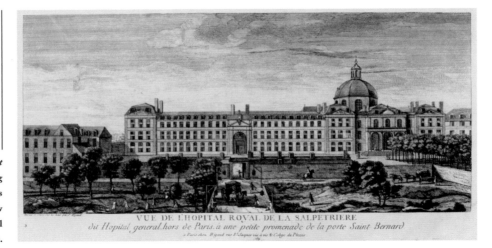

VUE DE L'HOPITAL ROYAL DE LA SALPETRIERE
dit Hopital general, hors de Paris, a une petite promenade de la porte Saint Bernard

ever considered: he asked them about their conditions and listened to their answers.

From this emerged Pinel's revolution in therapy. 'There are few subjects in medicine', he wrote in his groundbreaking *Medico-Philosophical Treatise on Mental Alienation or Mania* (1801), 'where there are so many prejudices to be rectified and mistakes to be corrected.' The time-worn 'blind routine' of bloodletting and cold baths had no effect whatsoever on madness; its causes and even its cure could, however, be discovered through the 'keen attention of genuine observers'.[9]

Most of Pinel's treatise consisted of case studies in which the characters of his patients are carefully etched, and the sources of their mental conflict become readily apparent. Weaving together all these stories, he simplified the chaotic manifestations of madness, or 'mental alienation', into a handful of distinct species. 'Maniacal insanity', the old 'Bedlam madness' of English vernacular, tended to be periodic,

often chronic, but potentially curable. 'Melancholia' was often characterized by recurring ideas and manifested in 'a dreamy taciturn manner, touchy and suspicious, with a desire to be left alone'.[10] These were quite distinct from the incurable conditions of 'dementia', in which thought is abolished by degrees, and 'idiocy', in which the intellect has never developed.

The cures that Pinel recorded in his books took on the status of parables for his new doctrine of moral therapy. His most celebrated modus operandi was to discover the root of the mental distress (for example, a patient's fear that they were going to be guillotined) and then address it with a theatrical intervention (in this case, staging a mock revolutionary tribunal in which the patient was acquitted). The facts of these well-known cases are difficult to establish independently, and by Pinel's own account not every cure was successful or enduring, but they were memorable dramatizations of the new relationship

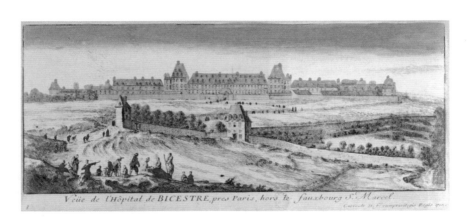

Veüe de l'Hôpital de BICESTRE, pres Paris, hors le fauxbourg S.t Marcel

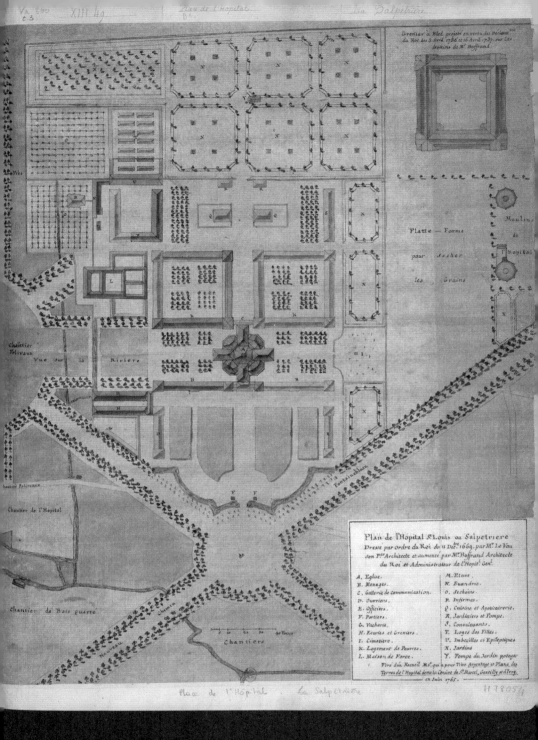

Grenier à Bled projeté en vertu des Déclar.
du Roi des 3 Avril 1786 et 16 Avril 1787. sur les
desseins de Mᵈᵉ Boffrand.

Platte — Forme

pour   Secher

les   Grains

Moulins
de
l'Hôpital

Chantier
Polivaux

Vue sur la Riviere

Chantier de l'Hôpital

Chantier de Bois guerre

Chantiers

Plan de l'Hôpital St Louis ou Salpetriere
Dressé par Ordre du Roi du 11 Déc. 1669. par Mʳ Le Vau
son Pʳᵉ Architecte et augmenté par Mʳ Boffrand Architecte
du Roi et Administrateur de l'Hôpitᵃˡ Genˡ.

A. Eglise.
B. Menages.
C. Gallerie de communication.
D. Ouvriere.
E. Officiers.
F. Portiers.
G. Vacherie.
H. Ecuries et Greniers.
I. Cimetiere.
K. Logement de Pauvres.
L. Maison de Force.
M. Etuve.
N. Buandrie.
O. Sechoirs.
P. Infirmes.
Q. Cuisine et Apoticairerie.
R. Jardiniers et Pompe.
S. Convalescents.
T. Loges des Filles.
V. Imbecilles et Epileptiques.
X. Jardins.
Y. Pompe du Jardin potager.

1   Tiré d'un Recueil Mˢᵗ qui a pour Titre Arpentage et Plans des
Terres de l'Hôpital dans la Censive de St Marcel, Gentilly et d'Ivry.
en Juin 1788.

above A plan of the buildings and grounds at Salpêtrière hospital in Paris, where Philippe Pinel was employed as chief physician from 1795 to his death in 1826.

next page Philippe Pinel *Freeing Mental Patients of their Chains in 1795 at the Hôpital de la Salpêtrière, Paris* (1876) by Tony Robert Fleury. In reality, the process of reform was more gradual.

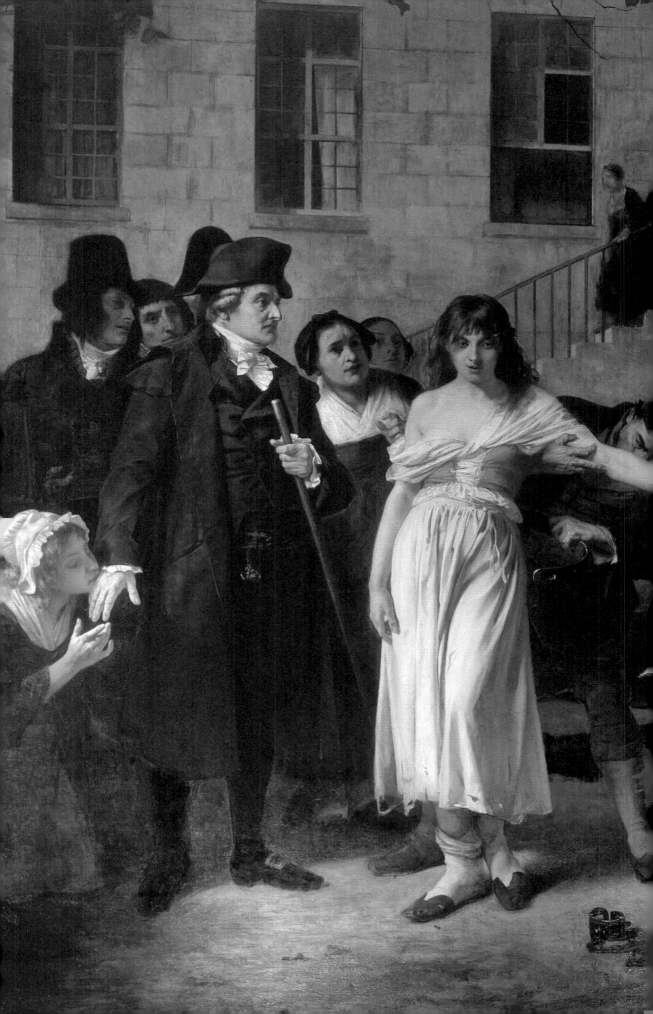

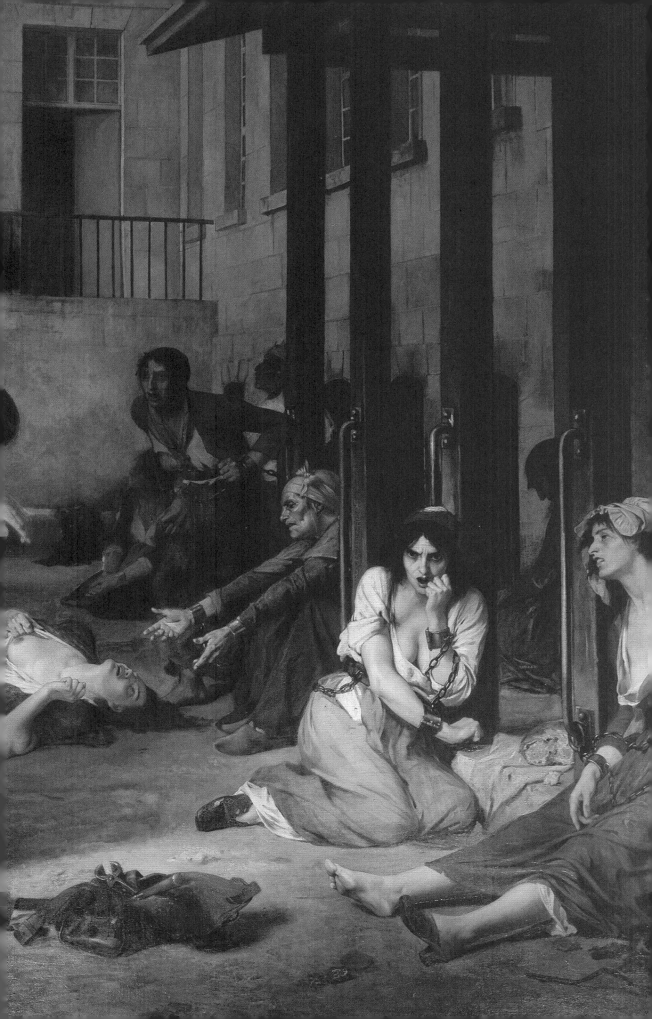

right
Engraving
after Swiss
physiognomist
J. C. Lavater,
who related
faces to
mental types.

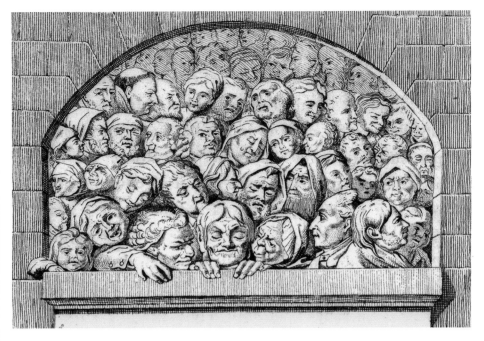

between doctor and lunatic. This was underpinned by a belief in their common humanity and expressed in 'kindly methods to gain the patient's confidence and convince him that one is only seeking to do him good'. Kindness alone, however, was an invitation to mischief and abuse of trust: it needed to be backed up by an 'apparatus of fear' in order to make the patient aware that resistance would be met, ultimately, with physical restraint or solitary confinement. When Pinel offered to unchain the most violent lunatic in Bicêtre hospital (so the story goes), the man promised to behave well but was sceptical of the proposal on the grounds that everyone was too afraid of him. Pinel assured him that he had six men standing by to enforce his commands if necessary.

Pinel paid close attention not only to his patients but also to his colleagues. Any hospital for mental patients, he observed, takes on the character of a 'miniature government', an enclosed world dominated by 'petty vanities and the ambition to be in charge'.[11] Bethlem at this point offered abundant evidence for Pinel's theory. The chief physician, Thomas Monro, had succeeded his father and grandfather to the post and took little interest in the day-to-day running of the hospital, which he rarely visited. Left to their own devices beneath him was an ill-tempered and frustrated apothecary, John Haslam, sharing the daily grind with an alcoholic surgeon, Bryan Crowther, who enlivened his routine of shaving and bleeding the inmates by performing post-mortem dissections of their

> **THE MADHOUSE
> WOULD BECOME
> A COMMUNITY IN
> WHICH EVERYONE
> HAD A STAKE.**

brains. Overworked and undermanaged, the keepers and attendants had fallen into the habit of keeping troublesome inmates in strait-waistcoats or chained to the wall. Furthermore, the state of the building was worse than ever: one wing had crumbled and was demolished in 1805, and the rest was dank and vermin-infested, its plaster rotting and its brickwork beyond repair. After years of petitioning the government, in 1810 the Bethlem governors finally were granted modest funding to acquire a new site.

This raised the question of the shape and design that would fit a new Bethlem, suitable for the 19th century and beyond. Lacking a clear vision of their own, the governors opened the question to a public competition advertised in *The Times*. Thirty-three designs were submitted, by far the most original of which came from within Bethlem's own walls. An inmate named James Tilly Matthews, who had been confined as an incurable lunatic since 1797, presented a set of finely drafted plans (see p. 86) for a tall and elegantly proportioned neoclassical block surrounded by generous green spaces and gardens. His new Bethlem was everything the old building was not: light, airy and salubrious, with spacious private cells, proper sanitation and extensive views of the outside world.

In the notes that accompanied the blueprints, Matthews expanded on his vision. The improved conditions he proposed were not only for the benefit of the inmates, but for everyone concerned. Rather than being confined uselessly in their cells and galleries, well-behaved inmates would be rewarded with rooms on the upper storeys and be given productive roles: engaging in maintenance work, caring for their fellows in the sickroom and producing their own food in the surrounding vegetable gardens. Residential staff, many of their burdens lifted, would spend more time at leisure in attractive new lodgings facing the outside world. The madhouse would become a community in which everyone had a stake, rather than a tyranny where the authorities were obliged to keep order through fear and punishment. Under this harmonious regime, recovery rates would naturally rise. The new Bethlem would be therapy in stone.

The Bethlem governors offered Matthews a small reward for his ingenious plans, but declined to submit them for consideration by the Royal College of Physicians. The medical world was not ready to take advice from a lunatic. But Matthews's vision anticipated the future with uncanny precision. Although he could not have known it, locked away as he was in Bethlem's crumbling cells, the

next page **Lithograph, late 19th century. The basic elements of phrenology, physiognomy and palmistry, with diagrams of heads and hands, and portraits of historical figures.**

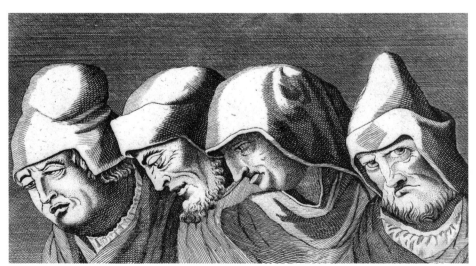

left **Heads demonstrating points of physiognomy. From** *Essays on physiognomy, calculated to extend the knowledge and the love of mankind* **(1797) by J. C. Lavater.**

LA PHRÉNOLOGIE est un système sur lequel les savants sont très-partagés, et que l'on définit la science de l'homme au point de vue de son organisation naturelle, ou l'explication des fonctions du cerveau.

Selon quelques savants, le cerveau n'est point un organe unique : c'est un assemblage d'organes particuliers qui ont des fonctions différentes.

Le cerveau est divisé en deux hémisphères, qui sont mis en rapport par des commissures, et les organes sont doubles.

Chaque organe a son *but*, son *excès* ou son *inactivité*.

Ainsi, par exemple, l'organe de l'ALIMENTAVITÉ, dont le but est la nutrition, et qui produit le désir de nourriture et l'appétit, porte, lorsqu'il est trop développé, à la gourmandise, à la gloutonnerie ; et s'il est inactif, à l'abstinence et à l'indifférence pour le choix des aliments.

Les facultés AFFECTIVES (les INSTINCTS) sont celles dont la nature essentielle est d'éprouver des désirs et des émotions. Elles agissent du dedans et ne sont nullement acquises par les impressions extérieures.

Les facultés INTELLECTUELLES sont celles dont la nature essentielle est de procurer des connaissances ou des idées.

Il est certain, néanmoins, que si l'on prenait pour absolues les conclusions de ces systèmes, on tomberait le plus souvent dans des erreurs graves et dangereuses ; et que mille circonstances, l'éducation, le genre de vie, l'entourage d'un homme, modifient toujours ses dispositions premières, quand elles ne les transforment pas complètement.

On a adopté dans le tableau suivant la nomenclature de SPURZHEIM, plus complète que celle de GALL.

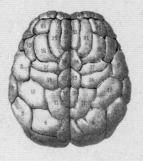

CERVEAU
vu en dessus

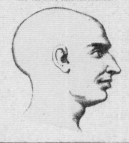

Prédominance
des facultés intellectuelles

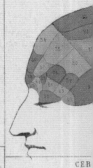

CER

NOMENCLATURE DES FACULTÉS.

A. — ALIMENTAVITÉ. Faim. — Voracité, Gourmandise. Sobriété, Tempérance.

N. — AMOUR DE LA VIE. Instinct de la conservation.

1. — AMATIVITÉ. Libertinage, Amour du plaisir. — Pudeur, Décence, Chasteté.

2. — PHILOGÉNITURE. Amour des enfants et de la famille.

3. — HABITAVITÉ. Nostalgie. — Amour des voyages.

4. — AFFECTIONIVITÉ. Amitié, Attachement, Tendresse.

5. — COMBATIVITÉ. Instinct de la défense de soi-même et de sa propriété. — Penchant aux rixes, Courage, Audace, Témérité. Lâcheté, Peur, Timidité, Poltronnerie.

6. — DESTRUCTIVITÉ. Instinct carnassier, Meurtre, Assassinat, Cruauté. — Dégoût de la vie.

7. — SECRÉTIVITÉ. Ruse, Duplicité, Fausseté, Discrétion, Mensonge, Tromperie. — Sincérité, Savoir-faire.

8. — ACQUISIVITÉ. Sentiment de la propriété, Instinct de faire des provisions. — Convoitise, Penchant au vol.

LA PHYSIOGNOMONIE est une science ou plutôt un système qui cherche dans certains signes l'indication des facultés à l'état de repos ; elle préjuge l'intérieur de l'homme par son extérieur : c'est l'étude des rapports du physique au moral.

Malgré toute l'analogie qu'il y a dans la multitude innombrable des figures humaines, il est impossible d'en trouver deux qui, mises l'une à côté de l'autre et comparées exactement, ne diffèrent sensiblement entre elles. Il est certain qu'il serait tout aussi impossible de trouver deux caractères d'esprit parfaitement ressemblants.

Tout le système repose sur cette présomption : que la différence extérieure de la figure doit avoir un certain rapport, une analogie naturelle, avec la différence intérieure de l'esprit et du cœur. Tout homme, qu'il s'en doute ou non, fait de la physiognomonie ; il n'est pas une seule créature intelligente qui ne tire des conséquences du moins à sa manière, de l'extérieur à l'intérieur et qui ne prétende juger d'après ce qui frappe les sens, ce qui leur est inaccessible.

L'appréciation des qualités morales d'un homme dépend plutôt de l'ensemble de ses traits que de la forme de chacun d'eux ; mais il est certains signes plus caractéristiques dont on donne ici des exemples, en avertissant toutefois que *l'on se tromperait étrangement si l'on prétendait en tirer des conséquences rigoureuses et absolues.*

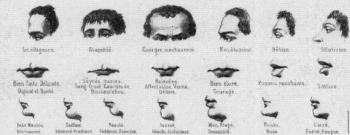

Intelligence. — Stupidité. — Énergie, méchanceté. — Entêtement. — Bêtise. — Idiotisme.

Bien faits, Délicats, Dignité et Bonté. — Lèvres minces, Sang-froid, Exactitude, Dissimulation. — Relevées, Affectation, Vanité, Dédain. — Bien close, Courage. — Mauvais penchants. — Sottise. — Prudence. — Bonté, Sensualité.

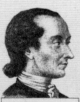
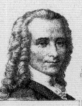

Petit Menton, Méchanceté. — Saillant, Fermeté, Prudence. — Reculé, Faiblesse, Frivolité. — Incisé, Résolu, Judicieux. — Nez étagé, Sensualité. — Pointu, Ruse. — Carré, Force, Fougue.

OREILLES rouges ; Sa... DENTS avancées, Ca... petites et courtes... longues ; Faibles...

TYPES

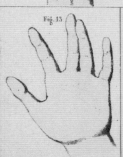

VINCENT DE PAUL
Bonté, Charité

LAVATER
Observation, Appréciation

VOLTAIRE
Esprit, Causticité

STERNE
Esprit de Saillies

DE TALLEYRAND
Finesse, Ruse

Fig. 1   Fig. 2   Fig. 3   Fig. 4   Fig. 5   Fig. 6

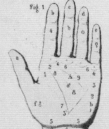

Fig. 13

LA CHIROMANCIE n'est, en réalité, qu'un jeu de l'esprit et n'a aucune portée scientifique ; on a pourtant voulu en faire un art au moyen duquel on prétend deviner le tempérament, les inclinations de l'âme et la destinée humaine par l'inspection des signes de toute espèce que la nature a tracés dans les mains de l'homme.

C'est ce qu'on appelle plus communément *Art divinatoire* ou *Bonne Aventure.*

Voici, *comme curiosité*, les principaux signes dont on prétend tirer des conséquences et qu'il suffit d'énumérer pour en faire voir toute l'absurdité.

DIVISION DE LA MAIN (fig. 1re).

a Pouce ; — *b* Index, Jupiter ; — *c* Moyen, Saturne ; — *d* Annulaire, Soleil ; — *e* Auriculaire, Mercure ; — + Montagne des doigts ; A Palme ; — *f* Montagne du pouce ; — Vénus ; — *g* Jointures ; — *h* Percussion, ⚏ Lune.

Lignes. — 1. 1. Ligne de Vie ou du Cœur ; — 2. 2. Moyenne naturelle ; — 3. 3. du Foie ou Hépatique ; — 4. 4. Mensale ou de Fortune ; — 5. 5. Restreinte ; — 6. 6. Mensale imparfaite ; — 7. 7. Sœur de la ligne de vie ; — 8.8. Id. ; — Triangle de Mars ; — 9. Table ou Quadrangle.

LIGNE DE VIE, 1. 1 (fig. 1re).

Longue, droite, luisante, indique : Santé, Longue vie. — Diffuse : Mauvaise santé, Brièveté de vie, Pas de réussite. — Large, grosse, confuse : Désordre. — Étroite, bien colorée : Courage, Droiture. — Marquée de points et variant de couleur : Malice, Finesse, Amour-propre, Bavardage. — Très-large et rouge : Inconstance, Méchanceté. — Couleur plombée : Mauvais caractère, Colère. — Sinueuse : Caractère cauteleux, Poltronnerie. — Accompagnée de deux lignes : Gaieté, Prodigalité, Libertinage. — Avec rameaux

tournés vers les doigts : Succès, Honneurs, Richesses ; — vers le bas : Malheur, Misère. — Semée de petits points : Querelles. — Une croix attenant à la ligne de Vie et accompagnée de petites lignes, a (fig. 2), annonce une grande propension au dérèglement. — *b* avec rameaux vers le pouce : Exaltation, Douleurs de tête, Mauvaise santé.

LIGNE MOYENNE NATURELLE, 2. 2.
(FIG. 1re).

Droite, longue, nette, bien sentie : Esprit délié, Entendement vif. — Quand elle va jusqu'au mont de la Lune : Courage. — Courte : Craintif, Lâche, Avare, Déloyal. — Arrêtée entre le doigt moyen et l'annulaire : Mœurs corrompues. — Courbée vers le bas, *a* (fig. 3) : Pauvreté ; — vers le haut, *b* : Malice, Impudence. — Inégale de forme et de couleur : Tendance au vol. — Droite, égale et luisante : Bonne conscience, Justice. — Large et grosse : Imprévoyance, Rusticité. — Mince et blême : Faiblesse et bêtise. — Avec petit, rayons : Colère. — Mêlée de nœuds (fig. 4) : Cruauté. — Formant un angle avec la ligne de Vie : Mémoire, Bonté. — Inégale et ne sortant pas du creux de la main : Avare, Craintif. — Avec une croix, *a*

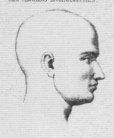

Prédominance
des facultés intellectuelles.

TOPOGRAPHIE
des facultés

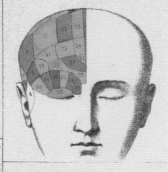

23. — CONFIGURATION. Forme, Ligne, Dessin, Géo-
métrie, Mémoire des figures.
24. — ÉTENDUE. Appréciation au Coup d'œil.
25. — PESANTEUR. Appréciation du poids des
objets.
26. — COULEURS. Sens du coloris.
27. — LOCALITÉ. Mémoire des lieux, Espace,
Orientabilité, Amour des voyages.
28. — CALCUL. Arithmétique, Mathématiques.
29. — ORDRE. Méthode, Propreté.
30. — ÉVENTUALITÉ. Éducabilité, Mémoire des faits,
Analyse.
31. — TEMPS. Mesure, Rhythme.
32. — TONALITÉ. Sens des sons, Musique, Mélodie.
33. — LANGAGE. Mémoire des mots, Éloquence,
Loquacité, Noms propres.
34. — COMPARAISON. Sagacité, Jugement, Raison,
Intelligence, Entendement, Allégorie.
35. — CAUSALITÉ. Esprit métaphysique, Spécu-
lation, Paradoxe, Sophisme.

9. — CONSTRUCTIVITÉ. Adresse, Mécanique, Sens
des arts.
10. — ESTIME DE SOI. Élévation, Orgueil, Fierté,
Ambition, Dignité personnelle. — Mo-
destie. — Humilité.
11. — APPROBATIVITÉ. Vanité, Ostentation, Indé-
pendance.
12. — CIRCONSPECTION. Prudence, Réserve, Rete-
nue, Prévoyance.
13. — BIENVEILLANCE. Bonté, Douceur, Charité,
Dévouement, Sensibilité.
14. — RELIGIOSITÉ. Sentiments religieux. Vénération, Mysticité.
15. — FERMETÉ. Persévérance, Énergie, Entêtement.

16. — CONSCIENCIOSITÉ. Justice.
17. — ESPÉRANCE. Projets, Sentiment de l'avenir.
18. — MERVEILLOSITÉ. Visions, Rêves.
19. — IDÉALITÉ. Imagination, Poésie.
20. — GAIETÉ. Saillie, Causticité.
21. — IMITATION. Gestes et Pantomime.
22. — INDIVIDUALITÉ. Distinction d'un objet d'un
autre objet.

Certaines facultés sont communes à l'homme et aux ani-
maux ; d'autres sont particulières à l'homme seul.

Suivant les degrés d'énergie d'une faculté, il en résulte
ce qu'on désigne par les noms de disposition, d'inclination,
de penchant, de désir, de besoin, de passion ; c'est-à-dire
que chaque faculté fondamentale est susceptible de ces
différents degrés de manifestation.

Les manifestations des facultés sont modifiées par la
disposition des organes et l'influence mutuelle des facultés.

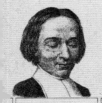

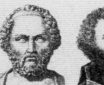
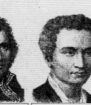
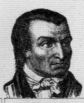

COU court et fort, Colère.
gras, Sottise, Gourmandise.
long, Faibles facultés.
bien fait, Dignité.

TEINT brun jaune foncé,
Tempérament bilieux Coloré;
Sanguin, Blême, Lymphatique

VISAGE, LAVATER divisait le Visage en trois régions :
1° Supérieure ; le front qui reflète les facultés de l'intelligence
2° Moyenne ; les yeux et le nez, les facultés morales.
3° Inférieure ; la bouche et le menton, les facultés physiques.

ANGLE FACIAL DE CAMPER.

Tirer, le long du bas du nez, une ligne droite
horizontale ND qui passe par le trou auditif extérieur C ; puis une autre droite verticale GM,
depuis les incisives supérieures jusqu'au point
le plus élevé du front.

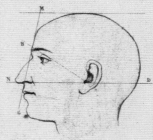

NOMIES.

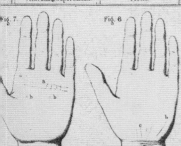

DIACRE-PARIS
Vénération, Superstition.

HOMÈRE
Poésie.

KLÉBER
Courage.

CARTOUCHE
Perversité.

FOUQUIER-TINVILLE
Méchanceté, Cruauté.

Plus l'angle MND que font entre elles les lignes
MG et ND est ouvert, plus l'animal ou l'homme
a de facultés intellectuelles ; plus, au contraire,
cet angle est aigu, moins l'animal ou l'homme a
d'intelligence.

Une simple ligne CB donne un résultat analogue

Fig. 7   Fig. 8   Fig. 9   Fig. 10   Fig. 11   Fig. 12

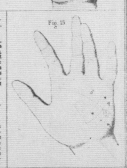

Fig. 15

(fig. 4) : Opiniâtreté, Chicane. — Croisée de petites
lignes b b : Orgueil, Médisance.
LIGNE DU FOIE, 3. 3. (FIG. 1re).
Ne se trouve pas sur toutes les mains, et est surtout
un signe de bonne et forte santé.
LIGNE MENSALE, 4. 4. (FIG. 1re).
Longue, droite, égale : Bonne qualité de nature. —
Touchant la montagne de Jupiter : Esprit. — Avec
rameaux vers le doigt de Jupiter : Ambition. — Avec
trois lignes à la fin, a (fig. 5) : Gaieté, Douceur, Libé-
ralité. — Se terminant en b : Tromperie, Mensonge.
— Angle avec la Moyenne : Esprit désordonné. —
Jointe à la ligne de Vie : Danger d'accidents. —
Droite et fine en c : Amour de la famille. — Inter-
rompue : Inconstance, Ineptie. — De forme a (fig. 6) :
Être dangereux ; — b, Force et vigueur de tempéra-
ment. La disposition a (fig. 7) : Bonnes qualités. —
Avec deux croix bb : Dignités spirituelles.
LIGNE RESTRAINCTE, 5. 5. (FIG. 1re)
De belle couleur : Bonne complexion. — Composée de
2 lignes : Richesses ; — de 4 lignes, a (fig. 8) : Honneurs,
héritages. — Une ligne b : Adversité. — Des lignes c :

Dignité, Orgueil. — Tranché de petites lignes : Famille
nombreuse. — Petites étoiles : Mauvaise Vie. —
h Richesses. — Mont du doigt moyen, uni : Raison ; —
avec une ligne joignant la mensale : Mélancolie ; —
plusieurs incisions : Chagrins ; — ligne courbe joignant
l'Annulaire : Paresse ; — Mont de l'Annulaire, uni, avec
des lignes allant à la Mensale** : Gravité, Éloquence,
Savoir ; — traversé de lignes fines : Prudence et Gaieté ;
— deux lignes allant à la Restrainte i : Bonheur. —
Mont de l'Auriculaire, uni et plat : Bon signe, Pureté,
Innocence. — Une ligne colorée joignant la Mensale k :
Liberalité ; — rouge seulement l : Mensonge, Rapacité.—
Ligne m : bonté naturelle, Fortune. — Petites lignes irré-
gulières et recourbées, chez les femmes : Mauvaises
langues. — n Studieux, Appliqué. — Renversée en forme
de V : Passions vives. — o Aptitude, Vivacité. —
p Misère.

RÉGION DE LA LUNE (FIG. 15).
Unie : Bon signe. — Ridée ou marquée d'étoiles q :
Mauvais sort, Vue faible.

TRIANGLE DE MARS (FIG 1re).
S'il est formé de doubles lignes : Méchanceté. —
Très-ouvert dénote : Opiniâtreté, Présomption.

Vie joyeuse et heureuse. — a (fig. 9) Fortune incon-
stante. — b Prospérité. — c (fig. 10) : Voyages lointains.
TRIANGLE DE LA MAIN, (FIG 1re).
Formé par les lignes de Vie, Moyenne et du Foie.
— L'angle a (fig. 11) : Liberté. — Angle b, bien
marqué : Bonnes qualités du corps, Courage, Dignité ;
— fortement prononcé : Audace, Générosité ; — étroit
et court : Avarice et lâcheté ; — tranché par des plis :
Mauvaise complexion. — Angle c, bien formé : Bonnes
qualités, Innocence de mœurs. — Si les deux lignes
ne se joignent pas : Mensonge, Fausseté. — (fig. 12)
Signe d'infidélité. — L'angle à très-aigu : Parleur et
...queur.

QUADRANGLE, 9 (FIG. 1re).
Bien formé : Jugement, Esprit, Courage, Libéralité. —
Croix au milieu (fig. 13) : Bonheur, Tendresse.

MONTAGNES DES DOIGTS (FIG. 14).
La Montagne du pouce a, unie et de belle couleur :
Penchant à la coquetterie ; — quatre lignes c : Prospé-
rité, — des étoiles d, Penchant pour le jeu, la musique
et la Vie joyeuse ; — rayée inégalement et confusément :
Ivrognerie, Méchanceté. — Anneau e, bien marqué :
Mort violente. — Plusieurs croix f : Dévotion. — Le
mont de l'Index uni : Honnêteté, Bonté. Une croix

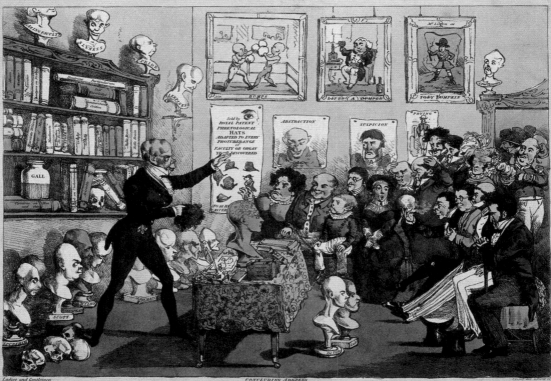

CALVES' HEADS AND BRAINS OR A PHRENOLOGICAL LECTURE.

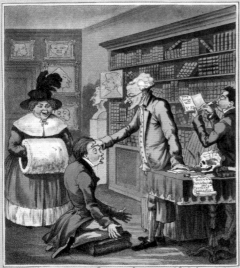

Bumpology

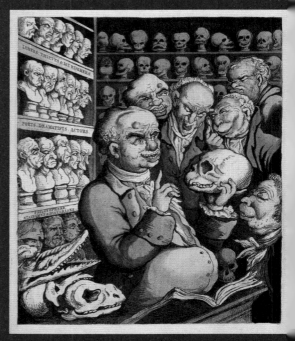

The theory of phrenology developed from the idea that faces displayed mental types: *top* Leading British phrenologist George Combe lecturing at Edinburgh, 1826; *above (left)* 'Bumpology' (1826) by George Cruikshank, a caricature of phrenologist J. De Dille examining a patient; *above (right)* Coloured etching by Thomas Rowlandson, 1808, in which Franz Joseph Gall leads his colleagues in a discussion of phrenology; *right page* Gall is satirized: measuring the head of an elderly patient (*above*) and feeling the bumps of William Pitt and King Gustavus of Sweden (*below*), 1806.

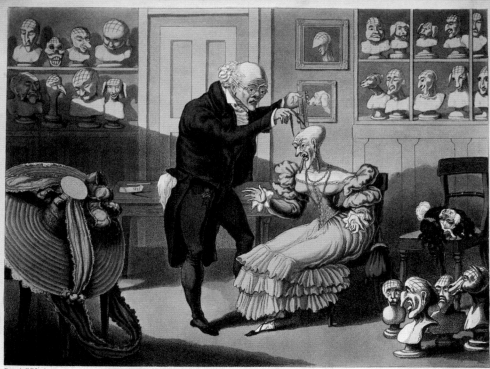

Drawn by E.F. Lambert. Engd by F.C. Hunt.

AN OLD MAID'S SKULL PHRENOLOGISED,

Old Maid :— *Doctor S.* when you have examined all my bumps, *I'll trouble you to explain the* faculties, sympathies & propensities *of my dear* Poodle Pompey.

Doctor S. *Miss Strangeways!* I can distinctly enumerate thro' the aid of my Patent Skullometer, *that your cranium contains* 16.542 ½ *Mental Faculties which I shall by my Scale of individuality describe on a future occasion.* As for your Poodle Pompey *his prominent bumps are* Veneration[s] *and* Philoprogenitiveness!!!

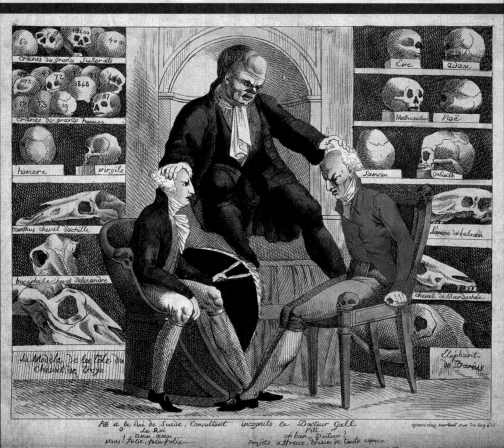

Pitt & le Roi de Suède, Consultant incognito le Docteur Gall
Pitt
le Roi
Ah bien, Docteur?
ainsi, ainsi......
Vous! Folie, folie folie...... Projets affreux, Crimes de toute espèce.

aparochez marbret rue Du Coq &15

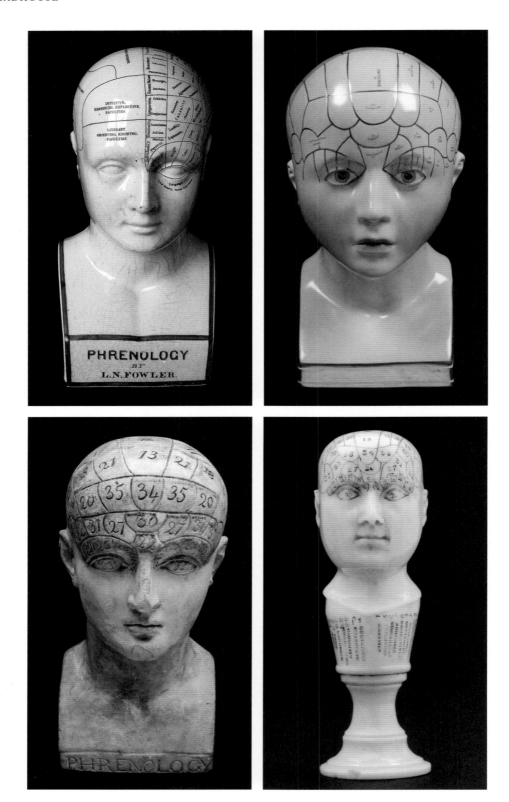

top (left)
Phrenological head
by L. N. Fowler, in the
Wellcome Historical
Medical Museum.

top (right)
Porcelain phrenological
bust, tinted skin colour,
with divisions and
numbers marked in gilt.

above (left)
Earthenware
phrenological bust with
areas marked off by an
impressed line, 1821.

above (right)
Ivory head marked off in
sections for phrenological
consultations,
1910–1925.

right page
Phrenological skull
with brain sections
labelled in French,
1801–1900.

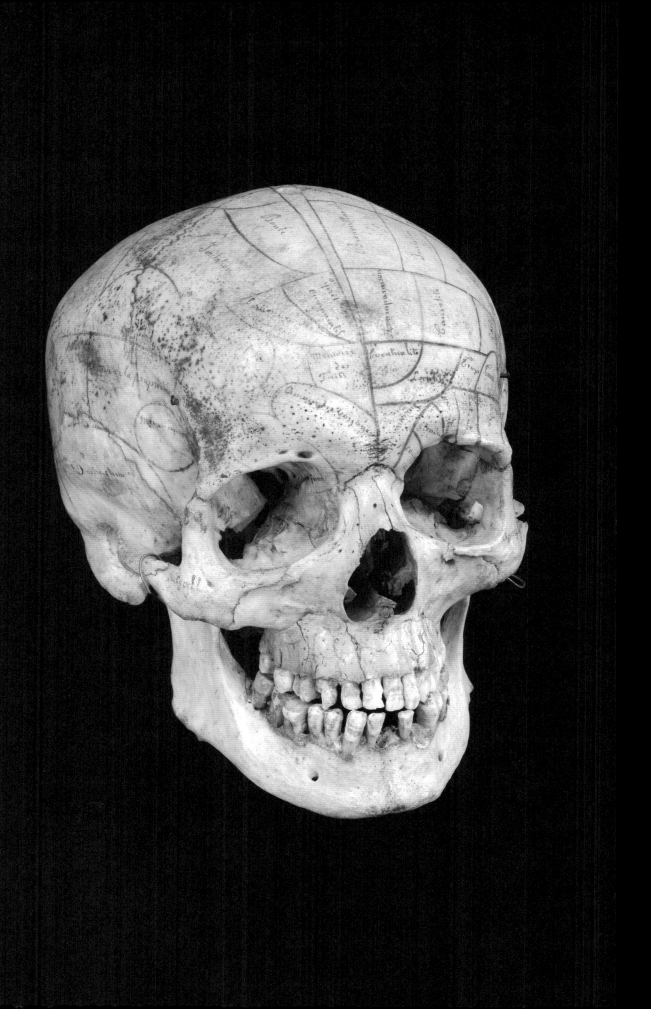

right
A collection
of commonly
used instruments
of restraint,
including
wrist cuffs and
chains, collars,
muffs and
ankle bands.

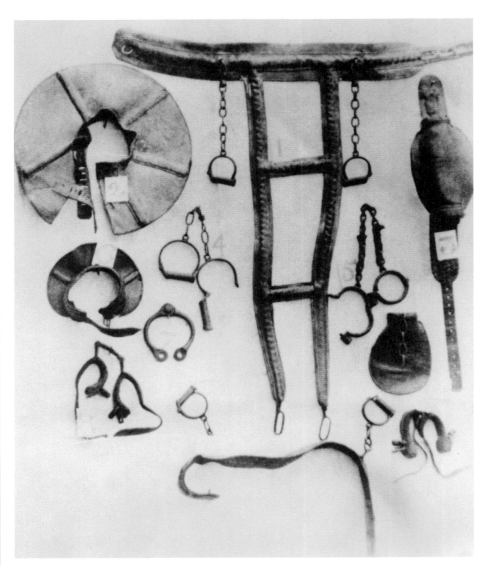

type of institution he imagined was already emerging. Within a generation, it would be taking root across the world.

In republican France, Pinel and his successors were already transforming the medical profession into a significant arm of the state. Madness became the business of physicians, usurping the authority of the Church: in 1790 Pinel lent medical support to the abolition of monasteries by classifying religious experiences as forms of hysteria or delirium. 'Alienists', as mad-doctors styled themselves, claimed legal jurisdiction by creating a new category of 'monomaniacal homicide', which only they were competent to diagnose. They insinuated themselves ever more widely into politics: in the delicate phrasing of Pinel's protégé Jean-Etienne-Dominique Esquirol, 'the physician enlightens the

government about mental tendencies'.[12] Esquirol successfully embedded these new powers in the constitution in 1838 with a law that created a specialist asylum for each of France's *départements*, independent from the general hospital system and working directly with the Ministry of the Interior to monitor and control dangerous individuals.

Revolution finally came to Bethlem in 1814 in the person of Edward Wakefield, a Quaker philanthropist whose mother had been confined in a madhouse and who dedicated himself to campaigning for reform. He was part of a growing movement of social reformers, many of them at this point drawn from the Evangelical and dissenting communities, for whom the humane treatment of lunatics had become part of a crusade that encompassed the improvement of prisons and workhouses

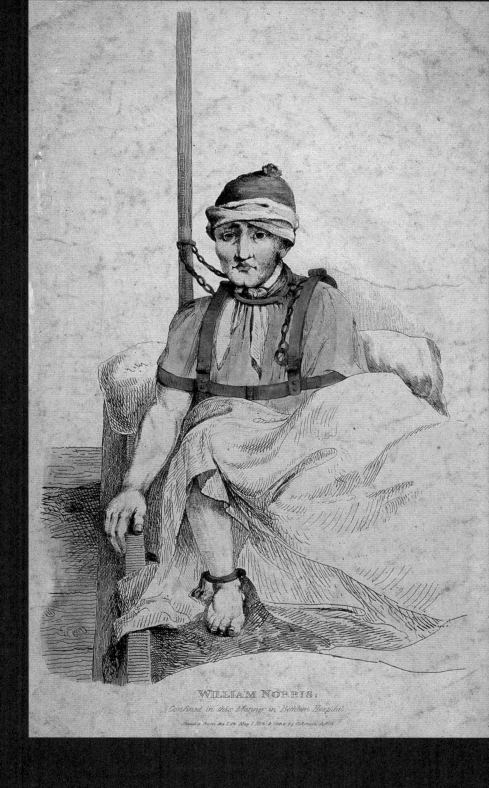

WILLIAM NORRIS:

Confined in this Manner in Bethlem Hospital.

Sketch'd from the Life May 1.1814 & Etch'd by G. Arnald A.R.A.

above Etching by George Cruikshank, *c.* 1820.
James Norris (misnamed as William) was the
most notorious case of mistreatment in Bethlem.
He was chained in this device for ten years.

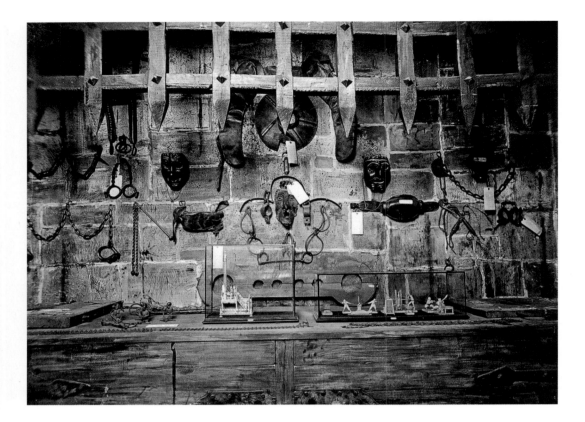

and the abolition of slavery. They shared the growing belief that the mad were not beings bereft of reason and responsive only to fear or punishment, but - like slaves, criminals and the poor - common members of humanity who could be redeemed by reason, justice and kindness. It was the same assumption that Pinel's therapy framed in medical terms: madness could be addressed by reason and by engaging its sufferers in their own cure.

On Wakefield's first visit, the Bethlem staff sullenly denied him entry from behind a locked door. When he returned accompanied by a Member of Parliament, he was appalled to discover patients neglected, poorly clothed and shivering with cold, and in one particularly distressing case chained to the wall by an iron ring riveted around the neck. Wakefield's report caused a public scandal, and a House of Commons committee elicited damning evidence of a regime in which brutality and neglect had become endemic. The staff blamed one another, and the physician and apothecary were both dismissed. In the meantime, the new Bethlem had risen on the south bank of the Thames, and Bethlem's 122 lunatics were transported, on 24 August 1815, across London in carriages, to the hope of a new beginning.

1   Thomas Brown, *Amusements Serious and Comical, Calculated for the Meridian of London* (London: 1700) p. 29
2   Thomas Tryon, *A Treatise of Dreams and Visions* (1695)
3   Thomas Tryon, *Discourse on the Causes, Nature and Cure of Madness, Phrensie and Distraction* (1689)
4   Ward, *The London Spy* (Folio ed. 1955, pp. 48–50)
5   *ibid.* p. 407
6   John Monro, *Remarks on William Battie's Treatise* (1758) in *Three Hundred Years of Psychiatry 1535–1860* (London: 1963) p. 415
7   Evidence of Dr Richard Warren, court physician, 13 January 1789
8   Thomas Erskine, *Proceedings on the Trial of James Hadfield at the Court of the King's Bench for High Treason*, June 26 1800
9   Philippe Pinel, *Medico-Philosophical Treatise on Mental Alienation* (2nd ed. 1809, tr. Gordon Hickish, David Healy, Louis C. Charland; Wiley-Blackwell, Oxford: 2008) p. xxix
10   *ibid.* p. 62
11   *ibid.* p. 84
12   Quoted in Jan Goldstein, *Console and Classify* (Chicago: University of Chicago Press, 1989) p. 158

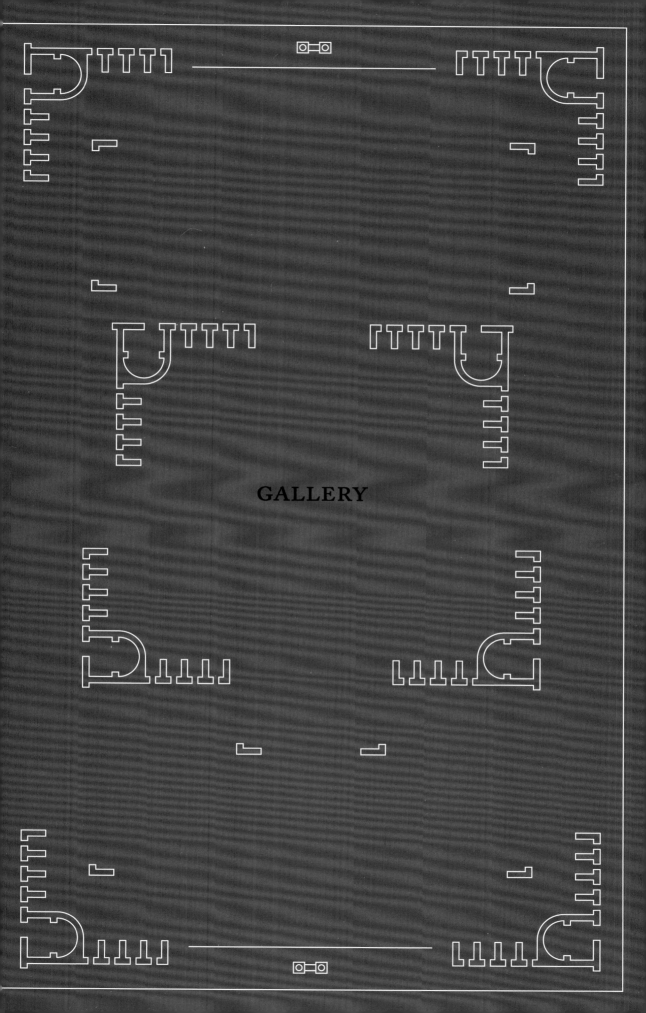

GALLERY

Hadfield (see p. 62) was confined in Bethlem hospital as criminally insane in 1800. He escaped in 1802, was recaptured at Dover and remained in the criminal wing at Southwark until his death in 1841.

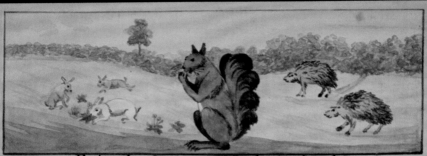

Epitaph, of my poor Jack, Squirrel.

Here are the remains of my poor little Jack.
Who, with a little fall; almost broke his back.
And I myself was the occasion of that.
By letting him be frighten'd, by a Cat.
I then picked him up, from off the floor;
But he, alas! Never danced a hornpipe more;
And many a time, have I laugh'd, to see him So cunning;
To Sit and Crack the nuts I gave him So funny;
Now in Remembrance of his pretty tricks.
I have had him Stuff'd, that I might not him forget.
And So he is gone; and I must go, as well as him;
And pray God, Send I may go, but wi the little Sin;
So there is an End, to my little dancing Jack.
That will never more, be frighten'd, by a Cat.

Died Sunday
Morning   James Hadfield.   Bethlem
July 23rd 26.   Hospital.

Epitaph, of my poor Jack. Squirrel.

Here are the Remains of my poor little Jack,
Who, with a little fall; almost broke his back;
And I myself was the occasion of that
By letting him be frighten'd, by a Cat;
I then picked him up, from off the floor;
But he, alas! never danced a hornpipe more;
And many a time have I laugh'd, to see him come,
So Sit and Crack the nuts I gave him So funny;
Now in Remembrance of his pretty tricks;
I have had him, Stuff'd, I might not him forget;
And So he is gone; and I must go; as well as him;
And pray God; Send I may go; best with little Sin;
So there is an end, to my little dancing Jack;
That will never more be, frighten'd, by a Cat.

Died Sunday
Morning   James Hadfield
July. 23. 1826.

JAMES TILLY MATTHEWS

UNKNOWN—1815

Matthews (see p.71) was a tea merchant who became caught up in political intrigues during the French Revolution. He was admitted to Bethlem after publicly accusing members of the British government of treason.

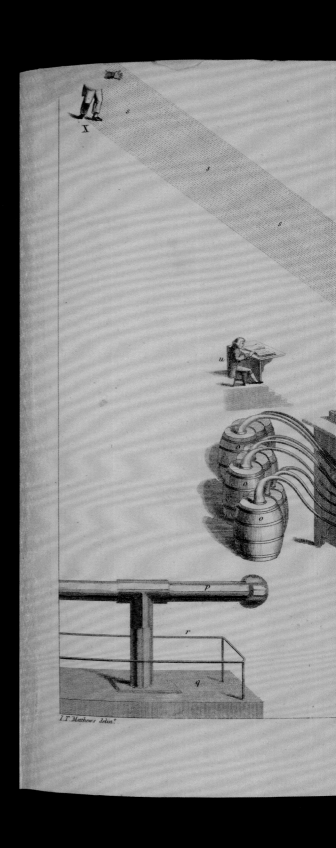

right
The Air Loom by James Tilly Matthews, from John Haslam's *Illustrations of Madness* (1810). The artist believed that his mind was under the control of a terrifying machine called the Air Loom.

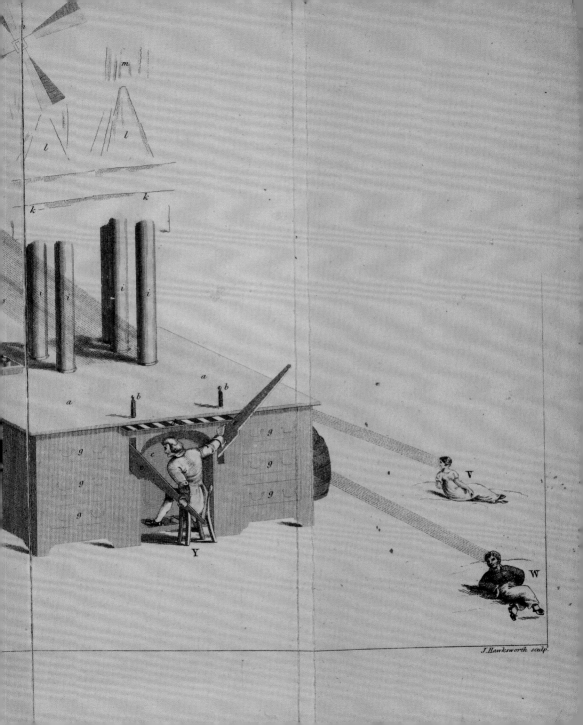

so made to project sufficiently, in length equal with the 4 Innermost Pilaster Plinths, with next Ironwork arcades, it will form a handsome Balcony for the Governors

to take View of the whole length of the Front Gardens, &c from. The Entrance Court is supposed raised above the Grounds general Level, as the Black line denotes —

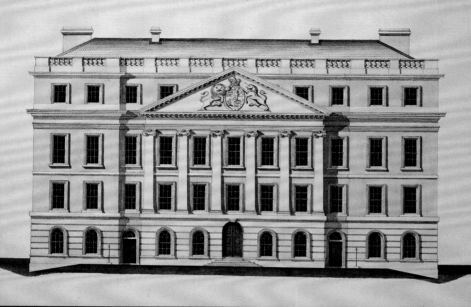

This Sheet shows the Principal Front Elevation at **A**. The Criminal Lunatics Asylums at **B**; with the Laundry, &c, in its proportion of height, between

but beyond them. The Steam from the Washouse, and Smoke from the Chimneys and Straw Shaft, does not rise within full 100 feet of the nearest parts of such Asylums.

The Plan Score shews the Recesses for View in the Back Front of the Hospital **C**. with the passages, Arcades &c to the Asylums,

to the Laundry, to the Back, Straw Shaft &c as they lie and apply to and between the Hospital, the Asylums & the mid Buildings.

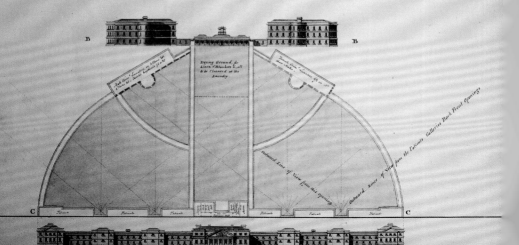

B   B

Drying Ground, for
Linen &Blankets &c all
to be Cleansed at the
Laundry

Outward Line of View from this opening

Outward Lines of View from the Patients Galleries Back Front Openings

C   C

Patients   Patients   Patients   Patients   Patients   Patients

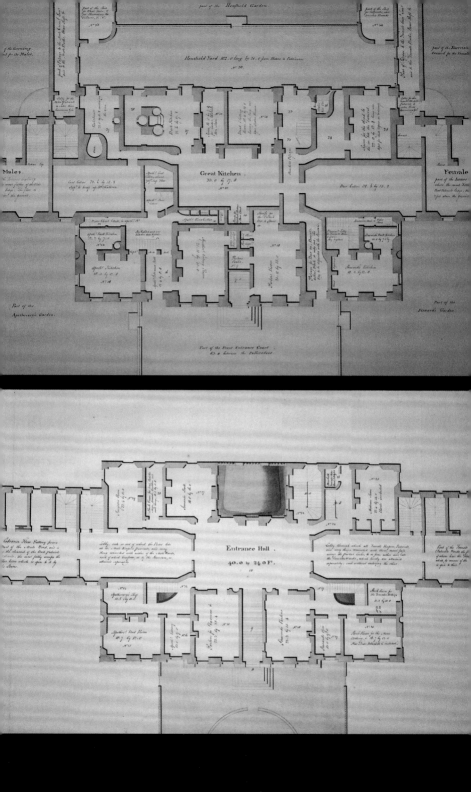

left page
From James Tilly Matthews's *Architectural Plans and Explanatory Notes* (1810–1811), which he submitted to the governors in a public competition. The front elevation (*top*) was included in the design plans for the rebuilding of Bethlem. Matthews' view of the spacious grounds (*bottom*) featured a kitchen garden, where patients would work

above
Two extensive floor plans. Matthews's designs and proposals also included detailed notes that described how the new hospital regime would operate.

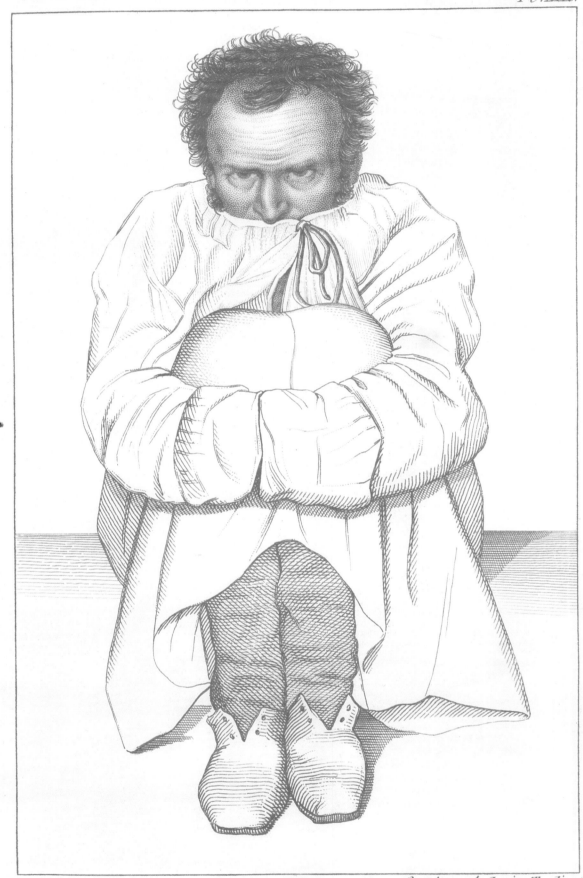

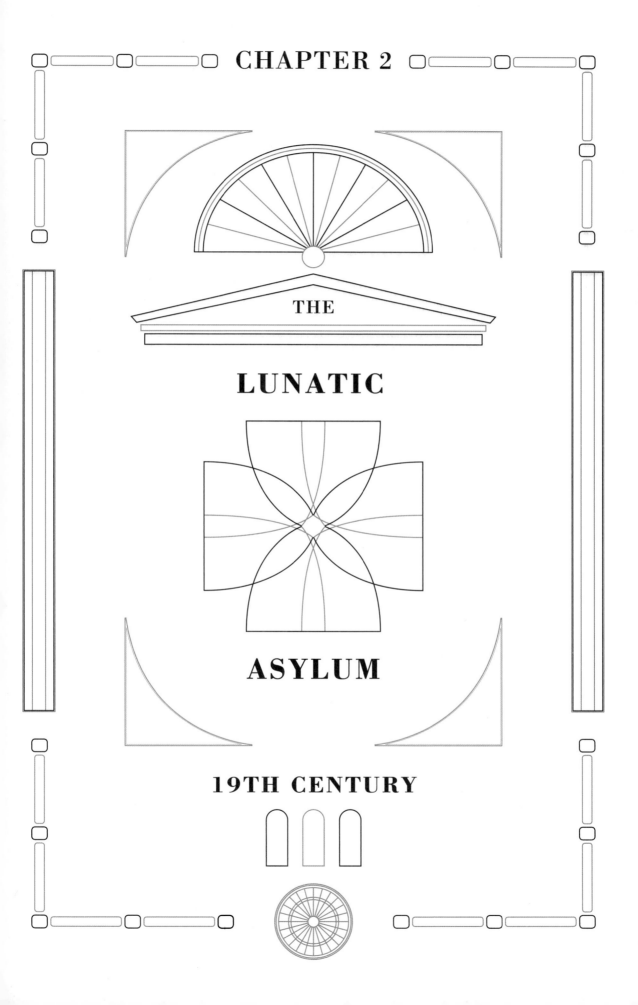

CHAPTER 2

THE

LUNATIC

ASYLUM

19TH CENTURY

RIGHT
COLOURED
ENGRAVING BY
JOHN PASS, 1814
THE NEW BETHLEM
HOSPITAL AT
ST GEORGE'S FIELDS,
SOUTHWARK.

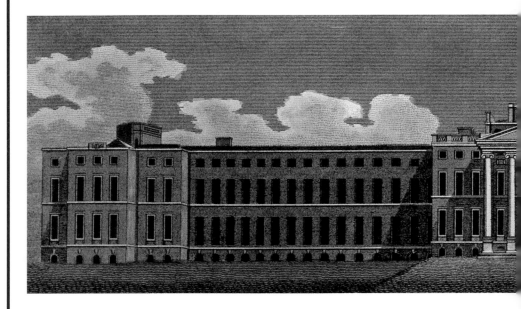

90

The old Bethlem was demolished to a chorus of sentiment for 'the only building which looked like a palace in London',[1] but its theatrical grandeur belonged to a bygone age. The new building was plain and serious, resembling a barracks or administrative block, sited on the south bank of the Thames in a cheap district mostly given over to slum housing and industries, such as tanning, brewing and vinegar distilling, that were only permitted outside the city proper. Its facade was an unadorned neoclassical rectangle; the signature figures of *Raving* and *Melancholy Madness* (1676) had been removed from public view and placed discreetly in the entrance hall. With the exception of a solid central portico, the sole ornamentation – added to address concerns that the building erred too far on the side of plainness – was a central cupola, later replaced with a taller dome that resembled a birdcage. The dome still looms over Southwark today, and the building now houses the Imperial War Museum.

Bethlem received extra funding for a purpose-built wing for criminal lunatics, as mandated by the legislation that was passed hurriedly in the wake of James Hadfield's acquittal. It was designed for maximum security and to protect the other inmates from the violently insane; it was also intended to offer a more therapeutic environment than the county jail cells in which criminal lunatics were at the time confined for life, despite their technical innocence. Hadfield was among the wing's first intake of twenty men and two women, and he remained there until 1841, living an existence he described as worse than death. The other new galleries were little improvement on the previous building: they were damp and gloomy, with open sewers and unglazed windows set too high to allow views or direct sunlight. A novel but inefficient steam heating system in the basement failed to circulate the little warmth it generated, and the inmates froze through the winter much as they had in the palatial ruins at Moorfields.

The abuses exposed by the parliamentary committee persisted under the new regime. In 1818 Urbane Metcalf, an itinerant hawker who believed he was heir to the throne of Denmark, published a pamphlet

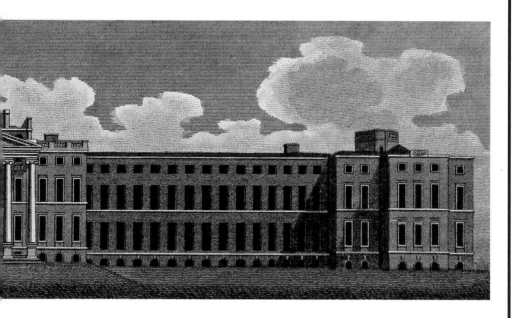

describing the time that he had spent in both Bethlem buildings. He found in the new one 'many alterations in the provisions, and in other things that greatly added to the comfort of the patients', but the same culture of corruption and malpractice among the staff. Metcalf was, according to the hospital, a far more troublesome inmate than he admitted and some details of his story seem unlikely, but its broad outlines would be recognized by asylum patients throughout history. The keepers operated with impunity and covered up for one another, demanding bribes for basic provisions and stealing the food of those who complained. Inmates became desperate for the favour of the keepers, who set them against one another for their own amusement; the wardens had no compunction about doling out vicious beatings and no trouble covering up fatalities. The result was 'a total abuse to humanity', a system in which those with power contrived to make it absolute and those without became permanent victims. Anyone who tried to appeal for justice was refused outside visits: when Metcalf mentioned the abuses to the physicians or to visiting gentlemen, they 'treated them with indifference and neglect'.[2]

«THE NEW BUILDING WAS PLAIN AND SERIOUS, RESEMBLING A BARRACKS»

By this time an alternative form of care for the mad had emerged, much closer to the Bethlem that James Tilly Matthews had envisaged. In 1813 *Description of the Retreat: Institution Near York for Insane Persons of the Society of Friends* announced to the world a quiet revolution that had been taking place among the Society of Friends, more commonly known as the Quakers, in the north of England. Its author, Samuel Tuke, was a member of a Quaker family who had become wealthy in the tea trade and, motivated by the appalling conditions in York's public asylum, opened their own hospital in 1796.

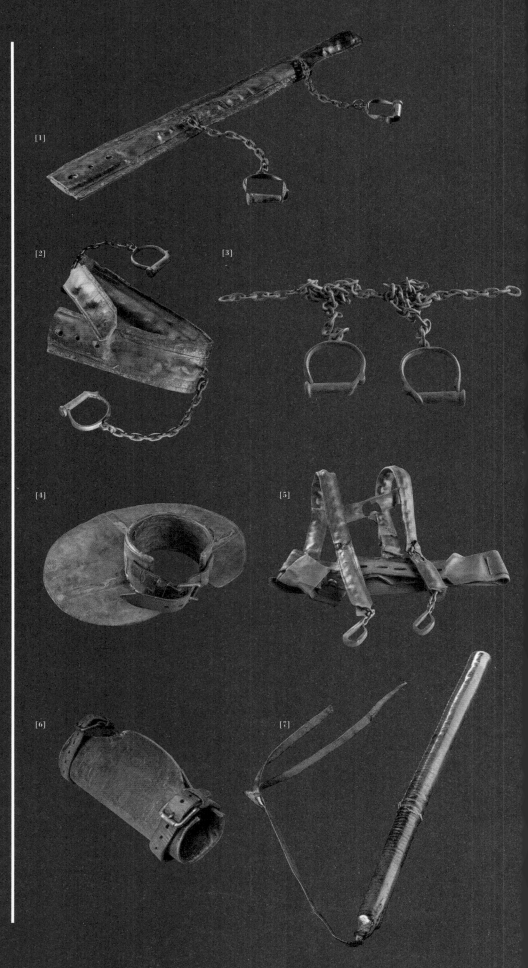

RIGHT
A CHEST OF LEATHER RESTRAINT HARNESSES WAS FOUND AT THE HANWELL ASYLUM IN MIDDLESEX IN 1930. THE DEVICES WERE USED TO RESTRICT THE MOVEMENTS OF MENTALLY ILL PATIENTS WHO WERE CONSIDERED TO BE VIOLENT. COPIES OF THE RESTRAINTS WERE POSSIBLY CREATED TO ILLUSTRATE THIS FORMER TREATMENT OF INMATES.

THESE ITEMS ARE REPLICAS OF THE 19TH-CENTURY RESTRAINT HARNESSES FOUND AT HANWELL. THEY INCLUDE A REPLICA OF A WIDE-BRIMMED LEATHER RESTRAINT COLLAR (4), WHICH MAY HAVE BEEN USED IN CONJUNCTION WITH MANACLES OR A STRAITJACKET, AND A FOREARM RESTRAINT (6), WHICH WOULD HAVE HELPED TO CONTAIN A VIOLENT OR UNRULY PATIENT.

[1]

[2]

[3]

[4]

[5]

[6]

[7]

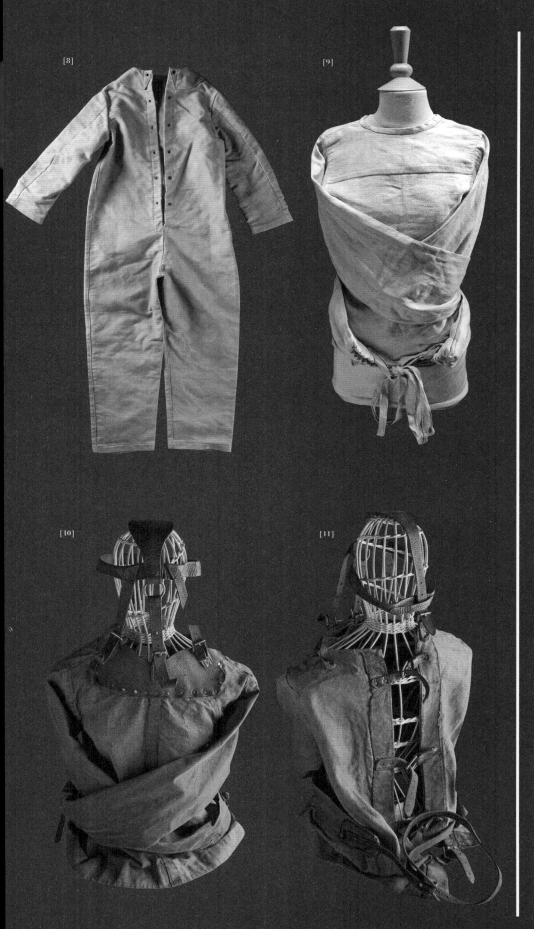

[8]

[9]

[10]

[11]

LEFT
THE STRAITJACKET
WAS NOT ONLY USED
FOR RESTRAINING
PATIENTS BUT ALSO
AS A 'TREATMENT'.
THE RESTRAINT
OR WARMING
SUIT (8) IS FROM
BRIGHTON COUNTY
BOROUGH ASYLUM,
FORMERLY SUSSEX
LUNATIC ASYLUM,
1890–1948, WHERE
IT MAY HAVE
BEEN USED LIKE
A CONVENTIONAL
STRAITJACKET (9).
HOWEVER, THERE
ARE NO VISIBLE
BELTS OR BUCKLES
SO IT IS MAY HAVE
BEEN A WARMING
SUIT FOR PATIENTS
IN THE INFIRMARY.

LEFT
CANVAS AND
LEATHER REPLICAS
OF A STRAITJACKET
(RESTRAINT SUIT)
WITH HEAD STRAPS,
EUROPE, 1925–1935.

RIGHT
PLANS OF THE
GROUND FLOOR
(*ABOVE*) AND
SECOND FLOOR
OF THE RETREAT
NEAR YORK. FROM
*DESCRIPTION OF
THE RETREAT,
AN INSTITUTION
NEAR YORK, FOR
INSANE PERSONS
OF THE SOCIETY OF
FRIENDS* (1813) BY
SAMUEL TUKE.

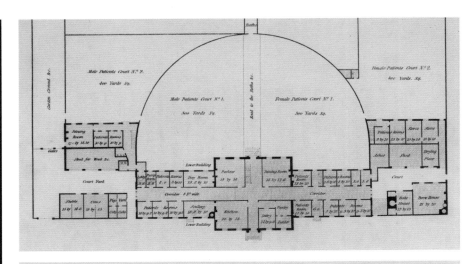

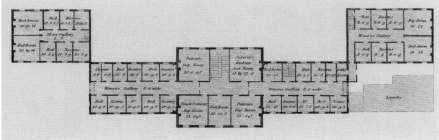

The York Retreat was a purpose-built mansion on high, open ground, surrounded by gardens and woods criss-crossed with pleasant walking trails. There were no doctors: the superintendent was a charismatic lay preacher from the local Quaker community. The building was designed to resemble a family home as much as possible. Window bars and door locks were concealed discreetly behind hand-carved panels and soft furnishings, and the galleries were comfortable day rooms in which tables were set for communal dining in the evening. Female patients polished the furniture, churned the butter and sat in sewing circles; men repaired the building and tended the vegetable plots.

Tuke utilized the term 'moral treatment', borrowed and translated from Philippe Pinel, to describe the York Retreat's regime. 'Moral' is misleading to modern ears – we would probably say 'social' – but its significance was as an alternative to 'medical'. Initially, the Tuke family had tried various medical therapies, but they rejected them and decided instead to create an environment with as little whiff of a hospital as possible. Moral treatment was therapy for the whole person, not for any supposed mental defect. In place of bleeding and purging, it offered individual care that was designed to nurture a stable personality through useful occupations and religious devotion, with the aim of restoring the patient to normal society. York Retreat was also, in a phrase that would not be coined until much later, a therapeutic community. Patients and staff lived, worked and ate together; the bonds of family replaced the hierarchy of control. Instead of languishing in bare galleries and becoming ever more raving or melancholy while waiting for a cure to materialize, patients were subsumed into a life that was as normal as possible, with the hope that they would one day find themselves recovered without having noticed any therapy taking place.

In some respects, the new model asylum – the term preferred to 'hospital' or 'madhouse' – replicated Pinel's reforms in France, but in other ways it rejected them. Like Pinel, it treated madness as a misfortune that could be remedied, and it embodied the conviction that a specially designed institution was better suited to promoting recovery than the household in which the condition had arisen. However, medicine was central to Pinel's model: he was transforming the old madhouses into clinics where madness was treated without moral judgment as a curable illness. The energetic network of reformers who took *Description of the Retreat* as their blueprint saw medical authority as part of the problem, not the solution. As the York Retreat's reputation spread, the Tukes and their fellow reformers were invited onto the governing boards of old madhouses eager to rebrand themselves as enlightened and humane. Physicians found themselves on the defensive, pressed for evidence that madness

benefited from medical intervention. They were on firmer ground in jurisprudence, in which the demand for expert medical testimony in insanity pleas was growing. As mad-doctors were sidelined on the statutory bodies of asylum licensing and inspection, they were called on more often in the courts to define concepts such as 'unsound mind', 'lucid intervals' and 'imbecility'.

However, the new model of care described so inspiringly by Tuke proved hard to replicate. It required passionately dedicated staff, who were happy to spend their entire lives caring for demanding patients, many of whom were by no means docile or on a smooth road to recovery. Even in the most enlightened asylum, recovery rates remained stubbornly low and disruptive patients who upset their fellows needed to be kept under control for the general good.

When keepers were overworked and poorly supervised, the old regime of bribes, rewards and punishments tended to reassert itself. Although locked cells, straitjackets and other restraints were kept discreetly out of sight, they remained all too tempting as a last resort. Moral treatment could succeed

«MORAL TREATMENT WAS THERAPY FOR THE WHOLE PERSON»

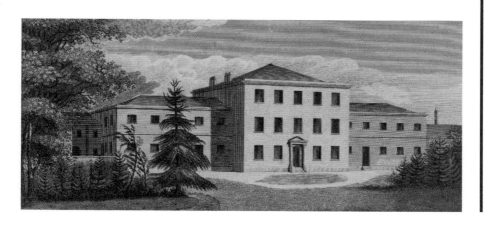

LEFT
A VIEW OF THE NORTH FRONT OF THE RETREAT NEAR YORK. FROM *DESCRIPTION OF THE RETREAT, AN INSTITUTION NEAR YORK, FOR INSANE PERSONS OF THE SOCIETY OF FRIENDS* (1813) BY SAMUEL TUKE.

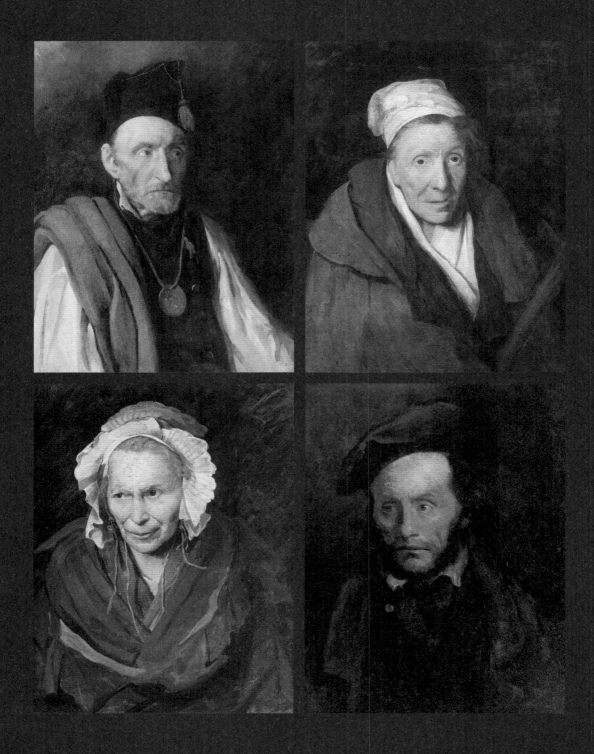

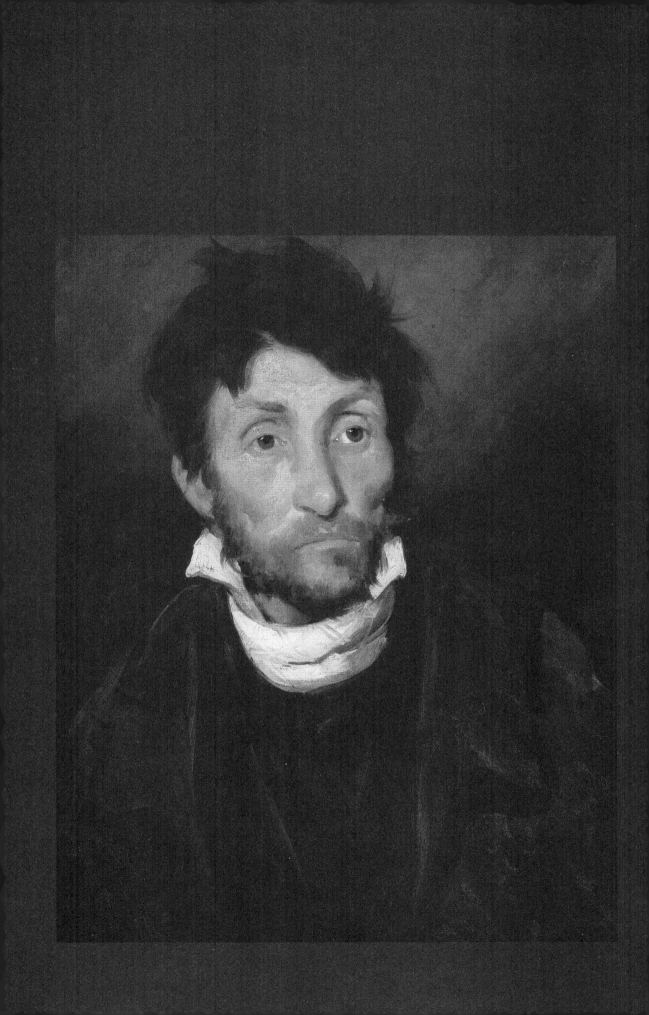

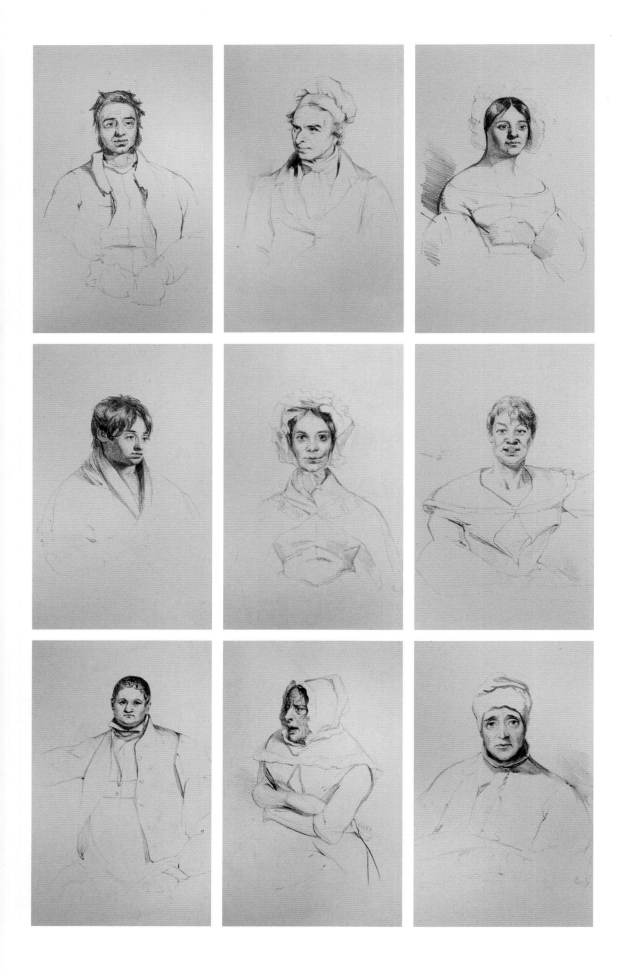

only when underpinned by considerable human and financial resources.

The tensions between moral and medical treatment played out around the globe. In the young United States, physicians such as Benjamin Rush – signatory to the Declaration of Independence (1776) and officially designated 'Father of American Psychiatry' by the American Psychiatric Association – aimed to put the treatment of insanity on a firm medical footing. Rush believed that most mental diseases were caused by disruptions to blood circulation, and he devised elaborate mechanical restraints, including a 'tranquillizer chair' complete with straps and head brace, to reduce the blood supply to the brain. But effective medical treatment was very limited, and physicians who recorded the causes of insanity found them to be more often social or religious than biological. The roots of madness might ultimately lie in lesions of the brain, but the search for a cure needed to consider the constitution of American society, too.

Traditionally, pioneer and settler communities had taken care of their mentally distressed relatives at home, but the ideas of moral therapy inspired a growing network of charitable asylums. Friends Hospital was founded outside Philadelphia in 1813 after local Quakers visited the York Retreat, and Tuke composed a guide for effective moral treatment to be circulated through the Religious Societies of Friends across the United States. Moral and medical therapies were combined gradually: the physician at Massachusetts General Hospital in Boston adopted moral treatment in 1818 after reading Tuke's *Description of the Retreat*, while the

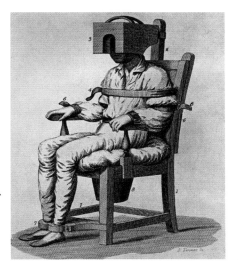

founders of Hartford Retreat for the Insane in Connecticut employed a medical superintendent, having been persuaded by local physicians that many cases of insanity had a physical component. Bloomingdale Asylum in New York was one of many institutions that had begun by keeping lunatics in basement cells, but these were replaced by spacious, light and airy buildings and a working farm.

As the 19th century progressed, the asylum became an emblem of social progress. It embodied the new sensitivity towards suffering that manifested itself in many forms: campaigns against child labour and animal cruelty, the growing distaste for public hangings and the introduction of anaesthetics into surgery. The impoverished, homeless, disabled and mentally disordered were a reproach to a feeling society, and also a blemish on the proud neighbourhoods of the new middling classes. Asylums flourished alongside the other progressive institutions that defined the age: cooperative and benefit societies,

THE LUNATIC ASYLUM

99

boards of philanthropy and committees for cultural improvement. At the same time, the demands and pressures on them were growing fast. The market economy and industry that were transforming both rural and urban life made families less able to care for their unproductive members. Madness spilled out from homes and families, as the breadwinners abandoned the household to become live-in servants or to lodge in factories and workers' cottages. Furthermore, as the asylums expanded, they became worlds unto themselves. The voices of their patients receded, muffled both by the regimes that ran them and the wish of the public to believe they were humane. Occasionally, protests made themselves heard and exposed the realities of life behind the high walls. In Britain, the most prominent was that of John Perceval for whom, like Alexander Cruden, madness was a tragic thread in a remarkable life story. His father, Spencer Perceval, had been the British prime minister until a deranged lunatic assassinated him in the House of Commons in 1812, when his son was only nine years old. John subsequently attended Oxford University where he became an ardent Evangelical, devoting himself to prayer and fasting. In 1830 he travelled to Scotland to visit a rural congregation well known for speaking

«MADNESS SPILLED OUT FROM HOMES AND FAMILIES AS THE BREAD-WINNERS ABANDONED THE HOUSEHOLD»

in tongues; it was an experience that shook him profoundly and imbued him with Pentecostal fire. He moved on to Dublin where, as his spiritual crisis deepened, he contracted syphilis from a prostitute and began to hear voices.

John Perceval's social class made his voice more audible than those of most asylum patients, but it also showed – as the madness of George III had done previously – that ultimately the stubbornly disruptive are dealt with in much the same way, whatever their background. When Perceval became unmanageable, he was confined in a succession of private asylums culminating in Ticehurst, the most exclusive and expensive in the country. Set in a large expanse of parkland in the Sussex countryside, it was the destination of choice for distressed aristocrats throughout the 19th century. Their personal servants attended many of those confined there. The grounds, scattered with gold and silver pheasants, included a summer house, bowling green, pagoda, archery field and cricket pitch, as well as enough countryside for hunting with hounds. The main residential block was a stately home with a reading room and theatre as well as a regular programme of concerts and lectures.

By the time Perceval arrived at Ticehurst, the most severe phase of his

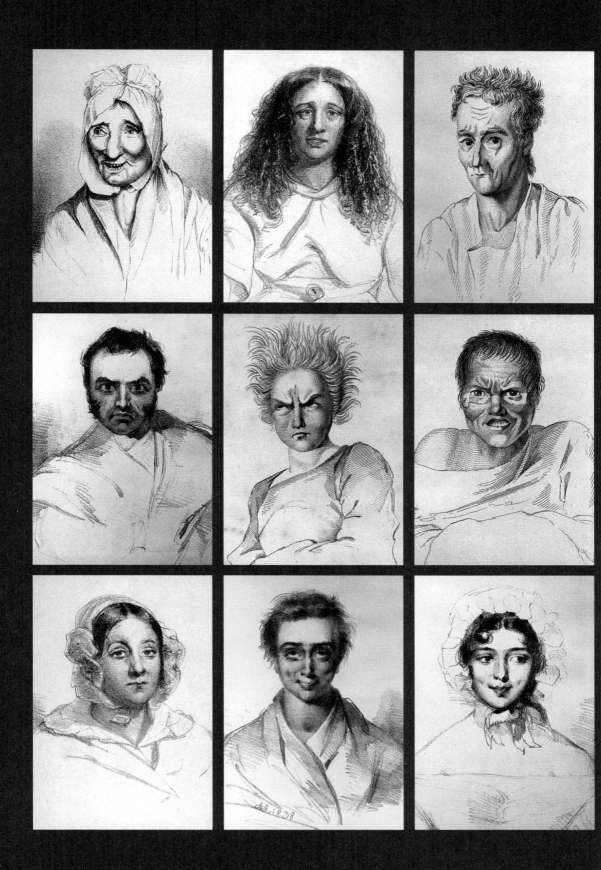

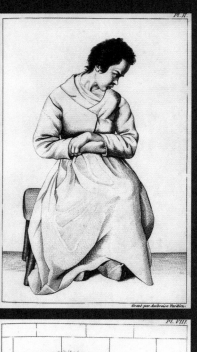

Pl. II.

Gravé par Ambroise Tardieu.

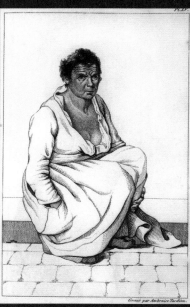

Pl. XV.

Gravé par Ambroise Tardieu.

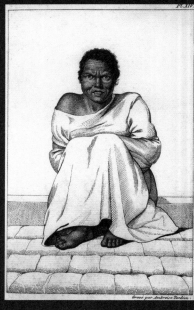

Pl. XIV.

Gravé par Ambroise Tardieu.

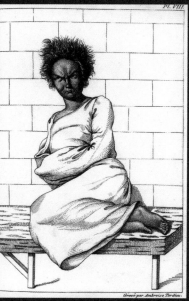

Pl. VIII.

Gravé par Ambroise Tardieu.

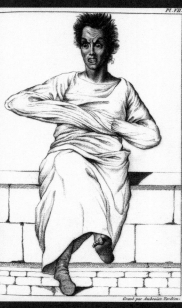

Pl. VII.

Gravé par Ambroise Tardieu.

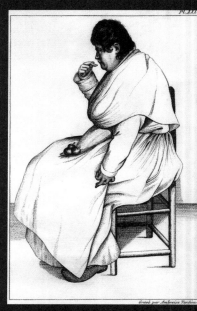

Pl. XXI.

Gravé par Ambroise Tardieu.

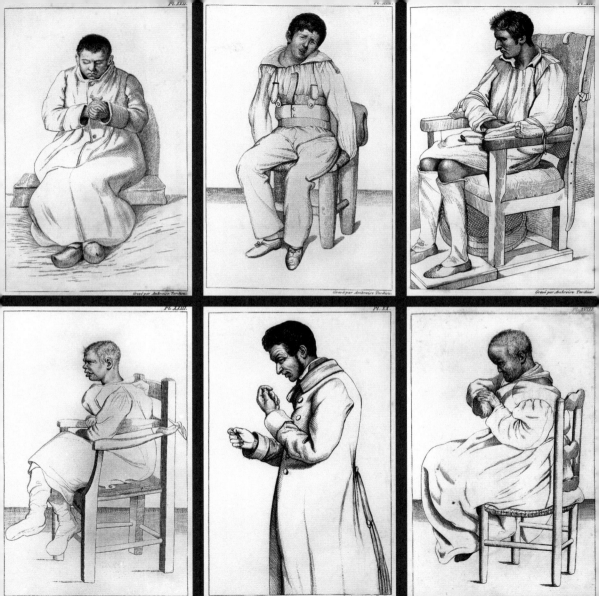

THIS PAGE AND
OPPOSITE
FROM A
PHOTOGRAPHIC
PROJECT BY JANE
FRADGLEY TITLED
'HELD'. THESE
IMAGES DEPICT
TWO TYPES OF
RESTRAINING
GARMENTS WORN
BY PATIENTS IN
LONDON COUNTY
ASYLUMS.

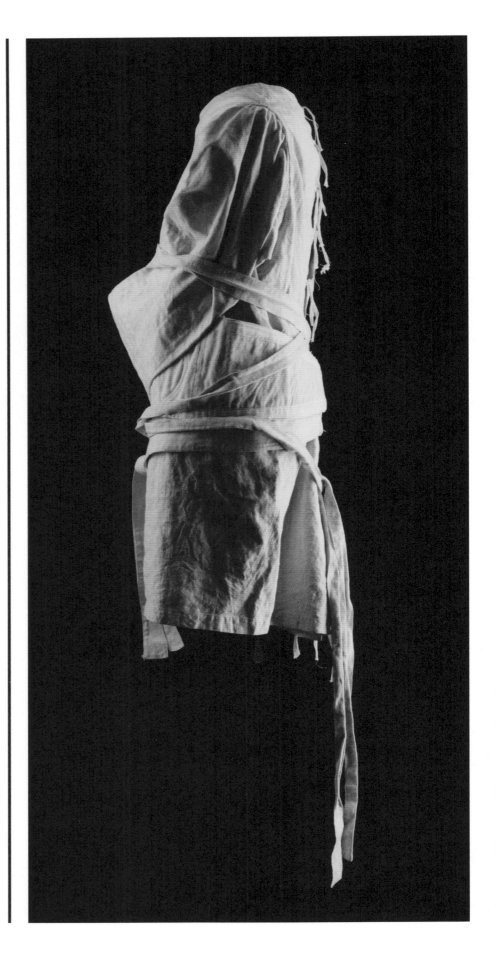

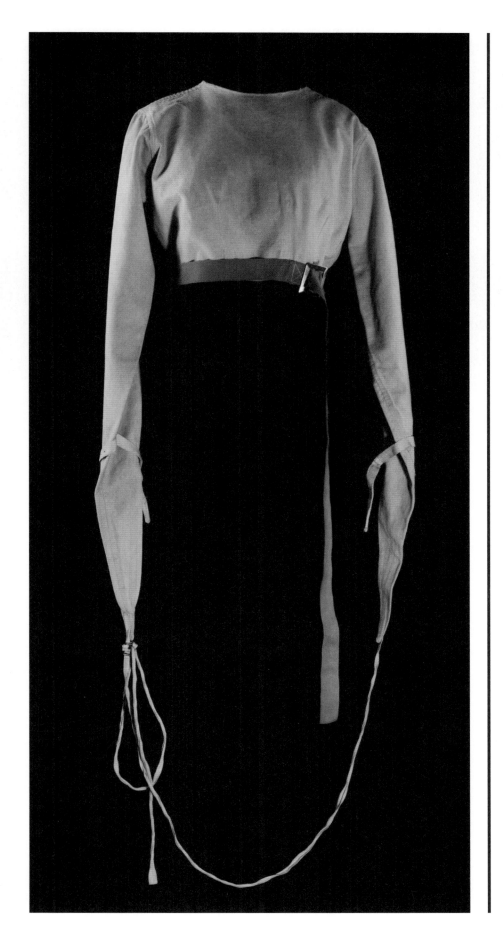

FRADGLEY
SAID OF THE
CLOTHING:
'I WAS FASCINATED
BY THE AESTHETIC
CONSIDERATIONS
POSSIBLY INTENDING
TO PROTECT AND
CARE FOR THE
WEARER WHILST
MAINTAINING
THEIR DIGNITY.'

THE LUNATIC ASYLUM
105

mania had lifted, but in other institutions his imperious and violent behaviour was treated, in his opinion, with deliberate cruelty. He was strapped into beds and straitjackets, and the 'incomprehensible demands, injunctions, insinuations, threats, taunts, insults, sarcasms' directed at him by the staff merged with the tormenting voices in his head.

On his remission, he published a two-volume work titled *A Narrative of the Treatment Experienced by a Gentleman, during a state of Mental Derangement* (1838–1840), a catalogue of beatings, cold showers and inedible food that took him back to his schooldays at Harrow. For much of the time, he was not 'aware that I was a lunatic' but believed he was undergoing a series of spiritual trials, perhaps a form of crucifixion. He was appalled at his heavy-handed treatment by servants and keepers who were his social inferiors, and adamant that 'the greatest part of the violence that occurs in lunatic asylums is to be attributed to the conduct of those who are dealing with the disease.'

Across Britain, the world of the asylum became as stratified and class-ridden as the society that had created it. By mid-century, the rest of Europe was a patchwork in which every phase of the asylum's history coexisted. Under the influence of Pinel's energetic successor Jean-Etienne-Dominique Esquirol, French law had mandated the replacement of the *ancien régime*'s squalid hospitals with a national network of state-run asylums managed by a cadre of specialists. In Vienna, as recently as 1784, a *Narrenturm* (Fool's Tower) had been built, in which lunatics were locked up in solitary cells in the manner of the old madhouses; throughout the surrounding countryside, a number of private retreat-style asylums emerged as humane alternatives to it. In many of the German states and in Russia, medieval cloisters and church-run priories were still the only public provision for the mad.

The Belgian town of Geel, where the church of St Dymphna had since medieval times allocated the lunatics who turned up there to the care of local families, became a focus of the debates between competing systems, and it provoked a long-running controversy that became known as 'the Geel question'. For some, the town was a dismal relic of the dark ages where the boarders were condemned to lives of drudgery, without any hope of treatment or cure. However, others saw in it a glimpse of the future. Esquirol, visiting in 1821, was astonished to see the mad wandering freely around the town and praised the tolerance of a system in which they were 'elevated to the dignity of the sick'.[3] Pinel declared that 'the farmers of Geel are arguably the most competent doctors': by treating their wards as normally as possible, they were practising what 'may turn out to be the only reasonable treatment of insanity'.[4] In its stolid practicality, Geel

«BY MID-CENTURY EVERY PHASE OF THE ASYLUM'S HISTORY COEXISTED»

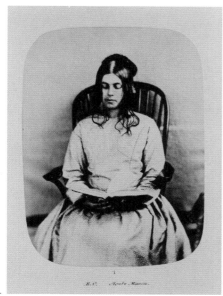

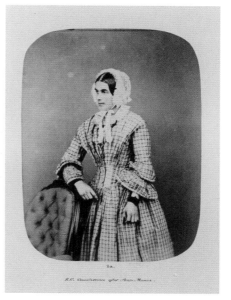

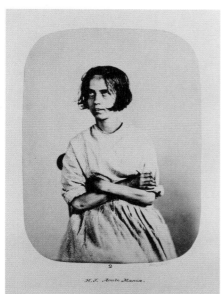

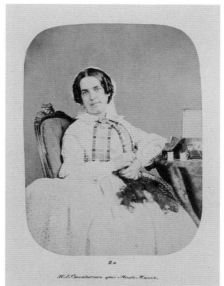

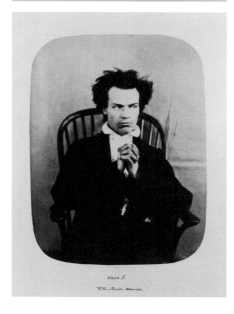

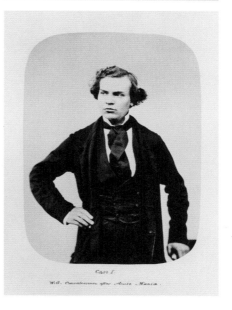

LEFT
HENRY HERING'S
STUDIES OF
BETHLEM PATIENTS
(1857–1859)
INCLUDED PAIRED
PHOTOGRAPHS
IN WHICH INSANE
PATIENTS WERE
CONTRASTED
WITH A LATER
IMAGE OF THEIR
'CURED' SELVES.

THE LUNATIC ASYLUM

107

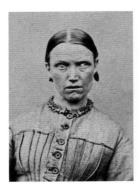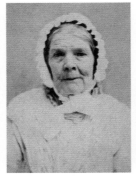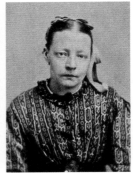

THIS PAGE AND
OPPOSITE
ALBUMEN PRINTS
c. 1869, ATTRIBUTED
TO HENRY CLARKE.
THESE IMAGES
OF PATIENTS AT
THE WEST RIDING
LUNATIC ASYLUM,
WAKEFIELD,
YORKSHIRE
INCLUDE PRISONER
NO. 9743, WHOSE
HEAD IS SUPPORTED
BY A WARDEN, AND
MALE PATIENTS
STRAPPED INTO
CONVICT CHAIRS.

pointed to a future beyond the asylum, in which moral treatment was patched into society at large.

Across the world, the reform of asylums went hand in hand with their expansion. In the United States, the most powerful advocate for both was Dorothea Dix, a schoolteacher from Boston who, as a sickly and depressive young woman, was sent to England to recover her fragile health. A family intimately connected with the Quaker network of asylum reformers cared for her, and she met progressive luminaries, including Samuel Tuke and the prison reformer Elizabeth Fry. The model of the York Retreat became the inspiration for her own recovery, and for what became a lifelong obsession with asylum reform.

On her return to the United States in 1840, she launched an indefatigable crusade against abuses in private asylums, venturing into the poorest and most obscure to uncover terrible scenes where, as she declared on the title page of her first 'Memorial to the Legislature of Massachusetts' (1843), lunatics were 'chained, naked, beaten with rods and lashed into obedience!' Dix worked her way state by state from New Hampshire to Louisiana, forcing through appropriation bills for more and better regulated asylums. She regarded insanity as eminently curable, and therefore, even the bad asylums, despite their horrors, were preferable to being cared for at home. The new institutions for which she campaigned filled and overflowed; the old barbarities of beatings and chains were condemned and outlawed, but all too often replaced with the familiar petty tyranny of bribes and threats, rewards and punishments.

In Britain, the network of reformers that had inspired Dix was growing. Its figurehead was Anthony Ashley-Cooper, 7th Earl of Shaftesbury and later Lord Shaftesbury, who in 1828 had been appointed to the government committee supervising London's pauper asylums. He was appalled to find patients sleeping naked on filthy straw, just as Edward Wakefield had in the unreformed Bedlam. Meanwhile, John Perceval began a campaign against the conditions in private asylums, and in 1845 he became a founder member of the Alleged Lunatics' Friends Society: a campaigning group formed largely of respectable gentlemen who had found themselves detained as lunatics – in several cases in connection with financial

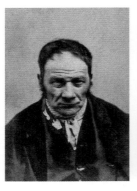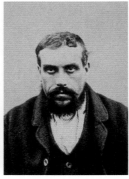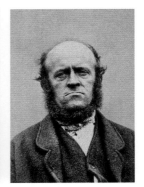

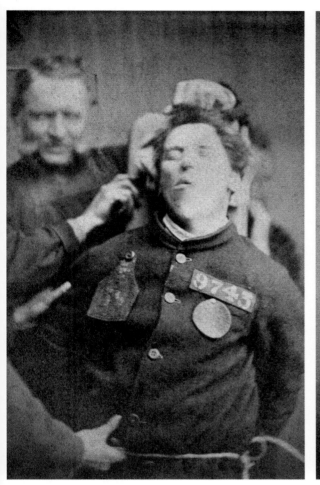
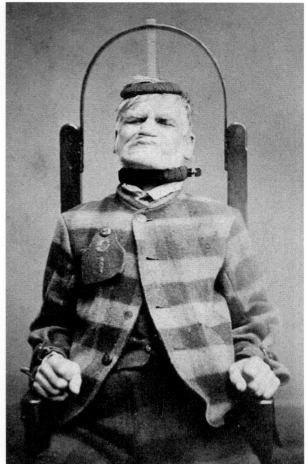
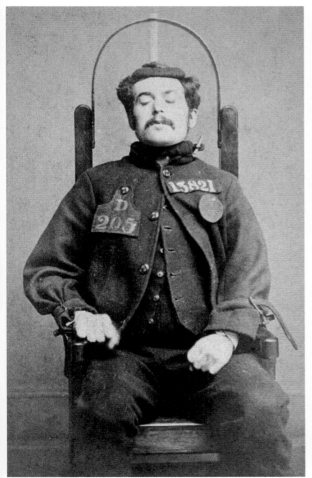
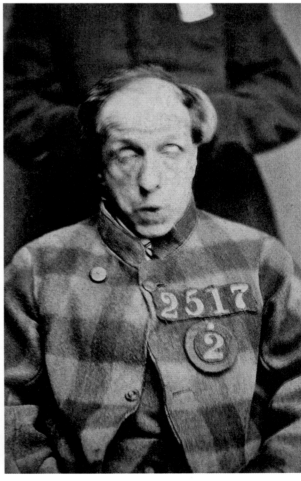

disputes – and had shocking tales to tell of their cruel and unjust treatment.

Such exposures tarnished the image of asylums and fed a public hunger for their reform. The most inspiring vision for an alternative came from Dr William Browne, superintendent of the Montrose Lunatic Asylum in Scotland, who had instituted a regime of moral treatment that drew equally from the York Retreat and Pinel. Browne was a pioneer of group drama, music and art therapy, and perhaps the first doctor to

had not been done away with. Recent developments had come mostly from fear of parliamentary investigations and statutory inspections; the genuine revolution was yet to come.

Browne dreamed of the perfect asylum, not as a utopia but as a practical goal. 'The whole secret,' he believed, 'may be summed up in two words: kindness and occupation.'[7] Medicine was a valuable tool, but care of the insane should never be entrusted to 'the mere drug exhibiter'. The perfect

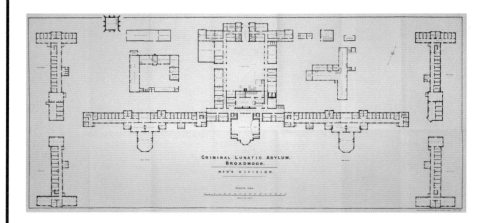

CRIMINAL LUNATIC ASYLUM.
BROADMOOR.
MEN'S DIVISION.

collect the artworks of asylum patients. Since the 1830s he had been delivering passionate lectures on his vision for the asylum, which were collected in a hugely influential book, *What Asylums Were, Are and Ought to Be* (1837). Pinel, he argued, had rescued the asylum from its long dark ages, where 'the great objects were – confine, conceal'.[5] Prisons had been used as asylums and asylums as prisons, 'with this important difference, however, that in the latter case the prisoner was guiltless'.[6] Much had improved, but the old Bastilles

asylum needed to be conceived from the ground up, with the interests of the patient at heart. It would be beautiful and open, with complete freedom inside its walls: 'There is in this community no compulsion, no chains, no whips, no corporal chastisement, simply because these are proved to be less effectual.' The main building would be a mansion, 'airy, and elevated, and elegant, surrounded by swelling grounds and gardens', containing 'galleries, and workshops, and music rooms', a 'hive of industry' with patients weaving, baking, playing music, reading, drawing and bookbinding'.[8] It was the vision that James Tilly Matthews had conjured in his Bethlem cell a generation earlier, but now the world was glad to listen.

In 1845 Lord Shaftesbury presented to Parliament two pieces of legislation that aimed to consign the old Bastilles to history. The Lunacy Act obliged all

trade. The new asylums would provide a place of safety for the mentally fragile, who previously had been forced into the workhouse system, and would put an end to the miserable conditions in public asylums and unscrupulous practices in private ones.

The immediate effect of the two acts was to accelerate both the growth in

LEFT
PLAN OF
THE WOMEN'S
DIVISION BLOCKS.
THE HOSPITAL WAS
DESIGNED AS A
SELF-SUFFICIENT
COMMUNITY IN
QUIET RURAL
SURROUNDINGS.

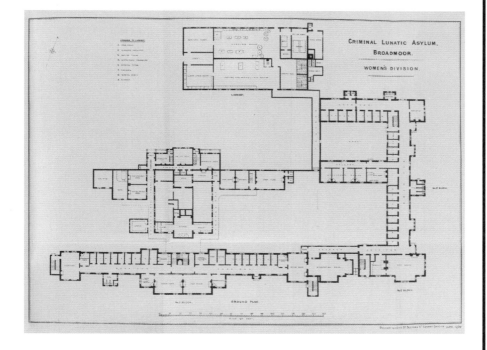

public and private asylums to register for inspection and to have a resident physician (although not a specialist mad-doctor); the County Asylums Act, passed with it, mandated that a public asylum be built in every county. These acts were presented as a landmark for enlightened reform, the closing of a barbaric chapter of history to be compared with the abolition of the slave

asylums and the numbers confined in them. Medical voices warned that the insane should be kept segregated, and some suggested that their conditions might be contagious or connected to other forms of infectious disease. Women in particular who were not suitable for employment were more frequently diagnosed with insanity, a category into which social ills, such as poverty and

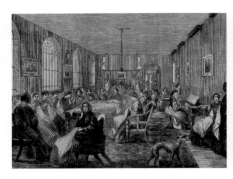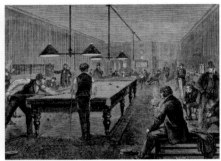

illegitimacy, were subsumed. Typically, the 'stark Bedlam mad' had been male, but now the stereotype was reversed: prison for men, the asylum for women. The true picture was more complex – the ratio of female patients also reflected the fact that they lived longer and were less likely to be discharged – but new asylums began to be constructed with more wards for women than for men.

The increase in county asylums closed the shabby pauper wings of some private asylums, as Lord Shaftesbury had hoped it would, but it also led to more of the rural poor being diagnosed as insane. Prophecies that madness was on the rise became self-fulfilling, creating new diagnoses and categories of those at risk, while at the same time public contact with it declined. As the asylums expanded, care fell into mechanical routines. The architecture of the new institutions was standardized around staff priorities, with intensive and acute care concentrated at the front near the main entrance. The more chronic and severe cases were housed in 'back wards', where patients were visited less often, lost contact with the outside world and became ever less likely to rejoin society. Insanity pleas were received more sympathetically in the courts, and

« CONOLLY WAS CONVINCED THAT ASYLUMS WERE CAPABLE OF BEING MOULDED INTO IDEAL SOCIETIES »

the criminal lunatic wards in the new county asylums filled and overflowed. Like prisons, asylums became a powerful economic sector adept at arguing for their own expansion. All these upward pressures were enough to suppress, though not silence, the inconvenient arguments against them: that they were not kind but cruel, and that their recovery rates were extremely poor.

In 1839 the huge new county asylum at Hanwell in London took on a resident physician named John Conolly, an idealistic supporter of the Chartist movement for working men's rights and, like William Browne, of the social entrepreneur Robert Owen. Conolly was appalled to discover in the staff rooms a collection of hand-cuffs, leg-locks, res-traint chairs and screw-gags that seemed more appropriate to a torture chamber. He promptly announced that all restraints were to be banned, and within three months the asylum had dispensed with them. In their place, he instituted a regime of moral treatment that included improved diet, classes in literacy and arithmetic, and regular bible study.

Conolly was convinced that asylums were capable of being moulded into ideal societies, free from the malign influences of modern life. He recognized that non-restraint made harder work for staff and persuaded the governors to reward them with better conditions, higher wages and specialist training. He led tirelessly from the front, always on duty, listening and attending to his patients' needs. In a summation of his practice, *The Treatment of the Insane without Mechanical Restraints* (1856), he stressed that the physician must 'mingle with, and partake of, all that constitutes the daily life of his patients', making it impossible for staff or governors to undermine the system behind his back. The asylum must become an extension of its superintendent, 'an harmonious system of which he is the very soul'.[9]

Conolly's achievements were celebrated widely and won him a public profile that enabled him to talk over the heads of an often sceptical or dissenting medical profession. He became the public figurehead for the 'non-restraint movement', delivering the message that the reformers and the wider public all wished to hear: the asylum did not need to be synonymous with cruelty and neglect. However, like Tuke's regime at the York Retreat, his example proved difficult to emulate. Few asylum superintendents had the passionate commitment that his system demanded, which amounted to a lifelong personal martyrdom to the institution. Without constant inspection and correction, the old habits were always liable to creep back, following the path of least resistance.

As the searchlight of the non-restraint movement swept across the asylums, Bethlem came under investigation once more, this time from the Lunacy Commission that had been set up as an official regulator by the Lunacy Act of 1845. In 1852 it reported to Parliament that patients in the female wards were neglected and abused, washed down with cold water and mops, and freezing at night in straw-filled cots. In response, the governors appointed for the first time a resident physician-superintendent, who it was hoped would become the compassionate soul of the asylum, as Conolly had at Hanwell. Their hopes were well founded. William Charles

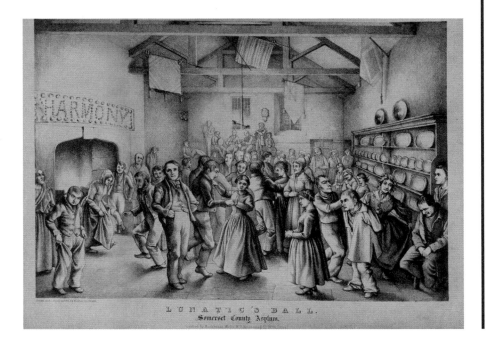

LUNATIC'S BALL.
Somerset County Asylum.

PLANCHE VII

FIG. 1.

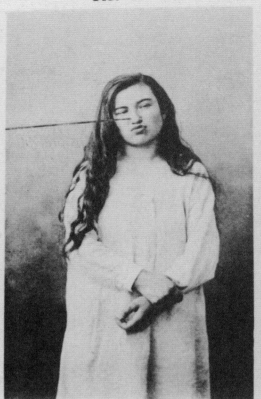

FIG. 2.

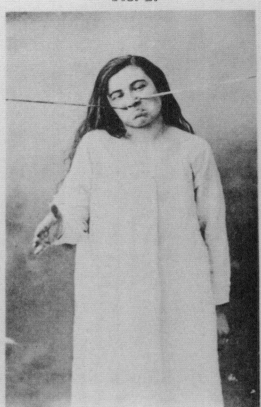

FIG. 3.

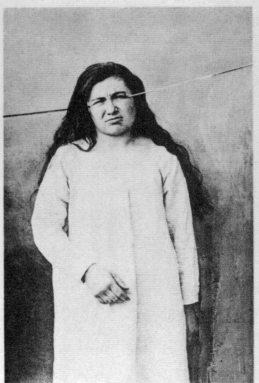

FIG. 4.

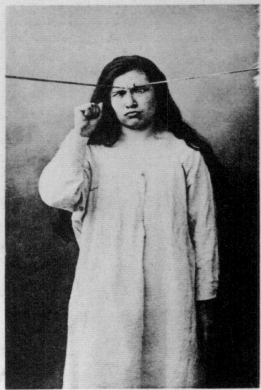

Cliché de F. PANAJOU, chef du service photographique à la Faculté de médecine de Bordeaux.

Hood was both a medical specialist and a devout Christian, and he overhauled the running of Bethlem with inexhaustible energy and saintly devotion.

Citing the example of his hero Pinel, he abolished restraints and reduced the number of locked doors; he installed new windows, cleaned the wards and upgraded the bedding. Hood also left flowers, books and pictures in the galleries for the patients' enjoyment and installed a magic lantern for their evening entertainment. Well-behaved

public were encouraged to attend. The 'lunatics' ball', often held in high summer or at Christmas, was an eye-catching initiative adopted by many asylums to highlight the aspiration of returning their patients to normal society. Visiting journalists were frequently enraptured by the spectacle of patients carefully dressed for the occasion and absorbed into a masquerade of the outside world. Others, such as Dickens when he attended St Luke's Christmas Ball of 1851, found 'much that is mournfully

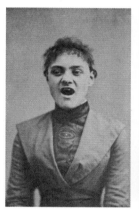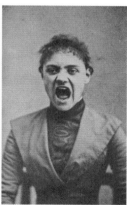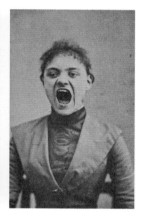

patients were taken on outings to the National Gallery and Kew Gardens.

In the climate of optimism inspired by Browne and Conolly, asylum success stories were always good newspaper copy. Hood's management raised Bethlem's profile and improved its image: Charles Dickens's *Household Words* magazine ran approving and sentimental coverage, and the paupers on parish support were joined by more of the middling classes whose families were able to pay the relatively modest fees. Hood began to hold Monday night balls, which the

affecting in such a sight'. Amid the odd stares and faltering steps, it was all too obvious that 'to lighten the affliction of insanity by all human means, is not to restore the greatest of Divine gifts'.[10]

Among Hood's patients in the criminal lunatic wing was the artist Richard Dadd (see p. 140), who in his youth had been an outstanding talent at the Royal Academy, known for his detailed and fantastical scenes of fairyland. In 1842 Dadd had become mentally unbalanced while travelling in Egypt and the Holy Land on a painting

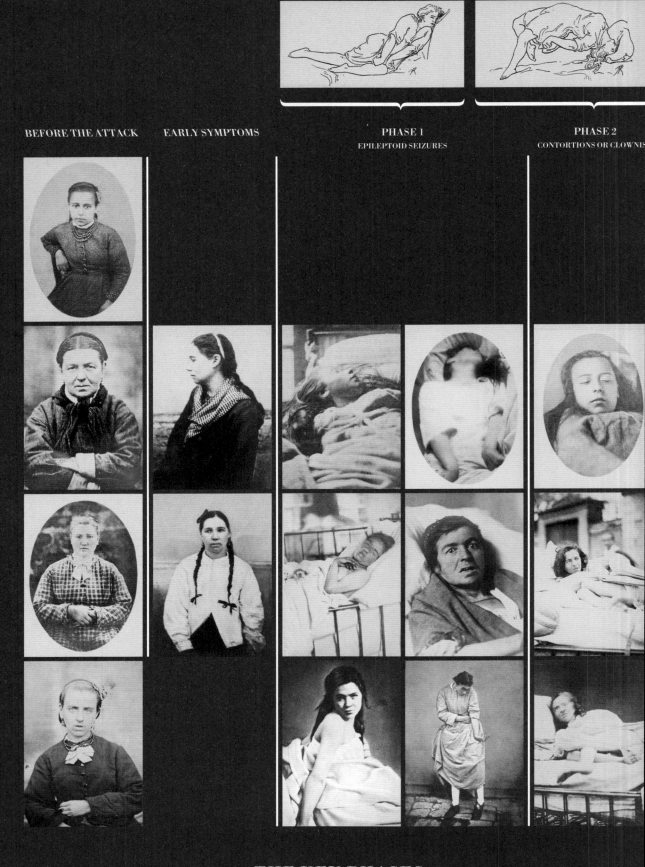

BEFORE THE ATTACK

EARLY SYMPTOMS

PHASE 1
EPILEPTOID SEIZURES

PHASE 2
CONTORTIONS OR CLOWNIS

THE KEY PHASES
OF A MAJOR HYSTERICAL ATTACK
JEAN-MARTIN CHARCOT

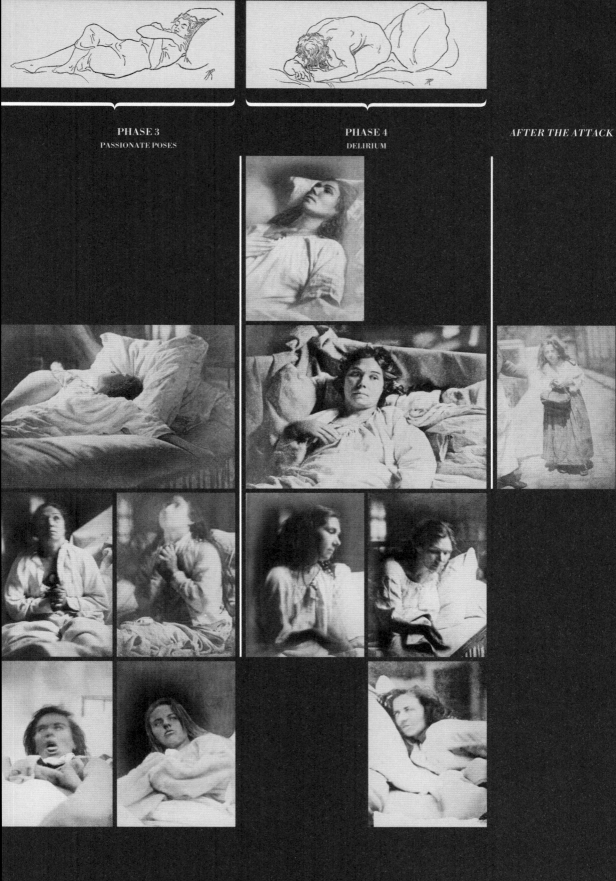

PHASE 3
PASSIONATE POSES

PHASE 4
DELIRIUM

AFTER THE ATTACK

THIS PAGE AND OPPOSITE
FRENCH DOCTOR JEAN-MARTIN CHARCOT, KNOWN AS 'THE EMPEROR OF THE NEUROSES',
ILLUSTRATED HIS THEORY OF HYSTERIA WITH PHOTOGRAPHS OF PATIENTS UNDER
HYPNOSIS AT SALPÊTRIÈRE HOSPITAL.

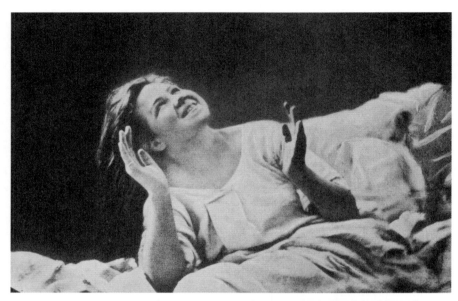

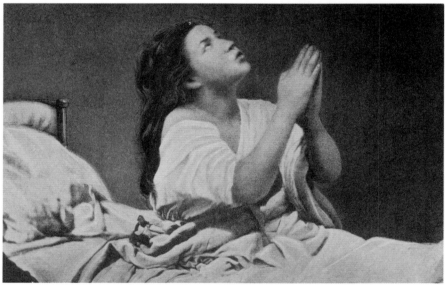

THIS PAGE AND OPPOSITE
FROM *ICONOGRAPHIE PHOTOGRAPHIQUE DE LA SALPÊTRIÈRE* (SERVICE DE M. CHARCOT), THESE
PHOTOGRAPHS WERE TAKEN BY PAUL REGNARD BETWEEN 1876 AND 1880 AND DEPICT PATIENTS AT
SALPÊTRIÈRE HOSPITAL IN VARIOUS STATES: ECSTASY (TOP), SUPPLICATION (ABOVE) AND EROTICISM
(OPPOSITE). AUGUSTINE GLEIZES, ONE OF CHARCOT'S FAVOURITE AND MOST DRAMATIC SUBJECTS,
WAS EVENTUALLY RELEASED FROM CONFINEMENT AND EMPLOYED.

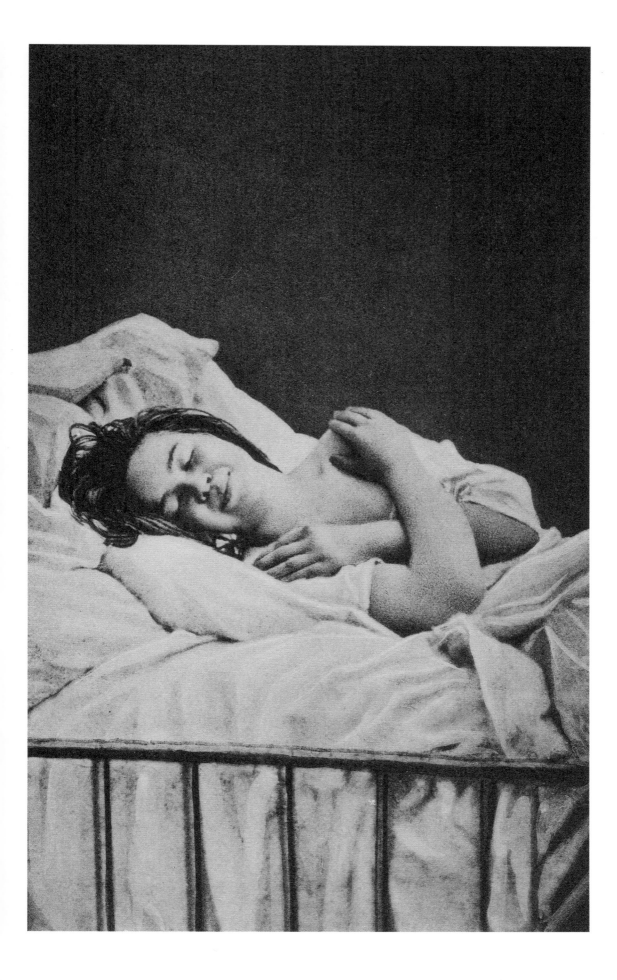

assignment, and on his return he had stabbed his father to death. In court, it transpired that he believed himself to be under the command of the god Osiris. Dadd was found guilty but insane and confined in Bethlem's criminal wing, where Hood took a close interest in him. He recorded his belief in spirits, his lack of remorse, and his occasional violent and indecent behaviour, but also noted that 'he can be a very sensible and agreeable companion, and shew in conversation, a mind once well educated'.[11] Hood arranged his transfer to a larger, brighter ward away from the troublesome convict patients, and Dadd dedicated his late masterpiece, titled *Contradiction: Oberon and Titania* (1854–1858), to him.

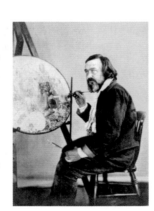

In 1864 Dadd became part of the first intake into Broadmoor, the specialist asylum for criminal lunatics that had been promised since James Hadfield's day. In contrast to the congested and polluted environs of Southwark, Broadmoor was set in pleasant countryside to the west of London. It had large grounds and a 12-acre (4.8 ha) kitchen garden, and it was intended to be a self-sufficient community, providing its own food and clothing. However, the high proportion of aggressive inmates confined under lock and key limited these ambitions. Dadd continued to paint and decorated the in-house theatre in the main hall, reverting from his crowded and hallucinatory canvases back to simpler bucolic scenes from classical myth.

Inspiring physicians such as Conolly and Hood improved the public perception of asylums and the lives of their patients, but they made little impact on the rates of recovery. Under Hood's benevolent regime, recovery fell by six per cent: one of the effects of making Bethlem more congenial was to shift the balance towards long-stay and incurable patients. Even at Ticehurst, with the best facilities that money could buy, rates of remission in the 1870s were no better than five per cent a year. At Hanwell, the number of patients under Conolly's obsessive care grew relentlessly until nearly a thousand were crammed into a complex designed for five hundred. But Conolly remained at its heart. He had developed an irritable skin condition that gave him insomnia, and he prowled the wards and corridors day and night. The asylum was his world, and gradually it became his solution to the problems of society at large. His list of those who would benefit from it grew ever longer: the eccentric, the unhygienic, the drunk, the dishonest, the ill-tempered, the disobedient. For all these, the 'protection, and seclusion, and order, and systematic treatment as can only be afforded in the asylum, are often indispensable'.[12] The logic of the perfect asylum, taken to its conclusion, was that the entire world should become one.

The larger the asylums became, the harder it was for the idealists to hold onto them. The Middlesex county magistrates,

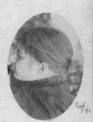

Oct: 1891.

Sep 91

Oct. 30. The above photo gives an idea of her condition about this time. She obstinately resisted every thing that was done for her, was constantly on the watch prepared to bolt through doors. Her arms were generally in a state of extreme muscular tension. She occasionally endeavours to destroy her things & invariably required about 4 nurses to dress & undress her.
                                                    D.R. Henderson.

Nov. 7. Was today transferred to
St Luke's Hospital. "Not improved."

---

refuses her food, because she says it is poisoned. She is at times noisy, incoherent & rambling & offers much resistance to nurses.

30 July. She remains in the same rather agitated state as on admission - she refuses to shake hands with, or enter into detailed conversation with reporter (this has occurred every morning for past week) - She now denies she said her food was poisoned - Is rambling & almost incoherent in conversation at times, & offers violence to the nurses.
Health fair.

10 August. There is no improvement to be noted in mental state, but her bodily condition is improved. She is taking [Ft Ohss ℥ XV / M. labor℥ ℥ XV / aqua ℥j ☧]

24 Aug. She is quieter & less resistive to nurses than on admission but is taking her food much better - She refuses however to enter into any conversation or shake hands with the medical Officer, is entirely unoccupied the whole day, & shows no disposition to be friendly with anyone - Health slightly improved -

28 Sept. Unchanged -

Oct. 31. She remains in a suspicious weak-minded condition, refuses to converse with, or enter on friendly terms with any one in the building, will neither shake hands, or protrude her tongue. When addressed she has a peculiar, nervous method of shrinking backwards away. Sept 6 1890

April [TEMPERATURE CHART] June [TEMPERATURE CHART] June [TEMPERATURE CHART]

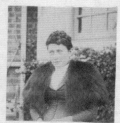

Oct: 1891. D.B.

Gheel   L'Entrée de l'Infirmerie

alarmed by the ever-increasing running costs of Hanwell, forced Conolly into retirement in 1852. By this time, a new era of grand asylum building was in full swing.

In 1851 Middlesex opened a new county asylum, Colney Hatch, designed to hold 1,250 patients and boasting the longest corridor in Europe. Its spectacular facade, crowded with towers, cupolas and baroque ornamentation, recalled the old Bethlem; like the old Bethlem, the cracks began to show almost immediately and by 1859 the county magistrates were suing the architects for negligence. In these oversized and under-resourced institutions, it became virtually impossible to prevent patient care from hardening into blank routine.

Against this background, the family care system at Geel became increasingly popular as an alternative to the asylums. In 1850 the town had been absorbed into the Belgian state hospital system, designated as a 'colony of the mad' inside the limits of which boarders were free to roam. Oversight of the ancient system was transferred from the church to a group of physicians who devised an innovative system that preserved

«THE FAMILY CARE SYSTEM AT GEEL BECAME INCREASINGLY POPULAR»

the best aspects of the tradition. The church had kept a register of boarders, but left families to look after them as they saw fit. Under local by-laws, families were responsible for any laws broken by their guests, and this had sometimes led to disruptive ones being beaten or restrained with leather straps. In exchange for a small state payment to the families, restraint and corporal punishment were banned. In 1861 Belgium's leading specialist in asylum care, Dr Joseph Guislain, built a new hospital on the edge of Geel into which patients were received and assessed on arrival, and to which they could be taken if they became unmanageable. Later, three bathhouses were built on the edge of town to which boarders were taken twice a week for basic hygiene and health checks, and this also allowed for discreet supervision outside the family sphere.

In the local parlance, care took place 'outside' – in the town, among local families – wherever possible. 'Inside' – the hospital – was a resource to be used only when absolutely necessary, and everyone worked to make visits there as short as possible. This 'mixed

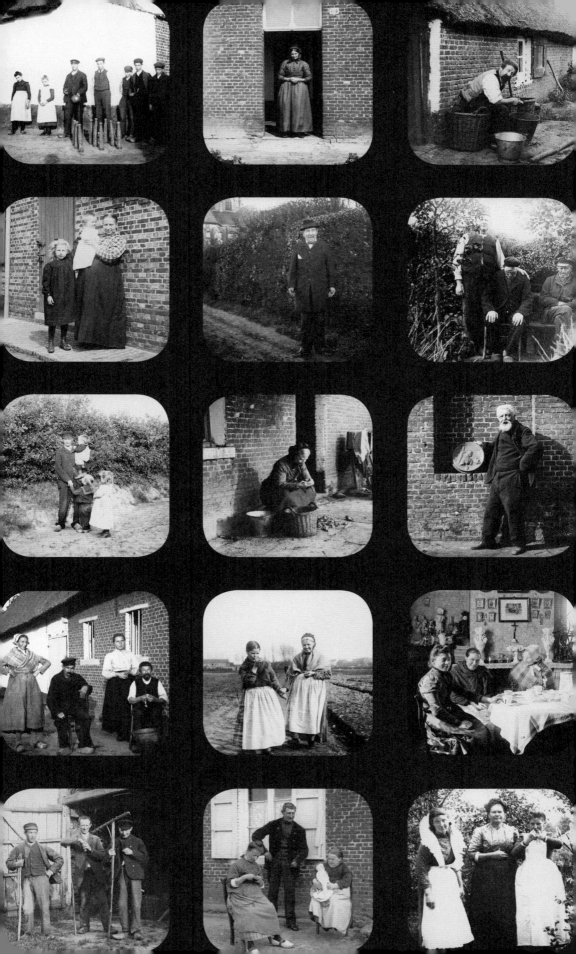

RIGHT AND
OPPOSITE
TICEHURST ASLYUM
IN SUSSEX
WAS AMONG THE
MOST EXCLUSIVE
PRIVATE ASYLUMS
IN BRITAIN. BY
1900 ITS GROUNDS
HAD EXPANDED
TO 300 ACRES. THE
ILLUSTRATIONS
OPPOSITE SHOW
(TOP LEFT TO
BOTTOM RIGHT)
THE PAVILION,
ITALIAN GARDEN,
MAIN BUILDING,
ENTRANCE TO THE
HIGHLANDS ANNEX,
CHAPEL, MUSEUM,
DRAWING ROOM
AND MUSIC ROOM.

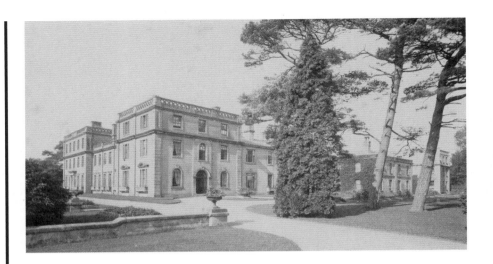

system', as it was known, was studied by visiting physicians and adopted in dozens of small towns in France and Germany and also as far away as Japan, where a similar tradition had evolved independently. The 'Geel question' was formally resolved in 1902 when the International Congress of Psychiatry declared it an example of best practice, to be emulated wherever possible.

Elsewhere, the rapid advance of medical science promised new solutions. In Germany in particular, a new generation of mental specialists had made striking progress in mapping the brain areas connected with functions such as movement and speech, and in developing physical tests that correlated with certain nervous conditions. Universities established clinics where the pathologies of brain and nerves could be studied, usually in subjects drawn from the asylum population. Insanity was reconceived as 'mental disease' and connected to the infections and deformities of the brain and spinal cord that were being revealed under the microscope. The term 'psychiatry', originally coined by physician Johann Christian Reil in 1808, came into wider use to designate this new generation of laboratory-based specialists.

Unusually among his colleagues, Emil Kraepelin, who in 1888 became professor of psychiatry at the University of Heidelberg, studied asylum patients in their thousands, not as physical specimens but as living examples of the behaviours and symptoms common to different forms of delusional insanity or 'psychosis'. Like William Battie and Pinel before him, he made a primary distinction between curable and incurable forms, which evolved over a series of influential textbooks into ever more complex subcategories. The curable form, which cycled through distinct phases and sometimes went into remission altogether, he named 'manic-depression' and the incurable form, which he believed to be a degenerative brain disease, *dementia praecox*. The symptoms of the latter were later subsumed into a new diagnostic category – schizophrenia – and Kraepelin's categories remain the basis of psychotic disorders today.

'Psychiatry' was adopted slowly in the English-speaking world to identify a new breed of scientifically minded specialists with higher professional ambitions than 'asylum superintendent'. Their doyen in Britain was Henry Maudsley, an ambitious asylum doctor from Yorkshire, who corresponded with German neurologists and psychiatrists, joined their learned societies and introduced their ideas to the British

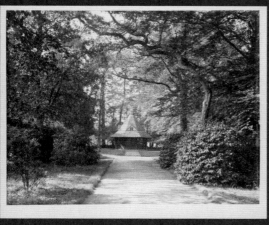

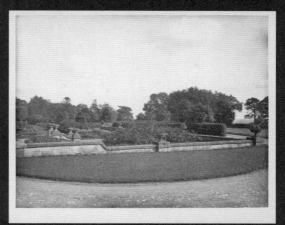

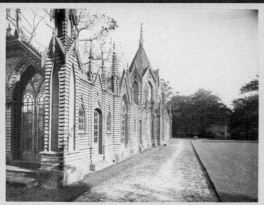

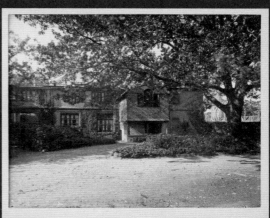

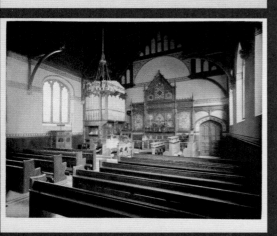

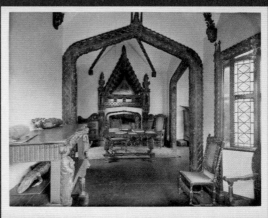

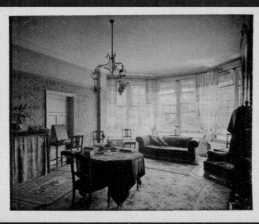

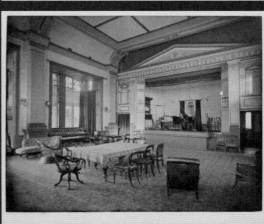

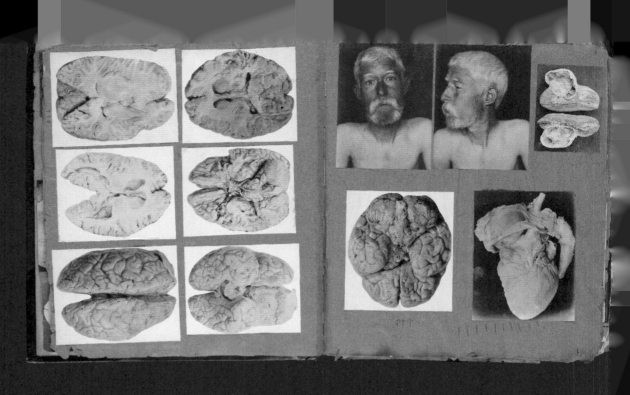

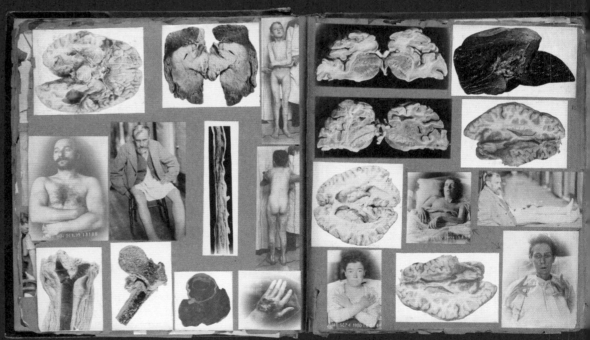

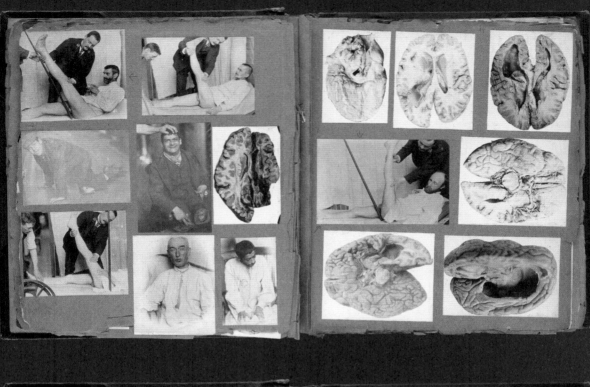

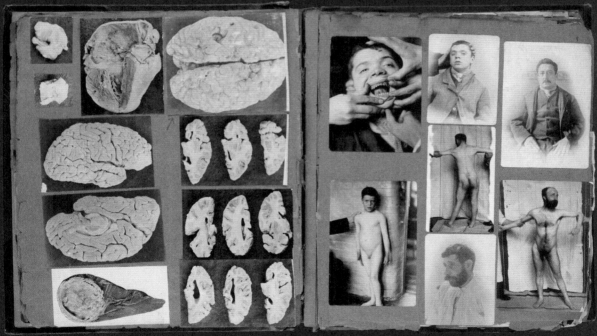

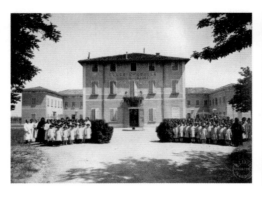
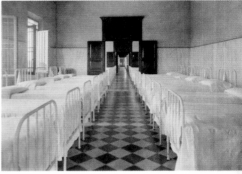

medical profession. In 1863 he was appointed co-editor of the *Journal of Mental Science*, rising to senior editor in 1870 and turning it into the profession's most influential voice. In 1866 he married Conolly's daughter, Ann, and took over the running of Lawn House, the private asylum for wealthy ladies that Conolly had set up on his retirement from Hanwell.

Maudsley's ideas drew heavily on Darwinism, and Charles Darwin in turn would later draw on Maudsley's work on the biological basis of human and animal behaviour. He believed that mental disturbances were physical in origin, and in most cases hereditary. In this view of insanity, asylums could be little more than care homes, and Maudsley regarded them predominantly as a worse option than remaining with the family. He withdrew early from asylum doctoring and devoted the rest of his life to writing and treating a wealthy private clientele. His cold and gloomy disposition, the product of a grim upbringing blighted by the death of his mother, was the very opposite of that of his father-in-law. Although Maudsley was too politic to criticize Conolly's optimism and zeal while he was

alive, he described him witheringly in his obituary as 'of a feminine type; capable of a momentary lively sympathy' but 'prone to shrink from the disagreeable occasions of life'.[13] Maudsley's later writings gave scientific support to those who opposed asylums on humanitarian grounds, but also to those on the opposite end of the spectrum who argued that the insane were biologically unfit and should be sterilized.

As medical science probed the biological causes of madness, it also redefined the condition, shifting the focus away from the asylum and into the general population. Nervous disorders and hereditary weaknesses might reveal themselves in the form of homosexuality or radical politics, perversions or suicidal tendencies, avant-garde art or hysteria. Constitutional weaknesses were exposed and exacerbated by the stresses of modern life: commuting, intellectual burnout, breakdown of the family or immersion in the ethnic melting pots of the new cities. Psychiatrists found careers beyond the asylum in the expanding world of private practice, with its greater status and earning power. Those who could afford it withdrew their relatives from the vast

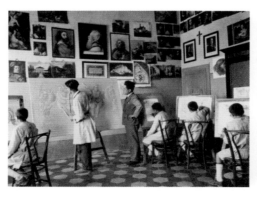
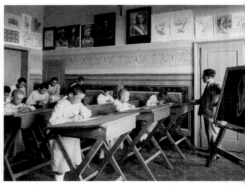

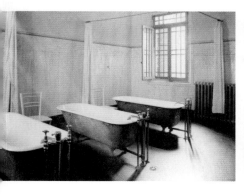

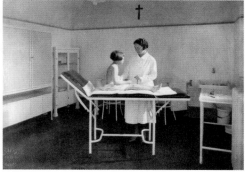

and bleak public asylums and presented them to the private 'nerve doctors'.

The new diagnosis of neurasthenia – exhaustion of the 'nerve force' – became an emblem of the age, rather as melancholy had during the Renaissance or anxiety would in the 1950s. In the United States in particular, it was seen as the inevitable corollary of national vigour and the fast-paced, competitive business world: in the words of US neurologist George Beard, who coined the diagnosis, 'American nervousness is the product of American civilization.'[14] Particularly in female cases, the recommended treatment was complete rest in a controlled environment, isolated from friends and family. However, neurasthenia was typically diagnosed among the wealthy and professional classes who could afford alternatives to the public asylum. Private clinics and sanatoriums flourished, and asylum admissions narrowed to those who had no alternative. Many of the older hospitals and retreats such as Bloomingdale gave up their state funding and turned themselves into upmarket clinics for the new wealthy clientele.

Across Europe, the bourgeois flight from the asylum created a new golden age of the spa. In the mineral springs of the French Pyrenees and the German resorts of Baden-Baden and Carlsbad, where the wealthy of the 18th century had taken the waters while convalescing, the neurasthenics, insomniacs and neuralgics of the *fin de siècle* arrived in their hundreds for rest cures, diet and exercise regimes, and hydrotherapy. The new nervous conditions created a fashion for electromedical devices, which delivered low voltage tingles or bursts of static that were believed to stimulate or recharge the neurasthenic constitution worn out by modern life. In the upmarket sanatoriums, these were delivered by impressive machines with brass knobs and glowing vacuum tubes; the classified pages of magazines were filled with advertisements for electropathic belts and vibro-massagers.

Some sanatoriums developed ambitious regimes for the type of serious mental disturbance that had usually led to asylum committal. The Bellevue in Switzerland, on the wooded slopes above Lake Constance, was a luxuriously appointed complex offering rest cures, hydrotherapy and rehabilitation for nervous exhaustion. In 1911 it was taken over by Ludwig

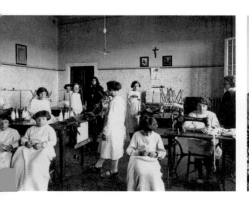

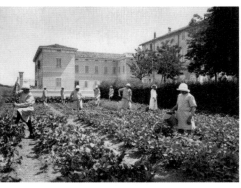

NEXT PAGE
AT THE HIGHER
END OF THE
MARKET, PRIVATE
SANATORIUMS FOR
THE WEALTHY,
SUCH AS BATTLE
CREEK SANITARIUM,
MICHIGAN,
RESEMBLED
LUXURY HOTELS.
POSTCARDS FROM
THE 1900S TO 1930S.

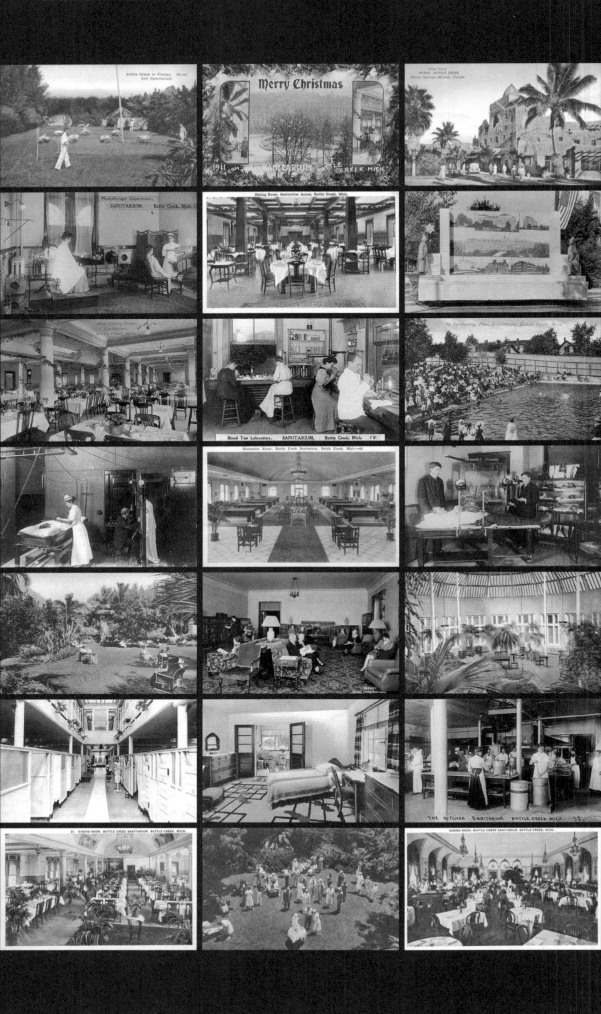

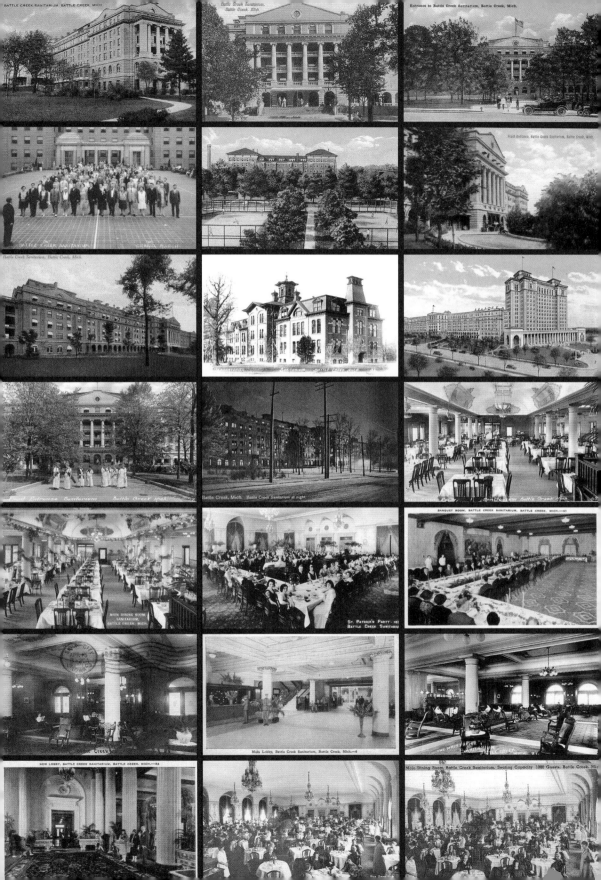

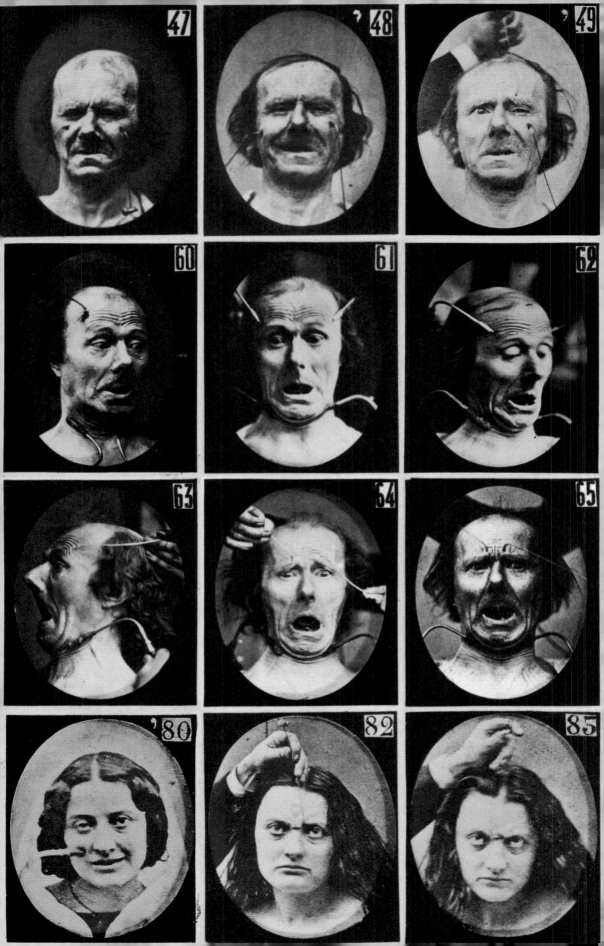

Binswanger, the son of the previous director, who had trained with Carl Jung in Vienna and was a close friend of Sigmund Freud. Binswanger accepted that mental illnesses had their roots in the brain but believed they needed to be treated as existential conditions and explored through psychoanalysis, art and group therapy.

The core of the daily routine was a midday meal taken together by doctors, staff and patients, in which clinical formalities were dispensed with and therapeutic pathways freely explored. Binswanger took in several of Freud's patients and occasional celebrity cases, too, including the ballet dancer Vaslav Nijinsky. Increasingly fragile and disturbed after his break with Sergei Diaghilev, Nijinsky arrived at Bellevue with a diagnosis of 'catatonia', his behaviour alternating between blank paralysis and violent bursts of leaping and twisting. Binswanger persuaded him to perform a dance recital and rolled back the Persian rug in the main villa's drawing room. Nijinsky pounded discordantly on the piano until one of the audience took over, at which point he danced himself into a trance and performed 'a suicide-madness scene'. Afterwards he was wrung out, trembling and chain-smoking; Binswanger was unable to decide whether he had witnessed a spontaneous burst of madness or simply an artful performance of it. To judge by his private diaries, Nijinsky

shared the confusion. However, the question was soon answered by others: he was diagnosed as schizophrenic, spent the next thirty years in and out of mental institutions and never danced in public again.

The sense that madness had escaped the asylum and taken root in the culture at large was confirmed in 1914, when an entire generation was thrust into the horror and insanity of war. Previously healthy young men in their thousands developed symptoms that formerly had been seen only in those with acute nervous illnesses: hallucinations, paralysis, uncontrollable tremors and even hysterical blindness. 'Shell shock', as it was referred to in the ranks, was treated initially as cowardice and malingering; hundreds of soldiers were executed before it became obvious that even the ultimate deterrent had no effect. The symptoms were reinterpreted as a neurological response to the deafening volume of exploding shells; soon, though, they appeared in soldiers who had never been near an explosion. Alternative physical causes, from concussion to pressure changes to toxic gases, were ruled out one by one. Psychiatrists proposed a series of biological explanations, including compression of the central nerves and hereditary weakness, but they were unable to offer practical therapies.

Army doctors on all sides were forced eventually to accept that such extreme

OPPOSITE
FROM *MÉCANISME DE LA PHYSIONOMIE HUMAINE, OU, ANALYSE ÉLECTRO-PHYSIOLOGIQUE DE L'EXPRESSION DES PASSIONS* (1862) BY GUILLAUME BENJAMIN AMAND DUCHENNE DE BOULOGNE. DUCHENNE USED ELECTRIC CURRENTS TO STUDY THE MECHANISMS OF FACIAL EXPRESSION.

LEFT
DAVIS AND KIDDER'S PATENT ELECTRIC-MEDICAL MACHINE, 1870-1900. THESE DEVICES WERE WIDELY ADVERTISED FOR RESTORING HEALTH TO EXHAUSTED NERVOUS SYSTEMS.

RIGHT
PHOTOGRAPH
OF A VICTIM OF
'SHELL SHOCK' IN
THE TRENCHES
DURING THE
BATTLE OF FLERS–
COURCELETTE IN
1916. THIS DAZED
EXPRESSION WAS
REFERRED TO AS
THE 'THOUSAND
YARD STARE'.

134

THE LUNATIC ASYLUM

OPPOSITE
PHOTOGRAPHS OF
THE MAUDSLEY
NEUROLOGICAL
CLEARING HOSPITAL,
DENMARK HILL
SHOW (TOP LEFT
TO BOTTOM RIGHT)
THE OFFICE,
DINING HALL, 'E'
BLOCK SCHOOL,
PATHOLOGICAL
LAB, LOUNGE,
TREATMENT ROOM,
WARD 4 AND THE
WARD MASTER'S
OFFICE.

physical symptoms could be produced by psychological and emotional stress. They were the consequence, it seemed, of the conflicting imperatives of self-preservation and patriotic duty in a situation where thousands were being sacrificed senselessly and randomly.

Across Europe, public and private asylums were requisitioned to house the psychic casualties of war, in numbers that often approached those of the physically wounded. For many, the symptoms vanished once they were removed from the combat role that was the source of their inner conflict, as they almost always did in prisoner-of-war camps. For some of those whose physical symptoms persisted, talking therapies were strikingly effective. These ranged from motivational

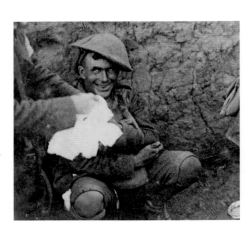

'pep talks' and positive thinking to hypnosis and psychoanalysis. The last was used only in a minority of cases but it became an inspiration for new models of asylum treatment.

At first, casualties were sent to regimented wards where discussion of the battlefield was suppressed, but some psychiatrists adopted more relaxed regimes at country retreats where – for a few privileged patients at least – the traumas of war could be recalled gently and their terror dissipated. The asylum that became the emblem of this transition

was Craiglockhart War Hospital for Officers, a grim Victorian building in the hills outside Edinburgh, where Siegfried Sassoon – a brave and dashing officer who had rebelled against the inhumane strategies of the British command – was dispatched with a diagnosis of shell shock.

Under the compassionate guidance of psychiatrist William Rivers, Sassoon explored his dreams and through them the tensions between his military role and his private feelings. He came to recognize that his weaknesses were inevitable, not to be denied or repressed but accepted and understood. He concluded that he was not suffering from shell shock but an 'anti-war complex'. The world had become a great Bedlam, and the rest of his life would be a journey towards sanity. In the wake of the Great War, the 19th-century asylums took on the tragic aspect of relics, their crowded back wards filled with the mute and forgotten survivors of a world now consigned to history. Medical, social and psychological therapies were all on the march, and the outlines of another revolution were taking shape.

In 1918 Rivers and his Cambridge colleague Charles Myers, who had been the first to use the term 'shell shock' in medical literature, took stock of

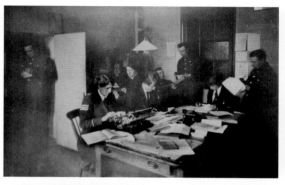
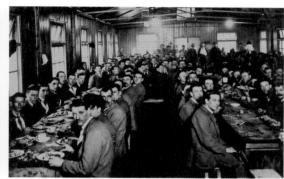
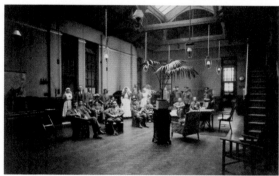
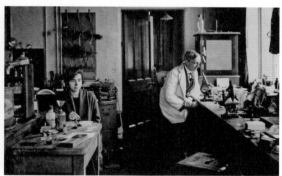
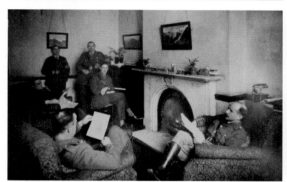
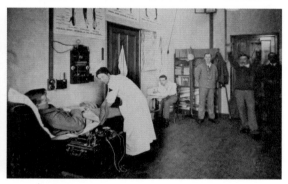
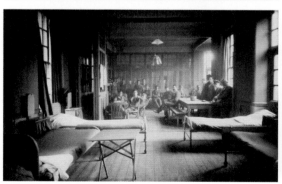
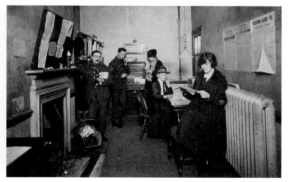

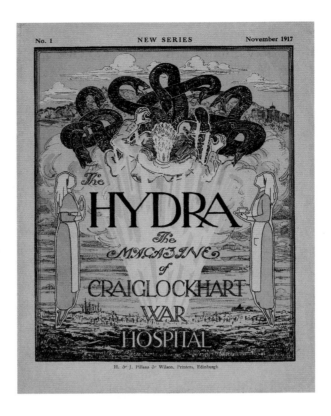

the new situation. The war had shown that most people would manifest some form of mental instability when put under enough emotional pressure. Rather than labelling a section of the population as mentally unfit and locking them away, psychiatry should bring its skills and theories into schools, the workplace and the domains of normal life. In order to do this, a new type of institution would be needed: not an asylum shut off from the world, but a new kind of clinic patched into the community to watch over its mental health. It would offer everything from educational visits to drug prescriptions, psychotherapy sessions to residential care, ministering to the mind as flexibly as a general hospital does to the body. Madness and sanity would no longer be opposites, but a spectrum on which everyone could find their place.

◄ FOOTNOTES ►

1 *An Historical and Descriptive Account of the Royal Hospital...at Chelsea* (London: T. Faulkner, 1805) p. 46

2 Urbane Metcalf, *The Interior of Bethlehem Hospital* (1818), repr. in Dale Peterson (ed.), *A Mad People's History of Madness* (Pittsburgh: U. of Pittsburgh Press, 1982) pp. 77–91

3 Eugene Roosens, *Geel Revisited* (Antwerp: Garant Uitgevers, 2007) p. 27

4 Rolf Brüggemann & Gisela Schmidt-Krebs, *Locating the Soul: museums of psychiatry in Europe* (Frankfurt: Mabuse-Verlag, 2007) p. 81

5 W. A. F. Browne, *What Asylums Were, Are and Ought to Be* (Edinburgh: Adam and Charles Black, 1837) p. 101

6 *ibid.* p. 113

7 *ibid.* p. 176

8 all *ibid.* p. 229

9 pp. 172-3

10 Charles Dickens, 'A Curious Dance around a Curious Tree', in *Household Words*, 17 January 1852

11 Richard Dadd case notes, reproduced in Nicholas Tromans, *Richard Dadd* (London: Tate Publishing, 2012) pp. 195-6

12 John Conolly, *A Remonstrance with the Lord Chief Baron touching the case Nottidge vs Ripley* (London: Churchill, 1849) pp. 6-7

13 Henry Maudsley, *Journal of Mental Science*, 12 (1866) p. 173

14 George M. Beard, *American Nervousness: its causes and consequences* (New York: 1881) p. 96

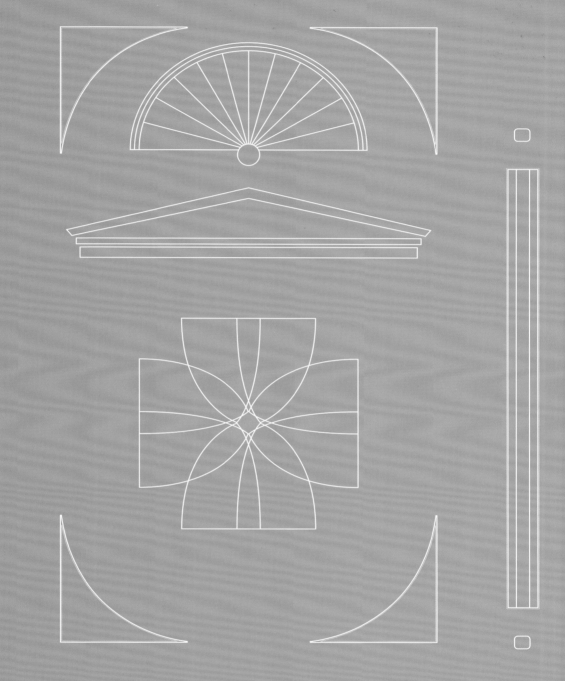

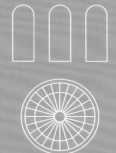

JONATHAN MARTIN

1782 · 1838

Martin was confined in Bethlem as a criminal lunatic from 1829 to 1838 after setting fire to York Minster cathedral. His art depicts the prophetic visions he experienced throughout his life.

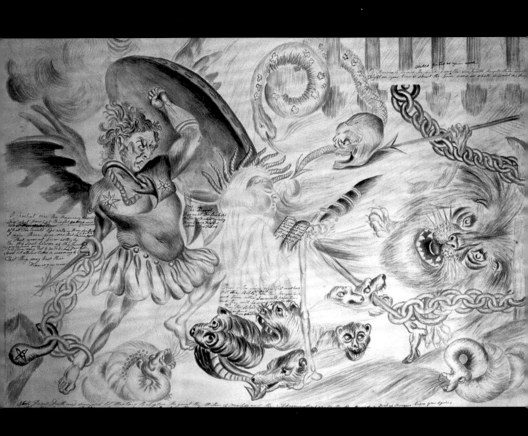

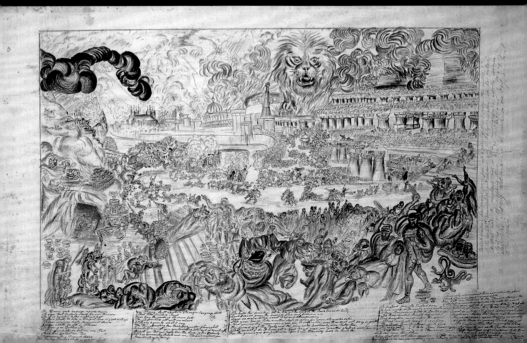

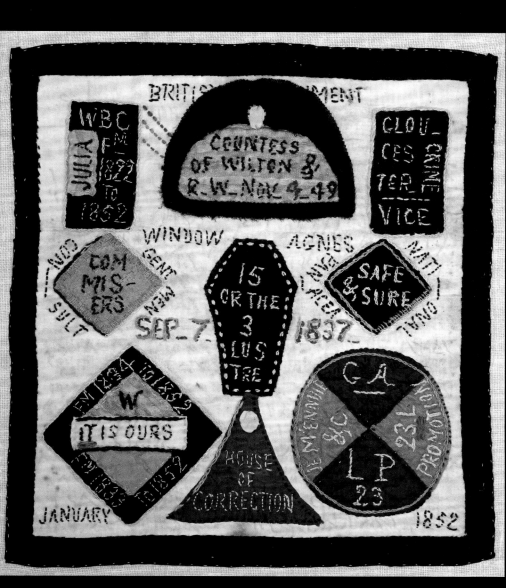

MARY FRANCES HEATON

• UNKNOWN – 1878 •

Mary was admitted to Wakefield Asylum in 1837
and remained there for thirty-six years. During
that time, she produced a number of samplers
intricately embroidered with text and images.

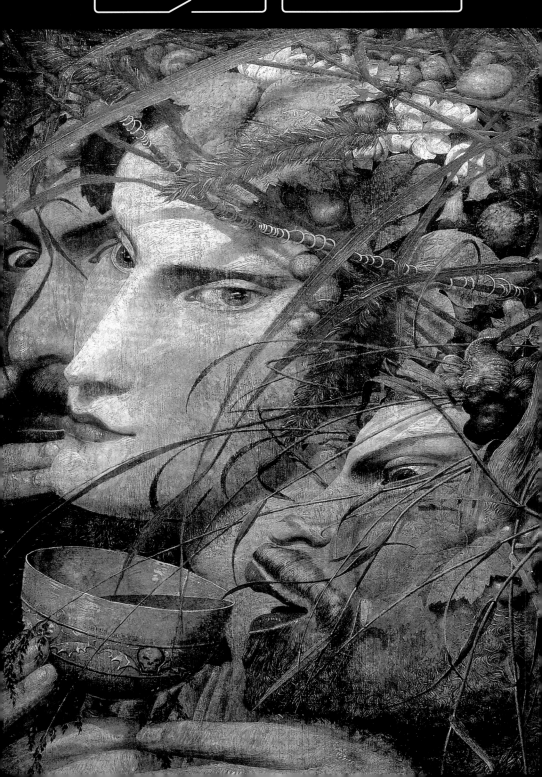

Dadd (see p.115) was a promising young artist who became mentally ill during a visit to the Holy Land. On his return, he stabbed his father to death and was confined in Bethlem as a criminal lunatic.

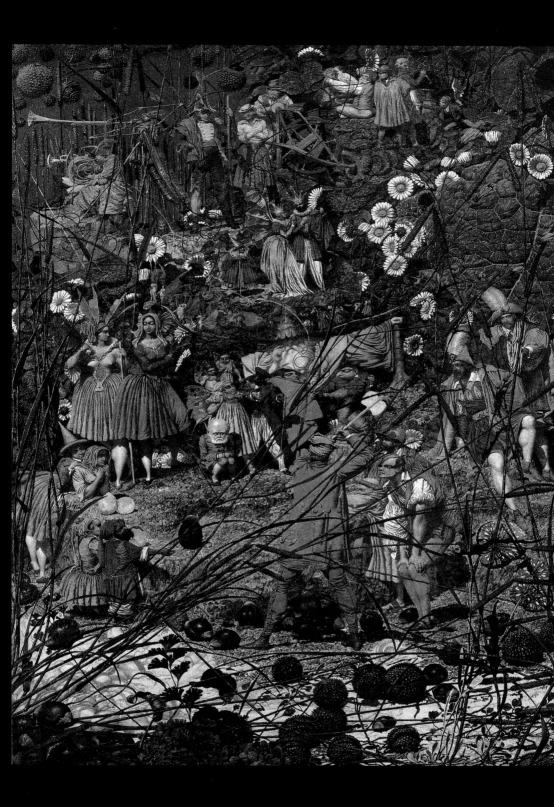

opp.
Bacchanalian Scene
(1862), oil on wood,
by Richard Dadd.
This work was painted
in Bethlem and has
an inscription, or
incantation, in Latin
on the reverse.

above
The Fairy Feller's
Master-stroke
(*c.*1855–1864),
oil on wood, by
Richard Dadd. This
work was donated
to the Tate in 1963
by Siegfried Sassoon.

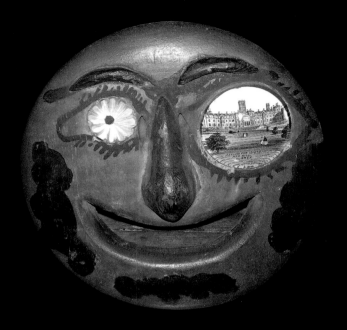

JAMES
HENRY
PULLEN

1835–1916

During the sixty years he spent in Earlswood Asylum, Pullen produced a remarkable body of paintings, drawings and sculptures, including a series of fantastical model boats. He became known as the 'genius of Earlswood Asylum'.

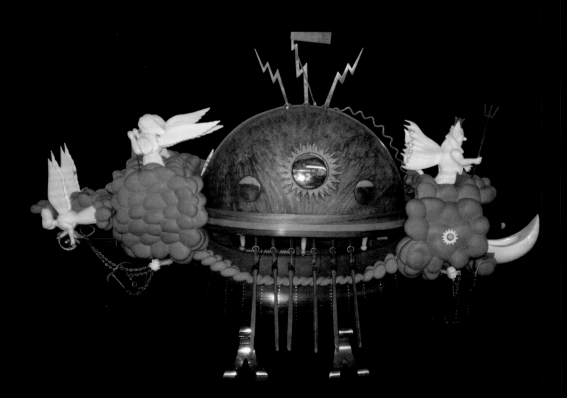

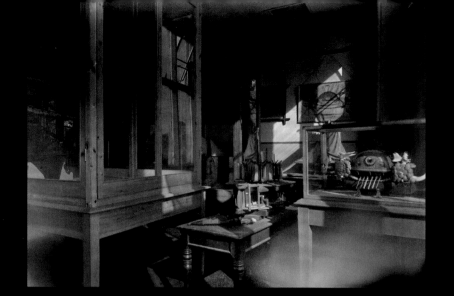

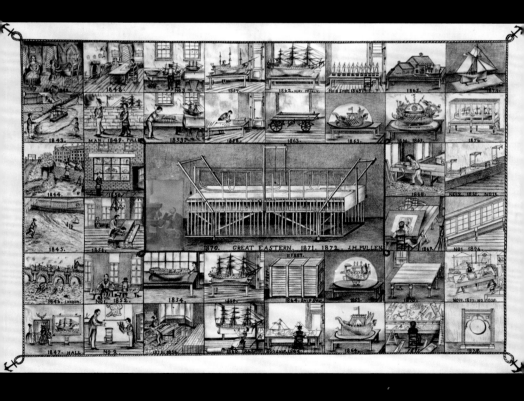

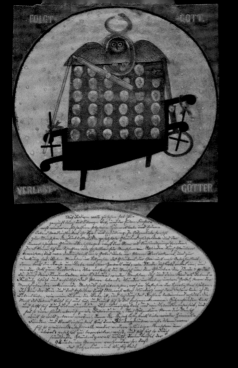

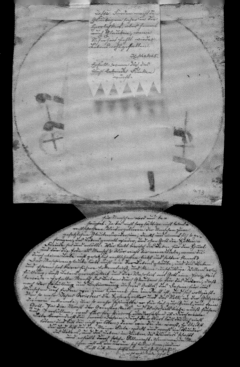

HEINRICH HERMANN MEBES

· 1842–UNKNOWN ·

A watchmaker by trade, Mebes was admitted to Eberswalde Asylum, Germany, diagnosed with *dementia praecox*. He died in the asylum.

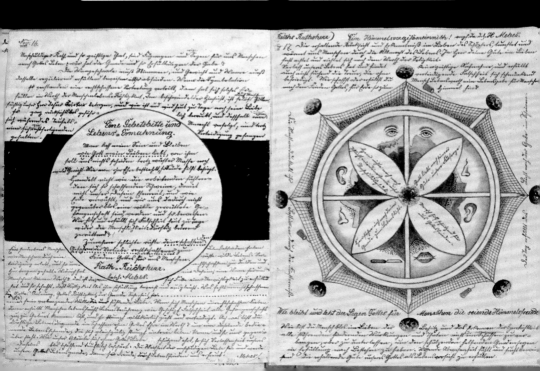

Mebes produced tiny and intricate depictions of the religious and mystical epiphanies he experienced. Like many asylum artists, he combined text with images in his work.

FRANZ JOSEPH KLEBER

• 1857–1909 •

Kleber was confined from
1880 to 1896 at Prüll, a former
Benedictine Abbey in Regensburg,
Bavaria. He was diagnosed
with 'primary insanity'.

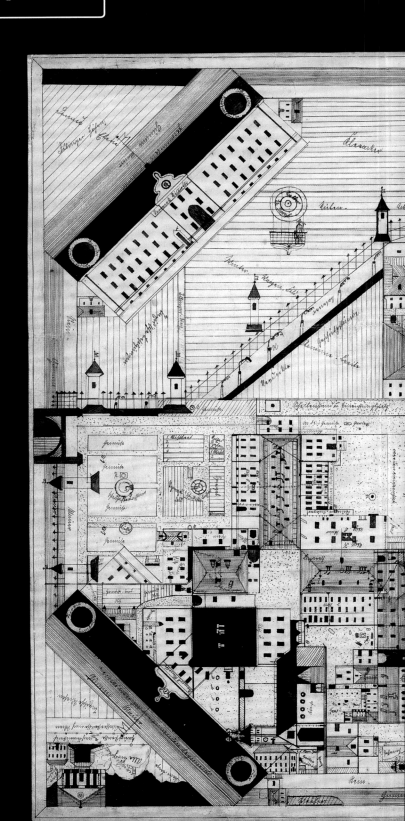

right
Franz Joseph Kleber:
Plan of the Regensburg
Institution, Kartause
Prüll (1880–1896).
Pen on cardboard.
Now held in the
Prinzhorn Collection
in Heidelberg.

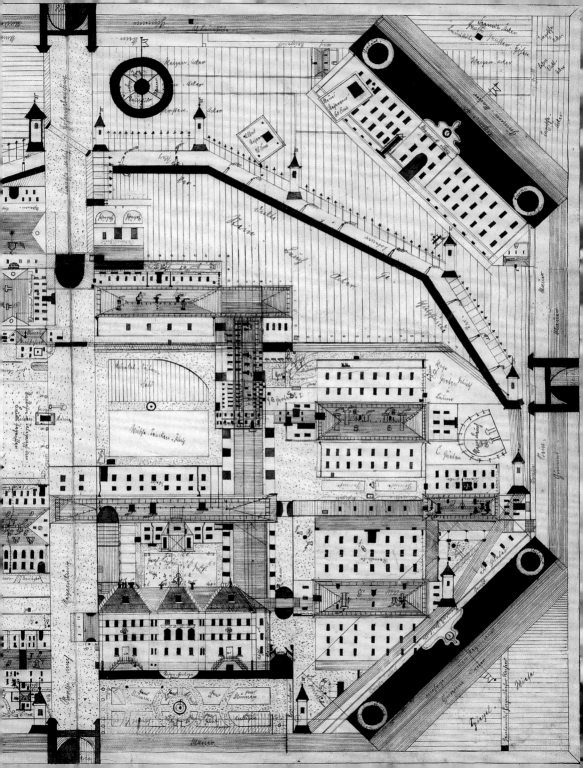

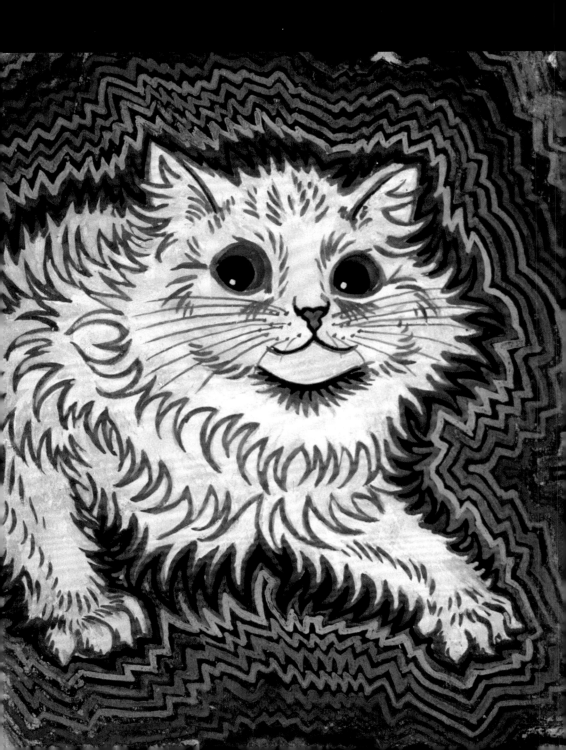

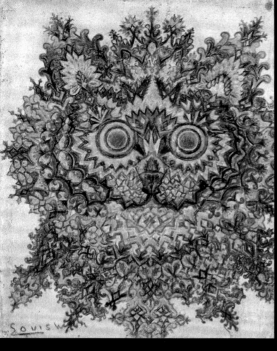

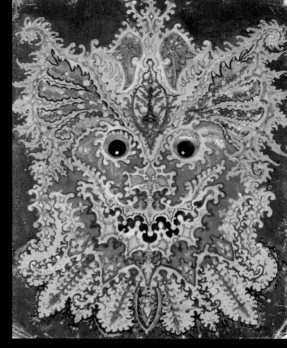

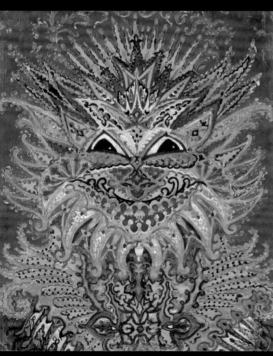

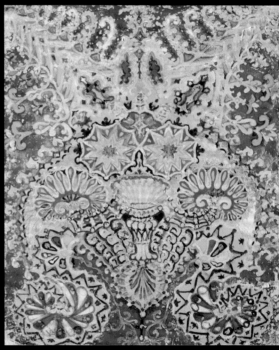

*opp. and above
Kaleidoscope Cats
III to VII* by Louis
Wain (late 19th or
early 20th century).
Gouache on paper.

Wain had been
well known and
loved for his

paintings, and
he continued
to depict cats
in Bethlem and
elsewhere. In
addition to his
comic, sentimental
and satirical
treatments,

jewelled and
abstract feline
forms. Some people
have attempted to
identify these works
with his periods
of florid insanity,
but this cannot be
proved because

undated. It seems
that Wain produced
these striking
experimental
works occasionally
throughout his life,
regardless of his
mental state. He
referred to them as

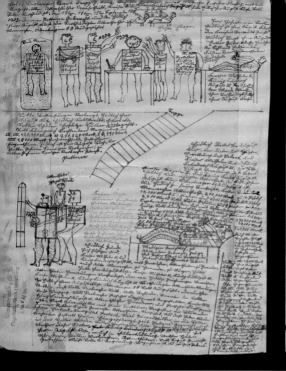

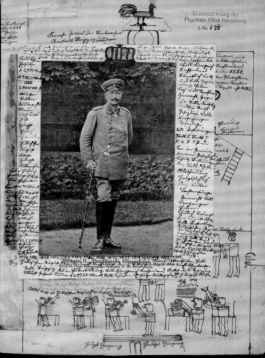

AUGUST JOHANN KLOSE

• 1862–1942 •

Diagnosed with *paranoia querulans*,
Klose spent much of his extensive time in
Hubertusburg Asylum, Germany writing his
Autobiography and History of the Institution.

*above and below
Autobiography
and History of the
Institution* (1918) by
August Johann Klose.
Pencil, pen and paint,
booklet made from
war pamphlets, paper
from the institution
and toilet paper.

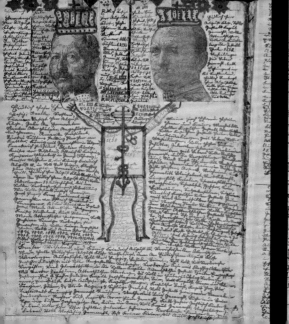

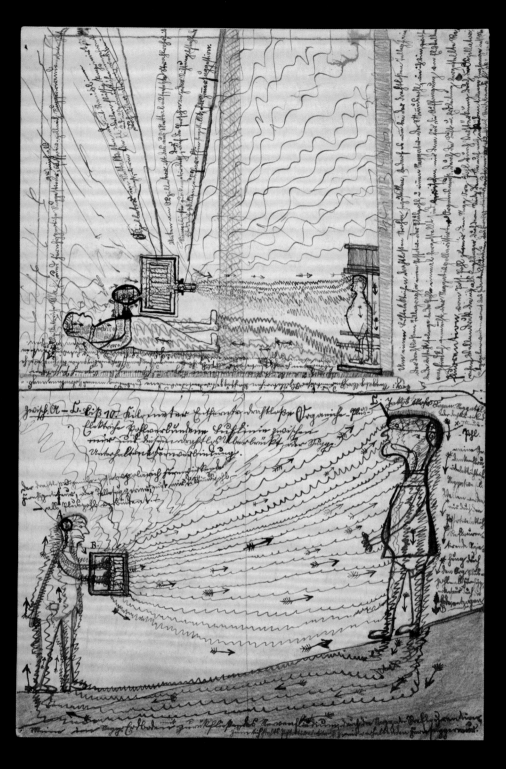

JAKOB MOHR

1884–1935

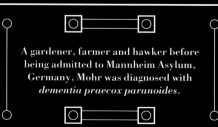

A gardener, farmer and hawker before being admitted to Mannheim Asylum, Germany, Mohr was diagnosed with *dementia praecox paranoides*.

above
Proofs (*c.* 1910) by Jakob Mohr. Pencil and pen on office paper. A psychiatrist operates an 'influencing machine', wearing headphones to listen in to Mohr's thoughts.

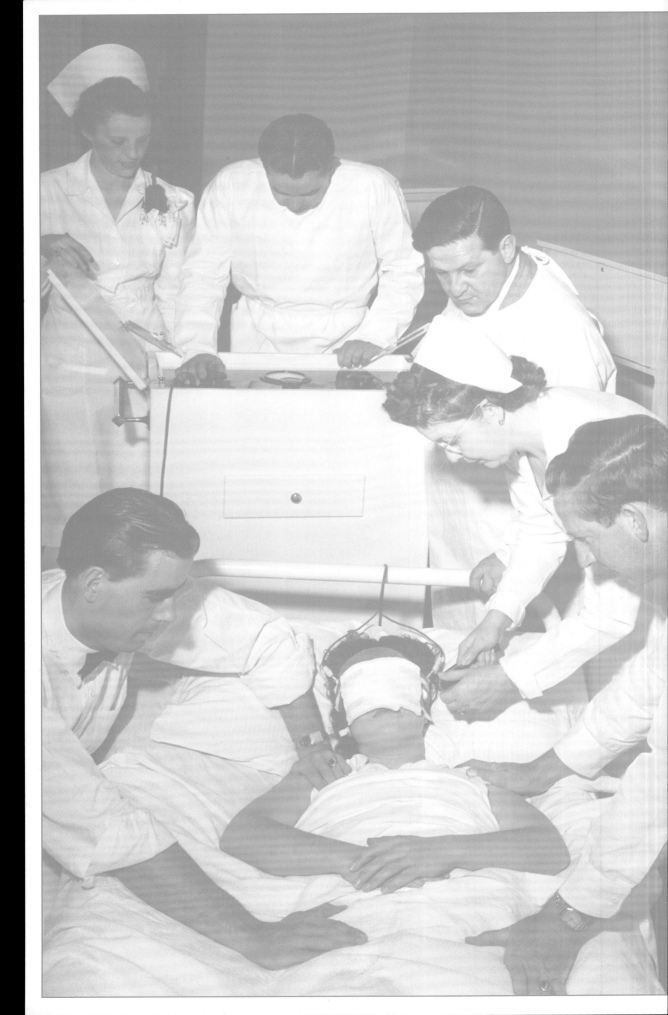

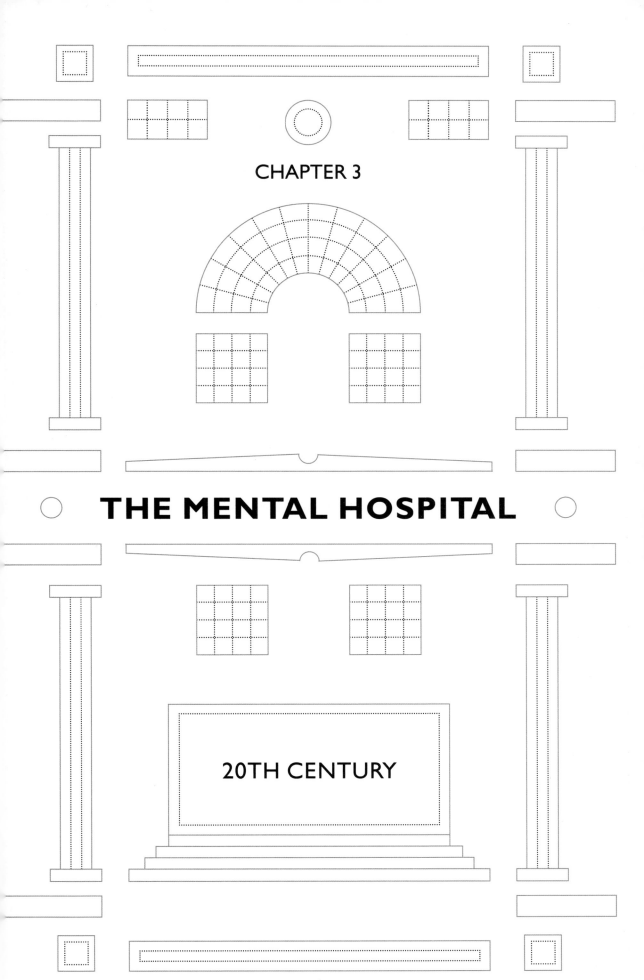

CHAPTER 3

THE MENTAL HOSPITAL

20TH CENTURY

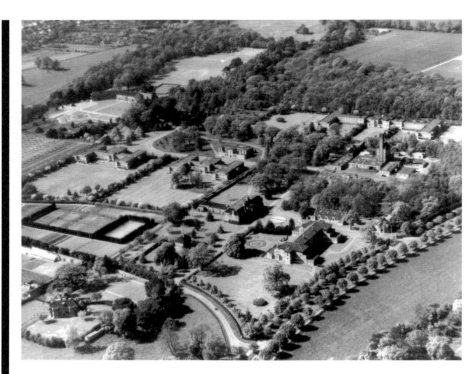

On 9 July 1930 a thousand guests were delivered by specially chartered train to celebrate the grand opening of the new Bethlem Royal Hospital at its site in Monks Orchard, a semi-rural estate on London's southern outskirts. Befitting its royal charter, the honoured guest was Queen Mary – wife of King George V – who was followed by a gaggle of reporters and photographers as she strolled the closely mown lawns in blazing sunshine, admired the airy and brightly painted rooms and planted a tree in the grounds.

Bethlem's 20th-century incarnation was a complex of ultra-modern design, incorporating elements of Scandinavian and Bauhaus styles. It was a conscious turn away from the barracks-style asylum at Southwark, just as that building had distanced itself from the baroque madhouse of the previous century. The imposing Victorian mansion that had been the centrepiece of the old Monks Orchard estate was demolished, and the hospital buildings were dispersed among the surrounding parkland in the newly fashionable 'villa system'. Discreet low-rise residential wards, their floors laid with the thick Axminster carpet more usually associated with hotels, were connected by neat brick paths and edged by verandas that allowed patients to sit outside in the shade. The villa system was more than a modern aesthetic: it embodied the

RIGHT
Photographed in 1955,
the roadside chapel
at Monks Orchard,
positioned near the site
entrance, enhanced the
village and community
feel of the new hospital.

BELOW
The governor's block,
seen here in 1955,
was the most imposing
building on the Monks
Orchard site. It now
houses the museum,
archives and gallery.

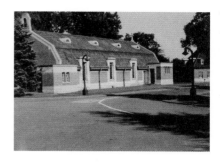

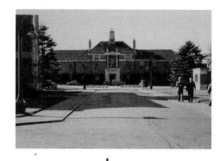

«'Lunatics' were now 'patients':
their condition was not their
destiny, but an illness from
which they could recover.»

BELOW
This photograph of
the new Bethlem at
Monks Orchard, taken
in 1955, shows the
'villa' design, which
incorporated four ward
blocks. Each one was
spaciously designed
with single-room
accommodation.

principles of the new mental hospital,
in which the uniform treatment of the
old asylum was to be replaced by a cluster
of departments offering a wide spectrum
of services.

The Mental Treatment Act of 1930,
passed after a first reform attempt had
failed eight years previously, jettisoned
the one-size-fits-all category of 'lunatic'
in favour of restoring to patients a measure
of choice in their treatment. They were
now assigned to one of three categories:
the 'certified', whose confinement was
mandated by the courts; the 'temporary',
who were held on medical authority with
their conditions regularly reviewed; and
the 'voluntary', who were free to check

in or out as they wished. The term 'asylum'
was discarded officially and replaced with
'mental hospital', in recognition of the
primacy of the psychiatric approach to
treatment. 'Lunatics' were now 'patients':
their condition was not their destiny,
but an illness
from which they
could recover.

At the same
time, the mental
hospital aimed
to incorporate
the best practices
of moral therapy.
The enlightened
asylum planners

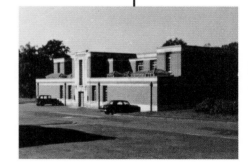

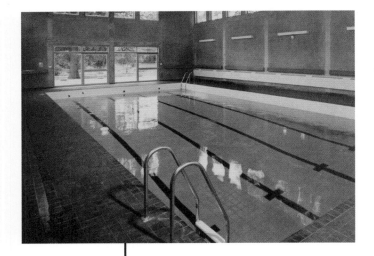

LEFT
In 1955 a community centre was built in the hospital grounds. It included a state-of-the-art swimming pool, with views to the gardens.

RIGHT
The facilities at Bethlem Royal Hospital at Monks Orchard included a small chapel, which was opened in 1930.

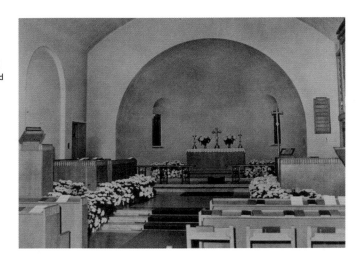

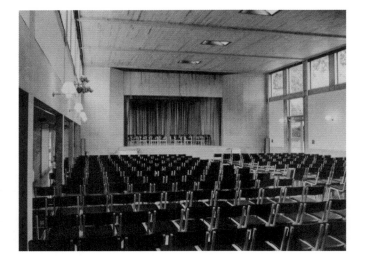

LEFT
Built to increase the hospital's range of recreational facilities, the community centre included an auditorium.

«Outside every block were ornamental flower beds and plenty of green spaces, where patients could stroll and relax.»

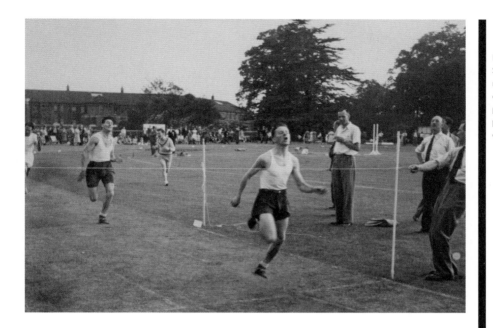

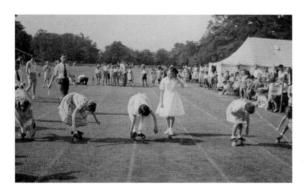

of the 19th century had stressed that this needed to begin with the site itself, and the Bethlem governors had wanted to relocate from the increasingly traffic-choked city to the countryside ever since Broadmoor had been established in its pleasant rural setting in 1863. Outside every block of the new hospital were ornamental flower beds and plenty of green spaces, where patients could stroll, relax and play cricket or bowls. Sunlight flooded into the day rooms, and patients were encouraged to occupy themselves with chess or billiards and to learn crafts such as woodwork and basket weaving.

One of the most popular occupations was art, which became a touchstone for the ideas that were transforming attitudes to mental illness. Drawing, painting and sculpture had been regarded as beneficial occupations since the era of William Browne and William Charles Hood, but they were now seen as therapeutic in more specific ways: tools for engaging with the patients who created them, or diagnostic tests through which psychiatrists could glimpse the workings of the patients' minds. In 1900 the resident physician at Bethlem, Theophilus Hyslop, had exhibited a selection of patient artworks in the common room of the old hospital, and at an international medical conference in London in 1913 he had curated the first public display of the art of the insane. It had garnered a great deal of attention,

«Psychiatrists began to collect what had been dismissed previously as worthless daubings.»

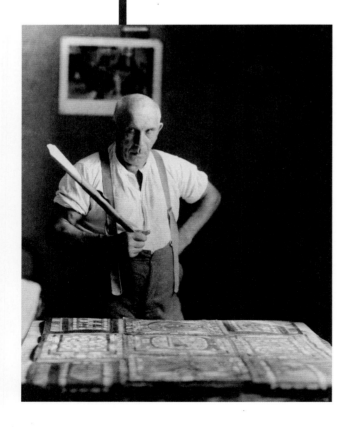

BELOW
Adolf Wölfli, violently insane but an artistic prodigy, is photographed in 1925 by his psychiatrist Walther Morgenthaler. His work is laid out in front of him and he holds a paper trumpet.

including a front page splash in the *Daily Mirror* that used their resemblance to works of the expressionists and cubists to deride the modernist fashions of the art world. The show sparked interest among psychiatrists, several of whom began to collect what had been dismissed previously as worthless daubings.

The most prolific of the early collectors was Hans Prinzhorn, who had acquired an art history doctorate before training as a psychiatrist. He was hired in 1919 by Emil Kraepelin's successor at Heidelberg, Karl Wilmanns, to work on the collection of art by psychotic patients that Kraepelin had assembled during his researches. Prinzhorn sent letters of request to other asylums and sanatoriums and rapidly amassed more than five thousand examples of spontaneous art by psychotic patients from across Germany, Austria, Switzerland and Italy. In 1922 he published a lavishly illustrated overview of his new collection, *Artistry of the Mentally Ill*. It was received by his fellow psychiatrists with mild curiosity but made a powerful impression on avant-garde artists such as Max Ernst and Paul Klee. Painter and sculptor Jean Dubuffet was influenced by Prinzhorn's collection and coined the term 'art brut', or 'raw art', to describe work produced by social outsiders without regard for aesthetic norms or conventions.

Prinzhorn believed that the art he was assembling had a great deal to teach psychiatry. He regarded the creativity of the mentally ill, with their often irresistible compulsion to draw and paint, as a window

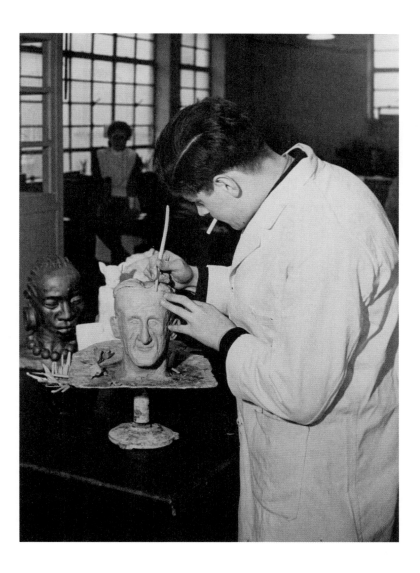

RIGHT
This patient is at
work in the art rooms
of the Maudsley
Hospital. Art was
encouraged for a
variety of reasons,
including occupation,
therapy and developing
craft skills.

into inner worlds that were otherwise inaccessible. It also opened up possibilities for therapy, since the drive towards artistic expression helped 'to actualize the psyche and thereby build a bridge from the self to others'.[1] Art was a common language through which patient and doctor could learn to communicate.

The most productive and intense early relationship of this kind was between Walther Morgenthaler, a psychiatrist at a private mental hospital outside Bern in Switzerland, and Adolf Wölfli (see p. 204), an incurable criminal patient in the nearby public asylum. Wölfli was unstoppably creative and prodigiously talented, turning out a constant stream of prose, poetry and music as well as paintings of dazzling colour, detail and intensity. Morgenthaler sat with him frequently as he painted, attempting to discern the connection between art and artist, and published a detailed study of his work. Wölfli had been arrested for a series of sexual assaults on young girls, certified as insane and confined to the asylum, where initially he had been brutal and unmanageable, in the grip of violent hallucinations. After five years, he finally settled in his small cell and began to elaborate his delusional world. Morgenthaler regarded him as schizophrenic, although he was less interested in the diagnosis than the individual. But he never cracked Wölfli's code. He came to understand that he was

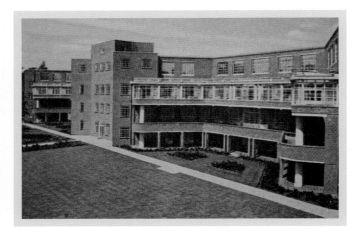

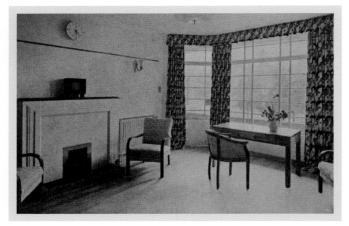

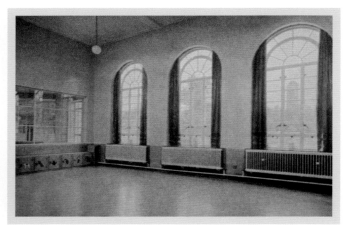

painting episodes from his personal history, abstracted into a jewelled symmetry, but the meaning of the endlessly repeated patterns was hidden from even Wölfli himself. When interrogated, he simply described them as 'decorations'.

In the 'sectorized' world of the mental hospital, Bethlem's new incarnation was a bid for the upper end of the market. The huge county asylums, such as Colney Hatch, had become the new Bedlams; the new Bethlem, by contrast, would resemble the spas and sanatoriums for nervous diseases that had emerged for those who could afford them. However, the old associations of Bedlam were not so easily overwritten. The hospital's notorious past reminded charitable donors of precisely what they were trying to eradicate, and fundraising efforts fell short of their targets. The Charity Commission offered limited government support but the new hospital found itself running deficits. Eventually, the solution was for Bethlem to merge with the Maudsley Hospital, a venture that had been launched with a donation from Henry Maudsley from the proceeds of his private practice. He had specified that it would not take chronic cases and would focus on medical research. It opened in south London in 1923 and established itself as the vanguard and teaching hospital for the medically orientated psychiatry that was at last transforming the treatment of mental disease.

ABOVE
Postcards of the Maudsley hospital in south London, established as a teaching hospital for the new cadre of medical specialists. Nurses were also trained in special therapeutic techniques.

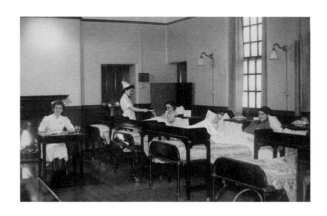

The first spectacular success of the new biological approach had come with general paralysis of the insane (GPI), a previously incurable form of neural damage and dementia that by the end of the 19th century was responsible for twenty per cent of male asylum admissions across Europe and the United States. German researchers had long suspected that GPI was caused by a bacterial infection, and that its symptoms might be connected to those of the tertiary stage of syphilis. In 1913 the connection was demonstrated conclusively with the discovery of syphilitic spirochaetes in the brains of sufferers. In a series of bold experiments in 1917, Julius Wagner-Jauregg, professor of psychiatry at the University of Vienna, infected GPI patients with malaria to induce a fever spike that would kill the spirochaetes. In several cases, their GPI went into remission.

Wagner-Jauregg's remedy was risky and traumatic for the patient, even with quinine to control the malaria, and its success rate is still disputed. However, it proved that one of the most terrifyingly destructive forms of insanity had a physical basis and, most significantly, a physical cure. More breakthroughs followed: the mental deterioration known as cretinism, which had been endemic in areas such as the Alps since ancient times, turned out to

---

BELOW
Nurses relax in the grounds at Maudsley Hospital. The institution became a leading centre for training psychiatric nurses, drawing many students from overseas.

ABOVE
Patients in the women's ward are attended by female nurses. The number of patients admitted to the Maudsley increased rapidly and the hospital also had a busy outpatient clinic.

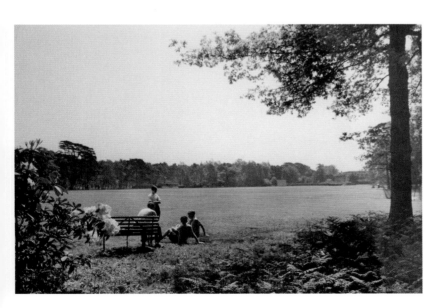

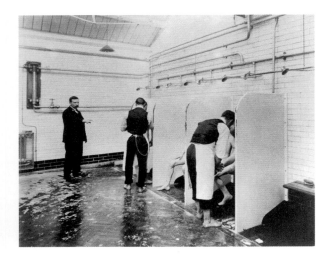

«These revelations initiated a worldwide search for 'magic bullets' to eradicate other mental illnesses.»

be the result of iodine deficiency; pellagra, a disease with severe mental symptoms that swept periodically across the Mediterranean and the southern United States, was caused by a lack of niacin. The dementias and deliriums of alcoholics, who comprised up to ten per cent of patients in many large asylums, had been commonly ascribed to hereditary weakness but they were now shown to be side effects of their addiction.

These revelations initiated a worldwide search for 'magic bullets' to eradicate other mental illnesses, particularly the chronic condition recently named schizophrenia. In the state hospital at Trenton, New Jersey, psychiatrist Henry Cotton developed a theory that not only GPI but all mental diseases were bacteriological in origin, caused by a hidden infection that dispersed toxins into the brain. He embarked on a massive experimental programme of excising possible sites of 'focal sepsis', which included teeth, tonsils, spleens, cervixes and colons. In Germany new sedative drugs known as barbiturates, marketed by the pharmaceutical giant Bayer, showed promise not only in calming manic behaviour but also as the basis of 'deep sleep' therapies: long periods of prescribed unconsciousness that seemed to benefit mood disorders.

In Vienna neurologist Manfred Sakel induced comas in schizophrenic patients by injecting them with the newly discovered hormone insulin, and reported that they re-emerged into consciousness with their mental disorders erased.

The younger generation of psychiatrists, who had begun their careers among the warehoused ranks of incurables in the old asylums, advocated these new therapies with a powerful sense of moral mission. The first medical superintendent at the Maudsley Hospital, Edward Mapother, had been a junior medical officer in the old asylums and subsequently had witnessed shell shock in France during the Great War; he also had an older sister who had ended her days as an incurable at Bethlem. He was passionately committed to the clinical and neurological approach, but concerned that some of the drastic new experimental therapies violated his professional oath to 'do no harm'.

Some of his protégés, however, believed that the question was too urgent for such scruples: if Wagner-Jauregg had not given malaria to his test subjects deliberately and without their consent, thousands more would have succumbed to syphilitic dementia. Mapother's student, William Sargant, idolized his teacher but was

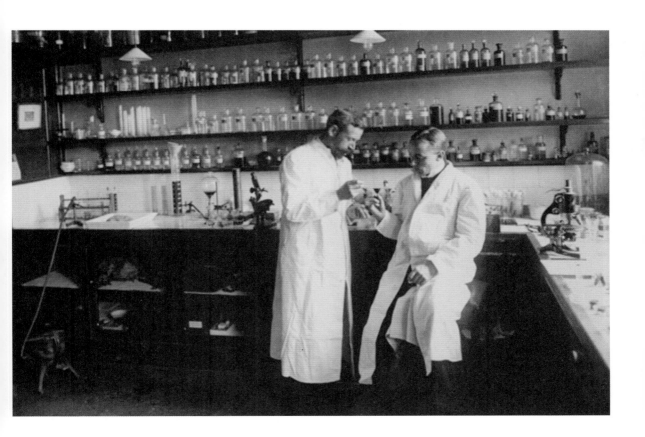

convinced that investigating new therapies such as insulin coma, sedative medication and electroshock was a matter of life and death. Sargant was haunted by his memories of the blank stares of catatonic patients whom he had been obliged to force feed at the county asylum at Hanwell, and by his own hospitalization for severe depression around the same time, although he never admitted the latter publicly. Mental illness was an enemy to be defeated, a stigma to be wiped away, both for his patients and for himself. Obtaining patient consent and keeping case notes were bureaucratic niceties that could only hamper progress.

In their search for new methods of targeting the brain, psychiatrists began to experiment with electricity. They discovered that high-voltage currents applied across the temples could induce epileptic seizures, which were believed at the time to diminish the symptoms of schizophrenia. In 1938 Italian neurologist Ugo Cerletti coined the term 'electroshock' for this practice, allegedly conceived after he witnessed the technique at a pig abattoir in Rome. In the first human trial, the voltage was not sufficient to produce a seizure, and the patient sat up with the words: 'Not a second. Deadly!' Cerletti dialled up the

OPPOSITE
Male patients are washed by hospital orderlies at Long Grove Asylum, Epsom in c. 1930.

ABOVE
Bethlem hospital's pharmacy c. 1900–1915. Psychiatry developed a wide range of medications

and pharmaceutical laboratories were incorporated into many residential mental hospitals.

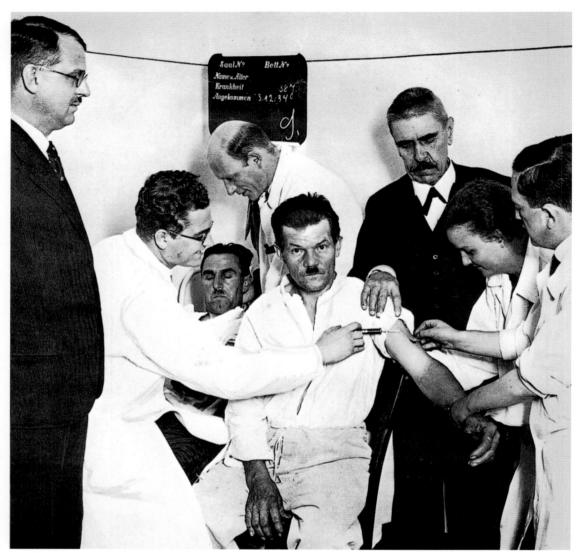

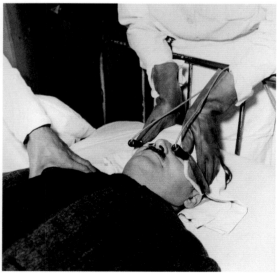

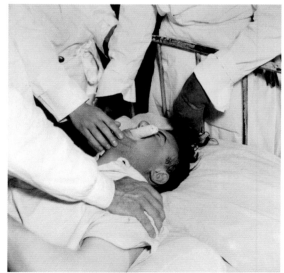

«Mental illness was an enemy to be defeated, a stigma to be wiped away.»

voltage and continued. According to his case notes, the patient improved rapidly and after eleven treatments went into 'complete remission'.[2]

Sargant immediately applied to develop this treatment at the Maudsley Hospital, but the Ministry of Health refused to support it. He found private funding and was soon reporting miraculous results. It was a pattern that became familiar among the new treatments: initial trials generated claims of spectacular success and the promise of large-scale studies to follow, but these often failed to materialize and, when they did, they were far less conclusive. Subsequent research has suggested that the early successes may have been influenced greatly by the increased levels of attention the trial patients were receiving and by the excitement and optimism of the doctors, both of which contrasted markedly with their previous experience on the back wards. The early reports also paid little attention to side effects, which in the case of electroshock commonly included dislocations and spinal fractures caused by the violence of the seizures induced. Science and advocacy were impossible to disentangle. For those who believed there was no alternative, reporting negatives could serve only to dampen morale and delay progress.

The new physical therapies recharged psychiatrists with the therapeutic optimism that the old asylums had ground out of even the most compassionate and idealistic. However, they depersonalized the patients, reducing them to test subjects in a vast experiment in which failure was of little interest. Typically, the recipients of electroshock and coma therapies were chronic cases from the public asylums, the residue of a failed system from which all who could afford to had escaped. The voice of the patient was recorded only when it conformed to the desired litany: 'I feel like a new person.' But other, darker perspectives survive. Antonin Artaud, the French poet and playwright who wore his madness as a badge of pride inseparable from his art, was certified and confined in the asylum

OPP. ABOVE
Julius Wagner-Juaregg, the developer of the malaria cure for syphilis, stands behind a patient and watches as the treatment is performed.

OPP. BELOW
Electroconvulsive therapy (ECT) became a standard treatment in mental hospitals from the 1940s. Here it is administered in the asylum in Rodez, France, where Antonin Artaud received treatment.

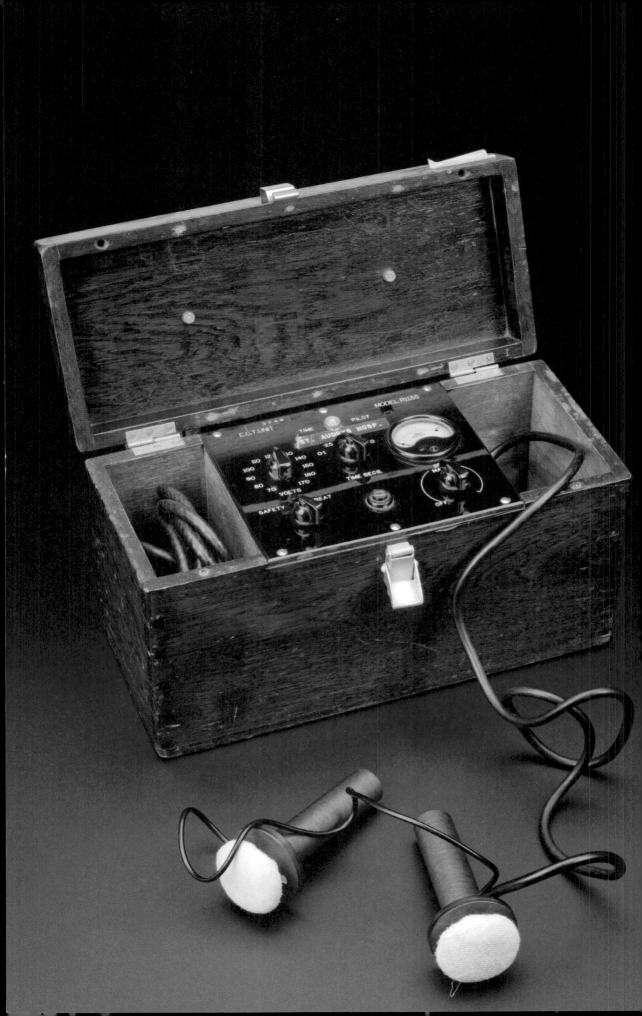

at Rodez near Toulouse in 1937, where he was subjected to insulin coma and electroshock therapy. The treatments left him a shell, his memory wiped and thoughts silenced. In his final works, he described them as a new form of black magic, the ultimate destruction of the individual by society's modern sorcerers.

In 1939 Sargant was awarded a grant from the Rockefeller Foundation to spend a year at Harvard University studying the latest psychiatric techniques. He had roared with laughter when told the previous year that a Portuguese neurologist, Egas Moniz, was claiming to cure mental illness by boring holes into the skull and destroying the frontal lobes of the brain by injecting alcohol into them. Yet, in Washington, Sargant was astonished to witness US neurologist Walter Freeman and his surgeon colleague, James Watts, severing the frontal lobes of a schizophrenic patient with a practised sweep, and the patient walking into their consulting room the following day with a broad grin. Freeman went on to become the most notorious proponent of the new psychiatry. He dispensed with Watts's surgical expertise and streamlined their lobotomy, as the operation was called, to the point where he could carry it out unassisted in minutes –

with an ice pick driven under the eyelid by a mallet – on a patient rendered briefly unconscious by electroshock. He toured the mental hospitals of the United States in a van he called his 'lobotomobile', charging $25 per operation.

Some doctors were highly sceptical of lobotomy from the beginning, and large-scale evidence for its efficacy was not presented properly. Nevertheless, even as accusations of malpractice and brain damage mounted, Moniz was awarded the Nobel Prize in Physiology or Medicine in 1949. Like the 19th-century asylums, the new physical therapies were a progressive solution driven by humane intentions. If they failed, the alternative was all too clear. Across the United States, many states were subjecting the mentally unfit to compulsory sterilization; in Britain, the respectable scientists of the Eugenics Society were insisting that those who carried the genes for mental deficiency should be sterilized, whether or not they exhibited any such traits themselves. In Germany, similar laws were passed in 1933 for hereditary diseases, a category that included schizophrenia and alcoholism. By the end of the Nazi era, some two hundred thousand people diagnosed as mentally ill had been systematically murdered. Those

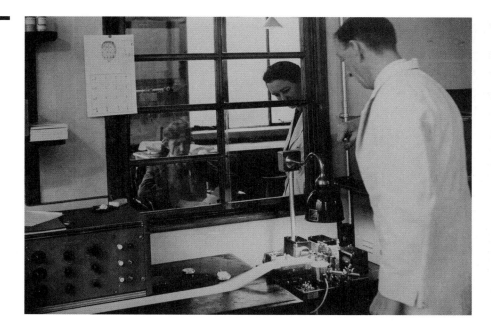

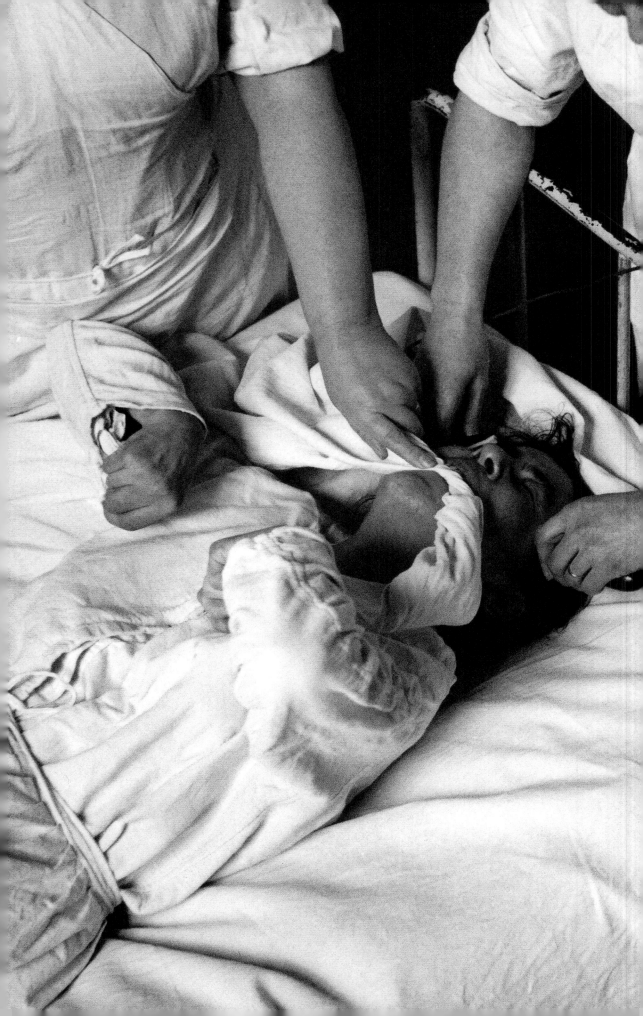

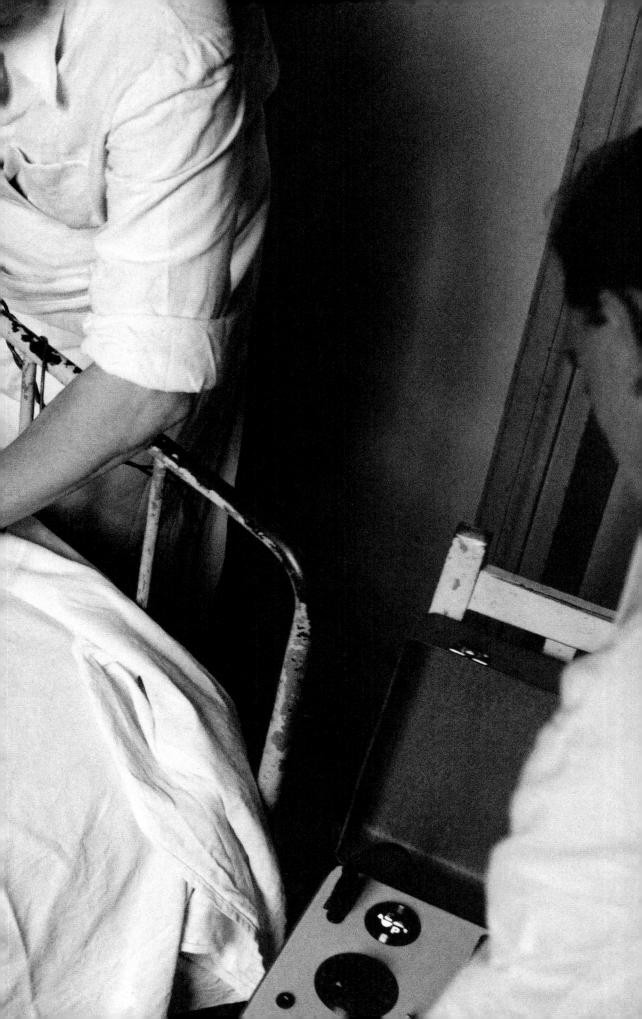

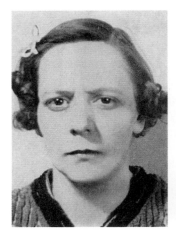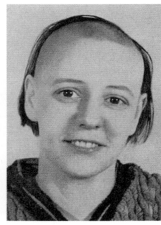

LEFT
Photographs of a patient shown before and after a lobotomy, reproduced in *Psychosurgery* by W. Freeman and J. W. Watts (1950). The 'before' photograph was taken on 23 March 1942 and is captioned 'Forever fighting . . . the meanest woman.' The 'after' photograph was taken on 4 April 1942, eleven days after the lobotomy, and is captioned 'She giggles a lot.'

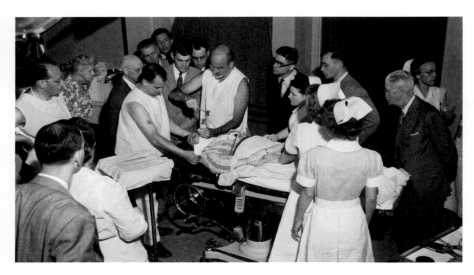

LEFT
At Fort Steilacoom, Washington, in July 1948, Walter Freeman performs a lobotomy using an instrument like an ice pick. Inserting the instrument under the upper eyelid of the patient, he cuts nerve connections in the front part of the brain.

pushing the boundaries of psychiatric medicine saw the new physical therapies not only as the alternative to the asylum, but also to far worse fates.

Yet there was another route of escape from the public asylum. There were still those who believed that the utopian ideal of asylum care envisaged by William Browne could be recovered. In the United States, the Progressive Era (1890–1920) produced idealistic experiments in living in which the disabled, socially deprived and mentally ill were invited to join self-sufficient religious communities. In 1913 William Gould, a devout Protestant and social reformer who had struggled with depression in his youth, founded a

farming community in the hills of Western Massachusetts. It was intended to be a residential home for troubled New York children from hospitals such as Bellevue, which had been established on the fringes of the city in the 18th century but was now in the teeming centre of Manhattan. By the time of its founder's death in 1925, Gould Farm – through shared hardscrabble labour and some support from social welfare societies in the city – had become a sustainable working farm and residence for a community that included the mentally ill, deprived children, recovering alcoholics and post-surgical convalescents.

In 1937 the Maudsley Hospital's clinical director, Aubrey Lewis, was sent with

Rockefeller Foundation funds to Europe to report on the state of psychiatry across the continent. He visited histology clinics in Amsterdam and inspected neurofibril cultures in laboratories in Turin; every conceivable avenue to biomedical treatment was being explored, although few were generating practical results. However, the longest section of his report was on the town of Geel, where he identified shortcomings in the data that recorded the duration of stays and rates of recovery but was struck, as so many doctors had been before him, by the calm coexistence of mental illness and normal life. The aspiration of the modern mental hospital had been a society in which, with discreet professional help, the boundary between madness and sanity could be dissolved. Here, such a society seemed to have existed forever.

As it had for Pinel and Esquirol a century before, the family care system at Geel presented itself to many psychiatrists as a beacon for the future. Faced with the choice of life in a shuttered ward or in the heart of a wholesome farming community, the families of Belgium's mentally ill and disabled were choosing the latter in greater numbers than ever before. Boarders were arriving from as far afield as Poland, and the Dutch community had built a Protestant church in the town for the four hundred of their compatriots who were now resident. The 'colony of the mad' was absorbing its guests in numbers that no psychiatrist would have thought possible: some four thousand among a native population of sixteen thousand. 'It seems,' Lewis concluded, that 'there will be more and more family care, if possible on the colony system. Gheel [sic] therefore is very valuable: it is the best experiment.'[3]

When war broke out in 1939, Lewis was posted to Mill Hill in north London to an evacuated school building that had been assigned to casualties of combat stress, the term now preferred to shell shock. He recruited a specialist in the biological basis of neuroses, Maxwell Jones, who had worked previously as a psychiatrist in Scotland. Lewis and Jones began with physiological testing, which quickly established that their hundred patients were all suffering from the same syndrome. They rapidly relearned the lesson of the Great War: confining traumatized soldiers to regimented wards was pointless when

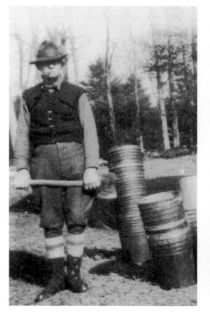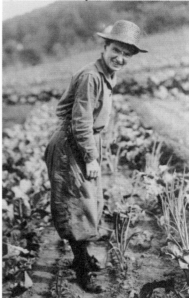

RIGHT
Gould Farm, photographed here in the 1910s and 1920s, is a farming community in the Massachusetts hills where the mentally vulnerable are welcomed and encouraged to participate in the tasks of daily life. The figure on the left is Lamont Brown; on the right is Carolyn Agnes.

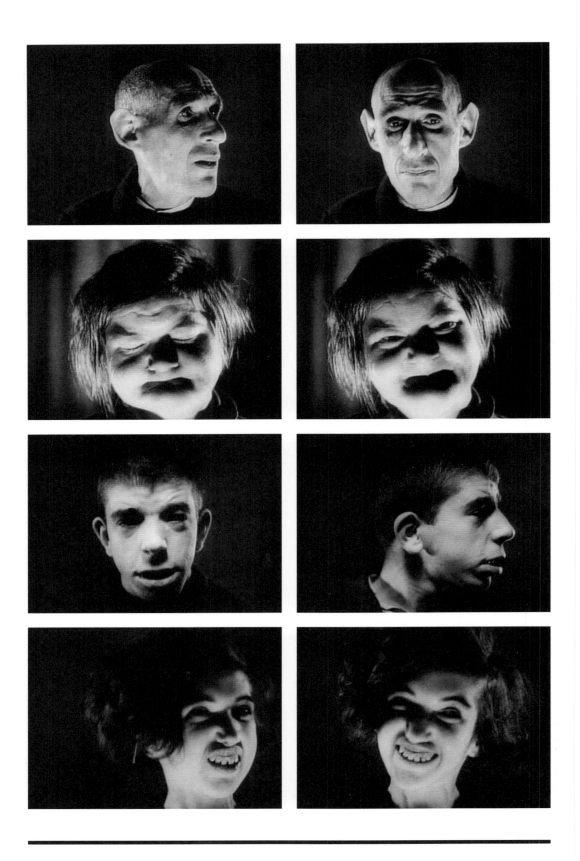

ABOVE AND OPPOSITE
These stills are from the Nazi propaganda film titled *Dasein ohne Leben* (*Existence without Life*, 1941),
which presented images of mentally and physically disabled people and proposed that they should
be euthanized. By the end of World War II, approximately 200,000 of those designated 'mentally unfit'
had been exterminated.

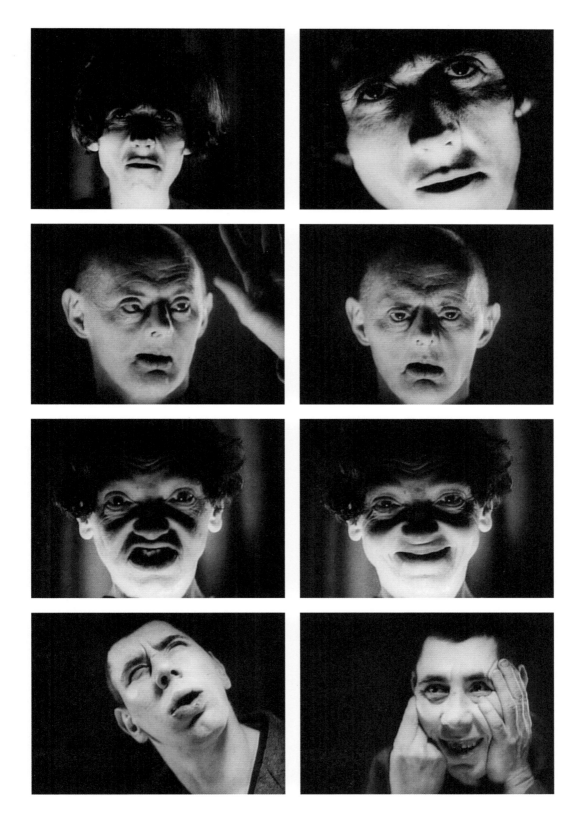

they were able and willing to help in running the place and designing their own therapies.

The patients' recovery proceeded rapidly once the physiological mechanism behind their symptoms was explained to them, and the hospital regime gave way to a more collegiate atmosphere in which patients took over staff roles. At Christmas, they all decided to transform the hospital into a medieval village named Maxwellton after their supervisor, with a festive banqueting hall, borrowed suits of armour and patients painting traditional Yuletide scenes. After this, regular group meetings were held on Mondays, at which the patients were encouraged to share suggestions and grievances; on other days, staff led discussion groups, showed films and ran drama workshops. A pass system allowed patients to leave the site and to spend time in the outside world. Jones began to formulate some principles to govern such experiments: they should be democratic and communal, with a presumption of permissiveness and a group commitment to 'reality confrontation' with patients who continued to manifest delusions or disordered thinking.

Similar arrangements evolved at other military hospitals, such as Northfield in Birmingham, where the term 'therapeutic community' was coined to describe them. Their theory and practice were developed further by Joshua Bierer, a psychiatrist who, like Sigmund Freud, had fled Vienna in 1938 and settled in London. Bierer began to teach the 'social approach'

and group therapy at Guy's and St Bartholomew's hospitals in 1942. The goal of his system was to make patients independent and 'self-deciding'; paradoxically, this could only be achieved if the individual was fully supported within a network to which they felt they belonged. The patient, Bierer taught, 'must be treated not only as a person but part of a community.'[4] When the war ended, Jones turned his experiment into a treatment centre in London, which later became the Henderson Hospital. In 1960 he moved to Oregon State Hospital and seeded his ideas in community clinics across the western United States.

The war also allowed more freewheeling experiments with physical therapies: Sargant treated combat stress with 'abreactive' shock methods, which included strapping down casualties, injecting them with amphetamines and urging them to relive their battlefield traumas. In 1943 a great medical breakthrough was achieved with the triumphantly successful trials of penicillin at the Venereal Disease Research Laboratory in Staten Island. Here, finally, was a 'magic bullet': a fast and universally effective remedy against a host of previously untreatable infections. The only problem was how to move it into mass production quickly enough. Hopes were renewed for the elusive penicillin for the mind, and it was not long before a candidate emerged. In 1951 Henri Laborit, a French neurosurgeon searching for anaesthetic compounds at the small pharmaceutical company Rhône-Poulenc, tried a modified antihistamine called

OPPOSITE
In these scenes from daily life at Mill Hill Emergency Hospital during World War II, patients are seen taking on staff roles and organizing their own activities, such as pottery and picture framing.

«The patient, Bierer taught, must be treated not only as a person but part of a community.»

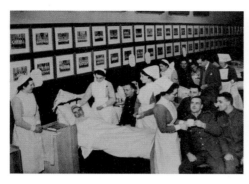

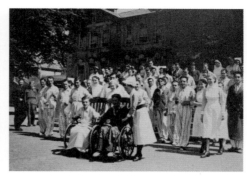

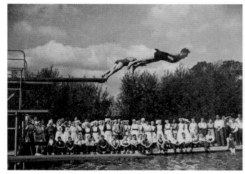

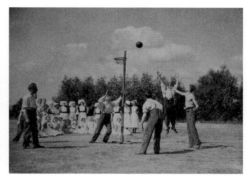

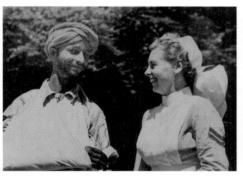

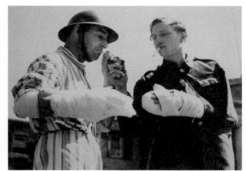

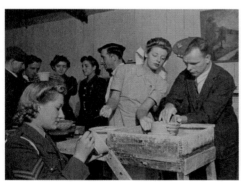

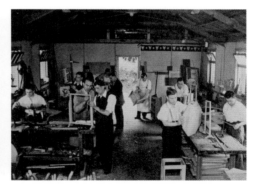

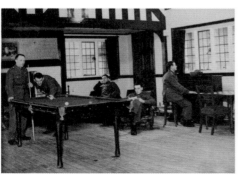

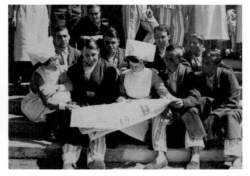

chlorpromazine on a few psychiatric
patients and reported that it relieved their
manic and psychotic states. By the end
of the year, it was being marketed across
France as Largactil, and within two years it
had effected an astonishing transformation
in Paris's public asylums. Violence, shouting,
disruptive behaviour and straitjackets had
all melted away, replaced by calm, silence
and daily injections.

Rhône-Poulenc licensed chlorpromazine
to Smith, Kline & French in the United
States, where it was branded Thorazine.

Other pharmaceutical companies, including
Ciba, Roche, Geigy and Sandoz, soon had
similar compounds on the market. The
new drugs were a clear advance on the
old narcotics such as chloral hydrate,
known as 'liquid cosh': rather than heavy
sedation they seemed to promote a calm,
disengaged state in which patients were
freed from violent mood swings. Some
early subjects reported a greatly improved
and lasting sense of well-being. Less
attention was paid to the side effects, such
as the blinking, grimacing and lip smacking
that often developed with regular use. It

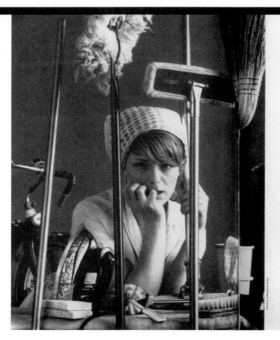

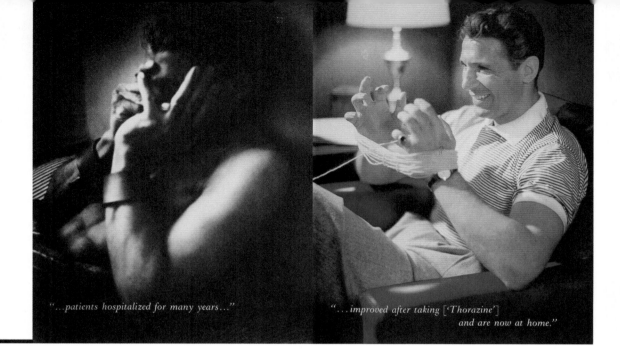

"...patients hospitalized for many years..."

"...improved after taking ['Thorazine'] and are now at home."

is a measure of the optimism with which chlorpromazine was received that it was given to around fifty million people before its side effects were recognized as symptoms of tardive dyskinesia, an incurable neurological condition that the drug was producing.

Early trials of chlorpromazine had promised a huge range of applications, which the brand name Largactil (large action) had reflected. Pharmaceutical companies pushed the new drugs vigorously, presenting them as a safer and more palatable alternative to ECT. But to be marketed effectively to psychiatrists, a more precise story about what they did and how they worked was needed: whether they acted on the causes of mental illness or merely suppressed some of its symptoms. The immediate solution was to coin new terms for the drugs. In Europe, they were referred to as 'neuroleptics' (taking hold of the nervous system) and in the United States as 'antipsychotics', suggesting that they had a specific effect on psychotic illnesses.

The neurochemistry of the new drugs was a work in progress, but they had a transformative effect on the mental hospital. They invigorated psychiatrists and nurses, freeing them from the need to administer restraints and solitary confinements, thereby making them feel more positive about their work

and optimistic for their patients' prospects. However, patients could be dehumanized by them: drugs that were believed to alleviate psychosis in the same way that penicillin removed infection made their feelings less relevant, and their protests easier to ignore. They also created new openings for the old problems of asylum abuse. Few patients took the drugs voluntarily: although they suppressed tension and reduced excitement, they created an unpleasant blankness, often accompanied by dizziness, drowsiness or muscle stiffening. Like the blistering and bloodletting of old, injections could be forced on troublesome patients or withheld as a reward for good behaviour. As routine medication took hold, patients became withdrawn, staring vacantly from their beds and chairs, passively awaiting the next meal or dose. The long-promised medical breakthrough had arrived, but it made mental hospital wards uncomfortably reminiscent of the old asylums.

The arrival of antipsychotic medication was expected to ease the pressures on mental hospitals, but in many respects it increased them. It sharpened the distinction between neurosis – mostly treated outside the hospitals by private psychotherapists and consultants – and psychosis, which demanded long-term and usually residential care, increasingly under chemical control. But this was also a distinction of class and wealth. As they had

177

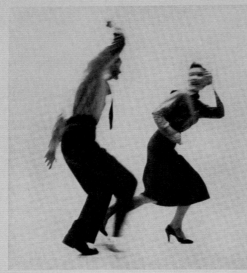

To control agitation—a symptom that cuts across diagnostic categories

Thorazine®, a fundamental drug in
brand of chlorpromazine
psychiatry—Because of its sedative effect, 'Thorazine' is especially useful in controlling hyperactivity, irritability and hostility. And because 'Thorazine' calms without clouding consciousness, the patient on 'Thorazine' usually becomes more sociable and more receptive to psychotherapy.

leaders in psychopharmaceutical research **SMITH KLINE & FRENCH**

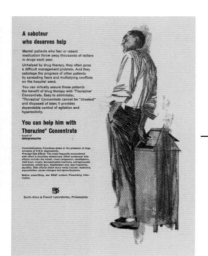

A saboteur
who deserves help

Mental patients who fear or resent medication throw away thousands of dollars in drugs each year.

Unhelped by drug therapy, they often pose a difficult management problem. And they sabotage the progress of other patients by spreading fears and multiplying conflicts on the hospital ward.

You can virtually assure these patients the benefit of drug therapy with 'Thorazine' Concentrate. Easy to administer, 'Thorazine' Concentrate cannot be "cheeked" and disposed of later; it provides dependable control of agitation and hyperactivity.

You can help him with Thorazine® Concentrate
brand of
chlorpromazine

Smith Kline & French Laboratories, Philadelphia

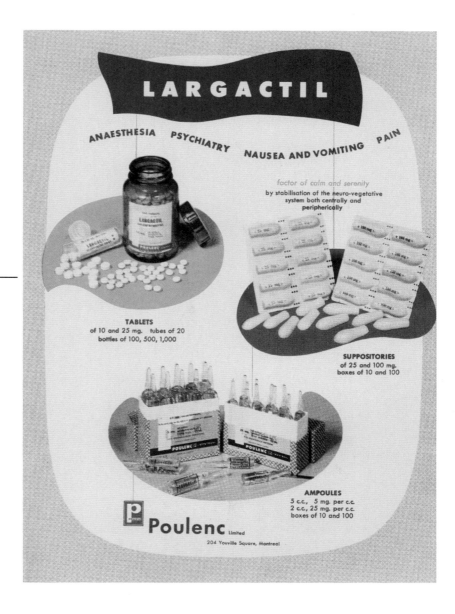

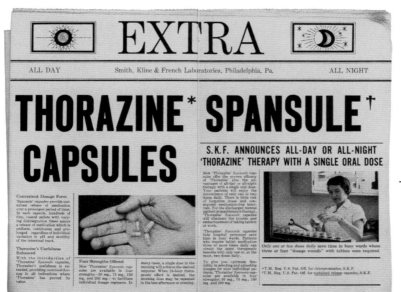

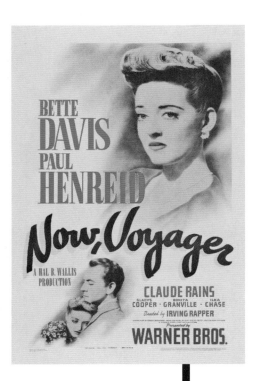

LEFT
In the blockbuster film *Now, Voyager* (1942),
Charlotte Vale, played by Bette Davis,
is a troubled spinster who regains control
of her life after a spell in a sanatorium.

BELOW
In *Dark Waters* (1944), directed by
André de Toth, a neurotic heiress with a
childhood phobia of water is tormented
by villains wishing to steal her inheritance.

at the end of the 19th century, those who
could afford to pay had many alternatives
to a life on the crowded wards, which filled
up and overflowed with those who had
no choice. In the United States, the larger
public asylums had already grown to the
size of small cities. By 1945 the Central
State Hospital at Milledgeville, Georgia,
was home to nine thousand patients, and
New York's Pilgrim State to ten thousand.

The sharp distinction between public
and private treatment was reflected
in popular culture and particularly in
Hollywood movies, in which the public
mental hospital became an archetypal
scene of horror much like 18th-century
Bedlam. Mary Jane Ward's autobiographical
novel *The Snake Pit* (1946), which became
a blockbuster film directed by Anatole
Litvak in 1948, portrayed a mental hospital
that would have been familiar to readers
of Alexander Cruden or Dorothea Dix: a
theatre of cruelty where resistance to the
all-powerful authorities was punished by
medical tortures, in this case electroshock
and sadistic 'hydrotherapy'. By contrast,
the psychoanalyst's sunlit office was
a scene in which terrors melted away,
tangled dramas were resolved and mental
burdens lifted. In Hollywood films of the
same vintage as *The Snake Pit*, including
Now, Voyager (1942), *Dark Waters* (1944),
Spellbound (1945) and *The Cobweb*
(1955), the private specialist – typically
a handsome male doctor ministering
to the female protagonist – is the source
of the insight that banishes the shadow
of the asylum.

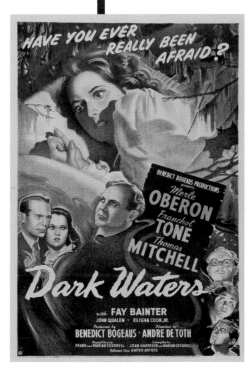

RIGHT
Alfred Hitchcock's
Spellbound (1945) is
set in an upmarket
sanatorium, where a
troubled and amnesiac
young man (Gregory
Peck) is restored to
sanity by the medical
skill (and love) of
psychoanalyst
Ingrid Bergman.

BELOW
In *The Snake Pit*
(1948), starring Olivia
de Havilland, the
overcrowded women-
only state mental
hospital is depicted as
a nightmare world of
oppression and mental
torture. One inmate
cannot remember how
she got there . . .

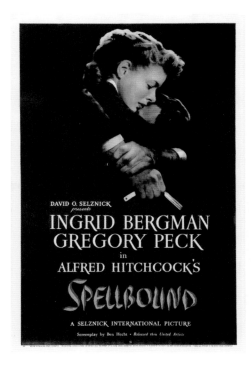

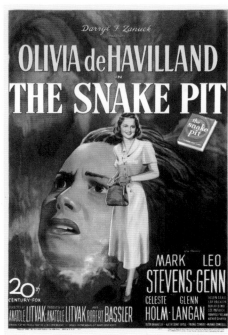

Outside the public hospitals, psychiatrists were moving away from the biologically based view that the mentally ill were a separate population from the sane for whom segregation was the only solution. At universities and teaching hospitals, the consensus was that most people might have episodes of mental ill health at some point in their lives: its roots lay not so much in the pathology of a deviant few as in the stresses of modern life. Soon after chlorpromazine emerged as a remedy for serious mental disorders, a new drug appeared for those dealing with 'minor' conditions in the world outside. In 1955 meprobamate, originally developed while searching for a preservative for penicillin, was marketed as Miltown by the Carter-Wallace company of New Jersey as a remedy for the anxieties that were a natural consequence of modern life. Concerned that the pharmaceutical market was already crowded with sedatives, Carter-Wallace adopted the term 'tranquillizer'.

Although the company had been concerned that there was no market for anxiety relief, Miltown was a runaway success. By reframing anxiety as normal, it avoided the stigma associated with mental illness and became an aspirational product for those who wished to smooth the rough edges of their busy and anxious lives. It took off most conspicuously in Hollywood – the epicentre of both the stresses and the luxuries of modern life – which became known as 'Miltown-by-the-Sea'. Soon pharmacies across the nation were hanging

«It was not long before
it became apparent that
the new tranquillizers were
dangerously habit forming.»

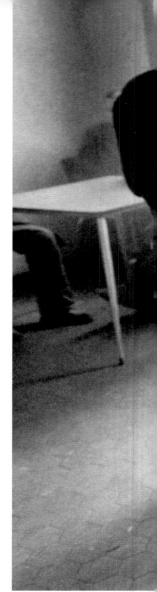

RIGHT
This photograph taken by French photojournalist
Raymond Depardon in 1979 depicts the
psychiatric hospital of San Servolo in Venice.
By the late 1970s, antipsychotic medication
had become a mainstay of hospital regimes.

'sold out' signs in their windows and announcing the time of the next delivery. Tiffany & Co sold ruby-and-diamond-studded pill coffers for ladies' handbags and charm bracelets with concealed pill compartments. There were Miltown cocktails: the 'Miltini', with a pill in place of the olive, and the 'Guided Missile', two pills in a double vodka. In 1958 Carter-Wallace commissioned Salvador Dalí, whose wife was a satisfied customer, to create a series of paintings illustrating the dream-like mental landscape the drug engendered.

Miltown and its many copycat compounds became known as 'anxiolytics' or 'minor tranquillizers', with the antipsychotics referred to by contrast as 'major tranquillizers'. Market surveys revealed that the strongest customer base was among suburban women. In her best-selling book *The Feminine Mystique* (1963), journalist Betty Friedan described the hidden malaise that tranquillizers seemed to be medicating. She surveyed female college graduates who had given up their careers for marriage and the suburban life, and discovered that many felt 'a strange stirring, a sense of dissatisfaction' that they struggled with alone: 'She was afraid to ask herself even the silent question – "is this all?"'[5] Women were prescribed tranquillizers at twice the rate of men, but the stresses of modern life were not

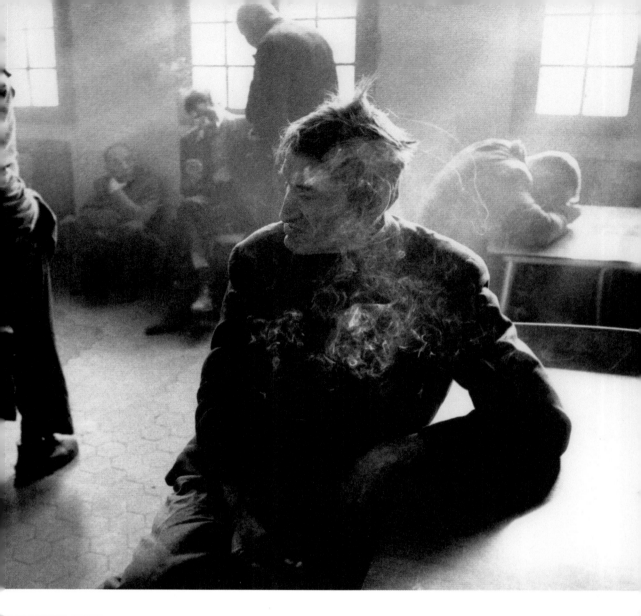

exclusive to them. A manual published by Roche pharmaceuticals enumerated the life stages when men were under 'particularly heavy stress': they included 'leaving the parental home, serving in the armed forces, marrying, becoming a father, getting ahead in business, growing older and retiring.'[6]

It was not long before it became apparent that the new tranquillizers were dangerously habit forming. Anxious customers came to depend on them, tolerance led to increased doses, and withdrawal was agonizing and potentially fatal. The danger was downplayed initially by the pharmaceutical industry and by doctors conscious that tranquillizers were a preferable alternative to mental hospitals. However, harrowing first-person accounts of addiction in popular television shows and magazines damaged their reputation and prompted governments to control their availability. In 1961 Germany limited the sale of tranquillizers to medical prescription only, and the following year the Food and Drug Administration (FDA) of the United States followed suit. Although only available from doctors, tranquillizers were still advertised in the mass media and their use continued to escalate. Hoffmann-La Roche launched valium, Miltown's best-known successor, in 1963; by 1978 it was selling 2.3 billion pills a year.

183

Nevertheless, the FDA's decision was a watershed. From this point onwards, the pharmaceutical industry and the medical profession, under government supervision, would be allied in managing a vast proprietary market and distribution monopoly. In order to qualify for sale, new medications were obliged to present themselves as specifics, targeted at closely defined diseases. This created a need to present mental illnesses in terms that were mutually intelligible with pharmacy, typically as a chemical imbalance that medication corrected. Neuroscientific research clustered around the theories that emerged from this dialogue. The monopoly on distribution transformed the role of doctors and psychiatrists, whose power to prescribe new drugs became central to their professional role.

As medication came to play a larger role in the treatment of mental illness, the rationale for public mental hospitals was called into question. Despite the new miracle drugs, the hospitals' population was still growing: by 1955 it had risen in the United States to 560,000. Long-term residential care on this scale was unsustainable, and many argued it was now unnecessary. The fast-expanding families of antipsychotics and tranquillizers were augmented by lithium compounds, which had dramatic effects in stabilizing mood, and by a new group of 'tricyclic' antidepressants, led by imipramine, which were presented as a major breakthrough in treating severe depression. The promise of the age of penicillin finally seemed to be shining its light into the darkest corners of the mind. William Sargant, who had become Britain's best-known psychiatrist thanks to his popular books

and articles about Soviet brainwashing, was experimenting with a 'deep narcosis' treatment, in which patients were kept asleep twenty hours a day for up to three months, and taken from their beds only for toilet visits and ECT sessions. 'How exciting it is to see one's dreams continue to come true,' he wrote.[7] The physical methods he had always championed were working their way through the mental illnesses one by one, banishing the ghosts of the asylum forever.

Across the United States and Britain, the mental hospital population was falling, but the new drugs were not the only reason for the decline. Throughout much of Europe, patient numbers continued to rise despite the drugs and in some respects because of them, because they made it more convenient to 'warehouse' patients in greater numbers and with fewer staff. In Britain and the United States, the decline was driven by policies that took advantage of the new treatments to discharge patients more promptly, to shrink the old asylums and to streamline their services. The Mental Health Act of 1959 signalled the British government's intention to start phasing out specialist mental hospitals and incorporating mental health care wards into general hospitals.

It was hard to imagine a modern world without huge public mental hospitals. Many of them had stood for more than a century in every county and city, a steady local employer for generations of doctors, nurses, managers, orderlies, cleaners, cooks, builders and tradesmen. In 1961 Enoch Powell, Britain's minister of health, confronted the problem in a forthright address to the annual conference of the

OPPOSITE
Suitcases left by former patients in the Willard Psychiatric Centre, New York, between 1910 and 1960. When the hospital closed in 1995, more than four hundred suitcases were discovered in an attic and placed in the permanent collection of the New York State Museum. In 2011, photographer Jon Crispin began the project of documenting them. He is archiving the images at www.willardsuitcases.com

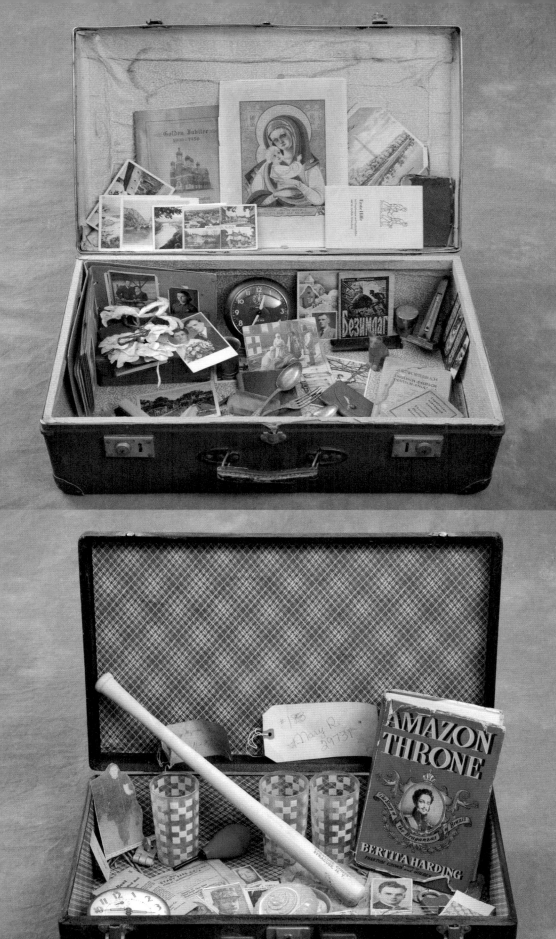

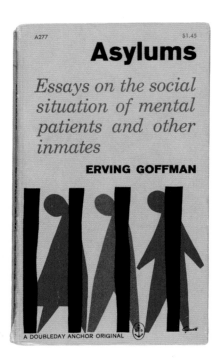

LEFT
In *Asylums* (1961),
sociologist Erving Goffman
argued that mental
hospitals had an inbuilt
tendency to operate for
the benefit of their staff
rather than of their patients.

«A consensus was
forming that once
the asylums were
gone, they would
not be missed.»

National Association for Mental Health
at Westminster. 'There they stand,' he
announced, 'isolated, majestic, imperious
. . . the asylums which our forefathers built
with such immense solidity to express the
notions of their day.' But the present day
was another world, and 'hospital building
is not like pyramid building, the erection
of memorials.' The asylums had been
reinvented and transformed in the past,
but now 'for the great majority of these
establishments there is no future use.'
Mental health care of the future would
consist of beds in general hospitals, at
roughly half the current number, with
care in the local community preferred
wherever possible.

Powell spoke in stirring and martial terms
about 'setting the torch to the funeral pyre'
and 'the defences we have to storm' to
an audience of many who had dedicated
their lives to the asylum (as the mental
hospital was once again becoming known,
particularly among its detractors). They
argued in response that community care
was limited to a handful of admirable but
modest ventures up and down the country,
and was entirely incapable of taking the
strain of the current hospital system.
Considerable new budgets would be
needed for local authorities to manage

the transition and to recruit and train
an army of social workers. But their
demands were given little attention.
Across psychiatry and politics, a consensus
was forming that mental illness was,
like infectious disease, finally yielding
to medical progress. Once the asylums
were gone, they would not be missed.

The following year, the mental hospital,
or asylum, was subjected to a series of
ideological challenges from which it would
never recover. In 1961 sociologist Erving
Goffman published *Asylums*, the fruits of
his research at St Elizabeth's Hospital in
Washington, DC, a vast mental institution
with more than seven thousand patients
(Goffman preferred the pre-medical term
'inmates'). His aim was to examine the
asylum from the point of view of those
who were confined there, and his analysis
described its mechanics with brutal clarity.
Like prisons, barracks, orphanages and
naval vessels, asylums were a type of
'total institution' — what Pinel had called
a 'miniature government' — in which
there was effectively no outside world.
The doctors and managers who believed
they ran them were, from the inmates'
perspective, distant figures; all such
institutions, however nobly intentioned,
tended in practice to end up organized

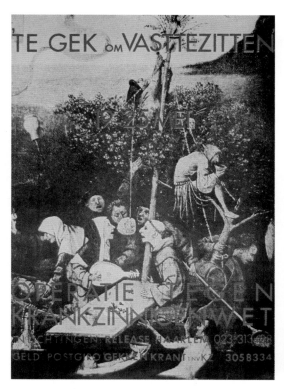

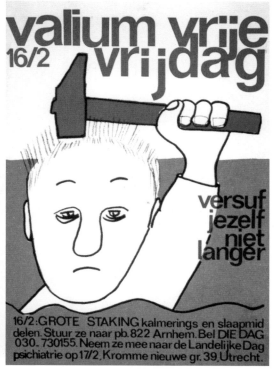

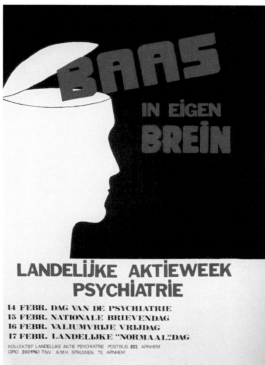

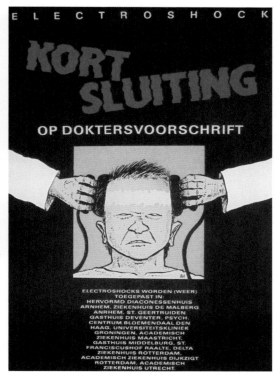

ABOVE

The writings of Erving Goffman, Thomas Szasz, Michel Foucault and R. D. Laing helped launch a popular movement against abuses of authority in the mental health system. These Dutch posters protesting against forcible incarceration, electroconvulsive therapy and neurosurgery are from the collection of the Dolhuys, the Dutch national museum of psychiatry in Haarlem.

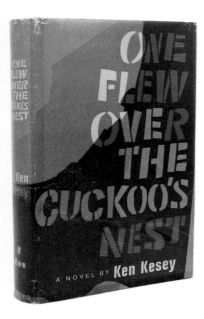

for the benefit of the lowly but all-powerful staff, who used the means at their disposal to divide and rule by reward and punishment.

It was an observation that had been made by countless inmates since the old Bedlam days of Urbane Metcalf, as well as by generations of reforming superintendents and psychiatrists. The effect on inmates was, in Goffman's term, 'institutionalization': all these pressures drove them towards becoming 'perfect patients' who conformed to the system and avoided attention and also gradually lost their life skills, their motivation to improve and ultimately their identity. The asylum was presented as a staging post to recovery, but in reality it was the opposite. Its internal logic systematically stripped away the inmates' personal resources and made it impossible for them to survive outside it.

Although Goffman's focus was the experience of the inmate, his critique extended to what he called the 'medical model', with its paradox that although everything was being done allegedly in the patient's interest, almost all the inmates were being held involuntarily and often explicitly against their will. This paradox formed the basis of another hugely influential book, also published in 1961, by New York psychiatrist Thomas Szasz, who extended it into a fundamental assault not only on the asylum but also on the reality of madness. In *The Myth of Mental Illness*, Szasz argued that the mentally ill were suffering genuine distress, but to say they were 'sick' was no more than a metaphor. Mental illness was defined by behaviour: people were said to be suffering from it only if they were troublesome or unproductive or refused to share the beliefs of those around them. Psychiatry was a modern priestcraft in which deviant behaviours were discussed as medical illnesses, much as priests once diagnosed those holding unacceptable beliefs as heretics or witches. Szasz delighted in reminding his readers that 19th-century doctors had created the diagnosis of 'drapetomania' for slaves who persisted in running away. Mental illness was the product of a moral consensus enforced by psychiatry and accepted by everyone except those to whom it was applied.

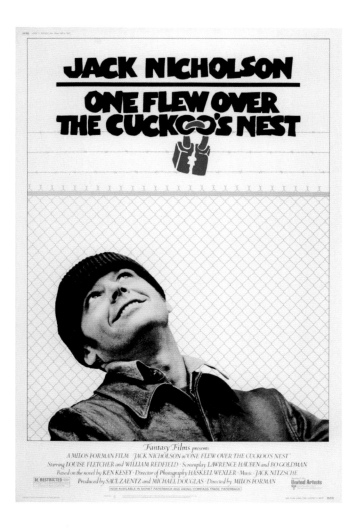

ABOVE
One Flew Over the Cuckoo's Nest (1975), Milos Forman's film of Kesey's novel, was a huge critical and commercial success. It is one of only three movies to win all five major Academy Awards: Best Picture, Best Director, Best Actor, Best Actress and Best Screenplay.

In the words attributed to 17th-century Bedlam inmate Nathaniel Lee, 'They called me mad, and I called them mad, and damn them, they outvoted me.'

In Paris, 1961 saw the first publication of Michel Foucault's monumental *Folie et Déraison: Histoire de la folie à l'âge classique* (published in abridged form in English as *Madness and Civilization: A History of Insanity in the Age of Reason*), an analysis of the asylum that became a springboard for the most influential critical theory of its era. For Foucault, the emergence of the asylum in the 17th century pointed to a rupture in history: the point at which reason assumed a cultural monopoly and the voices of the mad – previously seen as sources of allegory, wit and wisdom – ceased to be understood. Instead, the mad became undesirables, either forced into productive labour in the workhouse or confined in asylums. The 19th-century revolution in asylum care led by Pinel and the York Retreat was regarded as humane and progressive, but in reality it was just a more effective technique for coercion towards work and social norms. The language of psychiatry emerged as a way of speaking over the heads of the mad and insisting that they could only be discussed in the language of reason.

All these critiques emerged from specialized professional and academic worlds, but they fed into the currents of popular radicalism and dissent that gathered force through the 1960s. These were navigated most successfully by Scottish psychiatrist R. D. Laing, whose

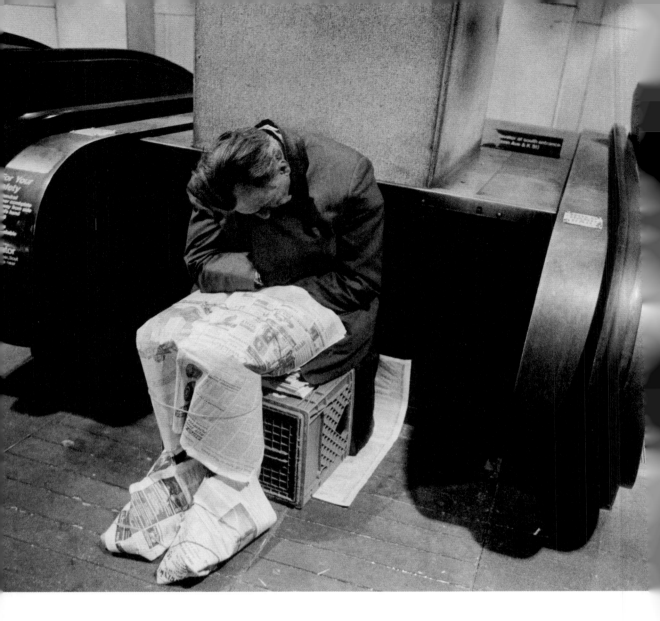

first book, *The Divided Self: An Existential Study in Sanity and Madness*, was published in London in 1960. It was an attempt to rescue the experience of mental illness — schizophrenia in particular — from the clinical language of his profession and to understand it in its own terms: as a solution to an insoluble problem, the last line of defence for the self when normal social relations have broken down. Laing cross-fertilized psychiatry with existentialism and later with eastern mysticism; his inspirations included *fin de siècle* therapists, such as Sigmund Freud and Ludwig Binswanger, alongside patients such as Artaud and philosophers from Jean-Paul Sartre to Karl Marx. The multiple

tracks of his thought — full of paradoxes, contradictions and renunciations — limited his direct influence within psychiatry, but its eclecticism and sense of revolutionary possibility made him an enduring icon of the counterculture.

These figures were broadly and often dismissively grouped together as the 'antipsychiatry' movement, a term that most of them roundly rejected. Their books were best sellers that spawned sequels, followers, social movements and new approaches, which reverberated through the worlds of academia, psychiatry, politics, protest and popular culture for decades. Their revolt against the asylum

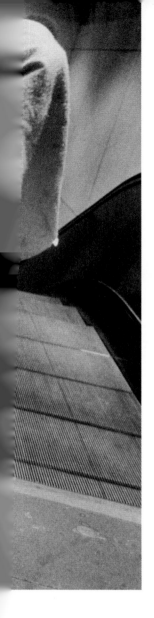

«By this time, public mental hospitals were closing at an astonishing rate.»

was fixed firmly in the public imagination by Ken Kesey's *One Flew Over the Cuckoo's Nest* (1962), a novel in the Jacobean tradition of feigned madness in which the protagonist, Randle McMurphy, fakes insanity to escape a prison sentence but finds himself ensnared in a total institution where his refusal to conform leads to the surgical excision of his identity.

Fact trumped fiction a few years later when psychologist David Rosenhan performed an experiment in which he asked seven of his perfectly sane students to request admission into various mental hospitals, claiming that they were hearing voices in their heads. All were admitted, diagnosed

with schizophrenia and released only after accepting their diagnosis. The world of psychiatry appeared to be a great Bedlam, in which the sane were mad and the mad sane. After the movie adaptation of *One Flew over the Cuckoo's Nest* (1975) won all five major Academy Awards, the asylum became all but impossible to defend. The film's most indelible scene showed Jack Nicholson crucified in agony as he receives ECT unmodified by anaesthetics or muscle relaxants; it mattered little that this practice had in reality been abandoned in the 1950s. The old meaning of the term 'asylum', a refuge from the world, had been overwritten by a new one: an institution of brutal social control.

By this time, public mental hospitals were closing at an astonishing rate. The shift in public attitudes may have made the process easier to manage but it was being driven by larger and more impersonal forces: economics, and the transfer of health care responsibilities from the state to the private sector. As the opponents of closure had predicted, the burden that the hospitals had been carrying, however

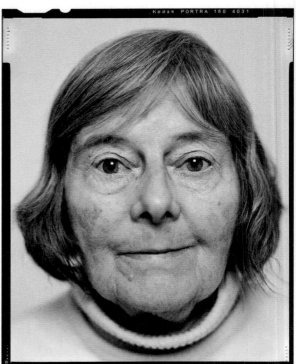
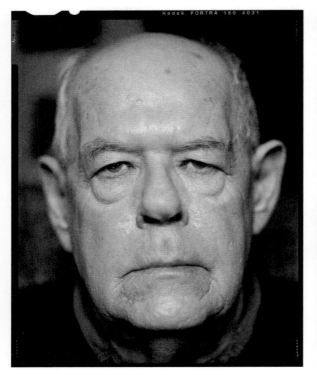
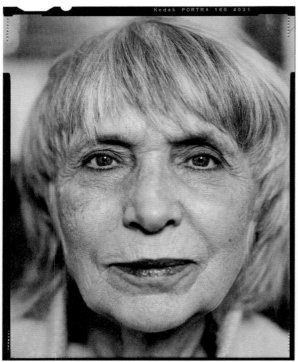
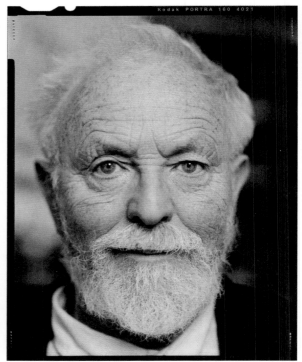

inadequately, was more than community and civil society could bear. In the United States, President Johnson's Great Society programmes, such as Medicaid and Medicare, gave federal support to community and activist groups who were organizing to provide alternatives to the unreformed and vastly expensive state hospitals. However, as insurance companies pared back their provision for mental illness to a maximum of thirty days and hospital budgets shrank, former patients without families to support them frequently ended up in grim hostels or on the street. They colonized the modern urban wastelands – skid rows, flyovers, subways, abandoned factories and empty lots – in the same way that the wandering Tom o'Bedlams of the pre-asylum era had holed up in the blasted heaths and hedgerows where nobody would whip them onwards.

The theorists who had undermined the old system had nothing to put in its place. Goffman had dissected the asylum with a sharp scalpel, but saw it as an inevitable consequence of how modern societies were organized. Szasz believed that mental health care should be a voluntary arrangement on all sides, without any support from the state or the taxpayer. Foucault regarded all institutions as repressive, and those constructed in a humanitarian spirit of reform as peculiarly blind to this tendency. Community activists such as Saul Alinsky recognized that ultimately the problem was not the asylum but society, and urged psychiatrists to become involved in the fundamental causes of mental distress: poverty, rootlessness, racism and unemployment. But the pressures on psychiatry were

pushing it in the opposite direction: towards maximizing limited resources by targeting the most acute and disruptive cases and managing symptoms with prescription drugs.

In Britain, as the wrecking balls swung through the old asylums, it became clear that care in the community, as the alternative was known, could be good or cheap but not both. Most of those 'decarcerated' from the old mental hospitals were without family or resources, and many had had their coping skills eroded by years of institutional care. By 1980 the number of psychiatric beds had been halved, just as Powell had planned, but mental illness was not fading away: on the contrary, psychiatric admissions were increasing. The only solution was to increase the 'throughput' of beds, shuttling patients back into the community as quickly as possible. But if the problems that had led to their admission were not addressed, it was only a matter of time before most of them returned. The 'warehousing' of the old asylums was replaced by the opposite problem: the 'revolving door'.

The post-war dream of the community hospital had survived in isolated pockets. In 1962 Maxwell Jones had returned from the United States and taken over the running of Dingleton Hospital on the outskirts of Edinburgh, where he had developed the principles evolved during the wartime experiment at Mill Hill. Scotland had a tradition of 'open-door' asylums, dating back to the era of William Browne, and had long been receptive to Geel's model of family care: in the 19th century, islands such as Shetland and

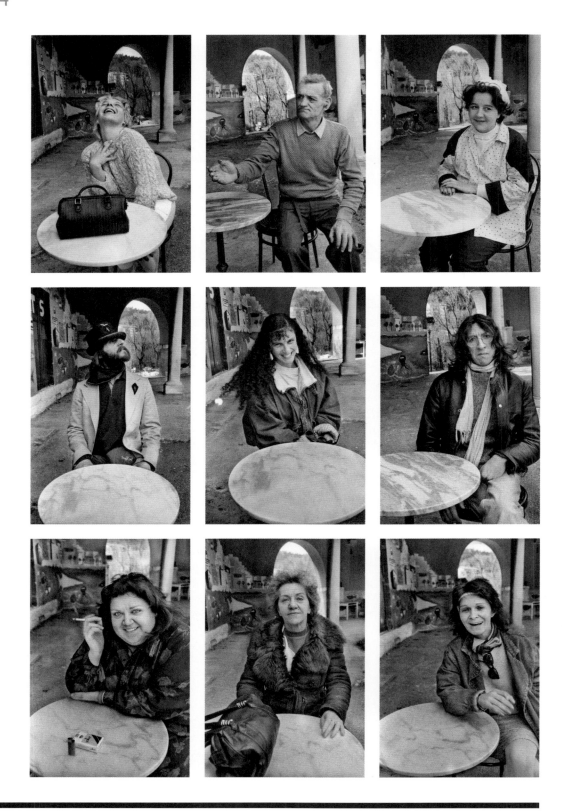

OVERLEAF
Photographs from *Asylum: Inside the Closed World of State Mental Hospitals* (2009) by Christopher Payne.
Patient toothbrushes, Hudson River State Hospital, Poughkeepsie, New York
Traverse City State Hospital, Traverse City, Michigan
Gurney (wheeled stretcher), Columbia State Hospital, Columbia, South Carolina
State records and files, Spring Grove State Hospital, Catonsville Maryland.

Arran were known as 'Geels of the North'. Dingleton already operated an open-door system, and Jones developed it into an equal society where doctors and patients sat together in weekly meetings at which the running of the hospital was decided and organized. Visitors were welcome and patients were allowed to roam freely. Jones had grown sceptical of the medical assumptions that defined his profession, according to which 'care' was second best to 'treatment' and the potential of patients to help themselves was largely ignored. Beyond the obvious biological and genetic conditions, he regarded mental ill health not as an illness but the result of adverse social forces, best treated not by medicine but by immersion in a well-constructed alternative society.

Such experimental societies were enthralling to be involved in and inspiring when they succeeded, but they were difficult to sustain in the post-asylum world. Dingleton Hospital's relaxed rules and open-door ethos went against the grain of a national policy that was increasingly driven by risk management. As resources shrank, they became concentrated on the minority of disruptive and criminal cases, and media coverage focused on exceptional stories of violence by the mentally unwell in the community (who were, then as now, far more likely to be the victims of violence than its perpetrators). In theory, open and permissive therapeutic communities were a desirable alternative to mental hospitals, but in practice they were resisted by local residents, councils and police forces. As they had since the birth of the asylum, the public wished the best for the mentally ill but also wanted as little contact with them as possible.

The therapeutic experiments that sprang up in the wake of the asylum were mostly short-lived. The most celebrated was Kingsley Hall in London's East End, which ran under the aegis of R. D. Laing from 1965 to 1970. Radical and chaotic, brave and exhibitionist, Kingsley Hall operated outside the state system and never claimed to offer a feasible alternative to it. Its freewheeling ethos generated dilemmas that were never resolved satisfactorily: the psychiatrists refused to exert their professional authority, but the patients still demanded it; the absence of all discipline ended with intolerable patients being violently restrained by their fellows. Its therapeutic worth remained unproven but it was hugely successful as public theatre, dramatizing an alternative relationship between doctor and patient, madness and sanity, the asylum and the world.

The most enduring examples of the therapeutic community were created in Italy by a movement driven by Venetian psychiatrist Franco Basaglia. In 1961 Basaglia was appointed director of the psychiatric hospital at Gorizia, a remote town on the Italian border with communist Yugoslavia, where he was confronted with the unreformed asylum in its full horror: patients abandoned for life behind prison bars, sedated with pills, threatened with ECT and force fed if they lost the will to live. Like John Conolly at Hanwell, Basaglia began by abolishing the use of all restraints and electroshock treatment. After a visit to Dingleton Hospital, he pushed forward with more radical approaches, unlocking wards and holding daily meetings in which the institutionalized patients

OPPOSITE
Portraits of former patients from the Trieste mental hospital, after its residential wards were emptied by Franco Basaglia and his team. Photographs by Uliano Lucas, 1988.

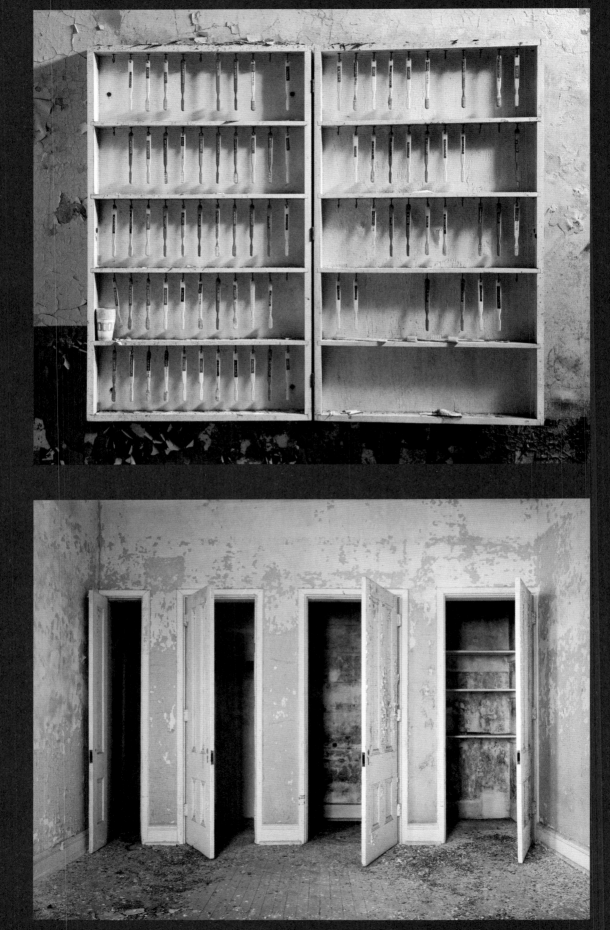

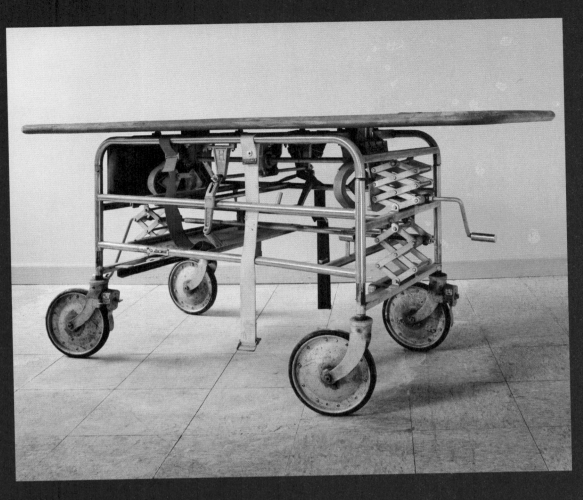

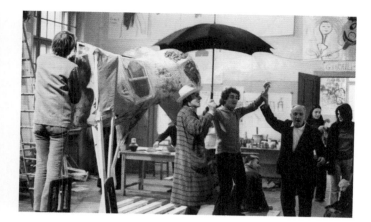

«The Basaglia Law made new admissions to mental hospitals illegal.»

could begin to take control of the hospital and of their own lives. A team of like-minded psychiatrists formed around him, visiting, volunteering and spreading his techniques through Italy's regions via their organization Psichiatria Democratica (Democratic Psychiatry). In 1971 Basaglia took over the running of mental health services in Trieste, where he closed the hospital amid mass celebrations, which turned his crusade into an exhilarating popular movement.

Basaglia's ideology was informed by Goffman and Foucault, and extended beyond asylum management into a fundamental critique of society and its authoritarian structures. However, he believed that it was vital to remain part of the system and to reform it from within. Unlike experiments such as Kingsley Hall, the Basaglians entrenched their methods in the national system, creating a professional network that

was dedicated to replacing asylums with community centres and to integrating the treatment of mental illness into general health care. In 1980 the Italian parliament passed a groundbreaking law that made new admissions to mental hospitals illegal and mandated community care for all mental illness. It was universally known as the Basaglia Law, although it received support from across the political spectrum, including from those primarily interested in cutting the state's burden of mental health care.

The outcome varied wildly between regions. In many areas of southern Italy, the health system was unprepared for its new burdens. Doctors were stretched to their limits and beyond by a disruptive and demanding new clientele. Patients were returned to families who were unable to care for them and legal loopholes were found to allow mental hospital admissions to continue.

ABOVE AND RIGHT
The icon of Franco Basaglia's closure of the asylum at Trieste was 'Marco Cavallo', a papier-mâché horse painted blue. The sculpture was constructed in 1973 by patients, staff and volunteers. They used a wooden frame to strengthen it, and when finished the horse stood 4 metres high. It was wheeled ceremonially out of the hospital grounds into the city streets.

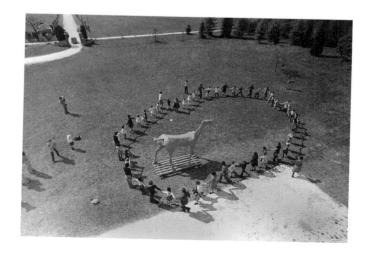

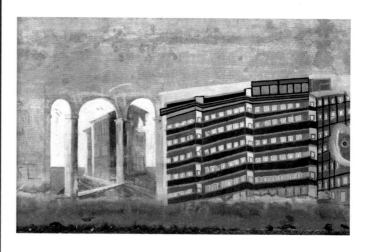

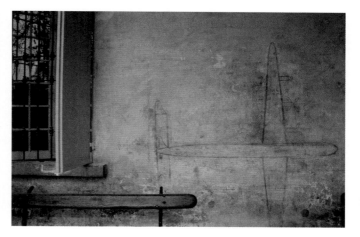

In other areas, such as Trieste, Perugia and Parma, Psichiatria Democratica had learned the harsh lessons of the Anglo-Saxon experience and laid the groundwork for success. Patients were housed properly and supported in leading independent lives, with medical care provided in neighbourhood day centres created through consultations and partnerships with the local community.

By this time, Bethlem Royal Hospital was being reshaped regularly by reforms of the British National Health Service (NHS), which aimed to organize it on a business-like basis for competition in an internal health care market. It had been broken down into its component parts and reassembled by a succession of new management regimes, and was struggling – as it had many times in its long history – to stay afloat and plan for the future. In 1994 Bethlem became an independent trust, part of the NHS but responsible for its own finances; in 1999 it merged once more with the wider NHS Trust of the South London and Maudsley mental health services.

Today, Bethlem offers a spectrum of services spread across the wards and blocks of its villa design: a medium secure forensic unit for criminal offenders, a mother and baby unit, a centre for anxiety disorders and a renowned psychosis unit with a national catchment that offers exceptional levels of care to a small number of atypical and problematic

ABOVE
The abandoned asylum buildings of San Lazzaro mental hospital in Reggio Emilia, covered with graffiti by former patients.

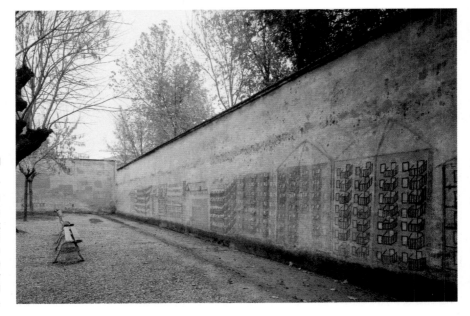

RIGHT
This wall of the abandoned San Lazzaro hospital is covered with a drawing of high-rise residential blocks. In many Italian cities the closing of the asylums placed huge new demands on residential housing and social welfare.

patients. Its residents are offered a variety of activities, from swimming to martial arts classes, visits to working farms and day trips to London. They can work towards qualifications in woodworking and textiles or develop their creative skills in an art workshop, with facilities for painting, pottery and sculpture, attached to a thriving gallery that exhibits the work of service users to growing interest from the public and the wider art world. A new museum at the entrance to the site houses the hospital's unique archives and showcases its historical and art collections.

Bethlem has achieved, and in a number of respects exceeded, the ideal of the mental hospital as envisaged by the optimistic generation of reformers in the years immediately after the Great War. Its tree-shaded brick villas house a quiet village of expertise and specialist services, far from the madding crowd but firmly patched into the community and the wider health care network. However, the psychiatrists of a century ago could not have anticipated how far its capacity has been outstripped by demand. Its patients are a small fraction of those in need, vastly outnumbered by those consigned to hospital waiting lists that stretch beyond their horizons, discharged into an outside world in which they are unable to cope or swallowed up in detention centres and prisons.

FOOTNOTES

1   quoted in John MacGregor, *The Discovery of the Art of the Insane* (Princeton: Princeton University Press, 1989) p. 197
2   Ugo Cerletti, 'Old and New Information about Electroshock', *The American Journal of Psychiatry*, Vol. 107, August 1950, pp. 87–94
3   'European Psychiatry on the Eve of War', *Medical History* Supplement No. 22 (London: Wellcome Trust Centre for Medicine at UCL, 2003) p. 77
4   Joshua Bierer, *The Lancet* (1959) p. 901
5   Betty Friedan, *The Feminine Mystique*, (W. W. Norton, 1963) p.15
6   *Aspects of Anxiety* (1968), quoted in Andrea Tone, *The Age of Anxiety* (New York: Basic Books, 2009) p. 158
7   William Sargant, *The Unquiet Mind* (London: Heinemann, 1967) p. 200

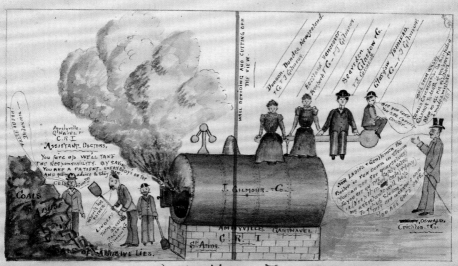

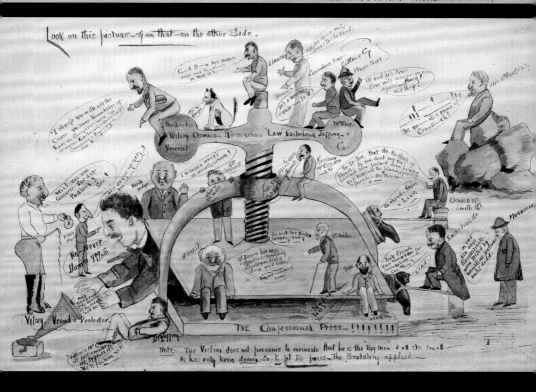

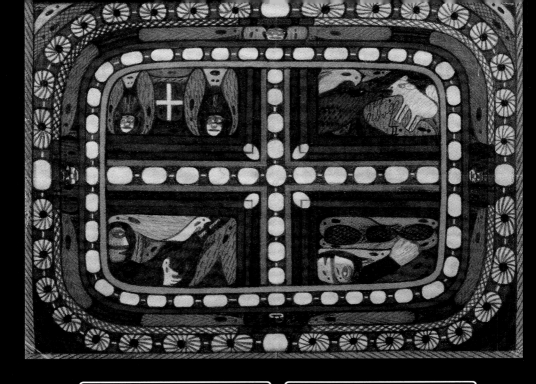

ADOLF WÖLFLI

1864—1930

Wölfli (see p. 159) was confined for life in 1895 in Bern. He was one of the first asylum patients to be noticed by the art world.

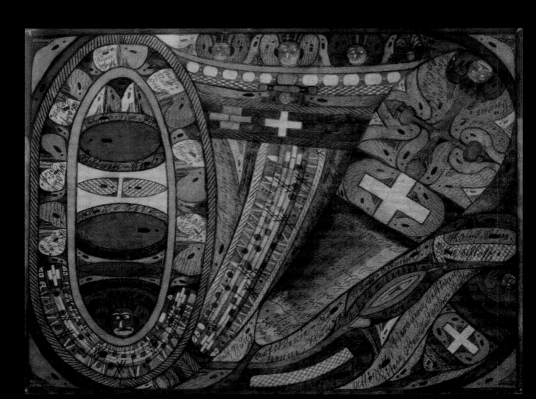

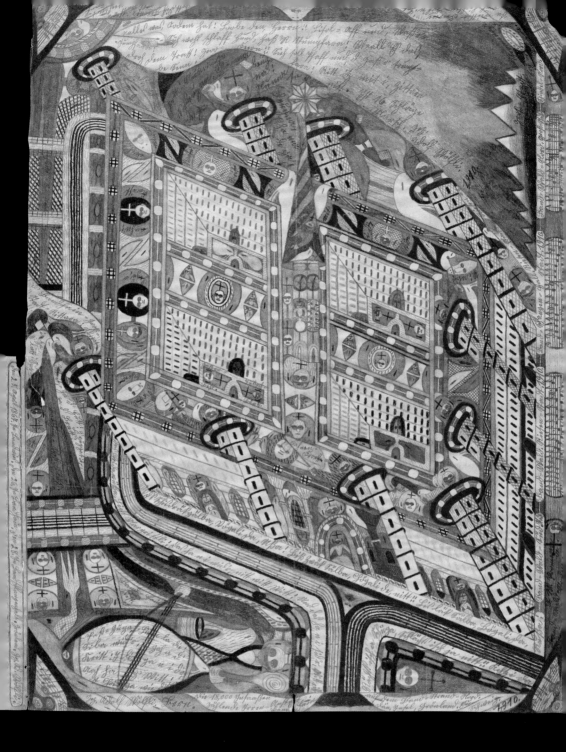

opp. above.
*Tschimberasso Forest
St Adolf-Throne* (1930)
by Adolf Wölfli. Pencil
and coloured pencil
on paper. Wölfli's art
was often accompanied
with texts and musical
compositions.

opp. below.
*The Kander Valley in
the Bernese Oberland*
(1926) by Adolf Wölfli.
Pencil and coloured
pencil on paper.
Wölfli's work was
admired by Surrealist
artist André Breton.

above
*Mental Asylum Band-
Copse* (1910) by Adolf
Wölfli, from Book 4
(the largest portion of
drawings) of *Cradle to
the Grave* (1908–1912).
Pencil and coloured
pencil on newsprint.

Russian aristocrat Pankejeff was better known as 'the wolf man'. The name was given to him by Sigmund Freud in one of his best-known case histories.

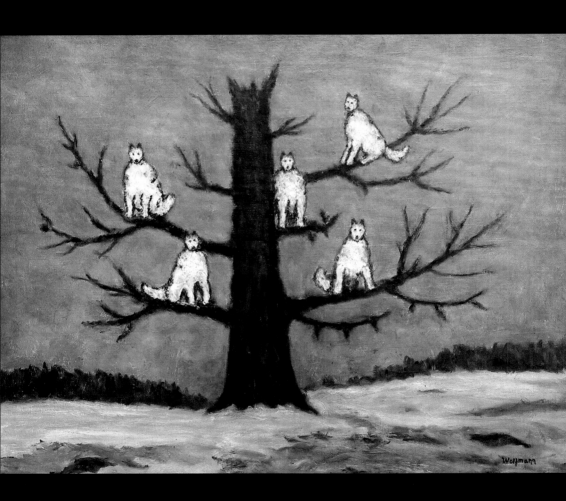

above
Painting of Wolves Sitting in a Tree
(1964) by Sergei Pankejeff. Oil on canvas. It depicts the dream about wolves that the artist first described to Freud in 1914.

opp.
Dudley Raymond Wilder produced these drawings in 1954. Held by the Wellcome Library, they are from a series of twelve satirical sketches of asylum life.

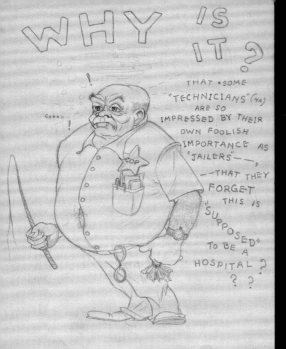

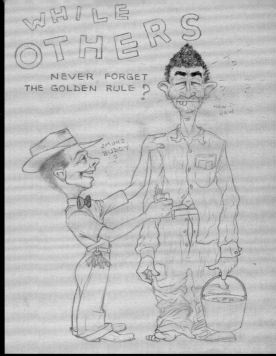

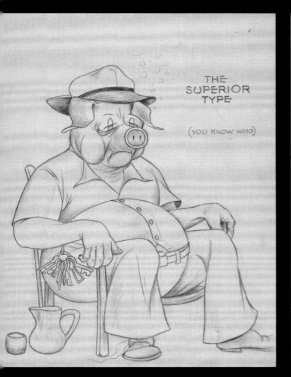

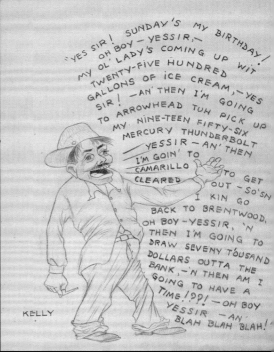

DUDLEY RAYMOND WILDER

• 1916 • • 1957 •

Wilder worked as a commercial artist in California and served in the US Marine Corps in World War II before being confined in Patton State Hospital, San Bernardino.

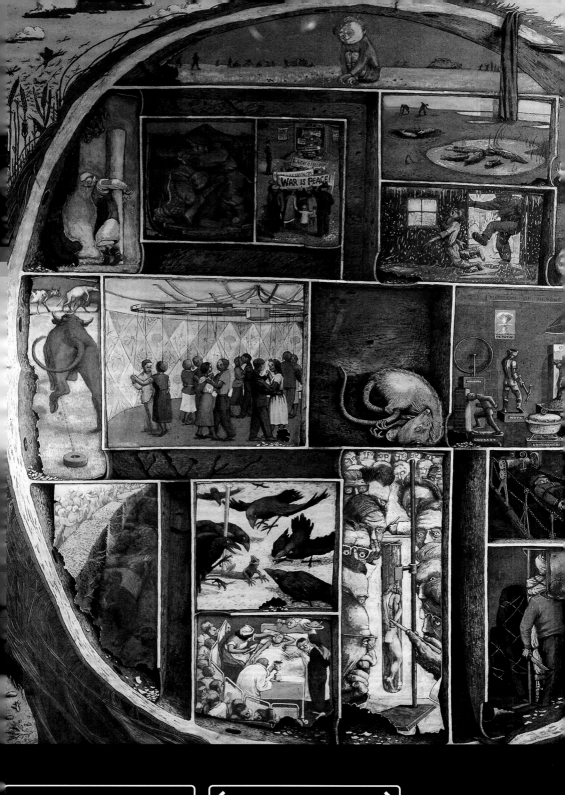

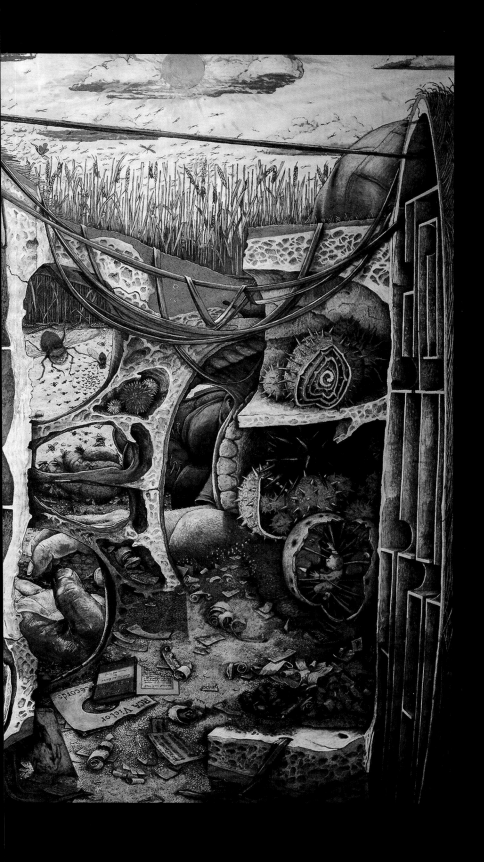

left
The Maze (1953)
by William Kurelek.
The head contains
scenes from his life,
including the ECT
to which, along with
his religious faith, he
attributed his recovery

Carlesi worked as a decorator
before being admitted in 1954 to
a psychiatric hospital in Florence.
In 1982 he joined La Tinaia artists'
collective for psychiatric patients.

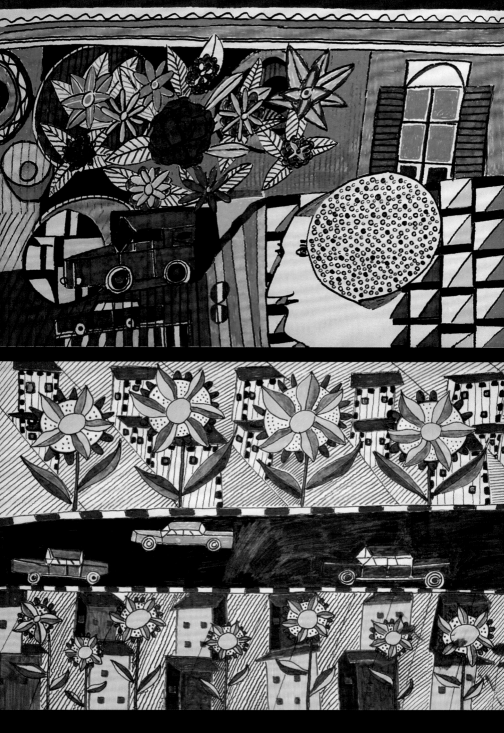

In all four works
shown here Vittorio
Carlesi has drawn
with marker pens
on paper. His works
feature depictions
of distant and recent
memories of people,
events and things.

Each picture contains
diverse elements
from different time
periods, creating
individual puzzles for
the viewer to explore.

opp. above
Untitled (1995)

opp. below
Untitled (1991)

above top
Untitled (1995)

above below
Untitled (1992)

CLAUDIO ULIVIERI

1947 — 2015

Ulivieri worked abroad before suffering a mental breakdown. In La Tinaia, despite having no artistic background, he began to produce highly acclaimed work.

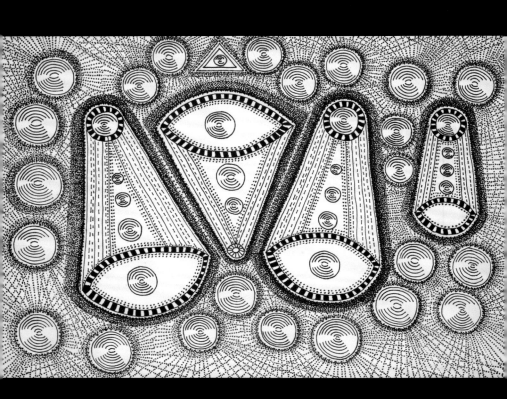

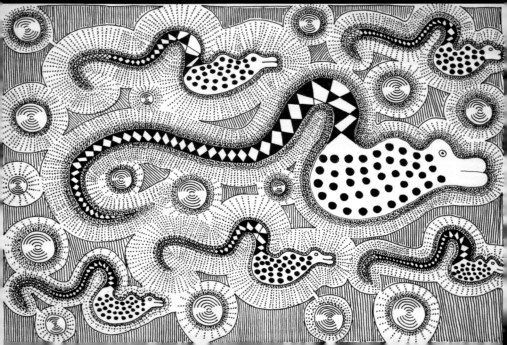

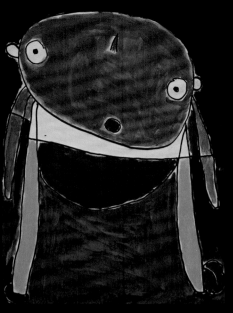

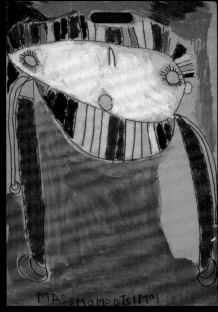

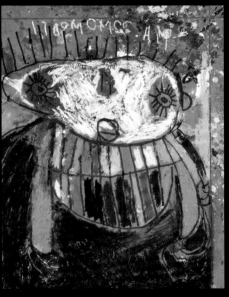

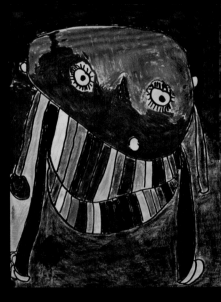

MASSMOMODISIMOI

1953   **PRESENT**

MASSIMO MODISTI

Modisti grew up in Florence and began attending La Tinaia in the early 1990s. He draws mostly with crayons and markers, but also watercolour and acrylics.

opp.
Ulivieri described his intricate drawings as 'surrealistic'. The works shown here are (top) *L'animale mai visto* (The Animal Never Seen) (1997) and (bottom) *Il frantoio* (The Mill) (1996).

above
The most often repeated subject of Massimo Modisti's work is the human figure. The forms are stylized but animated by suprising colour combinations.

The works shown here are, clockwise from top left:

Untitled (2011)
Untitled (2011)
Untitled (2002)
Untitled (2013)

Born in Florence, Raugei worked at La Tinaia artists' collective from 1986. Some of his work is held in the *Collection de l'Art Brut* in Lausanne.

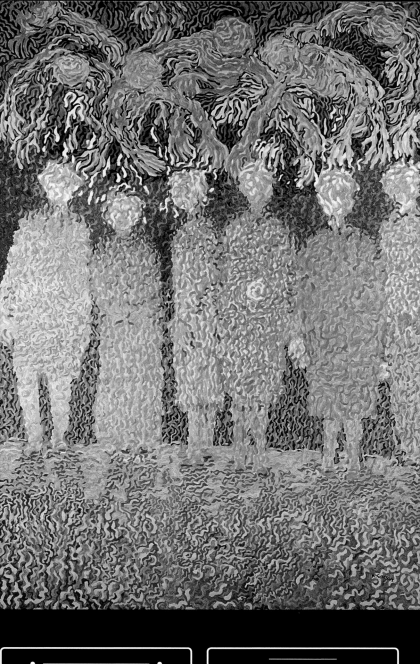

ROSEMARY CARSON

1962

PRESENT

Carson has spent periods in psychiatric hospitals and paints the spirits of fellow patients whom she encountered during her time there.

opp.
Untitled (1989) by Marco Raugei. Using felt pen on card, Raugei's work is characterized by repetition of figures or objects that fill the space rhythmically.

above
In this work from 1997, Rosemary Carson depicts a row of patients waiting to see the doctors. The figures hovering above them represent their fears.

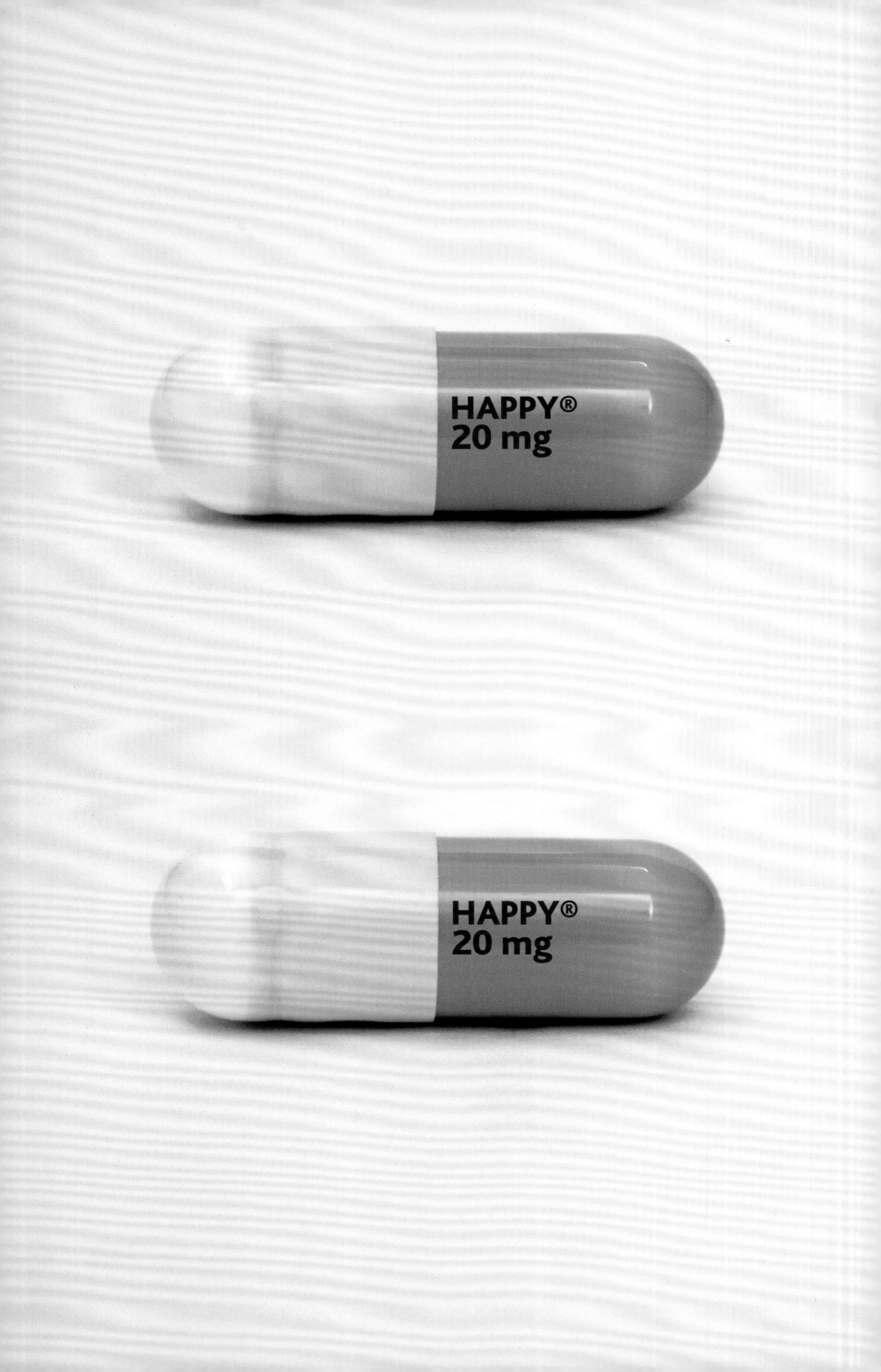
HAPPY®
20 mg
HAPPY®
20 mg

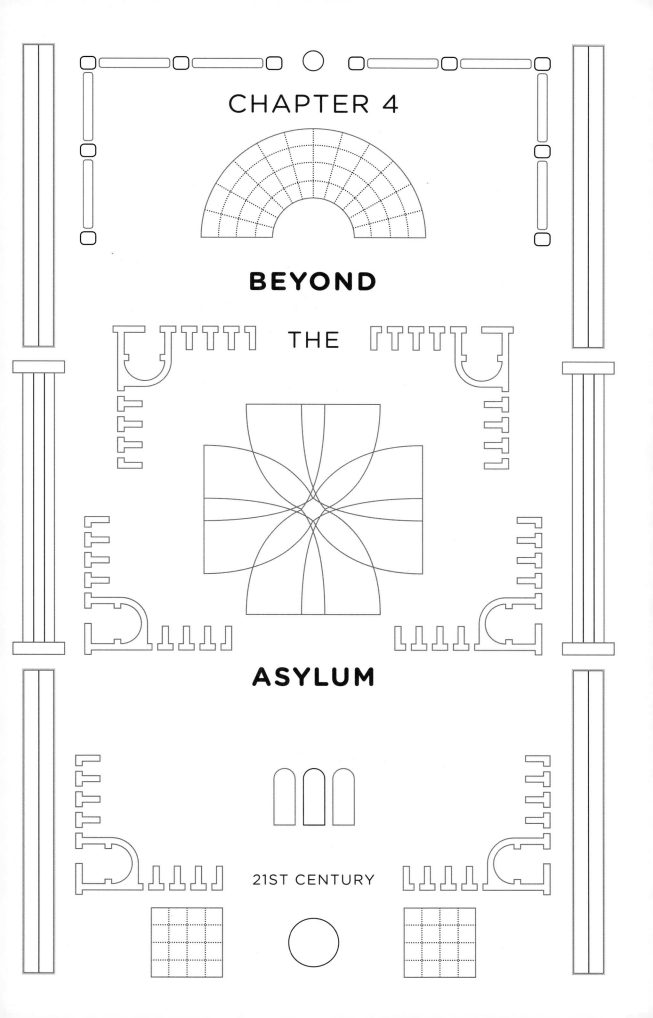

CHAPTER 4

BEYOND

THE

ASYLUM

21ST CENTURY

In the wake of the asylum, the world has become a great Bedlam. We know more about the brain and its workings than ever before, and we have created a galaxy of new medications to target mental pathologies. But we have not consigned mental illnesses to history. The death of the asylum was accompanied by predictions that mental illnesses would become largely invisible, managed routinely with tablets like diabetes or high blood pressure. Yet their prevalence is exploding across the globe, and particularly among the 21st-century natives of the younger generation. Most developed countries estimate that around ten per cent of those aged under fifteen have a mental health problem at any one time; in the United States around seven per cent of schoolchildren are on medication for mood or behaviour disorders, and diagnoses of juvenile bipolar disorder have increased forty fold since the century began.

The explosion in mental illnesses is matched by the growth in drugs to treat them. Antidepressants are now among the most profitable classes of pharmaceuticals, worth tens of billions of dollars a year; antipsychotics and sedatives are not far behind. But if they are combating mental illness, it is a battle that both seem to be winning.

When imipramine, the first tricyclic antidepressant, was developed in 1958, its manufacturer Geigy was concerned that depression – the more common clinical term at that time was 'melancholia' – was a relatively rare condition with a niche market at best. Today, across much of the Western world, around one in ten of the population has taken antidepressant medication, and depression has become a signature condition of our age, just as melancholy was for the Renaissance.

This is not simply a marketing trick: if the drugs had no beneficial effects, nobody would take them. Nor is depression a figment of our modern imaginations: its symptoms were described as clearly and consistently in the age of humours and demons as they are in the age of neuroscience. Yet there is an oddly symbiotic relationship between psychiatric medication and the conditions for which it is prescribed. Depression is a condition for which antidepressants offer relief, but by doing so they create more depression, shaping the distresses generated by modern life into medical form. Doctors are trained to look out for this condition because they can offer pharmaceutical treatments that, for some if not all, restore a sense of well-being.

OPPOSITE
Blister packs containing 20 mg capsules of Prozac (fluoxetine). Around twenty-five million Prozac prescriptions are filled per year in the United States.

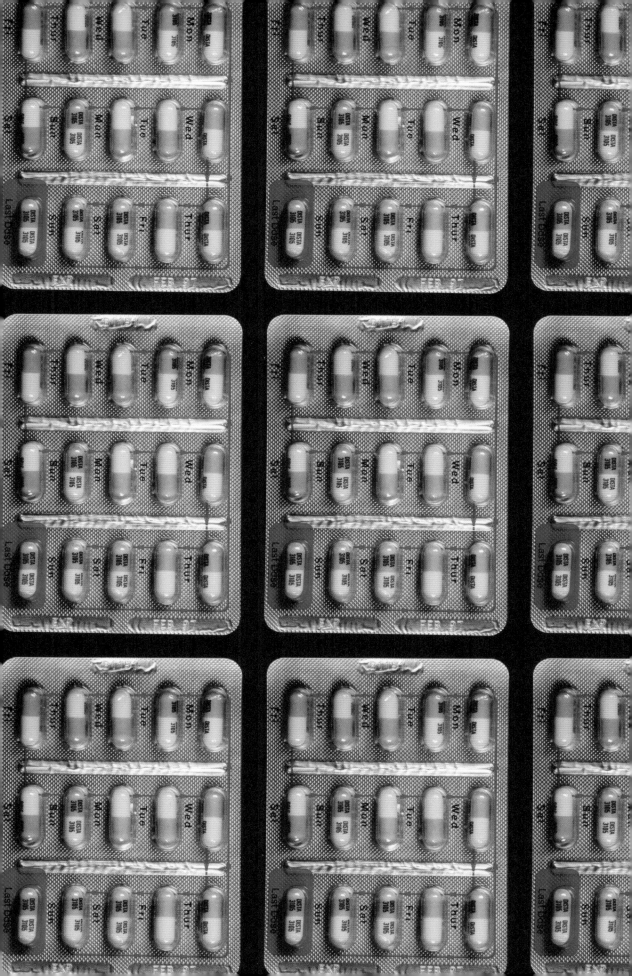

The prescription monopoly on psychiatric medication has created a de facto distinction that is the asylum's echo: a class of those whose mental health is recognized as requiring professional intervention. Yet the mentally ill are no longer a separate population, and mental health today encompasses far more than the transactions between service users and psychiatrists. Beyond the doctor's surgery and the psychiatric hospital lies a marketplace teeming with medicines, techniques and therapies for restoring meaning and balance to minds and lives. It is open all hours, its aisles crowded with self-help books and courses, spiritual practices, complementary medicines, traditional healers, meditation and mind tools, diets, creative therapies and magical rituals.

All this is often seen as a jumble of consumer fads, an indictment of our shallow and rootless postmodern lifestyles. However, a similar mix of modern and traditional, medical, psychological and spiritual therapies exists in most cultures around the globe today, and in many respects takes us back to our roots in the world before the asylum. In the 17th century as much as in the 21st, physicians, apothecaries, astrologers, preachers and folk healers competed with remedies that ranged from gentle herbs to powerful poisons, from horoscopes to exorcisms to cranial surgery.

The array of therapies that Robert Burton presented in *The Anatomy of Melancholy* (1621) is strikingly modern. He lists and evaluates hundreds of drug-based remedies – toxic chemicals including mercury and arsenic, exotic imports such as senna and tobacco, and gentle herbal potions from the hedgerow – alongside the other medical interventions of his day, such as bloodletting and blistering. Generally, he considered that strong medicine,

RIGHT
These viral skits for Prozac satirize how medicines for mental health are now marketed like a consumer product.

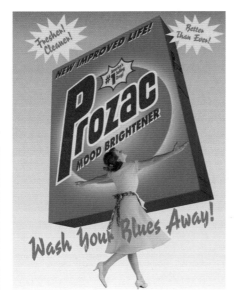

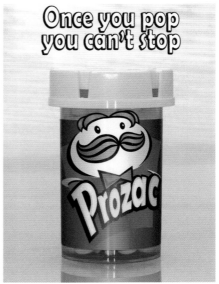

whether chemical or surgical, should be used sparingly. 'Those countries which use it least,' he observed, 'are the best in health.'

His world was equally rich in non-medical therapies. The use of music to calm the troubled mind reached back through the medieval Christian traditions to the classical era and the Old Testament, in which David soothed Saul's tormented spirits by playing his lyre. Burton believed that joyful music had great power to lift the spirits and invigorate the system, but equally that the 'pleasing melancholie' induced by sad music could bring profound mental solace. Sleep should be made as deep and prolonged as possible; exercise, bathing, a good diet and spring water could all restore body, mind and soul; fresh air lifted and invigorated the spirits. Calm and meditative mental states should be cultivated for their power to drive away anxiety. Everybody, melancholy or not, needed friendship, counselling and merry company. Faith and prayer were ever-present sources of strength. His prime directive was 'be not solitary, be not idle', the principle that would inform the moral and occupational therapies of centuries to come.

The medication of today is immeasurably more effective than that of Burton's era, but his principles still hold. Medicine is both a science and an art, and drugs alone cannot restore harmony and meaning to a life that has lost its balance. 'Recovery', in the view of many service users, is an unhelpful term for a lifelong process that cannot be reduced to success or failure. It involves not simply medicating the brain but finding a new purpose and focus, taking control of the circumstances of your life, becoming aware of your behaviour and its impact on those around you, nurturing your self-respect, finding a community in which you belong, learning to love yourself and others: in short, the challenges

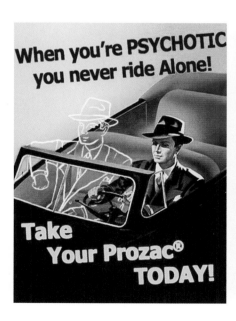

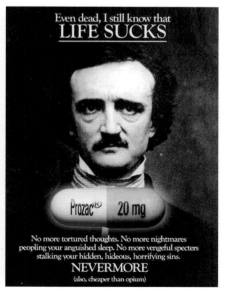

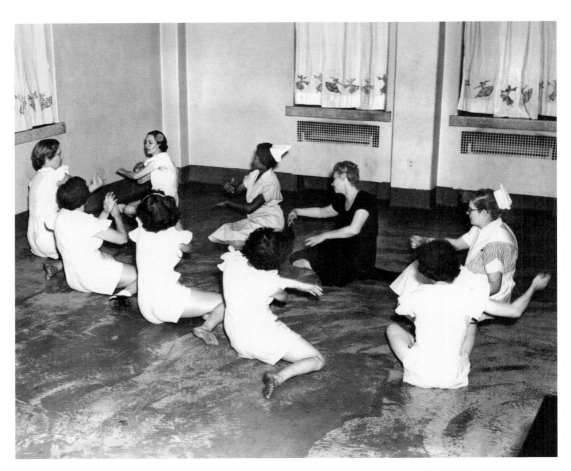

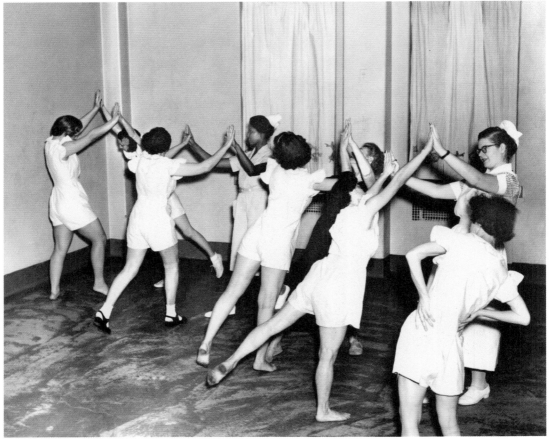

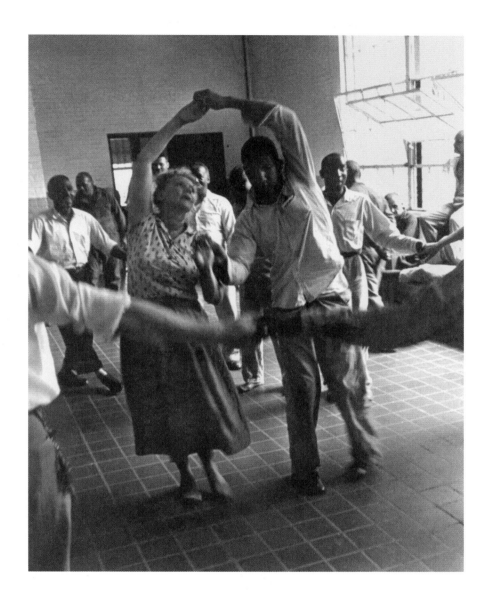

OPPOSITE AND ABOVE
Dance/movement therapy as pioneered by
Marian Chace in the United States in the 1960s.
The practice, used by Chace and other dance
educators such as Francesca Boas, can develop
communication skills, restore self-image and
allow patients to regain control of their physical
and mental identities.

RIGHT AND BELOW
Domestic scenes from daily life in Geel, where 'boarders' participate in and share family life today just as they have since medieval times.

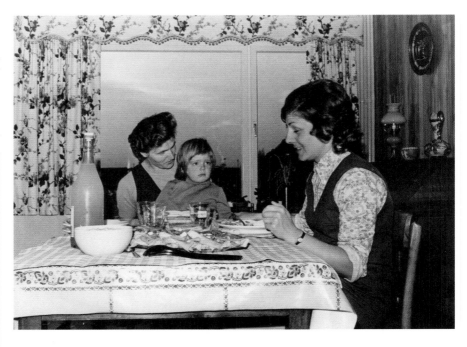

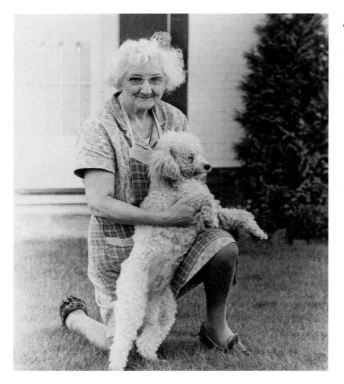

«Social psychiatry – the old 'moral therapy' – has proved its worth many times over the last two centuries.»

that everyone faces in trying to forge a happy and meaningful life.

If the medical approach has its limits, social and community therapies have also fallen short of their most optimistic claims. The clarion call of the Psichiatria Democratica movement was 'liberty is cure', but closing the asylums has not returned everyone to sanity, and 'community care' has too often become a synonym for neglect. The countercultural movements that coincided with the end of the asylum have helped to transform the relationship between madness and society: challenging the stigma of mental illness, listening to the voices of service users and winning them legal rights to privacy, dignity, informed consent and the investigation of abuses. But the radical claims that madness is merely a label constructed by psychiatry or an oppressive society have dovetailed all too neatly with the dismantling of mental health services.

As in the days of the asylum, the feeling public wishes to hear that the problem of madness can be resolved by humane intentions. However, the consequence of this belief is that its stubborn persistence goes unacknowledged, and troublesome cases are buried within the prison system from which the asylum was designed to rescue them.

Social psychiatry – the old 'moral therapy' – has proved its worth many times over the course of the last two centuries, but it has also shown itself to be extremely demanding. It requires levels of commitment that are hard to sustain and difficult to franchise beyond its charismatic and passionate leaders. However well we understand its biomedical underpinnings, madness – or mental illness – remains, in baldly pragmatic terms, what it was before the modern medical story began: a condition that has exhausted the capacity for support available from family and

BELOW
In Geel, the relationships that develop between boarders and children are believed to be particularly beneficial to both parties.

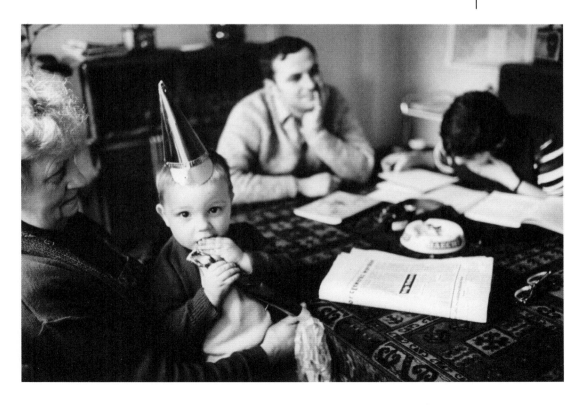

community. The asylum, through its many iterations, demonstrated that the remedy is in essence obvious: William Browne believed it could be reduced to two words, 'kindness and occupation'. But for those without support or resources, who have broken the ties that bind other members of society together, these are not so simply provided. Inside or outside the asylum, the solutions are the same: either money that can buy the support required, or carers who are prepared to dedicate themselves to providing support without financial reward.

Beyond the asylum lies a third option: a community in which the necessary support is part and parcel of the social contract. Geel is the most enduring example of such a community in the Western world, and a visit there today is both inspiring and sobering. It is a friendly, prosperous town with a thriving business park on its outskirts and a large, modern psychiatric hospital complex close to its historic centre. Its families still open their homes to the boarders who are a familiar and cheerful presence in the town, often to be seen sitting on benches or chatting in the cafe-lined main square. Several have spent upwards of fifty years living with the same family, making the transition from foster children to honorary uncles or aunts to elderly and beloved dependents. But nowadays there are only around three hundred of them, compared with three or four thousand a century ago. Most of Geel's families no longer work farms, where a day's labour was a straightforward exchange for a bed and an extra mouth to feed. They live in apartments, work shifts, travel and take holidays: all the freedoms taken

for granted in modern life make old-fashioned family care impossible. The people of Geel remain fiercely proud of their tradition, but they are not immune to the trends that are eroding traditional communities the world over.

The steepest decline in family care came in the 1970s, when new drugs became a central feature of psychiatric treatment. Families had always insisted that they were not doctors and most avoided the language of medical diagnosis altogether, preferring to refer to their boarders simply as 'different' or 'special'. The arrival of medication altered the relationship: boarders effectively became outpatients from the psychiatric hospital, their family care relegated to a residential arrangement. Hard-won patients' rights also eroded the old system: psychiatrists are now obliged to give boarders their diagnosis, which they can choose to share with their families or not. In recent years the hospital has expanded, with residential wards added for elderly, juvenile and acute care.

The decline in family care is not to be lamented altogether. Part of the reason for it is that, as elsewhere in the world, psychiatry has met the community halfway. The famous 'mixed system' that emerged at Geel in the 1860s has become today's model of best practice: care integrated into the community as far as possible, with a medical safety net deployed discreetly when necessary. In the post-asylum world, the community mental health team is psychiatry's vanguard, responding to crises in the home and supporting those who wish to remain there and maintain their independence. In doing

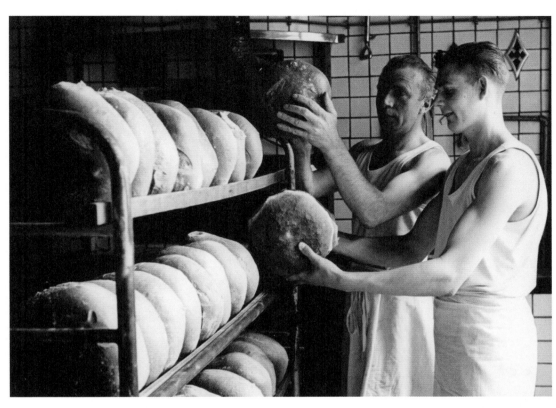

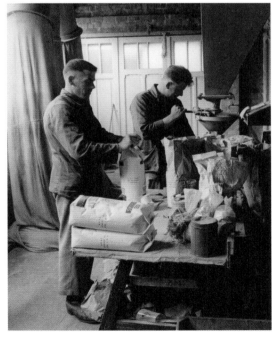

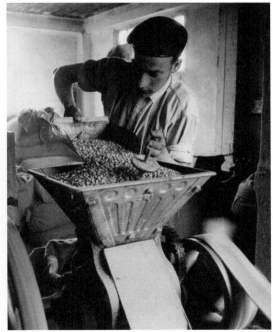

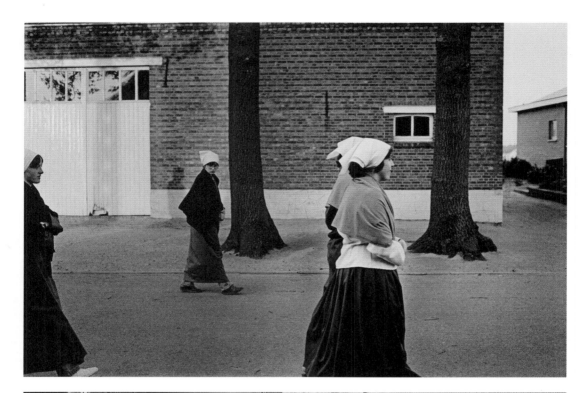

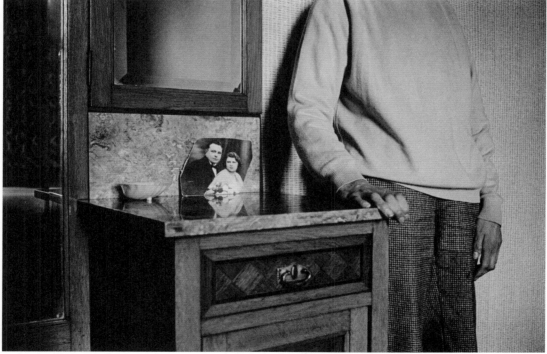

ABOVE AND OPPOSITE
These black-and-white
photographs are from the
series *Een gelaat van Geel*
(Faces of Geel) by Hugo
Minnen. They depict the
daily lives of the town's
boarders in 1980–1981.

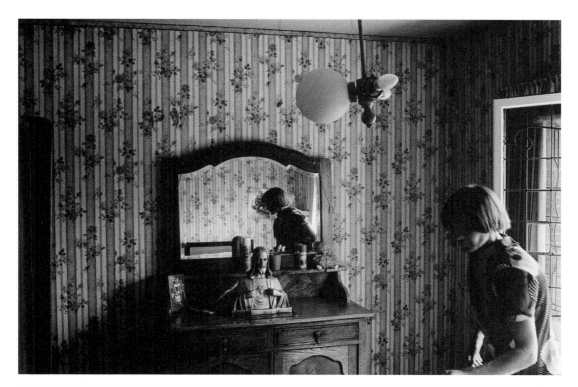

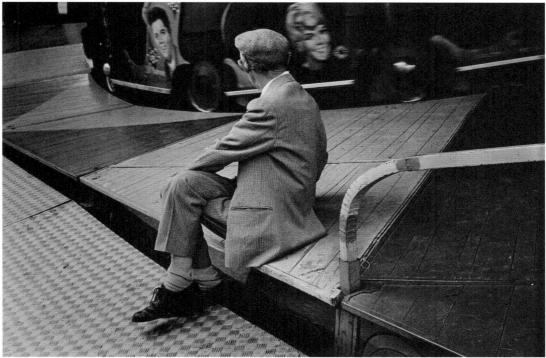

Boarders become members of the family, often for a lifetime. One boarder recently celebrated fifty years in his adoptive household. Although Geel has a large and modern psychiatric hospital, many boarders prefer to live 'outside' (in the town) rather than 'inside' (in residential care). On the streets of Geel, boarders are seen as part of a proud and distinctive tradition.

so, it must balance the benefits of freedom against the risks of the outside world, the immediate support of ambulance services against the deeper expertise of specialists units or the continuity provided by a single therapist, and it must manage the public's exaggerated perception of the danger that the mentally unwell represent.

The residential mental hospital, the asylum's final incarnation, has not been done away with. In forensic wings, acute care wards and other secure units, the locked doors, reinforced glass, regimented beds and smell of the hospital are still the norm for those detained under emergency sections or criminal sentences. In some respects, they are the modern equivalent of the 18th-century madhouse, segregating their inmates from society for the benefit of all. However, unlike their historical antecedents, they are highly professionalized and extremely expensive, with staff-to-patient ratios often at 1:1 or even higher. The calculus of risks and resources makes them the safest and most politically acceptable solution, but few would argue that they offer the best environments for recovery.

Most of those in crisis and severe distress want not a hospital ward but a home: a place of warmth and emotional safety, with housemates who can support each other as they regain control of their lives. Community refuges of this kind emerged in the dying days of the asylum, although usually as an alternative to the state system rather than a part of it. Where they exist today, they struggle to meet the criteria for statutory funding and are kept afloat by charitable donations and dedicated volunteers.

Yet the asylum in its most ambitious and generous incarnation aspired to be more than a safe place to weather a storm. In the ideal that originated at the York Retreat and was transformed into a utopian vision by the likes of William Browne, it was a self-sufficient community, a world outside the world, in which patients could remain citizens for as long as they needed or chose. It was a dream that never died. Gould Farm in Massachusetts, now more than a century old, has in recent decades come to specialize in the care of those with severe mental health problems, such as depression, bipolar disorder and schizophrenia, who have been decarcerated from the old mental hospitals. Today, around forty 'guests' live communally with a similar number of volunteers, discreetly supported by psychiatric and nursing staff. As Robert Burton recommended, they keep medication to a minimum and supplement it with psychotherapy, recovery work and useful occupation: working on the farm, growing vegetables, baking bread, maintaining the buildings, managing the adjoining tract of forestry, and socializing together in the evenings.

Such 'intentional communities', as they are now known, are spreading across the United States and beyond, often started up by the parents and families of those whose mental ill health consigned them to a lifetime in shuttered wards or living desperately on the streets. Foundations such as the CooperRiis Institute in North Carolina take over ranches and woodlands, turning them into self-sustaining mixed farming communities in which staff, volunteers and guest workers share their lives with those who would be unable to enjoy such

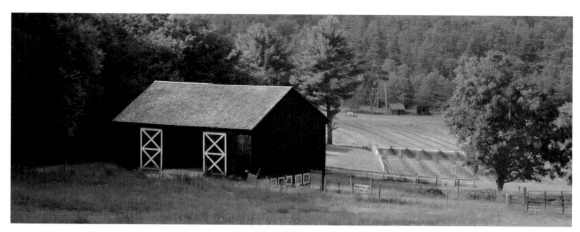

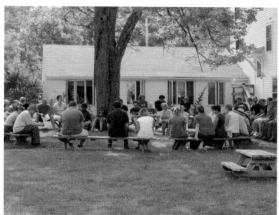

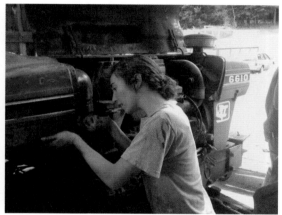

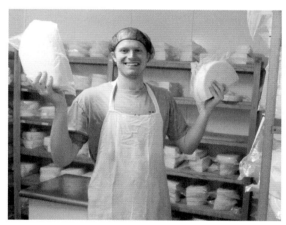

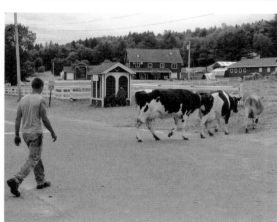

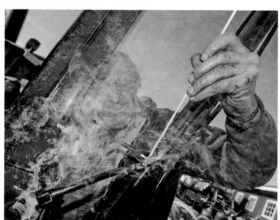

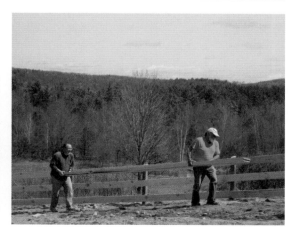

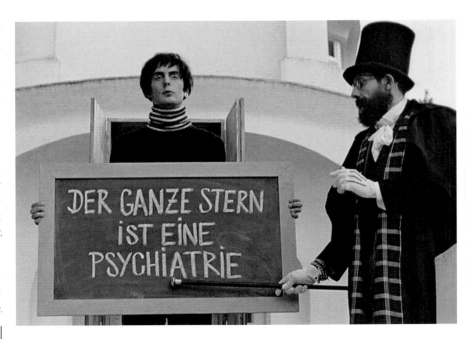

freedoms on their own. Meditation, group therapy, exercise programmes and work experience are open to all: the community can be experienced as an occupational therapy unit, training camp, workplace or ranch holiday.

Care of this kind is expensive, running to thousands of dollars a month. As such, it can be for a fortunate few only: if public mental health care is unable to cope with demand, such well-funded and dedicated communities can hardly be a universal solution. Like every private asylum from the York Retreat onwards, they set an unfair benchmark for the institutions whose state funding comes with a duty of care to the majority who have no alternative.

But they demonstrate the limits of the possible, and at best suggest ways of extending its reach. A recent trend is to combine the intentional community with the retirement village: a home both for the mentally unwell and for the elderly – often retired from the caring professions – who would rather spend their later lives engaged in communal activity and voluntary work than playing golf in a comfortable but atomized suburb. Their lifetime of experience in caring for others can be repaid by practical assistance from their able-bodied companions; together they can maintain levels of freedom that none of them could achieve alone. In the old adage of the people of Geel, 'care is cure', for everyone involved.

«'Care is cure' for everyone involved.»

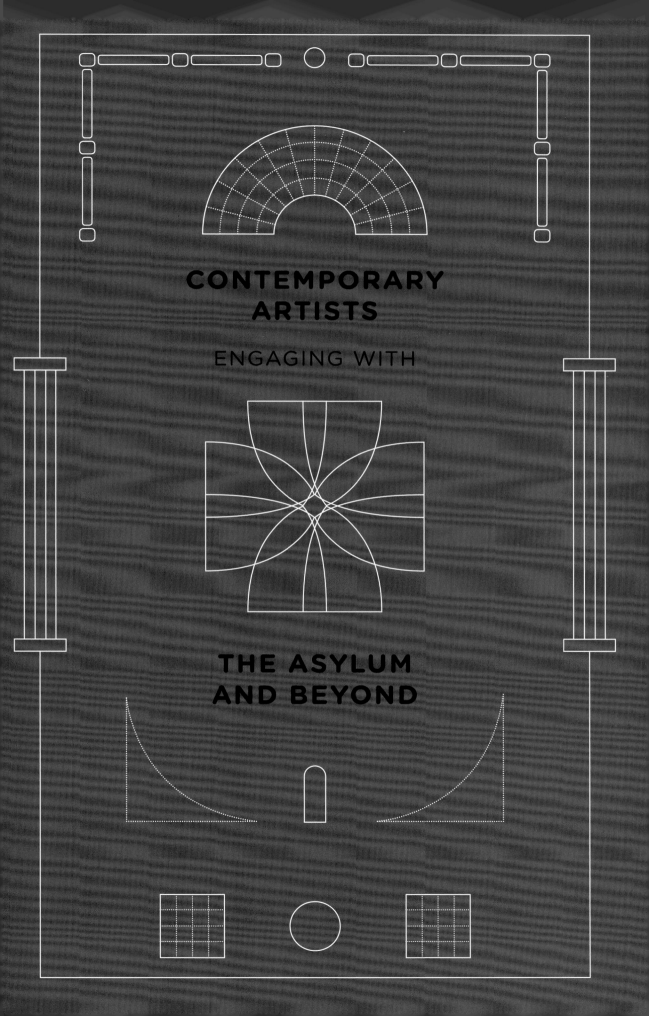

CONTEMPORARY ARTISTS

ENGAGING WITH

THE ASYLUM
AND BEYOND

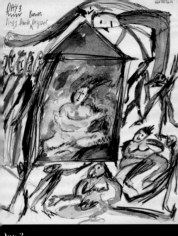

Day 3
My third day after starting at the day centre

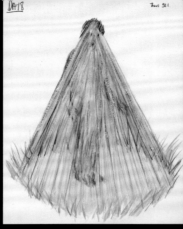

Day 8
I turn into a human waterfall, of tears

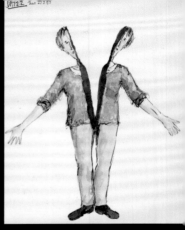

Day 22
Splitting in half with misery and fear

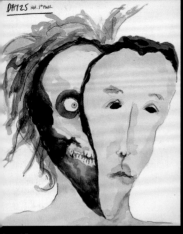

Day 25
A drawing experiment reveals hidden horrors

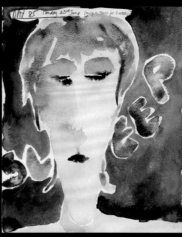

Day 85
Sleep can be a blissful break from anguish

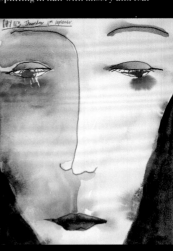

Day 113
Even weeping turns me to darker thoughts

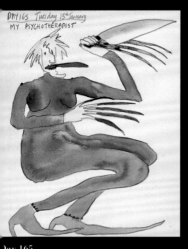

Day 165
My psychotherapist was annoying, so I drew this

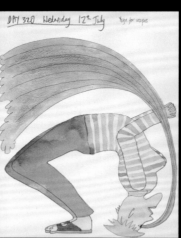

Day 320
Yoga for weepers is not terribly practical

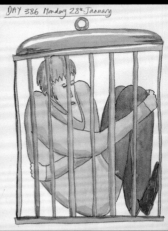

Day 386
Captured and defined by the mental health system

1950 — PRESENT

BOBBY BAKER

Baker is a female artist acclaimed for producing radical work of outstanding quality across disciplines such as performance, drawing and multi-media. She is the artistic director of Daily Life Ltd, an arts and mental health organization based in East London, funded by Arts Council England.

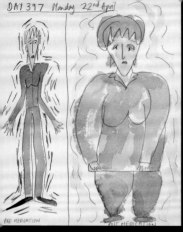

Day 397
The truth about side-effects

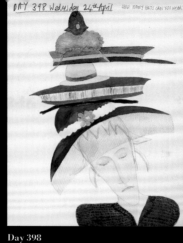

Day 398
Too much responsibility

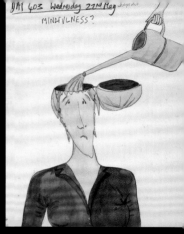

Day 403
Trying to learn 'mindfulness'

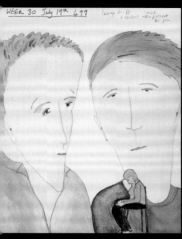

Day 499
Compassionate but dominating doctors

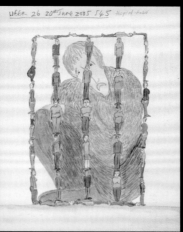

Day 545
Imprisoned by people

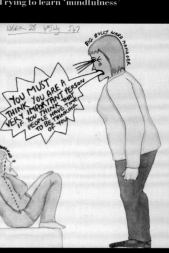

Day 547
This ward manager has lost control of hersel[f]

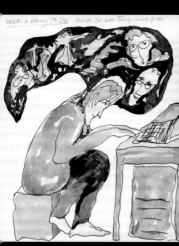

Day 630
Writing is the best way to tell my *own* story

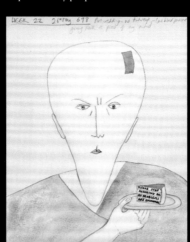

Day 698
'Stop assuming all my problems
are emotional – I have cancer'

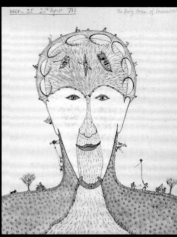

Day 711
The Daily Stream of Consciousness:
Resolution and peace - at last!

opp. and above
The exhibition *Bobby Baker's Diary Drawings: Mental
Illness and Me 1997–2008*, co-curated by Baker with her
daughter, a clinical psychologist, premiered at Wellcome
Collection in 2009. The accompanying book won MIND
Book of the Year 2011. A selection of 158 drawings was

The drawings cover Baker's experiences of day
hospitals, acute psychiatric wards, 'crisis' teams
and a variety of treatments. They chart the ups
and downs of her recovery, family life, work as
an artist, breast cancer and just how funny all

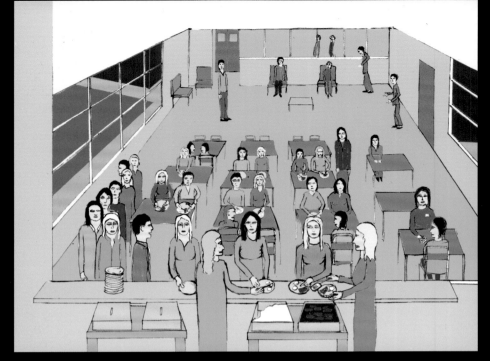

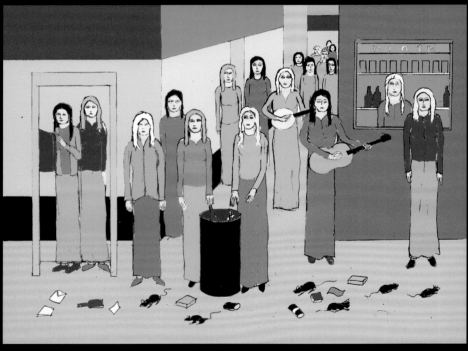

1957

PRESENT

DAVID BEALES

Beales has spent some twenty years in and out of hospitals. He is an artist and writer who regularly shows his work with Bethlem Gallery.

above
David Beales's art documents life in the psychiatric hospital of the 1970s. The works seen here are *Lunch Break* (top) and *High Street* (bottom).

Since 2006 Biffoli has attended the La Tinaia artists' collective in Florence, painting on canvas and specializing in contemporary portraits.

below
Biffoli's portraits are acrylic on canvas. Clockwise from top left: *Marilyn Monroe* (2010) *Chairman Mao* (2011), *Mona Lisa* (2010) and *Hugo Chávez* (2012).

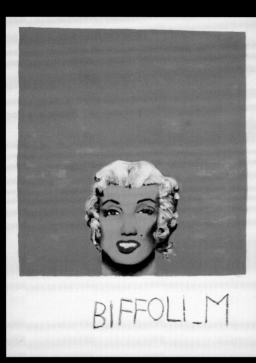

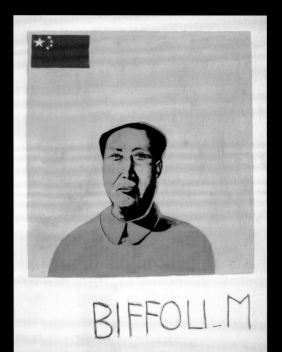

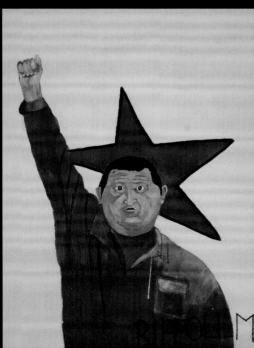

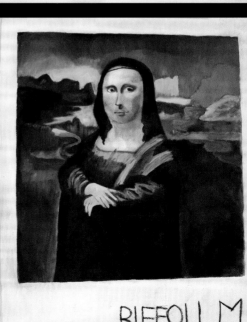

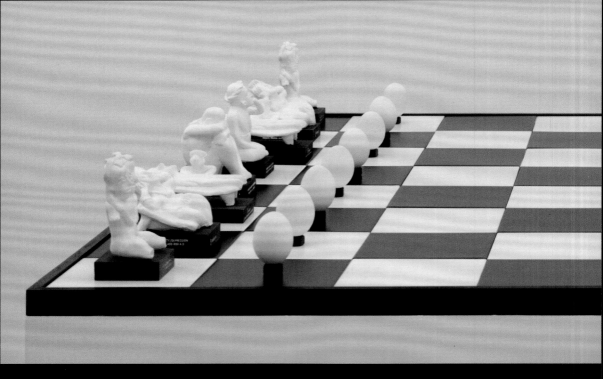

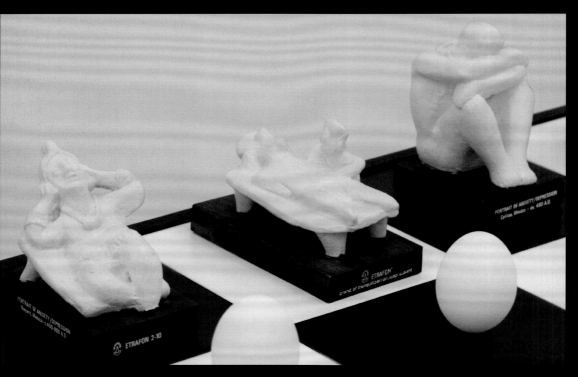

1969 • JAVIER TÉLLEZ • PRESENT

Téllez's work – developed often
in collaboration with psychiatric
patients – challenges the stereotypes
associated with mental illness.

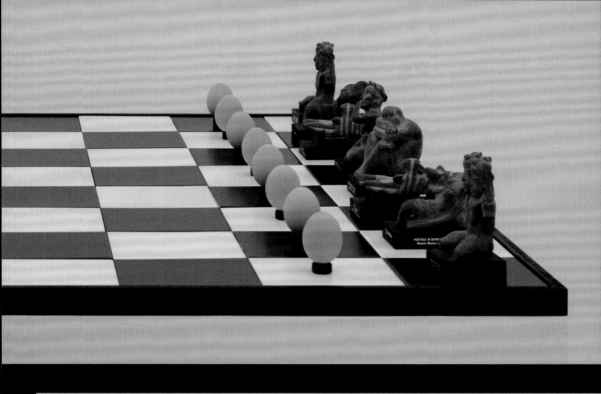

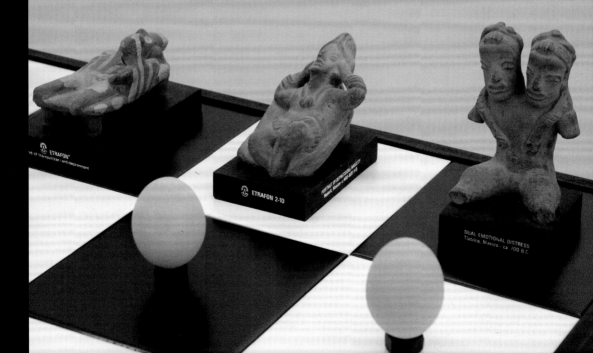

ANTONIO MELIS

1970

PRESENT

Melis has enjoyed drawing since childhood and now works with the La Tinaia collective, combining figure painting with geometric experiments.

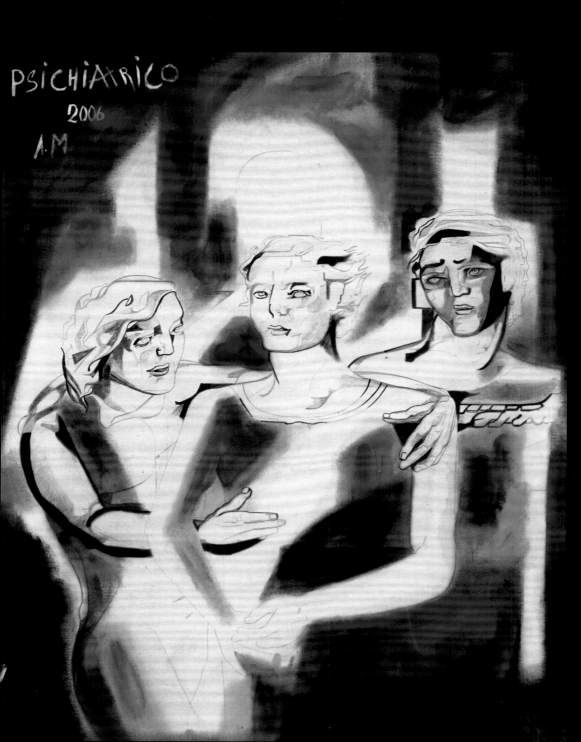

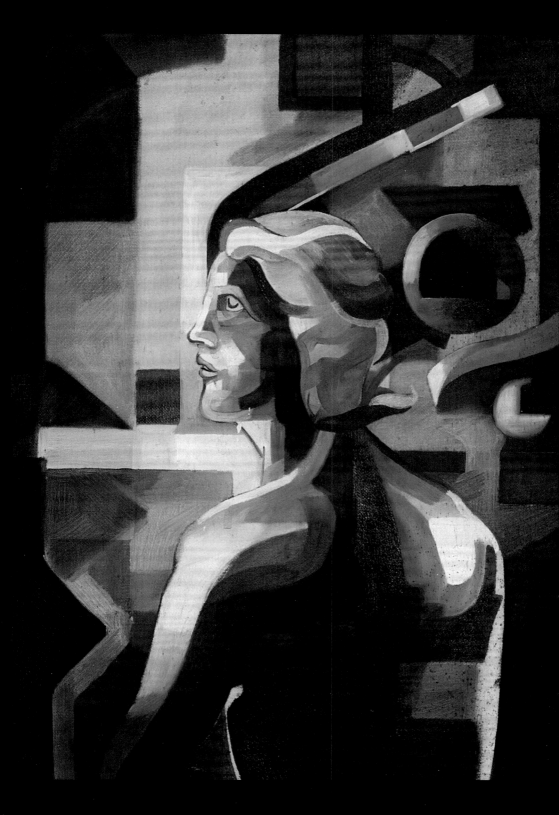

opp.
Psichiatrico (Psychiatric)
(2006) by Antonio Melis; acrylic
on canvas. The colours are
painted boldly on the canvas,
unifying the three figures.

above
Untitled (2007) by Antonio
Melis; oil on board. It features
the use of strong geometric
shapes characteristic of
nearly all Melis's work.

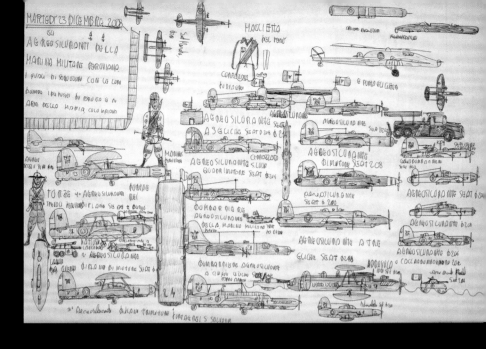

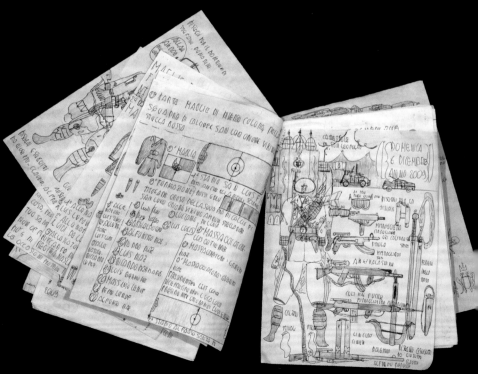

1971

**GUISEPPE
BAROCCHI**

PRESENT

Barocchi joined La Tinaia in 2008.
He weaves words and pictures together to
create dynamic narrative images, rendered
predominantly in pen and pencil on paper.

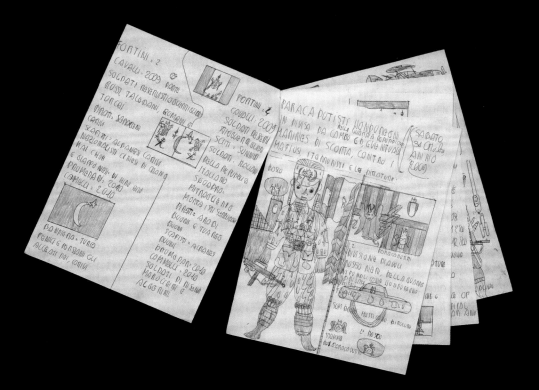

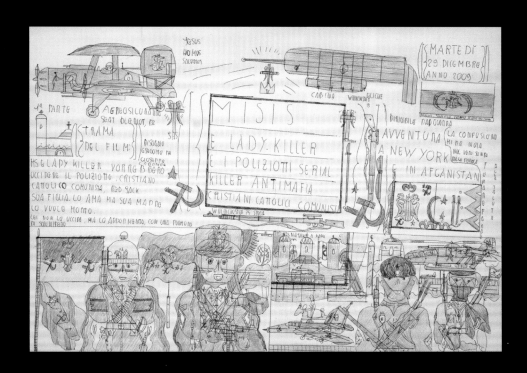

Giuseppe Barocchi's pen and pencil drawings feature many of the subjects he drew in childhood, such as aeroplanes, soldiers and weaponry. Each drawing is packed with annotation and narrative, integrated with the images.

opp. above
Untitled (2008)

opp. below
Untitled (2009), stapled sheets

above top
Untitled (2009), stapled sheets

above
Misis E Lady Killer
(2010)

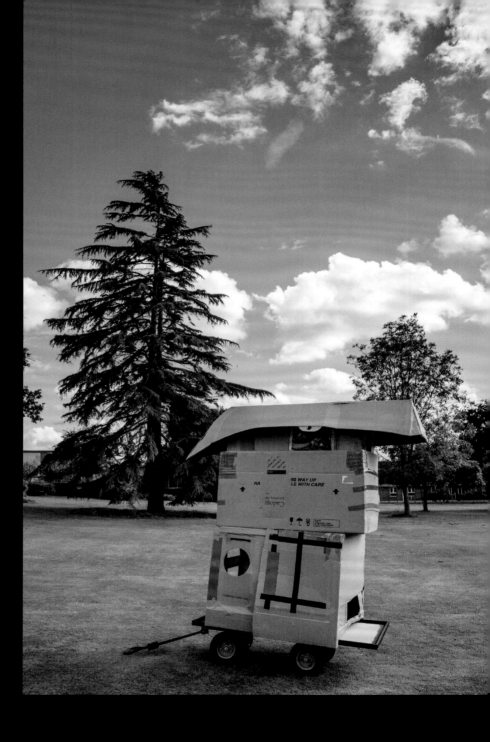

Mr X is an artist based at Bethlem
Royal Hospital, where he makes
cardboard structures and vehicles
that are repeatedly modified.

above
'The work is simultane...
of escape, a hiding pla...
a second skin – an alte...
of inhabiting the insti...
(Michaela Ross, art co...

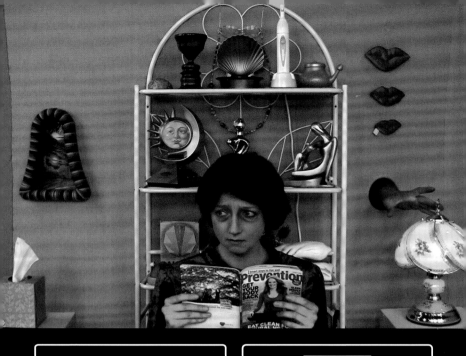

1976 · **PRESENT**

SHANA MOULTON

Moulton's films and colourful psychedelic performances explore contemporary anxieties through her alter ego, Cynthia.

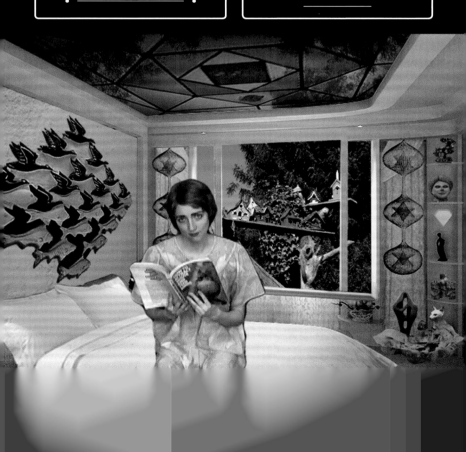

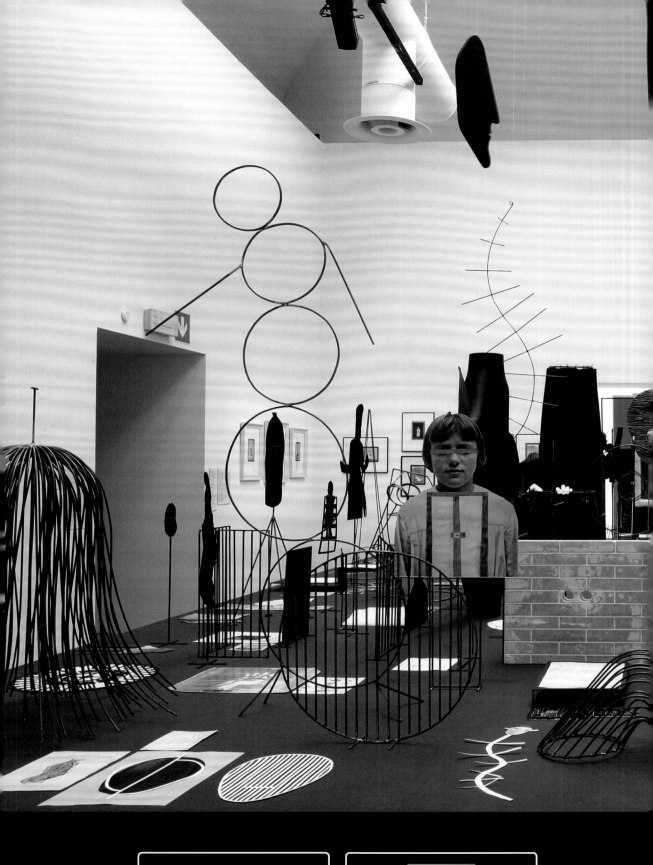

1982

PRESENT

**EVA
KOTÁTKOVÁ**

Kotátková's installations
and sculptures examine the
psychological and physical effects
of restraint and social pressures.

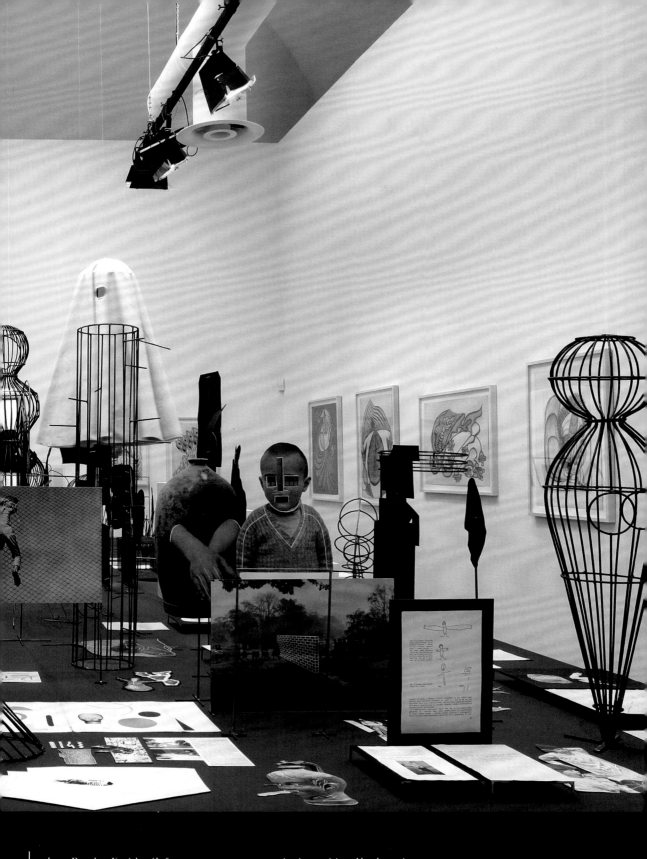

above Based on Kotátková's frequent
research visits to the Bohnice Psychiatric
Hospital in Prague, this mixed-media
installation is titled *Asylum* (2014).
Animated periodically by performers, it
attempts to capture both the institutional
constraints and the alternative mode of
communication envisioned by the patients.
In the words of the artist, '*Asylum* presents
a collection of fears, anxieties, phobias and
phantasmagoric visions of patients and
children suffering from communication
difficulties or struggling to fit within social
structure – a chaotic archive of inner visions.'

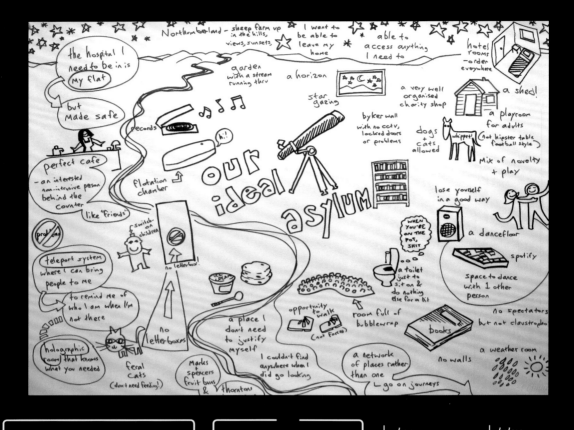

2014 — PRESENT

**MADLOVE
A DESIGNER
ASYLUM**

Madlove is an ongoing project led by the vacuum cleaner and Hannah Hull. It aims to re-imagine the notion of the asylum as 'a safe place to go mad'.

above
This sketch (2014) by Michael Duckett shows ideas for visually appealing, patient-centred spaces for mental health services.

below
Installation of the beta version of *Madlove: A Design Asylum* designed by Benjamin Koslowski and James Christian.

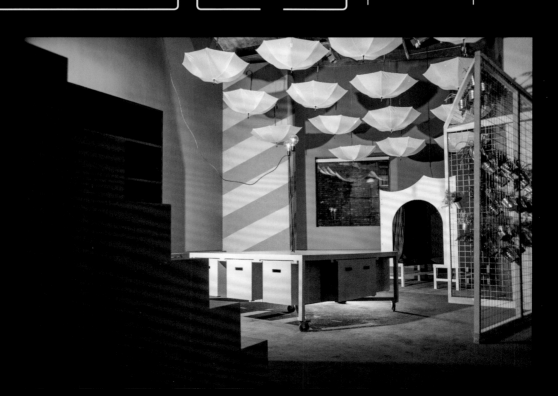

INTRODUCTION

—

The most recent and best single-volume history of madness is Andrew Scull's *Madness in Civilization* (London: Thames & Hudson, 2015). Roy Porter's *Madness: A Brief History* (Oxford and New York: Oxford University Press, 2002) covers a similar scope in condensed form; briefer still is Andrew Scull's *Madness: A Very Short Introduction* (Oxford and New York: Oxford University Press, 2011). The emergence of Western medical views of madness can be traced through the sources collected in *Three Hundred Years of Psychiatry 1535–1860*, edited by Richard Hunter and Ida Macalpine (London and New York: Oxford University Press, 1963).

For a summary of recent research into the social correlates of schizophrenia, see Tanya Marie Luhrmann's article 'Beyond the Brain' in *The Wilson Quarterly* (Summer 2012).

The History of Bethlem (London and New York: Routledge, 1997), edited by Jonathan Andrews, Asa Briggs, Roy Porter, Penny Tucker and Keir Waddington and produced to commemorate the hospital's 750th anniversary, has become the definitive account and is my main source throughout. The most popular and influential narrative for most of the 20th century was *The Story of Bethlehem Hospital from its Foundation in 1247* by Bethlem's chaplain Edward Geoffrey O'Donoghue (London: T. F. Unwin, 1914). These two are the prime sources for most popular histories.

Margery Kempe's narrative, *The Book of Margery Kempe*, is available in a modern translation from Penguin Classics (London: 1985).

The fullest English language source for the story of Geel is Eugen Roosens's *Geel Revisited after Centuries of Mental Rehabilitation* (Antwerp: Garant Uitgevers, 2007). There is a useful English language bibliography at faculty.samford.edu/~jlgoldst/geelbiblio.html

The role of Bedlam in Jacobean drama is the subject of Robert Reed's *Bedlam on the Jacobean Stage* (Cambridge, Mass: Harvard University Press, 1952) and Natsu Hattori's article 'The Pleasure of your Bedlam' in *History of Psychiatry*, VI (1995) pp. 283–308.

The various forms of madness recognized in 17th-century England are described in Michael MacDonald's *Mystical Bedlam* (Cambridge: Cambridge University Press, 1981).

Robert Burton's *The Anatomy of Melancholy* (1621) is available in a modern three-volume edition, edited by Thomas Faulkner, Nicholas Kiessling and Rhonda Blair (Oxford: Clarendon Press, 1990). An abridged version is edited and introduced by Kevin Jackson (Manchester: Fyfield Books, 2004). Another useful introduction is *Sanity in Bedlam: A Study of Robert Burton's Anatomy of Melancholy* by Lawrence Babb (Michigan: Michigan State University Press, 1959).

The history of Hamlet's psychiatric diagnoses is explored by William Bynum and Michael Neve in 'Hamlet on the Couch', in *The Anatomy of Madness*, ed. William Bynum, Roy Porter and Michael Shepherd, Volume 1 (London and New York: Tavistock Press, 1985). Don Quixote's madness is discussed in John Farrell's *Paranoia and Modernity* (Cornell University Press, 2007).

1: THE MADHOUSE

—

The emergence of the 18th-century madhouse in Britain is discussed by Roy Porter in various works, notably *Mind-Forg'd Manacles* (Cambridge, Mass.: Harvard University Press, 1987), and by William Parry-Jones in *The Trade in Lunacy* (London: Routledge & Kegan Paul, 1972).

For the wider European story see Erik Midelfort, *Madness in Sixteenth-Century Germany* (Stanford: Stanford University Press, 1999); David Lederer, *Madness, Religion and the State in Early Modern Europe* (Cambridge: Cambridge University Press, 2005) and Robert Castel, *The Regulation of Madness: The Origins of Incarceration in France* (Cambridge: Polity Press, 1988).

Alexander Cruden's *The London-Citizen Exceedingly Injured* (London: T. Cooper, 1739) is excerpted and discussed in *A Mad People's History of Madness*, a classic anthology edited by Dale Peterson (Pittsburgh: University of Pittsburgh Press, 1982).

Jonathan Andrews and Andrew Scull's *Undertaker of the Mind: John Monro and Mad-Doctoring in Eighteenth-Century England* (Berkeley: University of California Press, 2001) paints a vivid picture of practices in both public and private madhouses during that era. William Battie and John Monro's pamphlets are reproduced in Hunter and Macalpine (ed.), *Three Hundred Years of Psychiatry 1535–1860* (above).

The standard account of George III's madness is Ida Macalpine and Richard Hunter's *George III and the Mad-Business* (London: Allen Lane 1969). This is the source of the retrospective diagnosis of porphyria, which has become widely known through Alan Bennett's play and film, *The Madness of King George*. Recent scholarship has, however, brought it into question: see Peters, Timothy J. and Wilkinson, D., 'King George III and porphyria: a clinical re-examination of the historical evidence' in *History of Psychiatry* Vol 21; Issue 1; No 81 (March 2010).

Philippe Pinel's *Medico-Philosophical Treatise on Mental Alienation* (2nd ed., 1809) is published in an English translation by Gordon Hickish, David Healy and Louis C. Charland (Oxford: Wiley-Blackwell, 2008). The best English language account of the Pinelian revolution in psychiatry is Jan Goldstein's *Console and Classify* (Chicago: University of Chicago Press 1989); for an original treatment incorporating the patients' perspective, see Laure Murat, *The Man Who Thought He Was Napoleon* (Chicago and London: University of Chicago Press, 2014). On the legendary image of Pinel striking the chains from the mad, see Dora Weiner, 'Le Geste de Pinel: The History of a Psychiatric Myth' in *Discovering the History of Psychiatry*, ed. Mark Micale and Roy Porter (New York and Oxford: Oxford University Press, 1994).

James Tilly Matthews's remarkable story is the subject of my book *The Influencing Machine* (London: Strange Attractor Press, 2012), published in the United States as *A Visionary Madness* (Berkeley: North Atlantic Books 2014).

2. THE ASYLUM
—

The best starting point for the story of the 19th-century asylum is the work of Andrew Scull, particularly *Museums of Madness* (London: Allen Lane, 1979) and its revised version *The Most Solitary of Afflictions* (New Haven: Yale University Press, 1993).

On the York Retreat see Anne Digby, *Madness, Morality and Medicine* (Cambridge: Cambridge University Press, 1985) and Andrew Scull, 'Moral Treatment Reconsidered' in his edited volume *Madhouses, Mad-Doctors and Madmen* (Philadelphia: University of Pennsylvania Press, 1981).

On the growing importance of mad-doctors as expert witnesses in the 19th-century courtroom, see Joel Peter Eigen, *Witnessing Insanity: Madness and Mad-Doctors in the English Court* (New Haven and London: Yale University Press, 1995).

The most influential history of the emergence of the asylum in the United States is David Rothman's *The Discovery of the Asylum* (Boston: Little, Brown, 1971); see also Andrew Scull, 'The Discovery of the Asylum Revisited' in his *Madhouses, Mad-Doctors and Madmen* (above) and *Theaters of Madness* by Benjamin Reiss (Chicago and London: University of Chicago Press, 2008).

John Perceval's story is told by Roy Porter in *A Social History of Madness* (London: Phoenix, 1996). On Ticehurst Hospital, see Charlotte MacKenzie, *Psychiatry for the Rich* (London: Routledge, 1993) and William Parry-Jones, *The Trade in Lunacy* (above).

For 19th-century perspectives on Geel, see William Parry-Jones, 'The Model of the Geel Lunatic Colony and its Influence on the Nineteenth-Century Asylum System in Britain' in *Madhouses, Mad-Doctors and Madmen* (above).

On Dorothea Dix, see her biography *Voice for the Mad* by David Gollaher (New York: The Free Press, 1995). The Alleged Lunatics' Friends Society and the abuses of private asylums are the focus of *Inconvenient People* by Sarah Wise (London: Bodley Head, 2012).

William Browne's *What Asylums Were, Are and Ought to Be* (Edinburgh: Adam and Charles Black, 1837) has been reprinted as *The Asylum as Utopia* (London and New York: Tavistock/Routledge, 1991), edited with an introduction by Andrew Scull. On Browne and art collecting, see Maureen Park, *Art in Madness: W.A.F. Browne's Collection of Patient Art at Crichton Royal Institution, Dumfries* (Dumfries: Dumfries and Galloway Health Board, 2010).

On women and the asylum, see Elaine Showalter, *The Female Malady* (New York: Pantheon Books, 1985), a wide-ranging narrative of madness in the 19th and 20th centuries, and her article 'Victorian Women and Insanity' in Andrew Scull's *Madhouses, Mad-Doctors and Madmen* (above). Her arguments are discussed by Nancy Tomes in 'Feminist Histories of Psychiatry', in *Discovering the History of Psychiatry* (above). See also Lisa Appignanesi, *Mad, Bad and Sad* (London: Virago, 2008); for the story in France, see Yannick Ripa, *Women and Madness* (Cambridge: Polity Press, 1990).

Masters of Bedlam by Andrew Scull, Charlotte MacKenzie and Nicholas Hervey (New Jersey: Princeton University Press, 1996) includes valuable chapters on both William Browne and John Conolly. Elaine Showalter also considers John Conolly in *The Female Malady* (above). On non-restraint, see also Nancy Tomes, 'The Great Restraint Controversy' in *The Anatomy of Madness* (above) and Akihito Suzuki, 'The Politics and Ideology of Non-Restraint' in *Medical History* (Vol. 39, 1995).

On Bethlem under Charles Hood, and particularly on Richard Dadd, see Nicholas Tromans, *Richard Dadd: The Artist and the Asylum* (London: Tate Publishing, 2011).

Emil Kraepelin's *Memoirs* are published in English (Berlin and New York: Springer-Verlag, 1987; tr. Cheryl Wooding-Deane). Henry Maudsley's views are most fully expressed in his *The Pathology of Mind* (London: Macmillan, 1895). See also the chapter on him in *Masters of Bedlam* by Scull et al. (above), Elaine Showalter's *The Female Malady* (above) and Trevor Turner, 'Henry Maudsley – Psychiatrist, Philosopher and Entrepreneur' in *The Anatomy of Madness* (above).

On neurasthenia, see Edward Shorter, *From Paralysis to Fatigue* (New York: Free Press, 1993) and Janet Oppenheim, *Shattered Nerves* (Oxford: Oxford University Press 1991).

On the Bellevue sanatorium, Binswanger and Nijinsky, see Peter Ostwald's *Vaslav Nijinsky: A Leap into Madness* (New York: Lyle Stuart, 1991).

Ben Shephard's *A War of Nerves* (London: Jonathan Cape, 2000) is an excellent history of shell shock; see also Peter Barham, *Forgotten Lunatics of the Great War* (New Haven: Yale University Press, 2004) and Elaine Showalter, *The Female Malady* (above).

3. THE MENTAL HOSPITAL
—

On the early collectors of asylum art, see John M. MacGregor, *The Discovery of the Art of the Insane* (Princeton: Princeton University Press, 1989). Walther Morgenthaler's record of Wölfli is published in English as *Madness and Art: The Life and Works of Adolf Wölfli* (Lincoln: Nebraska University Press, 1992).

For contrasting views on the development of physical psychiatry in the early 20th century, see Edward Shorter, *A History of Psychiatry* (New York: John Wiley & Sons, 1997) and Andrew Scull, *Madness in Civilization* (above). Henry Cotton's career is examined in detail by Andrew Scull in *Madhouse* (New Haven and London: Yale University Press, 2007). The story of electroconvulsive therapy is told by Edward Shorter and David Healy in *Shock Therapy* (New Jersey: Rutgers University Press, 2007). On Artaud, see *Antonin Artaud: Man of Vision* (Chicago: Swallow Press, 1969) and Roy Porter, *A Social History of Madness* (above).

The story of Gould Farm is told in *Gould Farm: A Life of Sharing* by William McKee (Monterey, MA: Wm. J. Gould Associates, 1994).

On Mapother, Sargant, Lewis and the Maudsley Hospital in the 1930s, and for the text of Aubrey Lewis's Rockefeller Report of 1937, see *European Psychiatry on the Eve of War*, ed. Katherine Angel, Edgar Jones and Michael Neve (London: Wellcome Trust Centre for the History of Medicine at UCL, 2003). William Sargant relates his early career in his memoir *The Unquiet Mind* (London: William Heinemann, 1967).

Maxwell Jones discusses his early work in *Social Psychiatry: A Study of Therapeutic Communities* (London: Tavistock Publications, 1952), and the development of his ideas in 'The Therapeutic Community, Social Learning and Social Change', in *Therapeutic Communities: Reflections* and Progress, ed. R. D. Hinshelwood and Nick Manning (London: Routledge and Kegan Paul, 1979). His career is surveyed by D. W. Millard in 'Maxwell Jones and the Therapeutic Community', in 150 Years of British Psychiatry, ed. German Berrios and Hugh Freeman (London and New Jersey: Athlone Press, 1996).

On the discovery of antidepressants and antipsychotics, see The Rise of Psychopharmacology, ed. Thomas Ban, David Healy and Edward Shorter (Budapest: Animula, 1998) and David Healy, The Creation of Psychopharmacology (Cambridge, MA: Harvard University Press, 2002). For a critique of the biochemical claims made for them, see Joanna Moncrieff, The Myth of the Chemical Cure (New York: Palgrave Macmillan, 2004).

On psychiatry and the asylum in the movies, see Michael Fleming and Roger Manvell, Images of Madness: The Portrayal of Insanity in the Feature Film (London: Associated University Presses, 1985) and Stephen Farber and Marc Green, Hollywood on the Couch (New York: W. Morrow, 1993).

Andrea Tone's The Age of Anxiety (New York: Basic Books 2009) tells the story of Miltown and the impact of tranquillizers on American culture in the 1950s and 1960s. On the shift to medical prescription see David Healy, The Antidepressant Era (Cambridge, MA: Harvard University Press, 1997).

For a critical appraisal of Erving Goffman, Thomas Szasz, Michel Foucault and R. D. Laing, see Peter Sedgwick, Psycho Politics (London: Pluto Press, 1982). Norman Dain connects the antipsychiatry movement of the 1960s to earlier anti-medical traditions in 'Psychiatry and Anti-Psychiatry in the United States', in Discovering the History of Psychiatry (above). Szasz Under Fire (Chicago: Open Court, 2004) is a series of debates between Szasz and his critics, edited by Jeffrey Schaler. Foucault's work is critiqued in Rewriting the History of Madness, ed. Arthur Still and Irving Velody (London and New York: Routledge, 1992). On R. D. Laing, see Daniel Burston, The Wing of Madness (Cambridge, MA: Harvard University Press, 1998) and Elaine Showalter, The Female Malady (above).

On the closure of mental hospitals in the second half of the 20th century, see Andrew Scull, Decarceration (New Jersey: Prentice Hall, 1977) and Kathleen Jones, Asylums and After (London and New Jersey: Athlone Press, 1993). For a contemporary psychiatrist's perspective, see Tom Burns, Our Necessary Shadow (London: Allen Lane, 2013) and Oliver Sacks's essay 'The Lost Virtues of the Asylum' in The New York Review (September 24, 2009); for a patient's perspective, see Barbara Taylor, The Last Asylum (London: Hamish Hamilton, 2014).

The shift to community hospitals is discussed by Gerald Grob in From Asylum to Community (Princeton: Princeton University Press 1991) and Norman Dain in Discovering the History of Psychiatry (above). Kingsley Hall is documented in Peter Robinson's film Asylum (1972) and satirized as 'Meditation Manor' in the novel Zone of the Interior by R. D. Laing's former associate Clancy Sigal (New York: Thomas Y. Crowell Company, 1976).

On Franco Basaglia, see John Foot, The Man who Closed the Asylums (London: Verso, 2015) and Patrizia Guarnieri, 'The History of Psychiatry in Italy' in Discovering the History of Psychiatry (above).

4. BEYOND THE ASYLUM

—

The relationship between psychiatric medication and depression is analysed by David Healy in Let Them Eat Prozac (New York: New York University Press, 2004); Healy critiques the consequences of the modern prescription regime in Pharmageddon (Berkeley: University of California Press, 2012). See also Gary Greenberg, The Book of Woe (New York: Blue Rider Press, 2013) and 'Psychotropicana' by Mikkel Borch-Jacobsen in London Review of Books (11 July 2002).

For a lucid explanation of the role of the psychiatrist today, see Tom Burns, Our Necessary Shadow (above), which is also recommended as a readable history of psychiatry. There are many powerful and contrasting accounts of modern psychiatry from the patient's perspective. For a selection of recent books, see The Last Asylum by Barbara Taylor (above), which presents a personal memoir in parallel with a history of the asylum; Sectioned: A Life Interrupted by John O'Donoghue (London: John Murray, 2009); Henry's Demons by Patrick and Henry Cockburn (London: Simon & Schuster, 2011), which juxtaposes Henry's narrative of his mental breakdown with that of his father; and Imagining Robert by Jay Neugeboren (New York: William Morrow & Co, 1997), which describes a lifelong relationship with a brother with severe mental illness. There are many testimonies by those who have refused or abandoned psychiatric treatment, which can be found on activist sites such as igotbetter.org. The most influential advocate for this approach was Judi Chamberlin, who described her experience in On Our Own (London: MIND Publications, 1988).

The post-asylum world is considered by Sarah Payne in Outside the Walls of the Asylum, ed. Peter Bartlett and David Wright (London and New Brunswick: Athlone Press, 1999) and Kathleen Jones in Asylums and After (above).

The Philadelphia Association, which set up Kingsley Hall in 1965, still runs community homes that offer asylum for those in severe mental distress (www.philadelphia-association.org.uk). The Maytree, a charitable sanctuary in London for people in suicidal crisis, is profiled by Dara Mohammadi in 'Under the Maytree' (The Lancet, Vol. 2 No. 6, June 2015).

Present-day life in Geel is presented in the documentary film Geel (2007, Fish-Woestijnvis) and discussed in my article 'The Geel Question' (The Psychologist, Vol. 28 No. 9, September 2015).

In addition to William McKee's Gould Farm (above), see the website gouldfarm.org. For CooperRiis, see cooperriis.org.

254

ACKNOWLEDGMENTS

I wrote this book while developing and curating the Wellcome Collection exhibition *Bedlam: the asylum and beyond*. I'm very grateful to James Peto, the Wellcome's Head of Public Programmes, for his warm and generous support of my research throughout the process. Special thanks also to my co-curator on *Bedlam*, Bárbara Rodríguez Muñoz, who helped enormously with shaping these ideas and introduced me to so much fascinating material.

I've drawn heavily on the Wellcome Library and image collections, an unparalleled resource for the medical humanities in general and the history of madness in particular. I hope this book serves to highlight their richness. I received invaluable support from their staff during my researches: thanks in particular to Phoebe Harkins and Ross Macfarlane for their expert guidance in the early stages; to Crestina Forcina for assembling so many gems from the iconographic collection; to Stephen Lowther for enabling access to previously uncatalogued boxes of ephemera; and to Julia Nurse for her expertise and enthusiasm in unearthing early texts, manuscripts and book illustrations.

I'm very grateful to all the museums, hospitals, archives and other lenders who provided visual materials. My thanks in particular to Colin Gale, archivist at the Bethlem Art and History Collection Trust, and Bert Boeckx, archivist at Geel's psychiatric hospital, whose unique historical collections were essential to telling this story, and to Maria Rundle, for sharing stories and images from the history of Gould Farm. At Bethlem Hospital, I'd also like to thank Sukhinder Shergill and his team at the National Psychosis Unit for allowing me to observe their remarkable work, and Richard Morley for arranging access.

Special thanks to Andrew Scull, for taking the time to read an early draft of the manuscript and for his typically incisive comments; to Sarah Chaney, for sharing her prodigious knowledge of asylum history at an early stage; to Oliver Sacks, for introducing me to Gould Farm and much else besides; to Michael Neve, who has forgotten more about the history of madness than I will ever know; and as ever to Louise, for her boundless support and encouragement. I'm grateful to many others for conversations and insights along the way, including Rhodri Hayward, Nick Hervey, Rob Howard, James Leadbitter, John Marks, Victoria Northwood, Rowan Routh, Sonu Shamdasani, Victoria Tischler and Nick Tromans.

This book is the product of a remarkable team at Thames & Hudson: many thanks to Jane Laing, Tristan de Lancey and Maria Ranauro for their brilliant handling of its editing, design and pictures respectively. Thanks also to my agent Caroline Montgomery and to Kirty Topiwala, Publisher at Wellcome Collection, for their skill and commitment in helping to bring all the threads together.

Dedicated to Sarah Wheeler and Mental Fight Club, for furnishing such an inspiring example of what "care in the community" can and should mean.

This Way Madness Lies © 2016 Thames & Hudson Ltd, London

Text © 2016 Mike Jay

Design by Barnbrook

This book is published in partnership with Wellcome Collection for the exhibition "Bedlam: the asylum and beyond," curated by Mike Jay and Bárbara Rodríguez Muñoz, held at Wellcome Collection, London, from 15 September 2016 to 15 January 2017

www.wellcomecollection.org

wellcome collection

Wellcome Collection is the free visitor destination for the incurably curious. It explores the connections between medicine, life and art in the past, present and future. The Wellcome Trust is a global charitable foundation dedicated to improving health by supporting bright minds in science, the humanities and social sciences, and public engagement.

First published in 2016 in hardcover in the United States of America by Thames & Hudson Inc., 500 Fifth Avenue, New York, New York 10110

thamesandhudsonusa.com

Library of Congress Catalog Card Number 2016931244

ISBN 978-0-500-51897-7
Printed and bound in China by C&C Offset Printing Co. Ltd.

Cover artwork: Franz Joseph Kleber, *Plan of the Regensburg Institution, Kartause Prüll*, inv. 4506.
© Prinzhorn Collection, University Hospital Heidelberg

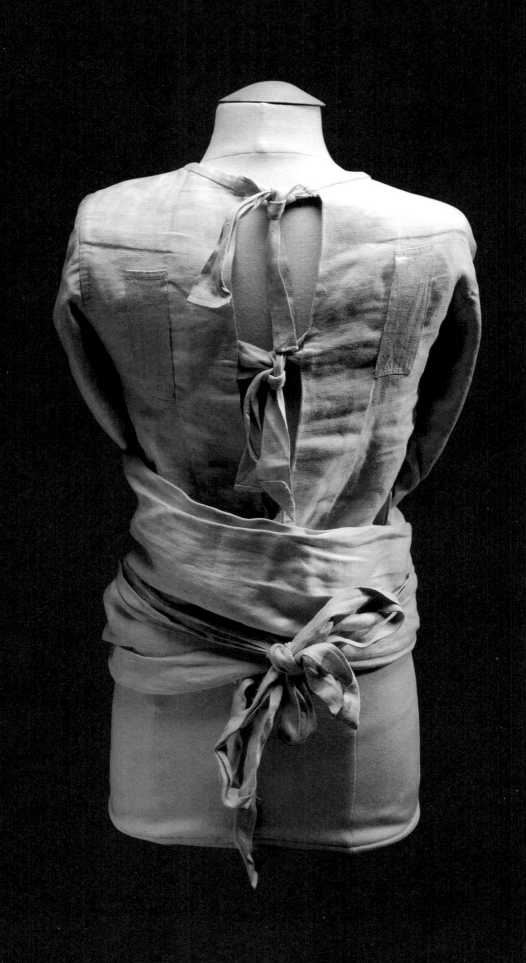

You Are Not
Forgotten

Also by Carol Jose . . .

Guerilla in Striped Pants: A U.S. Diplomat Joins the Italian Resistance
    with Walter Orebaugh
The Consul
The Sign of the Golden Grasshopper: A Biography of Sir Thomas Gresham
    with Perry Gresham
Evil Web: The True Story of Cult Abuse and Courage
    with Mary Rich
Saved by Love, A True Story
    with Evelyn Gaurino

You Are Not Forgotten

A Family's Quest for Truth and the Founding of
The National League of Families

Evelyn Grubb
and Carol Jose

Foreword by
Henry Kissinger

VANDAMERE
PRESS

Published by
Vandamere Press
P.O. Box 149
St. Petersburg, FL 33731
USA

ISBN 13   978-0-918339-71-3
ISBN 10   0-918339-71-5

Dedication

For Evelyn and Newk Grubb's sons: Jeffrey, Roland, Stephen, Roy, and their families.

For Evelyn's loved ones and friends, who remained steadfast through her ordeals and her life.

For the families, friends, and government officials who founded and aided the National League of Families of POW/MIA during the Vietnam War, and for the Veterans and dedicated Americans who have kept the POW/MIA flag flying high ever since.

For the National League of Families of POW/MIA—still active today.

For all who have served in our U.S. military forces and their families, our wounded veterans, and those who have gone to their eternal rest.

In loving memory of Evelyn Fowler Grubb, Lt. Colonel Wilmer Newlin "Newk" Grubb, and Captain Ray Harper . . .

We say from our hearts:

"Thank You—You Are Not Forgotten"

Advance Praise for
You Are Not Forgotten

Incredible events and great achievements are often the result of pure passion, determination, and great teamwork. You Are Not Forgotten *underscores this, and documents the indomitable power of the human spirit and family love to endure and triumph over adversity.* —The Honorable Jack Kemp, former Secretary of Housing and Urban Development, former Vice-Presidential Candidate, former U.S. Congressman

Reading this book, the memories came flooding back...those were tough times for all of us. Thank you for what you've done for the Grubb family, and for all of us, in recording this dark moment of our lives . . . and the history of the courage shown by our waiting families, that today still makes us proud. It's good to be free and back together again, in our own U.S.A. For those troops and POWs who gave their all, or are still missing, and their families, the POW/MIA flag and this riveting book tell it truthfully: you are not forgotten. —Marlene and Capt. John "Mike" McGrath, USN (Ret), POW/MIA historian, former Vietnam POW, author of *Prisoner of War: Six Years in Hanoi*

In You Are Not Forgotten, *you're along with them as Newk's wife Evie, my wife Helen, and thousands of wives and families of POW/MIA wage their incredible national and international battle to save, protect and repatriate captive and missing U.S. servicemen. From the depths of despair, the newly formed National League of Families of POW/MIA evolved into a force of great determination that had to be seriously considered in any negotiations. Their sacrifice should be a source of inspiration and enlightenment to all. They never gave up on us_and still haven't!* —Helen and Colonel Alan L. Brunstrom USAF (Retired), Newk Grubb's wingman, and a Vietnam POW 1966–1973

Over and over headlines have caused us to cry together. Ache together. We promise to remember, but move on as life moves on. The story doesn't move off the headlines into history, but into our hearts. Our days are spent determined to "live honoring America's fallen." Evelyn Grubb and Carol Jose's You Are Not Forgotten *is a poignant story of remembering those who live in history, reside in our hearts, and rest forever in the arms of God.* —Carmella LaSpada, Founder, No Greater Love

I found the book to be very gripping, with an astonishing amount of detail. We endured those times because, through the League, we were sharing our losses and fears together. —Joan Vinson, MIA widow, National Coordinator of the League of Families of MIA/POW, 1970–1971

Table of Contents

Acknowledgments

Sometimes it takes a village to birth a book. First, we thank Sybil Stockdale and salute the memory of her late husband, Vietnam POW and Medal of Honor recipient, Vice Admiral James Stockdale. Sybil began the National League of Families of POW/MIA in Southeast Asia, and aided Evelyn Grubb throughout their long ordeal. Sybil generously sent us documents and encouragement. She's a great lady in the truest sense.

Special thanks to the Ex-POWs, and their wives who were National League of Families activists: retired Air Force Colonels Al and Helen Brunstrom; Larry and Evelyn Guarino, John and Carolyn Finlay; retired Commander Paul and Phyllis Galanti; U.S. Navy retired Captain Mike and Marlene McGrath; and MIA widow Joan Vinson. All graciously helped with proofing, corrections, photos, and important information. Dedicated League members Joe McCain, William "Whitey" Lemmond, Carmella LaSpada, and Ann Mills Griffith, current Director of the League. Newk's boyhood buddy, author, and retired Air Force Sgt. Frank "Bud" Farrell and USAFR Colonel Sue Wisnom devoted many hours to finding facts, dates, and experts for us. Friends and family pitched in, too: Sarah Skirvin proofread, and did formatting and copyediting; Ivonne Isaias and Linda Downie read drafts, sorted and filed stacks of reference materials, papers, and letters; Evie's sons Roland, Van, Roy and wife Tina lugged boxes, unearthed photos, answered questions; Jeff and Elise Grubb provided photos, support, and the index. Mike Daly of CSI Creative Solutions, Inc. offered a strong shoulder and his PR expertise; CSI graphic arts wizard Scott Patrick worked magic with old photos, and created publicity pieces; and Matt Lutz of AP sleuthed out a very important photo. Retired U.S. Army Colonel Andy Byers, author of *The Imperfect Spy,* introduced me to Art Brown of Vandamere Press, whose faith in the manuscript and wise counsel have been an inspiration. Editor Pat Berger strengthened the book, and Victor Weaver created our book and cover design. Deepest gratitude also goes to a "wolf pack" of retired military experts, all combat veterans of Vietnam: USAF "Misty" fighter pilots Maj. General Don Shepperd, and Colonel Don Jones; U.S. Army Colonels Tom Delahunty, Todd Poch, and Gary Greenfield; and fiction author and Air Force Lt. Colonel Maynard Allington. Additional help came from my brother and retired U.S. Navy Chief Richard Lanza, and nephew, USCG pilot LCDR Craig O'Brien. As did these special people: Patsy Ketchum, Anita Greenfield, Lucylee Chiles, Sheila Delahunty, Dr. James Jacobson, John and Barbara O'Brien MSN, Joan Clawson, Ro and Don Thomas, Conrad Ottenhoff, and fellow authors Anna Flowers, Carolyn Cain, John Gourley, retired Air Force Lt. Colonel Eric Neitzke—so many friends, readers, and cheerleaders, kept me going, and Evie's memory alive.

Last . . . but definitely not least . . . my profound gratitude to Suzanne McFarlane, Executive Assistant to Henry Kissinger, to Dr. Kissinger for graciously writing the inspiring Foreword, and to my patient husband through all, Navy veteran Dale Jose.

This one's for Evie, her Newk, all American POW/MIA/KIA, and their brave and loving families. You have our deep respect, and thanks.

Preface

The story told here is but one aspect of my long and varied life. I have been girl and coed; wife and widow; mother and grandmother. I have experienced the depths of pain, the heights of joy, and I have drunk from the deep well of sorrow. I know personally about despair and frustration, loneliness, heart disease, cancer, and the tragic loss of family members and dear friends. Through it all, I have learned that the roughest experiences of life do toughen us up. They strengthen our spirit and solidify our determination to survive and overcome, but they do not make us immortal. It is important to preserve history in order to learn from it. My story is part of the national history of the United States of America and its military families during the Vietnam War era. I hope and believe that much can be learned today from this true account of my family's deep, albeit reluctant, encounter with that history, and the preserving of it in this book. **Evelyn Fowler Grubb, December 2005**

On December 28, 2005, before we were able to complete *You Are Not Forgotten*, my co-author and friend, Evelyn Grubb, passed away after a fight with cancer. I feel privileged to have worked with this amazing woman and to have helped her tell this powerful story. **Carol Jose, May 2008**

Foreword

The National League of Families of POW/MIA was, and remains, an organization very dear to my heart. During my years as National Security Adviser to President Nixon, and while serving as Secretary of State in the Nixon and Ford administrations, I came to know many of the concerned family members of American servicemen Missing in Action or being held as Prisoners of War during the Vietnam War. The courage, tenacity, and determination of these families to gain knowledge about their family member, to invoke the tenets of the Geneva Convention on humane treatment of prisoners, and to demand an accounting for them and the men missing in action, soon won my deep respect.

Often the greatest human sacrifices, and the most heroic deeds of humankind, are buried in the heat and dust of battle—or lost to history with the passing of the lives of those who experienced them. Fortunately, the preservation of the story of one such American family, and with it the recording of the genesis and growth of the National League of Families of POW/MIA, is accomplished in *You Are Not Forgotten*, as seen through the eyes of POW wife Evelyn Grubb. Following the photographed and publicized capture of her Air Force pilot husband, Captain Wilmer Newlin Grubb, in North Vietnam, Evelyn became closely involved with the formation of the League, and with the plight of the POWs and MIAs of the Vietnam War, and their anxious families. The attitude of these women was inspirational.

The League's mission, then as now, was dedicated to giving national and international voice to the plight of the POW/MIA of the Vietnam War, the longest war in American history. Many American POWs were held in barbaric conditions, suffering unspeakable deprivation and torture, some for more than seven years. Sixty-five American fighting men would perish while prisoners in those camps; many more Americans remained among the missing. With all their suffering, these women never lost faith in their government. They were deeply concerned but never permitted themselves to be influenced by pressure groups seeking to use their suffering.

When President Nixon appointed me as his National Security Adviser in 1969, I became his principal advisor on policy for extrication from Vietnam, and eventually the chief negotiator of the peace Agreement with the North Vietnamese. My Vietnamese counterparts were difficult, largely intractable negotiators. That meant that, much like our experience with the negotiations, the road for these families was destined to be a very long, difficult and frustrating one to travel, rougher by far than I imagined when I started on the task.

Sadly, we could not give them any guarantee in terms of a timetable for reaching the peace with honor that we all sought. But we were inspired by their fortitude to persevere.

In the course of negotiations with North Vietnamese Prime Minister Pham Van Dong, our discussions of the American soldiers and airmen who were prisoners of war or missing in action were frustrating. We knew of specific instances in which an American serviceman had been captured alive and had subsequently disappeared. The evidence consisted of either voice communications from the ground in advance of capture, or photographs and names published by the Communists. Yet none of these men was on the list of POWs handed over after the agreement was finally signed. I questioned him on this when I was in Hanoi in February 1973. Why? Were they dead? How did they die? Were they missing? How was that possible after capture? I called special attention to the nineteen cases where pictures of the captured had been published in the Communist press. (USAF Lt. Col. Wilmer Newlin "Newk" Grubb, was one of them.) Pham Van Dong replied noncommittally that the lists handed over to us were complete. He made no attempt to explain discrepancies.

We have not, at this writing more than three decades later, received an explanation of what could possibly have happened to prisoners whose pictures had appeared in Communist newspapers or to the airmen who we knew from voice communications had safely reached the ground.

No war since the Civil War in the United States has seared and divided the national consciousness to the extent that Vietnam did. Have there been answers to these complex questions posed by our involvement in Vietnam for nearly two decades?

Perhaps the reflections of President Abraham Lincoln near the end of the Civil War, in November 1864, might serve as a response:

> Let us, therefore, study the incidents of this, as philosophy
> to learn wisdom from, and none of them as wrongs to be
> revenged.

It is only through the recording of incidents like the ones you will read about here, in the pages of *You Are Not Forgotten,* that we can study them, and hopefully learn from that experience.

Henry A. Kissinger

1 The Taxi Driver

TIMELINE . . . 1966 . . . <u>WORLD</u> . . . UNMANNED SOVIET SPACESHIP MAKES SUCCESSFUL SOFT LANDING ON MOON . . . INDIRA GHANDI NAMED PRIME MINISTER OF INDIA . . . <u>VIETNAM</u> . . . PRESIDENT JOHNSON ENDS CEASE-FIRE JANUARY 31 . . . <u>USA</u> . . . SURVEYOR 1 MAKES SOFT LANDING ON MOON . . . CASSIUS CLAY HEAVYWEIGHT BOXING CHAMPION . . . BILLY CASPER WINS U.S. OPEN IN GOLF . . .

Nobody likes the man who brings bad news. —Sophocles

The volcano of the Vietnam War erupted on us in late January 1966 when we were in the middle of a blizzard in northern Virginia. I woke that morning to quite an accumulation of snow on the ground. Snowflakes were still coming down thick and fast. As I belted my robe across my expanding midsection, I felt the little one flutter slightly, just below my heart.

"Well, and good morning to you, too, Tinkerbell," I murmured, and sat down to drink my morning orange juice. Heidi, our four-month-old beagle pup, plopped down at my feet and started chewing on the toe of one of my slippers.

"Stop that, you silly pup!"

I smiled at her surprised look. Pulling my foot (and slipper) away, I got up and switched on the television to get the latest news. The reporter informed us that the blizzard was snarling traffic in and around Washington, D.C. He advised viewers that anyone who didn't absolutely need to go into the city today should stay home. A few snowflakes could bring our nation's capital, and with it our government, almost to a standstill. Things were not going well with the war in Vietnam either. In two minutes, I'd listened to enough discouraging reporting to ruin my day, so I switched the television off.

I knew that our three boys would be waking up soon, and the house would reverberate with kids' noise and activity. Reveling in a

1

brief period of hushed solitude on this snowy winter morning, I
went to peer out the window. A male cardinal perched on a snow-
clad branch of the leafless maple tree. He added a slash of bright
red to the spotless white wonderland our yard had become
overnight. Looking toward the road, I saw that no cars were moving on our street. There was snow piled atop the few I could see
parked by the curb, and neither the neighbors' driveways, nor the
road, showed any sign that anyone had been up and moving about
yet. That concerned me because with all that snow, and no snow-
plows out so far, there might not be a mail delivery today. That
would mean another day without any news from my husband,
"Newk," a U.S. Air Force pilot. Newk (officially Captain Wilmer
Newlin Grubb) was away, stationed in Saigon, the capital of South
Vietnam, flying reconnaissance missions in an RF-101.

In his last voice tape to us, he said he had just returned to
Saigon from his recent R&R (Rest and Recuperation) leave in
Okinawa. He had been flying a lot of "out of country" missions
lately, which he felt was good, though of course that worried me.
Out of country meant he was flying over hostile territories like
Cambodia, Laos, and North Vietnam. However, it also meant that
he'd soon wrap up his quota of 100 missions and could return home
to us. Newk was a career military pilot doing his job, and we were
at home doing ours. I was managing the kids and the home fires,
and we were keeping up his morale with cards, photos and tapes—
marking the days off the calendar until he would come home again,
and we could resume a somewhat normal life together.

This was his second assignment to Southeast Asia. The last one
had been a shorter stint away from us, flying missions out of
Thailand. Our oldest son Jeff, nine, had found the countries over
which his Dad was flying his reconnaissance missions now. Using
Newk's desk globe, he patiently pointed them all out to his two
younger brothers—Roland ("Roke"), four, and Stephen ("Van"),
two and a half. He'd point to Vietnam and patiently explain,
"Here's where Daddy is living, and where he mails his tapes and letters to us," he'd say. Then, drawing his finger along while turning
the globe, he'd tap Virginia on the map of the United States and tell
them, "and here's where we are, in Petersburg, Virginia, until Daddy
comes home." No sooner would Jeff put his finger on our home area

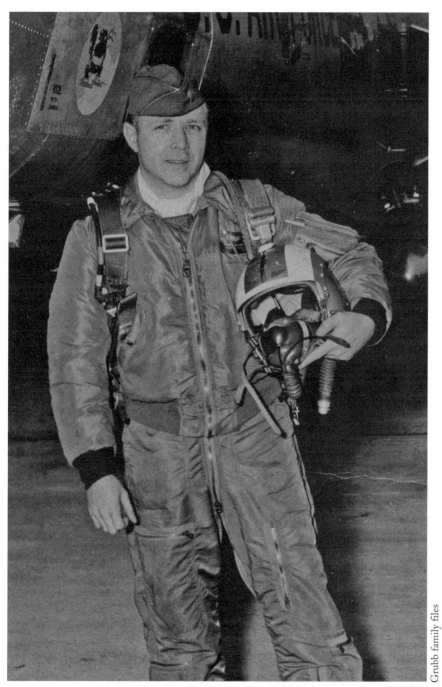

1st Lt. Wilmer Newlin "Newk" Grubb, USAF pilot, and the RF–101 Voodoo reconnaissance jet he flew, Laon AB, France, circa 1962.

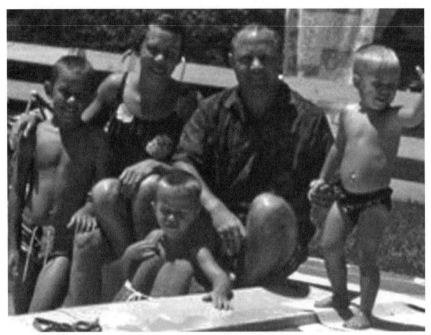

Newk, Evie and sons Jeff, Van, Roland, Summer 1965.

than Van would start chanting, "Daddy . . . Daddy! I want my Daddy to come home."

Van really missed his Daddy. Like Newk, Van was dedicated to the outdoors. He loved going fishing and hiking with his Dad and big brothers.

Well, Van wasn't alone—we all missed Newk. I was counting every month, every day, almost every hour until he came home again. Managing three energetic little boys alone every day, plus a new puppy and an unexpected but welcome pregnancy, was no picnic on the best of days. The last two things had been added just before Newk left—his "surprise" farewell gifts.

In Saigon, Newk and his buddies also were counting the days, ticking off missions as they negotiated the minefield of uncertainty that defined their role in this war. In an earlier tape to us, Newk had said,

> We've been apart three months now . . . seems like longer. Wish I had some of your Christmas cookies left . . . I still haven't gotten your letter you said you mailed me in mid-

December, with the promotion list enclosed . . . are you sure you mailed it? I'll be home as soon as I can, Sweetheart, soon as we do the job we have to do here. I'm counting the missions, and the hours . . . I love you, and the boys. Hug them and little Tinkerbell for me, and scratch Heidi's ears, so they don't forget me.[1]

I had written him about my pregnancy as soon as I found out. We were both from small families. I had only one sibling, my brother Bill. Newk had one sister, Beverly. We loved kids and wanted a big family. We'd talked about "at least six" kids. The way I felt this morning, "Tinkerbell"—our fourth child—would be plenty for me.

In Saigon, Newk returned from his missions to a rented French villa, where he shared a bedroom with three squadron mates. After every flight, they ripped another page off their mission calendars. I went to a drawer and pulled out a photo he had sent me recently. It made me smile. Newk had decided to grow a moustache again. I kept this picture in the kitchen drawer because of the art that was displayed on the wall behind him. It was the usual "guys away at war" decor—a collage of pin-up pictures of naked and nearly naked women torn from the more daring men's magazines.

We believed Newk would be home well before the new baby arrived in late July. Newk was surprised and delighted about our "Tinkerbell." He thought he'd left me with only the three boys and Heidi, the new puppy. Hah! As my thoughts turned to the boys, I realized school would definitely be closed today. That meant that Jeff would be home and could help me. He'd take Heidi the puppy and Van out to play in the snow. Four-year-old Roke was covered with chicken pox, and I knew he'd stage a major uproar when he learned he couldn't join his brothers outdoors. I sighed, then decided Roke's treat would be to listen to Daddy's last tape again, and help me get everything ready to make another to send him. It was a novelty for us to be sending and receiving talking letters instead of written ones. The tapes kept Newk closer to us. It was important for the boys to hear their Daddy's voice, and hearing it certainly was helping me get through this long separation we faced. It wasn't the first, and we knew that with the usual military routine, it wouldn't be the last.

Military life kept Newk away a lot. Often we couldn't go along, so we shared our lives by letter or tape to bridge those long and frustrating absences. There was so much of the "business" of family life to discuss and decide on: the day-to-day questions to be answered, like the kids' needs, or mine; the management of our separate finances; but most of all, tapes allowed us the simple pleasure of being a loving couple needing personal, occasionally intimate, conversation. Tape recordings also gave him the pleasure of hearing our voices over there. It was great for the kids, who grew so fast and changed so much while he was gone from them. Taping was better than letters on paper . . . or nothing. Live overseas telephone calls were usually difficult to arrange, and much too expensive. Personal calls to a war zone, where Newk was now, were impossible to contemplate except possibly for an extreme emergency, and even then there was no guarantee of success. I went over and clicked on the tape player to replay Newk's latest tape. Hearing his familiar deep, soft voice made my heart constrict with longing and wanting him, but it also calmed my nerves when I needed that.

> Hey there . . . it's me. I got three wonderful letters today, one from Mom and Dad, and I finally did get yours from the 17th of December with the Majors' list. I was glad to see that Charlie Shelton, who got shot down over Laos, was on the list . . . The other guys all got letters from around that same date, too, so I guess a sack of mail must have gotten lost somewhere for awhile . . . Wouldn't you know it would be just at Christmas time, when we're all so lonely and hungry for mail from home? I got your January 6th letter, too, at the same time. Hon, on the money question you had, I really don't like the policy of the bank not telling you in detail what deposits I'm making from here to our account each month—you should get a full detailed statement, and I'll write them and tell them so. Wish you could meet me for R&R in Okinawa next week . . . but I know it's just wishful thinking . . . I do a lot of that where you're concerned, as you know . . . I love you, and wish I could climb right into the envelope with this when I send it and be there with it when it arrives. Give my love to the boys. I'll be

home just as soon as I can, Sweetheart. I just can't tell you enough how much I miss you and love you, today, tomorrow, the next day and the next, ad infinitum, as you said in your letter . . . We'll get together again, one of these days soon, darling. I have to get up at 6 a.m. and so I'd better say goodnight and tell you again how much I love you all and miss you . . . Goodnight Evie, I love you . . . mwuh . . . . mwuh . . . mwuh![2]

I couldn't help smiling, remembering what had come just before that fond good-night and those kissy sounds—words that were for me alone. I knew he counted on me to listen to his tapes first, and edit them to erase any deeply personal commentary before playing them for the kids or our parents to hear.

I had settled on Petersburg, Virginia, to live while Newk was in Vietnam, to be closer to my mother and brother Bill. Also, Newk's parents were not far away, in Pennsylvania, and could visit us more often. Newk's sister Beverly, a missionary in Alaska, was the only family member who lived far away from all of us.

The house we had rented in Petersburg was small, cozy, and in a nice residential area. When Newk came back in a few months, we'd move to a new base and into bigger living quarters. We hoped we'd be assigned somewhere that offered plenty of outdoor activities we could enjoy as a family, like Mountain Home Air Force Base in Idaho.

In the meantime, being near my mother was a tremendous help to me. Dad had died ten years ago, so she was glad to have the boys and me nearby for company as well. I knew that helping me deal with them, and our pets, wasn't easy for her, but she was always willing, always there for me, and my brother and his wife Norma were, too. Even so, I deeply missed the camaraderie of our military friends and the lifestyle of being on a military base. Now I felt left out of the channel, and missed the "insider" news we always passed around at a base.

My pregnancy was progressing well, but it also brought mood changes, and my emotions stayed close to the surface. I couldn't wait to have Newk home again, to help me with the boys, the new baby, and the day-to-day problems. Actually, I needed and wanted his capable hands there in the evenings, and his strong arms wrapped around me at night. I needed more than just a voice on tape warming my ears. I wanted Newk—all of him, all that he was to us. We missed him terribly.

By the time I got the boys up and through the morning, and we'd finished lunch, Jeff and Van were worn out, and so was I. No wonder! They had spent the whole morning outside, playing in the snow with the neighborhood kids. Despite the chicken pox, I'd finally given in and let Roke go out long enough to help build the neighborhood snow fort. Now he was tired, whiny and cranky, and itching badly from the chicken pox.

"I think we all could use a nap," I declared, clearing the table. "Roke, you can come in and snuggle up with me. Then, later this afternoon, we'll make a tape for Daddy."

They all cheered up at that idea. Then, someone rapping hard at the front door startled us.

"Who could that be, on a day like this?" I grumbled.

I went to the door and opened it. The blast of cold air momen-

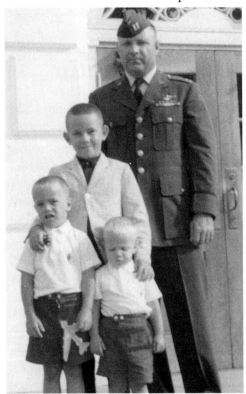

Capt. Newk Grubb with Jeff, Van, and Roland; Virginia, 1965.

tarily stunned me. Standing on the front porch was a stranger — a short, stocky man, all bundled up in a heavy jacket, scarf and gloves, holding a yellow envelope in his hand. Snowflakes were melting into beads of water on the dark blue beret he wore. A quick glance beyond him to the street revealed a taxicab with its engine still running at the curb in front of the house, and its top light on. He was probably lost en route to pick someone up. I smiled at him.

"Hello, there. Are you lost?"

"No. I have a telegram to deliver to Mrs. Wilmer Grubb. Is that you?" he asked.

I nodded yes, but my mind had frozen up on the word "telegram." TELEGRAM! It struck me like a physical blow. *Newk! Oh, God, No!*

"No, no, no, go away!" I shouted. "I know what that is. I don't want it! Just go!"

I hugged myself, bent over in agony, dizzy. I could dimly hear Jeff calling to me, "Mom, Mom, what is it? What does he want?"

The taxi driver stood there in the open doorway, holding out the telegram.

"I don't know what this is, but it says it's for Mrs. Wilmer Grubb. Please take it. It's for you, lady."

My mind was exploding in fragments of colors, thoughts, and memories . . . flash, flash, flash. They were going off like neon signs in my head.

Newk is dead. If I touch that telegram, Newk is dead.

"Not Newk, oh God, please, not Newk," I moaned.

"Look, can I maybe call somebody . . . a neighbor or someone, Missus? Look, you don't know what it is; you haven't even opened it yet. Maybe it's okay, eh? Please, if you could just sign here . . . " He held out a small card he'd pulled from his pocket.

"I already know what it says, so just go away!" *Why wouldn't this man leave? Why couldn't it be five minutes ago forever . . . ?*

Suddenly the colors stopped flashing in my head. I could see clearly again. *No. Newk just got back to Saigon from Okinawa; they wouldn't send him on a mission yet, He just got back there. He can't be dead. We're going to have a baby.*

It was like I was two people. One was watching what was going on. My other self was curled in a chair, protecting my stomach, avoiding all.

"Mom, Mom, what is it? Are you sick? Is it the baby? I'll get Mrs. Billingsley." Jeff ran past the man and down the front walk. I wanted to call for him to come back and get a jacket on, but I couldn't speak. Then Roke and Van were there, staring up at me, and they both started to cry.

The other me saw the neighbors from next door, the Billingsleys, young newlyweds, run up to the front porch with Jeff. They began talking to the taxi driver, who was still holding the yellow envelope and the signature card, looking confused.

The other me moved and spoke, calm and quiet, like a robot. "Here, I'll take it." That person crossed over to the man, took the envelope, and mechanically signed for it.

"Oh, I'm so sorry lady. This isn't fair!" he exclaimed, "I'm just a taxi driver, why me?" He muttered, "Never again! I quit!" and with that, he turned away and hurried back to his taxi, and drove off as if in slow motion, through the snow.

Meanwhile, the robot me tore open the envelope, while the other me—the one curled and hiding somewhere deep inside—screamed "NO, please!" But the robot me read every word of that telegram. It was all in capital letters that fairly shouted,

> "IT IS WITH DEEP REGRET THAT I OFFICIALLY
> INFORM YOU . . ."

Those words plunged the real me into a heart-constricting, pulse-pounding, flaming private hell. The robot me stood there and doggedly read on, each word a knife thrust into my heart.

> . . . THAT YOUR HUSBAND, CAPTAIN WILMER N.
> GRUBB, HAS BEEN MISSING IN A FLIGHT SINCE 26
> JANUARY, 1966, IN HOSTILE TERRITORY OVER
> NORTH VIETNAM WHILE ON AN OPERATIONAL
> MISSION.
>
> EXTENSIVE SEARCH IS NOW BEING CON-
> DUCTED. IT IS POSSIBLE THAT YOUR HUSBAND
> COULD HAVE BEEN TAKEN CAPTIVE BY HOSTILE
> FORCES BECAUSE OF THE AREA IN WHICH HE IS
> MISSING. IF THIS IS TRUE, IT IS SUGGESTED THAT
> IN REPLY TO INQUIRIES FROM SOURCES OUT-

SIDE YOUR IMMEDIATE FAMILY, FOR HIS WEL-
FARE, YOU REVEAL ONLY HIS NAME, RANK, SER-
VICE NUMBER AND DATE OF BIRTH . . . . WHEN
FURTHER INFORMATION IS RECEIVED, YOU
WILL BE NOTIFIED IMMEDIATELY . . . . A REPRE-
SENTATIVE FROM A NEARBY AIR FORCE BASE
WILL CALL ON YOU AS SOON AS THEY RECEIVE
THE OFFICIAL MISSING REPORT. SHOULD YOU
DESIRE ADDITIONAL INFORMATION, YOU MAY
CONTACT MY DUTY OFFICER . . .

PLEASE ACCEPT MY SINCERE SYMPATHY
IN THIS TIME OF ANXIETY.

MAJOR GENERAL G. B. GREENE, JR
ASSISTANT DEPUTY CHIEF OF STAFF, PERSON-
NEL, FOR MILITARY PERSONNEL, HEADQUAR-
TERS, UNITED STATES AIR FORCE.[3]

"Ohhhhh, not Newk. Poor Newk!" I cried aloud.

My two selves had merged into one again. Someone had gotten me to the couch and forced me to lie down.

"Poor Newk! Where are you now? Will we ever see you again?"

The room was eerily silent or else I was muffled in cotton wool and couldn't hear. Anne Billingsley, with Jeff's help, was putting the two little boys into their coats. Her husband started phoning other neighbors. The Wilsons from next door came, gathered my children together and took them home with them. The Billingsleys stayed with me.

I dragged myself up from the couch. I knew I needed to call my mother. I got her on the second ring, and just blurted out the awful news.

"Oh, Mother, I hate to tell you this, but I just got a telegram that Newk's plane was shot down, and he is missing."

"Oh Evie . . . oh dear . . . how terrible . . . I just can't believe this! Our dear, dear Newk! How awful for you, and the children. Hang on. I'll be right over."

"No . . . . please don't come if you're still not feeling well, Mother. The neighbors are here to help me. I don't want you catching more cold right now." She was just recovering from a nasty winter cold.

"Now, don't you worry about me, Evie. I'm not that sick that I can't come. I've been through a lot in my life. I can handle almost anything. I want to be with you and the boys. We'll get through this together, dear. Are the children all right?"

"Yes, they're at the Wilson's. Mother, Rob said he'll walk over to get you, so wait there for him, please. It's icy on the sidewalks. I don't want you to slip and fall."

When I hung up from talking to Mother, I called Mother and Dad Grubb, Newk's parents. They lived in Pennsylvania. I learned that they'd already heard the bad news. An Air Force officer had just left, after coming there to inform them. We offered each other mutual support but kept our conversation brief. We were now switching into a different mode, hoping and waiting for a follow-up call, either from Newk or the Air Force, to tell us that he'd been rescued and was safe.

Rob arrived with Mother. Then two military wives in the area with whom I was acquainted showed up. Their husbands were overseas, too, and they had come to do whatever they could to help me.

"Evie, please lie down for a little bit. You're white as a sheet," Mother said.

I tried to rest on the couch again. The phone kept ringing, and every time someone went to answer it, I'd jerk myself up, and call out, "Please . . . make it quick! We need to keep the phone line free! Newk might be trying to call me!"

I was truly frantic about anyone using the phone, because in my mind I was certain that Newk would be calling me "any minute now," as I said over and over to everyone. I willed him to call and tell me it had all been a mistake, that he was all right, and he would be coming home soon. It was an obsession—a fantasy of denial that I would cling to for weeks.

In what was probably a primitive protective shield, I simply couldn't permit the idea that Newk might be gone from our lives to register. The closest I'd come to it was when I thought about that taxi driver. I actually hated him, and I didn't even know him. What a horrible job he had, delivering telegrams like that. I kept praying out loud,

"Oh God, please let it not be true. Bring Newk back home." It was a mantra I'd repeat often over the next few weeks.

At the Wilson's, I learned later, the children were sitting down to a spaghetti dinner. Everyone there tried to keep the conversation light, but at one point Roke blurted out, very seriously,

"My Daddy is in a bad country and he doesn't have any money."

Startled, Betty Wilson asked, "What do you mean, Roke?"

"My Daddy's airplane was shot down, and he doesn't have any money!"

"Whatever gave you the idea that he hasn't any money, Roke?"

"Mommy . . . she said, 'Poor Newk, poor Newk!' "

A Note About Endnotes . . .
Grubb family originated correspondence, notes, and records excerpted or quoted in the balance of the book may be found in the Grubb family files unless otherwise indicated.

2 "With All My Heart . . ."

TIMELINE . . . 1950–1965 . . . <u>WORLD</u> . . . "COLD WAR" PERSISTS . . . KOREAN WAR . . . BERLIN WALL GOES UP . . . CASTRO TAKES OVER CUBA . . . VIETNAM SIGNS GENEVA CONVENTIONS . . . FRENCH DEFEATED AT DIEN BIEN PHU . . . <u>USA</u> . . . POST WWII BABY BOOM BEGINS . . . ELVIS, BUDDY HOLLY, BEATLES BRING ROCK AND ROLL . . . UNITED STATES SENDS MILITARY ADVISORS TO SOUTH VIETNAM . . . PRESIDENT KENNEDY ASSAS-SINATED . . . OSCAR WINNING FILMS INCLUDE *GOING MY WAY, SINGIN' IN THE RAIN, THE SOUND OF MUSIC* . . .

Time is dead as long as it is being clicked off by little wheels; only when the clock stops does time come to life. —Thornton Wilder

Although we had heard about each other all our lives, Newk and I didn't meet in person until we were both college students at Penn State University in 1951. Both our fathers and Newk's Uncle Roke were Penn State alumni and fraternity brothers in Alpha Chi Ro (AXP). They had remained close friends all their lives and attended homecoming at Penn State every year. Newk and I knew all about each other through them. So I felt comfortable calling Newk to ask him if he could arrange a date with one of his fraternity brothers for his Uncle Roke's daughter Betsy, who would be coming to Penn State with her parents for the 1951 Homecoming festivities. Newk sounded affable with a pleasant voice.

"Sure . . . I'll get her a date, Evie. What about you? Would you consider being my date? I've been wanting to meet you for a long time. I know a lot about you, as I'm sure you can imagine."

We both laughed. "Yes, I can imagine. Sure . . . I'll be your date, Newk. I've wanted to meet you, too."

"Well, great! I'll pick you both up on Saturday, okay?"

Wilmer Newlin Grubb, or "Newk" as everyone called him, turned out to be a really handsome guy. He had blonde hair, a cute nose, and a captivating smile. He was unpretentious, and like me, he loved kids, dogs, fishing, and the outdoor life. He was also sensitive, surprisingly romantic, and much more sentimental than I. He had the most mesmerizing deep blue eyes with thick, almost

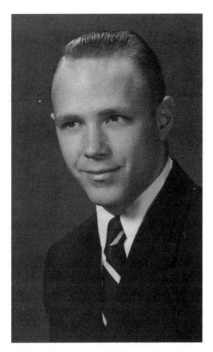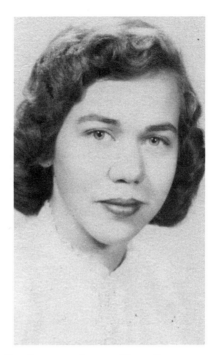

Wilmer N. "Newk" Grubb and Evelyn Fowler as students at Penn State, University, 1951.

double eyelashes, and bushy blond eyebrows. He was very athletic. He not only had a strong body, he had great strength of character, as I soon discovered. Because we were already somewhat familiar with one another through our families, Newk and I hit it off well on our first date, and were comfortable together. He was delighted that I liked the outdoors as much as he did. We had a lot of fun at homecoming and the dance afterward.

I think it was those eyes—honest, straightforward, but with a merry twinkle when he smiled—that first attracted me. He had a great sense of humor, too. He was never sarcastic. I found that he was mostly even-tempered. I also learned later that when angry, which was seldom, Newk could be formidable.

I was much more temperamental by nature, never afraid to say just what I meant or speak my mind when I was challenged. That was not always a good thing. My parents indulged my insatiable curiosity, too. Learning and experiencing new things continued to interest me all my life. When Newk and I first met that Saturday I was twenty. I had shoulder-length brown hair, blue eyes, and what was considered an attractive figure.

We started out as friends, but soon it became more than that. I loved the outdoors, and when I was growing up, we often went camping, fishing, and walking through the woods. So Newk started calling me "Jo," after the irrepressible tomboy sister from *Little Women.*

We attended the ROTC Military Ball together. In my senior year Newk gave me his fraternity pin. Being "pinned" meant you were serious. It was then that we began talking about "probably" getting married "some day."

During the summer break from school in 1952 we were working in different states. That was when our letter-writing career began. Newk wrote more often, and his letters were a great deal more openly romantic than mine. I still have this one from that summer:

> August 14, 1952
> Dearest Jo,
>
> Everything is wonderful, sweetheart. I love you with all my heart. I want you to wait until I get a start in life. Then I want you to marry me, Jo. I want you to be mine for the rest of our lives. Please don't answer yet, Darling. Just stay the way you are, and love me always. I'll try to be kind to you, honey, if you want me. I can't write letters very well, Jo, but my heart won't let me hold back the joy that is within.
>
> Yes, today is my birthday. I was hoping you would be here, but I guess you just can't make it. I love you Jo; I'll never get tired of saying so. I love you.
> Good night,
> Newk

When I received that note, any little insecurities I'd ever felt about us as a couple vanished. There was no need to set a wedding date yet, the future was ours. What I didn't reckon with was Newk's impulsive, romantic nature or his determination once he'd made up his mind about something. A few weeks later, we were at Niagara Falls.

"Let's go look at the falls from the bridge," Newk suggested one evening. Colored spotlights shining on the roaring falls created a thousand twinkling rainbow hues in that amazing backdrop—a fairyland atmosphere that was unbelievably beautiful and romantic. When we reached the middle of the bridge, Newk stopped, took me in his arms and kissed me. Then he said,

"I love you. I want us to get married soon, Jo. There's no sense waiting. We're sure this is it for both of us so why wait? I know it will be a financial struggle with both of us still in school. If our parents will continue helping us we'll get along fine. We can get part-time jobs. We'll manage somehow, you'll see."

I could read the strength of his feelings in his eyes. I said, "Yes." In April of 1953, during our spring break from school we were married. It was a simple but lovely ceremony at the United Presbyterian Church near my home in Pittsburgh. Both immediate families, plus myriad relatives and college friends were in attendance. When Newk's Uncle Roke came through the receiving line at the reception, he eyed us both and said,

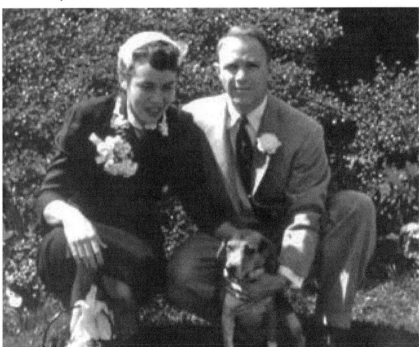

Newk and Evelyn on their wedding day with "Dandy," their beagle, April 1953.

"You two have a marriage made in heaven. Don't ever let it go to hell."

My father added, "You are always welcome to visit us any time, but your home now is with each other." Then, ever practical, he said, with a smile, "We hope marriage will improve your grades."

It did. I was graduated from Penn State University with honors and a B.S. in Art Education in August 1953, but Newk still had a year to go before he'd graduate. Unfortunately for me, there were no art teaching positions available in the Penn State area that fall. My father, wise in so many ways, but definitely of the persuasion that the man earned the living for the family, offered to finance another year for me to get my master's degree, which would allow Newk and me to remain together at Penn State

"I want your children to have a well-educated father *and* mother," he said. "I'm sure Newk will provide for you and I hope you'll never need your education to earn a living, Evie, but if that time ever comes I want you to be prepared."

Those early months and years of our marriage were a financial struggle every day. I also discovered that Newk had another passion

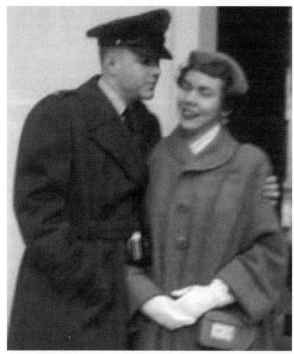

Newk and Evie at Newk's graduation from ROTC as an Air Force 2nd Lieutenant.

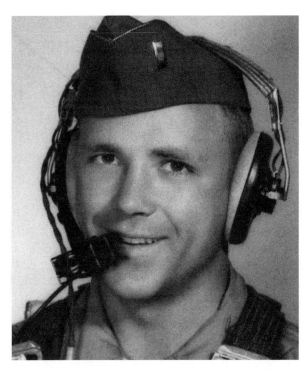

Lt. Newk Grubb, Air Force pilot, Mission, Texas, 1956.

besides me. He wanted to fly, to be a pilot. He had cherished that dream ever since he was a kid. Having been in the Air Force ROTC at Penn State he easily passed all the requirements for entering flight training following graduation.

In February of 1955, Newk received his B.S. degree in Agricultural Economics, and I got my M.A. in Education. Both sets of proud parents, and Newk's Uncle Roke, were in attendance at our graduation.

Later that same weekend, his mother and I pinned gold second lieutenant's bars on Newk's shoulders as he stood in his sharp Air Force uniform at the ROTC graduation.

Newk already had orders to report for active duty at Lackland Air Force Base in San Antonio, Texas, for basic training. When he left, I stayed behind at Penn State to pack up and vacate our apartment. I missed Newk terribly. When I was finally able to join him, both our mothers drove with me to San Antonio. They stayed with us for a week. They had barely left when Newk announced,

"Well, we're off to Mission, Texas, honey, and primary flight school."

He was so happy and excited to be training in the T-6 and T-28. His dreams of flying were about to come true. That was my first move as an Air Force wife, and before I knew it, we were way down in the southeastern corner of Texas, just west of Brownsville, practically into Mexico. Shortly after we arrived in Texas, I became pregnant. Six months later, Newk finished primary training.

We drove diagonally across the state to Big Spring, Texas, where he would transition into flying a jet, the T-33. Big Spring, west of Abilene on Route 20 in Texas, was a big cultural shock to me. It was really in the middle of nowhere. Available rentals for military families were almost nonexistent. Our first day there, we trekked from one dismal place to even more dismal places, looking for a rental in what I can only call stupefying heat. We even looked at a converted chicken coop that was advertised as "living space." I was seven months pregnant and felt like I was suffocating. We found nothing that was livable.

"I don't want to go home and have our first baby without you there," I said. This sagging old house had a scraggly rose bush climbing up a peeling front porch railing. Newk reached out to touch it and laughed, saying,

"Look, honey, the rose bush is in bloom. It's blooming for us."

"Yes, that's us," I agreed, and laughed with him. "We're just a couple of worn-out Texas roses." We rented the place, and moved in the next day. Newk was in his glory, flying T-33's, and I was happily contemplating my impending motherhood. Our first son, Jeffrey Newlin Grubb, was born in Big Spring on April 27, 1956. When the nurse came out to the waiting room to inform Newk he had a son, all the guys jumped up and threw their uniform hats in the air, cheering. Until Jeff, all the babies born during the previous four months had been girls. I was the heroine of the week for producing a boy and breaking the streak of girls.

When I came home from the hospital, my mother had arrived to help out and meet her new grandson. She couldn't believe the dust storms in Texas.

"How can you stand this heat and dirt, Evie?" she wanted to know.

"I have no choice, Mother," I replied. "This is where Newk is, so it's where we'll be for as long as he's assigned here."

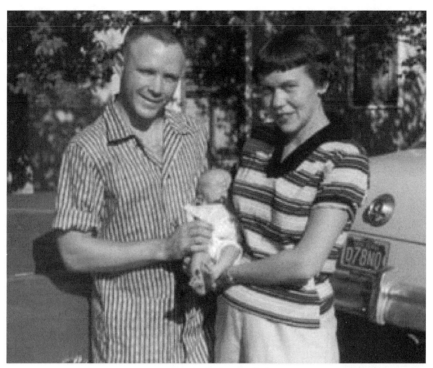

Newk and Evie, with Jeffrey Newlin Grubb, born Big Spring Texas, April 1956.

Three months later I pinned his new wings on his uniform, and we left Texas and made the long drive with baby Jeff to Tyndall Air Force Base in Florida's western Panhandle. It was hot there, too, but humid. Fortunately, we had a decent place to live. The base was on the beautiful Gulf Coast, near Panama City. I loved Florida at first sight, and vowed to come back there to live some day.

Newk spent the next couple of months transitioning into F-86 jets. It was while we were at Tyndall in 1956 that my dear father, who had been in failing health for some time, passed away. I worried a lot about Mother after that, but she weathered her loss well. We stayed in close touch by telephone and mail. Before I knew it, we were moving again. Newk was assigned to an air defense unit at Westover Air Force Base in Springfield, Massachusetts. We were overjoyed at the prospect of settling down into one place for three whole years and being a family again.

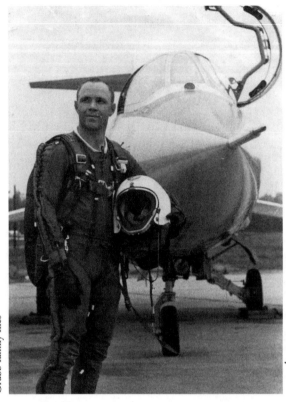

Grubb family files

*Newk flies the F-104
Starfighter, world's
fastest jet, at Westover
AFB, Springfield,
Massachusetts, 1957.*

Newk's flying career was a busy one at Westover, and he really
got into the whole idea of being in the Air Force while we were at
Westover. We were very happy there. Newk got a lot of "back home
in Pennsylvania" and other publicity when he flew the new F-104
Starfighter, which at that time was the world's fastest jet.

We had been at Westover two years when I finally became
pregnant again. We were ecstatic at the prospect of a baby brother
or sister for Jeff. I had an uneventful pregnancy, except for one time
when I bent over to pick Jeff up after he fell. I felt a lancing pain,
like a sharp tear, in my abdominal area, and went immediately to
the base hospital. The doctor on duty said he didn't find anything
amiss, nor did the doctor I saw at my next checkup. I carried the
baby to full term, and when I was admitted in labor, Newk was
given the usual instruction: "Go home and wait, we'll call you when
the baby is here."

I was in a lot more pain than I had been with Jeff at that point in my labor, but I received very little attention from the hospital staff. At one point I had to get up, but when I tried to do that, I was overwhelmed with pain and knew something was wrong. I rang for the nurse. She came in and looked at me and there was fluid or blood around me. She called for someone to page Dr. Allen. "We have a torn placenta here, and this baby needs oxygen . . . " They wheeled me to the delivery room. When the doctor did arrive, the baby came quickly. It was a little girl, and I was overjoyed when they announced that. Then everyone was suddenly rushing about and issuing orders and I was quickly anesthetized. Later, I was told that our baby daughter had died shortly after birth. I was shocked, beyond grief-stricken. Dr. Allen, the on-duty physician, had called Newk and told him, "Your wife's doing okay, but your baby, a girl, died at birth."

Newk was as shaken and upset as I was. When he questioned what went wrong, the doctor told him, "Just get here to the hospital as soon as you can." By the time Newk got there, the doctor had left. There was never an explanation about what had gone wrong at those final, critical moments. What did it matter? We'd lost our baby girl. There was no way to bring her back.

They moved me into a room where my bed was next to a new mother receiving visitors to celebrate the birth of her new baby. We couldn't believe they would do something like that to us.

"Please take me home. I just want to go home," I cried, when Newk appeared

I struggled to dress and we left. Newk called the hospital to tell them we'd gone home. I recovered quickly physically but not mentally or emotionally. A few days later, we buried our baby girl in South Hadley Cemetery in Massachusetts, with only Newk, me, and our minister present. Newk's parents and Mother arrived the following day, and they were wonderful to me. They took over with Jeff and helped pack all the baby things away. Afterward, our grief was internal, but remained constant. Inside, I was angry about our baby's death. I felt she had succumbed because of inattention and poor last-minute decision-making. We both tried hard to work our way through that terrible sense of loss and resume our normal daily lives again. Newk had to concentrate on flying his missions, and that probably helped him get past it. But there was no one at whom

I could direct my anger. In part, I felt that the Air Force didn't care much about us, the wives and children of the men, and the inattention I'd received in the hospital was part of that attitude. I showed no outward signs, but I had been deeply, grievously wounded by the death of our little daughter.

Meanwhile, life and the world went on. Outside our small nucleus in Westover, Massachusetts, communism and nuclear warfare had become much bigger threats.[1] In 1955, President Dwight D. Eisenhower had sent some of our military as advisors to Laos and South Vietnam, to help prevent the Communists from expanding outside North Vietnam and achieving a powerful base from which to spread their influence throughout all of Southeast Asia.

At that point few people in the United States knew much about Indochina or Vietnam, except for the handful of U.S. military men and women who had been sent there to advise the poorly trained South Vietnamese forces to defend themselves against the local Viet Cong Communist rebels and the menacing, well-trained and heavily armed North Vietnam troops. The rebels were intent on unifying all of Vietnam into a single, Communist-governed nation.

At the same time, serious confrontations erupted between the Communist forces of Mao Tse Tung in mainland China, and Chiang Kai Shek's Nationalist Republic of China on the island of Taiwan. President Eisenhower responded to this by stepping up the U.S. Air Force presence in Taiwan, and that directly affected us. In late 1958, Newk's squadron was ordered to Taiwan.[2] Since he wouldn't be with us for Christmas, Jeff and I went to Pennsylvania to be with Mother and the Grubbs. Newk's Christmas was a lonely one, far from home.

> December 28, 1958
> My Darling,
>   The days are getting longer and longer without you, sweetheart . . . I think of you and Jeff all the time and just can't imagine why I should be so lucky to have you both. Your letters make me so happy I could cry, and yet I am sad to be so far away. I will remember the last two weeks we had together for the rest of my life . . . Yes, we have a lot of memories, sweetheart, the good and the bad seem to melt into just goodness when they are recalled.

It was a happy surprise when on February 21, 1959, Newk wrote this:

> Dearest Evelyn,
>
> We are coming home!!! The movement starts on the first of March, and everyone should be gone from here by the 10th. . . . I'm just so happy I can hardly write this letter. . . . I just hope our life will be fuller and richer than ever before. I need you always Darling, you are my life. See you soon!
>
> Newk

He was right. Our lives *were* fuller and richer when Newk was around. After he returned to Westover from Taiwan, we tried to have another baby, but I miscarried—twice. That got me worrying that maybe I wouldn't be able to carry another child to term. Less than a year after he returned from Taiwan, Newk received orders to report to a tactical reconnaissance unit at Toule-Rosier Air Force Base in France. I was happy about that, as we would get to go with him this time. I was really looking forward to living in Europe with Newk. We had two weeks of leave before moving to Europe. We used it to visit our families, since major assignments overseas like this one were usually for three to four years, and that meant we wouldn't see them again for a long time. Mother was very upset that we'd be away for so long.

We drove down to Shaw Air Force Base near Sumter, South Carolina, where we crammed ourselves into a two-room furnished efficiency motel unit. Newk attended another training school for three months, then went to Survival School training out west. I decided that while he went there, Jeff and I would go and stay with Mother in Petersburg, Virginia, where she had settled after Dad's death. I was there when we learned that President Eisenhower had issued a directive curtailing all military family travel out of the country, because of the growing balance of trade deficit. I was stunned, and then outraged. That Executive Directive meant Jeff and I wouldn't be allowed to accompany Newk to Europe![3]

I'd just been given the wonderful news that we were expecting again. So this prospect of a long-term separation from Newk threw me into a major tailspin. Newk wouldn't be able to be with me for the new baby's birth.

All of our household furniture was in storage and I had no place to live. That was bad enough, but I also had other, deeper fears. Newk was young, attractive, and romantic by nature. With a separation that long I truly feared for our marriage. How could it survive such a long time apart? We'd been apart so much already! If we'd been at war, maybe I could have accepted it. We understood the need to sacrifice for a military crisis, but being separated in peacetime was a lot to ask. Such continuous lengthy separations, which entailed years of enforced celibacy and loneliness, not to mention the cost of maintaining two separate lives on separate continents, could destroy any young family. We were finally expecting another baby. We needed to be together! I knew what could, and did, happen when young men like Newk were alone, far from their wives and children, for long periods of time. There were affairs, fights, financial hardships, battles and ultimately—divorces. I'd already seen too many service families shattered from long, stressful separations. This was *not* wartime. I was mad as hell.

By the time Newk arrived in Petersburg after Survival School, I was ready to give up on the whole idea of married military life. We had a huge fight on that subject. Later that night, when we'd stopped yelling at each other, I tried to calm myself down. I wanted to be very calm when I told him my decision, so he'd see that I was being reasonable but determined. We sat down to talk. I worked to keep my voice level, and my tears at bay.

"I've thought a lot about this situation we're in, Newk, and I've decided I want a divorce."

At his stunned look, I wavered a bit. Then I sat up straighter and said,

"I mean it, Newk. I'm flying to Reno, Nevada, to apply for a divorce as soon as possible. It's best for both of us to be free of marriage while you're gone. If we still love each other when you come back from Europe, we can always get married again. But in the meantime, I want you to be free to go and do whatever you want. And the same for me. We don't need guilt to deal with after years of separation."

The word "divorce" had never entered our marital disagreements before. I could see that Newk was clearly shaken. He now realized I was serious, and he'd have to back away from the adamant, "you'll just have to deal with it, dammit . . . I'm under orders!" stance.

Newk kept his voice level and quiet, too. He reached out to take my hand. I resisted, drawing a deep breath, but he wouldn't let go of my hand.

"Evie, we're a team, you know, for better or worse. You promised, I promised. So let's just try to calm down and think about this problem. We'll figure something out. You're finally pregnant again. We just can't risk you getting all worked up like this. Neither of us wants to lose this baby, and I don't even want to hear about divorce. I love you all. I need and want all of you with me. I don't want to go to France without you. So trust me and let me work the problem, okay?" The sincere, heartsick look in his eyes did me in.

"All right, Newk . . . you handle it, because I sure can't. I'm not expecting miracles, though. They order us around like we're just cattle. Well, I'm a *pregnant* cow, and military life has cost us one baby. I'm not going to pay that price again."

I stormed out of the room, crying. Dammit, this problem *was* emotional. I was pregnant. We desperately wanted another child. I loved Newk, and he loved me. All we wanted was some family life. We'd had darn little of it, and I didn't foresee any help coming from the U.S. Air Force to give us more. So things remained tense between us as the time Newk was to leave for France drew closer, but he did work hard on solving the problem. One night, not long before his departure date, he said, "Evie, if you'll agree *not* to divorce me, I promise to figure out a way to get you and Jeff over to Europe to be with me, real soon. I know you have to trust me on that, and you don't like it, but *no divorce*, okay?"

"Okay, I'll trust you. I love you, Newk, you know that. I just cannot live married, but without you, for years. And that's what this assignment will be. It's just too hard on Jeff, on me, and the new baby needs its Daddy, too."

"I do understand, and I agree with you, honey. I'll move heaven and earth if I need to, so we'll be together somehow. It will be soon, I promise."

Newk put his arms around me, and we made up, and were soon a team again. I realized that our love for one another, and our marriage, could stand up under a lot of stress and strain without disintegrating—it just needed plenty of communication, and some heavy starch.

Newk had learned that some of the families had decided to ignore President Eisenhower's travel embargo. Their families were going to travel to Europe as private U.S. citizens. Newk decided Jeff and I would do that, too.

In November of 1960 young John Fitzgerald Kennedy was elected President of the United States and I was elated. President Kennedy had a young family. We were confident he'd understand us, and our needs, and would give the servicemen and their families some relief. Unfortunately, that didn't happen right away.

But Newk kept his word. In December of 1960, in spite of my obstetrician's objections, Jeff and I flew to Paris, and Newk. He had rented us a decrepit trailer home at Chambley, a de-activated French Air Force Base. It was located about 30 kilometers or so from Toule-Rosier, where he was stationed. I almost went into shock when I first saw it, but I kept my happy smile on and immediately set to work fixing it up as best I could. I cared only that we were there together and able to be a family. Newk would be with me for the new baby's arrival. Nothing else mattered. Our time there remained a happy and close time for us.

My pregnancy held, and on January 29, 1961, our second son Roland, named after Newk's Uncle Roke, was born at Toule-Rosier Air Force hospital. Newk was thrilled at having another son. He was a big help to me in caring for little Roke, who was sickly at the start, but soon perked up. Jeff was pleased to have a little brother, too. After so many disappointments in our desire for another child, I was ecstatic with Roke, and so pleased we were all there together with Newk as a family.

Newk loved to fly, loved the Air Force, and didn't want any other career. I knew that good, well-trained military men were scarce and sorely needed. Although I didn't like us being ordered to move around so much, or the too-frequent separations that military families faced, I came to enjoy and accept life as an Air Force wife and family while we were there in France.

The fallout from the Bay of Pigs in Cuba, the construction of the Berlin Wall by the Russians, and the Cuban Missile Crisis affected our lives in many ways during the years we were in Europe. "Brinksmanship diplomacy" was a common expression.[4] Several times, the United States put all of our armed forces, including those in Europe like Newk, on the highest alert status. Life shifted and became tense for us. Then Russian Premier Krushchev agreed to dismantle the Russian missile bases in Cuba, and once again, nuclear crisis was averted. President Kennedy also decided to commit more American troops to help the South Vietnamese fight off the continuing and growing Viet Cong threat. That decision meant little to us in Europe at the time. We had enough going on there between the Cold War confrontations in Berlin and with the Russians in general.

In truth, going to France on our own and living through those international crises contributed enormously to my personal growth. It also increased my knowledge and understanding of another country and of world affairs in general, as opposed to the relatively insular domestic preoccupation that had prevailed in the United States. I was able to mingle with the French people, learn some French, and enjoy a different lifestyle there. Every day there was something new and interesting to learn. Our love grew deeper, too, being there together, and watching our two boys grow. Newk took them everywhere with him when he was home and not flying.

By 1963 I was happily expecting our third child. Then Newk received orders to Ramstein Air Force Base near Landstuhl in Germany. We were pleased because families were now permitted to accompany the men. That meant we were eligible for military housing at Ramstein. That was a big improvement in our comfort and our finances. Newk was flying a lot there, so the boys and I had plenty of time by ourselves. I explored the surrounding area of Germany with the kids in tow and made friends with other Air Force wives there. We helped one another when our husbands were away.

Our third son, Stephen (Van), arrived in April 1963 without difficulty. It was hard to believe our three sons were each born in a different country: Jeff in the United States, Roke in France, Van in Germany. We were a truly international household.

Newk flew a lot of reconnaissance flights for the NATO mili-

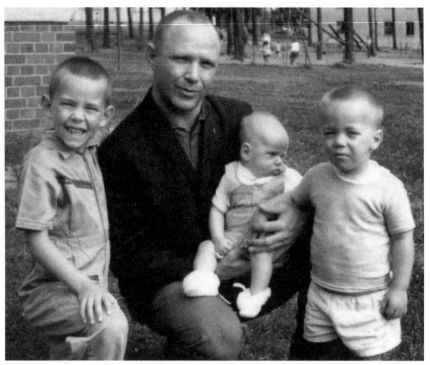

Newk holds third son Stephen (Van) born in Ramstein, Germany, April 1963, flanked by Jeff (left) and Roland (Roke, right).

tary forces. Eventually, the law of averages caught up with him. On one flight, his cockpit canopy imploded on takeoff. He was able to stabilize the plane and land it, but he received some nasty lacerations in the process. I was just grateful he got out alive. That accident brought to the fore the uneasiness and fear familiar to almost all pilots' wives. It also raised discussions between us again about whether he should stay in the Air Force or resign and apply for a commercial job back home that involved flying. I pointed out to Newk that we had three children to consider now, as well as ourselves.

Our discussions on the subject were lively ones, but not bitter fights. Newk definitely didn't want to give up flying. The family, Vietnam, and the general deterioration in international relations around the globe influenced my thinking more than it did his. Newk came home one day and stated his case with a sense of great finality.

"The truth is Evie . . . I want to continue to serve my country, and to fly. I really want to stay in the Air Force, and make it my career. I know how you feel, but I hope you'll agree, and continue to be a great Air Force wife at my side."

I'd learned by then that having your husband come home in a cheerful mood, happy because he is doing what he loves doing, and making a living at it as well, counts for a whole lot in a marriage. I had no control over the world situation, civilian or military. So I agreed to abide by his decision in this. For Newk's sake, I was determined we'd be a model Air Force family through and through.

In November of 1963, the assassination of President Kennedy plunged the world into deep gloom and Newk went on high alert again. We mourned for our young President. I could not imagine how it must have been for Jacqueline Kennedy, with those two adorable young children and a third child lost at birth, which inevitably reminded me of my own lost daughter. I felt grateful to have Newk and our three healthy boys.

Vice-President Lyndon B. Johnson was immediately sworn in as our new President and Commander-in-Chief, and eventually life returned to somewhat normal for us. Newk came off high alert status, and we were free to move around in the local area again. Jeff was eight and in school, and Newk taught him to fish. Roke was a busy, inquisitive three year old. He was trying to fish with Daddy, too. Van was almost a year old, and trying to walk.

That spring, in May of 1964, Newk had another flying accident, this time a serious one. Flying in stormy weather, his altimeter malfunctioned, and he had to bail out. During the ejection, one of his boots was torn off and two panels of his parachute simply disappeared. The plane crashed and was destroyed on impact. Fortunately, a German farmer saw the crash, spotted Newk's parachute coming down. When the farmer got to him, Newk was on the ground injured and bleeding, but alive. The farmer got him free of his chute and into his car. He drove Newk to the nearest medical clinic where a Turkish doctor and a German nurse initially treated him. Newk couldn't communicate well with them, but finally, someone arrived who spoke reasonable English and could translate for Newk. Newk had a long, deep gash down his calf, where his boot had been cut by a piece of metal as he ejected. He had a lot of smaller cuts and bruises, too. The doctor cleaned up the gash in his leg, and sent Newk in a World War II era ambulance to Weisbaden Air Force Base hospital, about 50 miles away. He was admitted and spent five days in the hospital. We felt extremely fortunate.

We were in our fourth year in Europe when Newk received orders in May 1964 to return home. He was again assigned to Shaw Air Force Base in South Carolina. That summer, we drove up to visit my family in Virginia, near Washington, D.C., for a week or so.

One night, while playing bridge with the radio on for background music, a newscaster interrupted with breaking news about the "Tonkin Gulf incident in North Vietnam."[5] We stopped the game to listen. Newk and I exchanged a meaningful look. We both sensed that Vietnam had just moved onto our radar screen.

On the morning of July 31, the Navy destroyer, *Maddox,* was cruising in the Tonkin Gulf near the island of Hon Me, when several North Vietnamese torpedo boats came out and fired at the ship. This attack by a small North Vietnamese boat on one of our large naval destroyers was about as successful as a mosquito attacking an elephant, but it was reported that fire from one of the torpedo boats struck the *Maddox.* A few days later, a second, similar incident was alleged to have occurred. These became the "Tonkin Gulf Incident" that Congress used to justify the Tonkin Gulf Resolution, allowing escalation of our military activity in Vietnam.[6]

Although we didn't know it until much later, Navy lieutenant Everett Alvarez, Jr., was one of the pilots flying air cover over our destroyers. His plane was shot down by the North Vietnamese, and he became the first American pilot to be captured in North Vietnam.[7] He was also the first of the American POWs, many of them pilots, who would eventually be held prisoner in and around Hanoi in North Vietnam.

Life at Shaw never returned to normal once the Tonkin Gulf Resolution was promulgated. We tried to keep it as pleasant as possible for the men and children, and Newk and I enjoyed a lot of family fun times with the boys. But for the two of us, tension and the knowledge he might have to leave for Vietnam on a moment's notice remained "the elephant in the room" in our daily lives.

Soon Newk was moved onto "constant alert" status. His departure suitcase remained packed, standing by the front door, ready for him to go at a moment's notice. It was a continuous reminder that

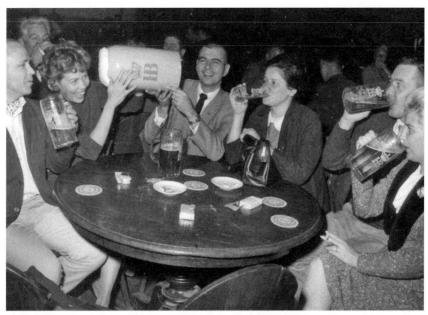

Newk and Evelyn enjoy an evening out with friends, Germany, 1964.

we'd likely be separated again soon, which kept me emotionally on edge.

In October 1964, Newk was sent to Fort Riley, Kansas, for something called "Operation Goldfire," a major war game and field training exercise. I got a few phone calls from him, and we exchanged letters. However, most of the time he was on "blackout," which meant not near any phones or other amenities, just slogging through the days in rain, mud, wet tents, wet gear, and dining on C-rations. I knew that all this field training meant Newk was getting closer to being assigned to somewhere in Southeast Asia in support of the escalating war. Fort Riley, an army base, wasn't known as "America's war-fighting center" for no reason.

Just before Easter 1965, we were at the movie theater at Shaw, watching *Around the World in 80 Days,* when a base alert interrupted the movie. The theater was evacuated, and the men were ordered to report immediately to their commanders. Very soon after that, Newk left us for temporary duty at a new base in Thailand to fly reconnaissance missions over North Vietnam. I remained at our home on Shaw AFB in South Carolina with the children, anticipating a long separation. However, barely two months after leaving for Thailand, Newk was back home again. We celebrated happily, believing that he wouldn't be called on to go back to Southeast Asia anytime soon.

We'd been married ten years, and Newk had been away from us for about half of that time. Our lives seemed to revolve around tearful farewells and joyous welcome homes for Newk. Meanwhile, in Vietnam, the drums of war were beating louder and faster, and soon they were thumping out Newk's name again. He was ordered to Saigon, Vietnam, in autumn of 1965. It was a "permanent change" assignment, which meant he'd be gone at least a year, maybe longer. Newk had enough advance notice to help the children and me make our move to Petersburg, Virginia. He was glad that we'd be close to Mother, with my brother Bill and his wife Norma close by, since this would be a longer assignment. Too soon, it was time for another tearful farewell.

My first shopping foray after he left us was to buy and mail Christmas gifts so they'd arrive in Saigon for the holidays. Mail was slow coming our way from Saigon, too. I read his first two letters to us sitting in the back yard. Piles of autumn leaves the boys and I had just raked were everywhere, and the first chill of oncoming winter made the air crisp. I had just experienced the first signs that I was pregnant again.

Over where Newk was, it wasn't crisp and cool, it was hot as Hell, in more ways than one. I called the boys over. "I have two letters from Daddy. Sit here on the ground and I'll read them to you." They were excited about letters from Daddy, and sat quietly to hear what he had written. I explained as I went, so they'd understand what Daddy meant, and skipped anything that was for me alone.

> Saigon, 15 November 1965
> Dearest Evelyn,
>
> We had a fast trip over here. The aircraft landed at Tan Son Nhut Air Base on Saturday night at about 1800 after 40 hours of flying time out of a total of 60 hours since we left home. Everyone was really beat and ready to collapse into the sack or anywhere. . . . This afternoon I flew my first combat mission. As you can see, there is no messing around—I'm still tired from the plane ride, but by tomorrow I hope to feel a little more human. It looks like we'll be

flying a mission every day . . . they have only about two a
week up north and the planning is such that everyone gets
an even share of those, so I will probably get one every two
months or so. I'm anxious to hear about you and the boys
and the new puppy. We moved right into the Chateau
house in Saigon, and I had to sleep in the living room the
first two nights. Smith and Bird left for home today, so
tonight I'll have a bed in an air-conditioned room. The
temperature here is about 90 degrees in the afternoon . . . I
had dinner last night on the floating restaurant in the river
. . . the one that was bombed last year. Very interesting
place. I had fried crab claws, fried rice, sweet and sour pork,
plus beer. Our house rent is about $900 US a month, so
someone is making money out of this war. [*Ed. Note:* Newk
then crosses out the word 'war' and 'sorry—police action' is
substituted]. I'm scheduled to fly tomorrow afternoon
again. That's about all from here, dear. I'll try to write again
tomorrow. I'm so tired trying to readjust my sleep habits.
But if you were here I still wouldn't get any sleep. I miss you
and the boys. Goodnight sweetheart.
Love,
Newk

19 November '65, noon
Dearest Evie,

I received your first and very warm letter this
morning. I bet Jeff's expression when he saw the pup was
priceless. He is such a good boy. We are very fortunate to
have such a nice family. I miss all of you. Life is empty
without you. I hope Heidi dog is taking over and directing
all of your lives by now. A 6-week-old pup is just the right
size to be a devil. I only wish that I could hold you darling
and tell you about it in every little detail, but I'm not
allowed to . . . I enjoy having the radio, they have an armed
forces radio station VietNam that even broadcasts games
from the states.

Thanksgiving arrived. I missed Newk and my Dad. We were a
traditional American family in many ways, and Thanksgiving was

something we looked forward to, especially when we were in the States. It brought memories of growing up, football games, college days and family closeness. We always prepared a big dinner, with all the trimmings, and the men watched football games on television, until I could finally drag them away from the TV and to the table, where Newk carved the Thanksgiving turkey. Newk's Thanksgiving Day letter from Saigon, when I finally received it, really brought me to tears. The pain of missing him, and the terrible realization of what he must be going through over there alone, with no family at all to comfort him washed over me.

> Thanksgiving Day, 1965
> Dearest Wifey-thing,
>   I flew mission number 11 today and number 32 total. We went up north a ways but everything was covered with clouds. We have had some low level flying also, so the missions are varied. The battle of Pleu Me was still raging today. Makes you wonder where all the Viet Cong come from. These V.C. were equipped very well . . . probably are direct from North Vietnam. I hate to think what might have happened without the air strikes that cut the heart out of the attack. The main thing that makes the flying easier down south here is the lack of medium and heavy anti-aircraft guns in the hands of the enemy. Their light weapons are only effective to about 3000 feet, and we take most of our pics well above that with the telephoto lens. Well, I'm going to miss carving the bird this year. I hope you all get enough to eat and enjoy the day. The temperature here is 90 degrees, and the electricity is off. This happens every other day. I think I'm feeling well enough to even chance an (ugh!) martini. I wish you could sip one with me Sweetheart, and get all warm and cozy . . . I can't say I'm thankful we're apart today, but I'm thankful for so many things we have, and have shared together. I just want to tell you how I love you in so many ways . . .
> Your Saigon Sweetie,
> Newk

We had a very lonely Christmas that year without Newk. He sent us the wonderful tape recorder with a tape of him talking to us,

which was a delight and special treat to all of us. This was an exciting new way for us to communicate when apart. I was happy when
a second tape arrived from him a couple of weeks later.

Then the counting of missions, counting of hours and days,
stopped suddenly, like a broken clock, on that snowy, cold January
afternoon when the taxi driver knocked on my door.

Somehow, the strength and determination I'd learned during
our time in Europe bolstered me for awhile following the telegram
saying that Newk had been shot down over North Vietnam and was
missing. I clung to hope that he'd be rescued very soon.

On that seemingly endless January day in 1966, as neighbors
and friends bustled about trying to help us, I nagged everyone to
keep the phone line free "in case Newk has been rescued, and wants
to call."

3 The Magic Elixir of Hope

TIMELINE . . . 1966 . . . <u>WORLD</u> . . . FLOODS IN ITALY DAMAGE PRICELESS BOOKS AND ART TREASURES . . . <u>VIETNAM</u> . . . HANOI THREATENS WAR CRIMES TRIBUNAL FOR POWS . . . HANOI MARCHES POWs THROUGH STREETS . . . <u>USA</u> . . . *NEW YORK HERALD TRI-BUNE* FOLDS . . . ELIZABETH ARDEN DIES . . .

Hope springs eternal in the human breast. —Alexander Pope

Newk hadn't called. Neither had the Air Force. That night, I fell into exhausted sleep in my bed. My dreams were chaotic. The next morning, I could tell by the glazed look in Van's eyes that he was coming down with chicken pox. Then, from the kitchen, I heard Jeff call,

"Mom, I don't feel so good. My head hurts and I'm itchy all over."

My brother Bill called to try and pep me up. He said they'd be coming that weekend to do whatever they could to help out.

"How's Roke doing?" he asked. "Still suffering with the chicken pox?"

"Yes, now he's got company—Jeff and Van."

"I hate to hear that, Evie. You sure don't need that right now. What does Roke want for his birthday?"

Oh, dear. This Saturday is Roland's fifth birthday!

"I'll have to ask him. I completely forgot about it."

"And no wonder, Evelyn! You're in shock right now. How can you remember anything?"

I had no answer for him. I didn't know myself what I was doing. My thoughts were all of Newk . . . where could he be? What might be happening to him? No one had answers for me, either.

Late that afternoon two enlisted men from Langley Air Force base visited me to offer sympathy and support. I was disappointed

38

that they had no further news about Newk to give me. Another long night passed. The next day, one of them returned with another official telegram:

> REFERENCE MY PREVIOUS COMMUNICATION(S) CONCERNING THE MISSING STATUS OF YOUR HUSBAND CAPTAIN WILMER N. GRUBB. THE ORGANIZED SEARCH HAS NOW BEEN SUSPENDED AS ALL ATTEMPTS TO LOCATE AND RESCUE HIM HAVE BEEN UNSUCCESSFUL. EVERY EFFORT WILL CONTINUE TO BE MADE TO DETERMINE HIS STATUS. ANY NEW INFORMATION RECEIVED BY THIS HEADQUARTERS WILL BE FURNISHED YOU IMMEDIATELY. YOUR HUSBAND'S COMMANDER IS WRITING YOU A LETTER WHICH WILL CONTAIN A SUMMARY OF THE CIRCUMSTANCES UNDER WHICH HE BECAME MISSING, AS WELL AS AN ACCOUNT OF THE SEARCH EFFORTS. MEANWHILE, CAPTAIN GRUBB WILL BE CARRIED OFFICIALLY IN A MISSING STATUS PENDING ANALYSIS AND EVALUATION OF ALL THE FACTORS PERTAINING TO HIS STATUS.
>
> MAJOR GENERAL G. B. GREENE, JR.
> ASSISTANT DEPUTY CHIEF OF STAFF, PERSONNEL, FOR MILITARY PERSONNEL,
> HEADQUARTERS, UNITED STATES AIR FORCE[1]

I felt full of despair. We didn't know if he was alive, injured, okay, or . . . I couldn't let myself even think the word . . .

Someone from the neighborhood brought us lunch. Mother coaxed me to eat, with a piece of banana nut bread.

"Here, Evelyn, try this. You have to eat something, you know, for the baby's sake. You haven't eaten one thing in two days."

She was right. I reached for the banana bread. After one bite, I practically swallowed it whole. It was the first food I could remember eating in the past 24 hours, and it was delicious.

Then the neighbor who had been handling phone duty for me hung up from a call and came hurrying over to me.

"Evie, that was a very strange call. From someone who says he's a friend of the family. He says there's something in the Philadelphia papers about the Chinese claiming an American jet was shot down, and the North Vietnamese captured the pilot, but he didn't have a copy of it right there. I asked him to please get a copy and call back to read it to you. He said he would."

My heart began to hammer in my chest, and I felt lightheaded.

"Somebody *please* turn on the television—maybe there's something on the news!" I cried. There was a strange ringing in my ears, and everything went gray. The next thing I knew, Mother was leaning over me, holding a wet cloth to the back of my neck. I knew someone else was there, too. It looked like a man.

"Newk?"

"*Shhh*. No, it's Mother, dear, and your neighbor. You started to faint. Here, bend your head down, Evie. You've gone deathly white. Don't pass out, my dear girl. Just be very still. Honestly, is there no respite for this woman?"

My head bent to my knees, I kept demanding, "The TV! Please . . . turn it on! There might be news."

Someone finally switched the television on and found a newscast. There was a brief comment that "a U.S. pilot" had been captured. They said it was believed to be a reconnaissance pilot since the bombing had been halted by President Johnson.[2] My hopes soared. I just knew that captured pilot had to be Newk, and praise God, he was alive! That one little shred of hope energized me. I felt better. I got up and telephoned the Air Force duty officer in Personnel at Randolph Air Force Base in Texas.[3] He said he couldn't confirm anything for me. I told him that the Philadelphia newspaper, and the TV newscaster saying that a reconnaissance pilot had been captured.

"Right now we have nothing positive to report Ma'am," he said.

"We'll let you know immediately when or if we have anything concrete to report to you about your husband's status, Mrs. Grubb."

"I think maybe you should watch the television news," I replied. "They seem to have better sources than the U.S. Air Force on what's happening over there!"

I tried to calm my anger and frustration. We all gathered and celebrated Roke's fifth birthday. When the mail came, there was a birthday card for him from Daddy. He had mailed it before that fateful flight. I took that as a good sign. Don't ask me why. We had hope . . . that the captive was Newk, he was alive, and all would soon be fine.

"There might be more mail still to come. Maybe another tape from Newk," I said, voicing that positive feeling aloud.

I received calls from several of the men Newk had flown with—friends of ours from Shaw Air Force Base. All of them cheered me up and expressed hope for the best, but none could confirm what I longed to know: Was that captured pilot indeed our Newk?

The next morning, an airman came with another telegram from Randolph Air Force Base.

> 1966 February 3, 4pm
> WE HAVE RECEIVED A REPORT FROM THE FOR-EIGN BROADCAST INFORMATION SERVICE . . . THAT RADIO HANOI HAS BROADCAST A STATE-MENT ALLEGEDLY MADE BY YOUR HUSBAND THIS DATE. WE HAVE REQUESTED A TAPE RECORDING OF THIS BROADCAST, AND WHEN WE RECEIVE IT, WE WILL NOTIFY YOU FURTHER. WE WILL CONTINUE TO CARRY YOUR HUSBAND IN A MISSING STATUS. AGAIN, PLEASE ACCEPT MY SINCERE SYMPATHY DURING THIS TRYING TIME.
>
> MAJOR GENERAL G. B. GREENE, JR.
> ASSISTANT DEPUTY CHIEF OF STAFF, PERSON-NEL, FOR MILITARY PERSONNEL,
> HEADQUARTERS, UNITED STATES AIR FORCE[4]

If that was true, then Newk was alive! I just knew I'd hear from him very soon. On February 9, I received a phone call from Altoona, Pennsylvania. It was one of our fathers' fraternity brothers from Penn State, John Hunter. Bless him, he got straight to the point.

"I've known Newk Grubb since he was a baby, and I was at your wedding, Evelyn. I have some news for you. There was a picture of your husband, as a captured prisoner of the Vietnamese, in the *Altoona Mirror* newspaper today. Have you seen that photo?"

I clenched the phone. At the look on my face, Mother hurried over to stand close.

"No, I haven't seen it," I replied. "Are you certain it is Newk in that picture, Mr. Hunter?"

"Absolutely. Recognized him right away."

"And he looked well?"

"Yup. Far as I could see, he did. Someone had a gun pointed at him; picture said it was a North Vietnamese. But Newk looked okay."

"Oh . . . oh . . . *thank you!* You can't imagine what the past few days have been like for us. If that is Newk, it's the first real evidence we have that he's alive! Can you please make a copy of that picture and send it to us?"

He said of course he would. "Want me to read you what it says now?"

"Yes. Oh, yes! Please do!"

"Says here, 'In Enemy Hands—A North Vietnamese soldier trains a gun on a captive identified as U.S. Air Force Captain Wilmer N. Glubb in this photograph released by North Vietnam's News Agency. The Communist report said Grubb's plane was shot down January 26.' That's about the gist of it. The Commies have got him, even if they call him Glubb."

I was relieved to learn Newk was alive, even though he was a captive. I hung up and hugged Mother joyfully. "Newk's alive! Dad's friend, Mr. Hunter, recognized him in the picture!" The tears flowed again, but this time they were tears of relief and happiness. My next thought was,

Why haven't I heard anything about this from the Air Force? They said they'd contact me immediately. There have been two reports about Newk being captured. Now Newk's picture is in the Pennsylvania papers as a captive, and I've heard nothing at all except a rumor of a tape from the Air Force. What is going on?

I called Randolph Air Force Base again and informed them of the picture in the Altoona newspaper.

"We haven't seen the photo, Mrs. Grubb. We'll check on it and get back to you as soon as we have anything confirmed on your husband's status."

"This is ludicrous. That I'm giving you the military this news. It should be coming from you to me. Something is very wrong with military communication with the families of men who are missing or captured!"

"We will contact you as soon as we know something, Mrs. Grubb."

Over the next week, clippings of newspaper articles, all containing the news photo Hunter told me about (it certainly *was* of Newk!) were mailed to me from people all over the United States. From people everywhere. But not from the U.S. Air Force or the American government.

Three different photos of Newk appeared in the press.[5] One was of Newk in his flight suit, sitting on the ground, with a Vietnamese woman tending to a superficial wound on his knee. A Vietnamese soldier was standing behind Newk. He was holding a rifle/bayonet, with the knife part of the bayonet pointed at Newk's head. The point of a second bayonet showed on the right, just behind his head, which meant there was definitely a second armed military person there guarding him. The caption that was a part of

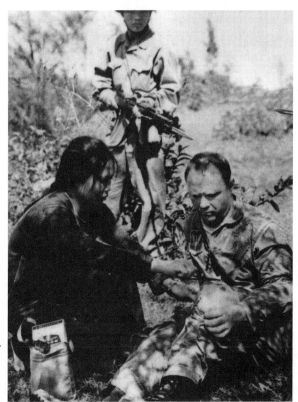

First photograph by North Vietnamese of Captain Wilmer N. "Newk" Grubb, following capture. Grubb shows no evidence of serious injury. Caption states: "But also…enjoy the lenient policy of the Vietnamese People."

Grubb family files

the photo misspelled his name "Glubb." That was how they pronounced it. The caption read:

> QUANG BINH PROVINCE, NORTH VIET NAM:
> In this photo released by an official Communist source,
> U.S. Captain Wilmer N. Glubb is shown as a captive of the
> local army after his jet plane was shot down here 1/26.
> Young girl at Glubb's side is said to be a rescue worker from
> a local militia unit, giving the American first aid.

The second photo was the one John Hunter called me about. In
that one, Newk was standing tall at attention, and a very petite
Vietnamese woman held a machine gun trained on him. What
wasn't shown in this photo, but showed up in others, were the six
armed military men just outside camera range. They were all holding rifles trained on Newk.

We pored over the news telephotos. We saw the positive proof
that Newk had been captured and was apparently okay. Meanwhile
letters were coming to me from various officials and commanders.
There was one from General Westmoreland, the commander of
American forces in Vietnam, and one from Major General Gilbert
Meyers, Vice-Commander of the 2nd Air Division. Both offered
their condolences and their deep distress over Newk's missing status. Well, he wasn't missing any more, he was a captive of the North
Vietnamese. His photos were now all over the world as such. Were
commanders not being notified that the North Vietnamese were
plastering photos of our captured troops in the media over there,
and our media were picking them up on the wire services? If they
could, why couldn't the military intelligence people do it?

I received a long, official, and somewhat personal letter from
Newk's boss, Ray Lowery, Commander of the 20th Tactical
Reconnaissance Squadron. Newk's nickname was confusing to
many people. The family all called him "Newk." The guys in the
squadron called him "Newt." His grade school pals had nicknamed
him "Nuggie," according to his childhood friend, Bud Farrell. I
guess the names "Wilmer" or "Newlin" didn't fit his personality.
They were serious old family names. Newk was fun, young, lively,
and outgoing as a person. "Newk" seemed to fit him perfectly.

Colonel Lowery's letter was dated February 5, 1966. He gave

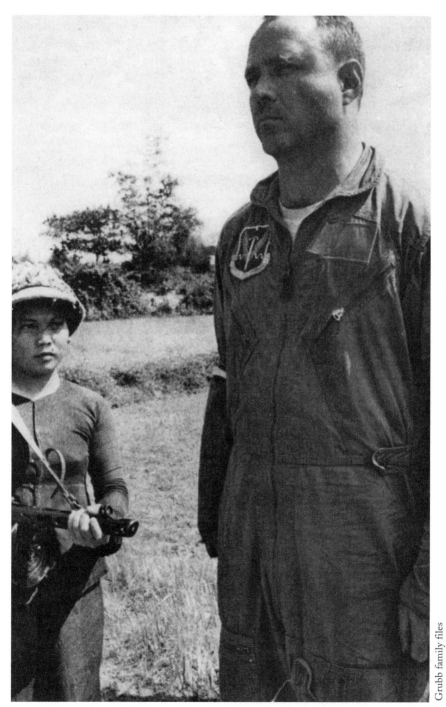

Capt. Newk Grubb fully upright, arms roped together behind him.

Grubb family files

me the circumstances and details of what had happened the day
Newk was shot down. Ray also said that Al Brunstrom, Newk's
wingman, had heard Newk's radio beeper on two separate passes
over the location. Lowery wrote:

> This Radio Beeper is designed to transmit only when the
> pilot's parachute has deployed, which in Newt's case is a
> strong indication he ejected from his disabled aircraft. . . .
> Unfortunately, neither Newt nor his aircraft could be locat-
> ed. Since this time, we have received several unofficial
> reports that further lead us to believe Newt ejected safely.
>
> The first report, a United Press International press
> release stating an American aircraft was shot down on 26
> January 1966 and the pilot captured. The second report was
> one I heard personally while listening to Radio Peking on
> Short Wave radio which reiterated the exact same informa-
> tion as the UPI press release. To my knowledge, I know of
> no other U.S. Aircraft shot down on this date, so I am con-
> fident it is to Newt both of these reports refer.
>
> I have appointed Captain George Wehling to
> inventory and package all of Newt's personal effects which
> by regulation we are directed to hold for thirty days before
> sending them on to you.
>
> Evie, if there is anything we can do to assist you in
> any way, please do not hesitate to let us know. I assure you
> that if we do hear anything further on Newt's disposition,
> we will keep you informed.[6]

Al Brunstrom also sent me a tape recording, describing everything
he could recall about that day, up to when he lost touch with Newk.
Al's tape said, in part,

> The sky was overcast and then we spotted a river thru a hole
> in the clouds. We went down thru the clear area and were
> not lined up on our target, so Newt made a 360 degree turn
> lining up on the river leading up to our target, the Xuan Son
> Barracks. On the turn to line up, Newt said he was pulling
> it in tight to stay inside the known defended areas. It's
> impossible to do any map reading and still stay in position
> going in that low and fast. So I knew we were in the target

area, but was unable to exactly pinpoint myself. Going down the river Newt called, 'Cameras on' and then shortly after started a pull-up and called 'I'm hit!' and then almost immediately disappeared into the overcast. At that time, I had assumed we had crossed over the target, started a pull up and then he'd gotten hit. When I looked at my film the next day, I found my film had stopped about 1 mile, or 7-8 seconds before the target. So from that it appears Newk had taken a hit prior to the target, started his pull-up and then called 'I'm hit' a couple of seconds later. It probably took him a couple of seconds to evaluate what had happened. So going on that basis, he probably bailed out and landed in or very near the Kuan Son Barracks and was probably captured before I had a chance to even come back around to look for him.[7]

It was at that point that some of my elation at knowing Newk was alive and a captive of the North Vietnamese troops turned to fear for what he might be enduring at the hands of the enemy. I immediately called several knowledgeable friends to ascertain whether North Vietnam was a signatory to the Geneva Conventions regarding treatment of Prisoners of War. Those would protect Newk. I was reassured when I learned that North Vietnam indeed had signed the Conventions. For my sake, and the children's, I tried to quell my fears and concentrate on the fact that Newk was alive.

"Where there's life, there's hope," I wrote in my replies to letters from our friends and family. But no matter what I felt about life and hope, I could get no official confirmation from the U.S. Air Force that my husband was actually a prisoner of the North Vietnamese. By then, photos of him as a captive had appeared in the *Washington Post* and on all major U.S. television networks, including a third photo, this one just a chest-to-head view of him, with three armed soldiers behind him, and what looked like the same petite woman whom I'd seen in the photo of Newk at attention. Since he was much taller than most Vietnamese, I could only assume from the other soldiers' positions behind and above him, that they were on a rise behind him, or that Newk was sitting, or kneeling on the ground, so that he would look shorter than those troops.[8]

However, as far as the Air Force was concerned, my husband, Captain Wilmer Newlin Grubb, was still classed as Missing in Action. It was most frustrating. I tried my best not to get upset. I tried to adopt a more positive attitude about the cold, indifferent way the Air Force had adopted in dealing with the families of men who had been shot down. Crying and being frightened all the time gave me a terrible headache and left me exhausted. Although hard to suppress, anger was also pointless. Days kept passing with no further news, no results, nothing from Newk, and little or no communication from the military authorities. I gritted my teeth and kept reminding myself that I had a baby growing inside me that I needed to nurture. Activity and a daily laugh out loud made all of us feel better. In private, when despair overwhelmed me, I allowed myself ten minutes of crying, anger, fear, or reflection. Then I

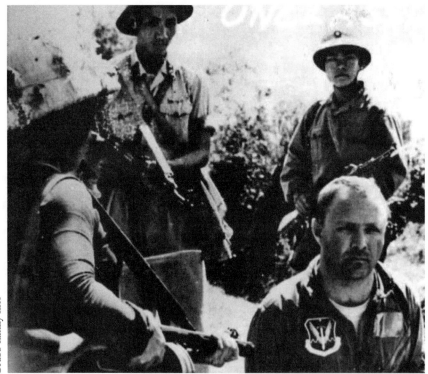

Grubb family files

Grubb with Vietnamese militia woman holding automatic weapon, two North Vietnamese military guards. Newk appears to be kneeling or sitting in this photo.

forced myself to go back to our regular daily life.

I sat down and wrote my first letter to Newk. Then realized I had not been given any information about how to send mail to him. I got no enlightenment from the Air Force, either. They gave me the same robotic answer they'd given to all my calls.

"We're sorry Mrs. Grubb, but we have no official information to give you."

I still have that first letter I wrote to Newk, which was never mailed, since I had no address to send it to. I also kept a copy of the second letter. I planned to mail them together as soon as I was given an address to write Newk. My first letter said:

> February 16, 1966
> Dearest Newk,
>
> I love you. Like so many of our crises in the past, things happened all at once here. The news that you were missing and probably a prisoner arrived the same day as the 'Blizzard of '66.' For over a week we were snowed in. Jeff and Roke had one day to play outside in the snow, then right on schedule, eleven days after Van; they broke out with chicken pox. Jeff didn't miss even a day of school, though, since it was closed because of the snow. Heidi just loved running and digging in the drifts but it was too deep for her to stay out very long. Now the snow is melted, the sun is shining, and everyone feels fine again. Tinkerbell is growing daily. Fortunately we have strong children, Darling. Mother and Dad (Grubb) have called often these days. So my thoughts and prayers are with you now, Newk. May they, and the knowledge that our love is ever present, give you the hope and the patience to endure.
>
> Yours always,
> Evelyn

On February 17, 1966, my brother Bill accompanied me to Washington, D.C., to hear a tape that the North Vietnamese alleged was made by Newk. A friend of ours from the CIA, who knew Newk well, accompanied us. We listened to the tape several times. The sound was grainy, the man's voice fast and unclear, and there was a lot of ambient noise. We agreed it was not Newk's voice on the tape. However, the personal information given by the person speaking on the tape, claiming he was Newk Grubb, was accurate.[9]

Then, in a private, handwritten letter to me dated February 20, 1966, Ray Lowery, Newk's commander, told me that he and George Wheling had listened to part of the tape 'over and over' . . . "it didn't, to either of us, really begin to sound like Newt talking. First of all, the rate of speech was way too fast, almost twice as fast as Newt would talk. Secondly, I can't conceive that Newt would voluntarily ever make a tape for the DRV under any circumstance. . . ."

It didn't occur to us then that the rapid rate of speech in the voice the North Vietnamese government claimed was Newk's on that tape might have been a result of savage torture.[10] It may also have just been poor electronics. I agreed with Ray Lowery that Newk wouldn't have made such a tape for the North Vietnamese. It never occurred to us, in those early days of Newk's captivity, that the North Vietnamese jailers might be torturing prisoners to force them to make such tapes of "confession."

On February 22, an Air Force staff car again pulled up out front, and yet another telegram was delivered. You'd think they'd just pick up a phone. It was nice to see that the Air Force had at last gotten around to acknowledging what the rest of us had known for more than two weeks!

> BASED ON RADIO HANOI REPORTS AND THE WIRE PHOTO OF YOUR HUSBAND, WE HAVE CHANGED HIS OFFICIAL STATUS FROM MISSING TO DETAINED. THIS ACTION WILL NOT RESULT IN ANY CHANGE TO ENTITLEMENTS WHICH YOU ARE PRESENTLY RECEIVING. PLEASE ACCEPT MY SYMPATHY IN THIS TIME OF ANXIETY.
>
> LT. COL JOSEPH G. LUTHER
> CHIEF, CASUALTY DIVISION
> HEADQUARTERS, UNITED STATES AIR FORCE[11]

The legal and bureaucratic nightmare of money, property, my status, our needs, and trying to sleuth out Newk's location in the Hanoi prison camps began. While Newk's status had been officially changed to "detained," *my* status with the military hadn't altered a bit. It appeared to me that our children and I were an unwelcome problem for the senior Air Force commanders in the United States. They didn't appear to have had much training in handling this kind of situation. I was expected to sit down, shut up, keep a low profile, and not bother them with questions. I had never been very good at doing any of those things on command, and nothing in this situation changed that.

Newk had obviously been taken prisoner in North Vietnam. There was photographic proof of that, which they'd just acknowledged. I felt I had a right to know where my husband was, how he was, and how and where I could write him. I made a note to look up the Geneva Conventions about Prisoners of War as soon as possible. At home, the boys and I began each dinner with a prayer of thanks that included an appeal: "Please watch over our Daddy and bring him home soon."

Shortly after Newk was reported missing, I was assigned an Air Force Sergeant from Langley Air Force Base as my "Casualty Officer."[12] To say that he was not happy with his assignment, and that I was incredibly unhappy with him, and his behavior toward me as Newk's wife and now interim head of our family, would be an understatement. He had little or no useful knowledge of how to deal with a situation like mine. From the outset, he adopted an attitude of suspicion and obstruction. It was as though his mission was to *protect* Newk from me and our children, as if we were the enemy, and he was there on a mission to save Newk from us.

One day I said, "I'm going to need to liquidate our boat savings account soon, to buy baby furniture, and I'll also need to get a bigger car after the baby arrives."

He couldn't believe that Newk had actually *told* me about the account we started to save money to buy a boat when he got back. I wanted to scream. With Newk gone so often I had to handle all the bills, the children, the banking, and our financial obligations, as did many other military spouses. We were the ones constantly left behind to take care of these things. Now I was expected to grovel to this cold stranger to access our own money! We had established the boat savings account together as a family project before we knew that we'd be having a fourth baby. I was flabbergasted that this sergeant thought men should keep things like boat savings accounts a secret from their wives. He made me so angry and frustrated that one day I dragged my tape recorder to our meeting. I couldn't believe I had to do this to get his permission to handle *our* money!

"Just listen to this, and you'll hear for yourself that my husband and I are totally together on how our finances are managed when he's away."

I played Newk's last tape for him, the part where Newk talked about having the bank give me detailed statements of his deposits every month. The sergeant stared at the tape recorder in disbelief, as if he'd heard Newk utter some kind of blasphemy.

I wrote another letter to Newk, telling him that photographs of him being treated for knee scrapes had been published in the newspapers. I gave him all the news about what the boys were doing, and closed with a paragraph that let him know about our finances, saying,

> Your affairs are all in order darling. I'm going to transfer our savings to here, more interest and much easier for me. Fort Sam is the same as always for us, but I closed out the Special account. Hope that's okay. I hope to hear from you, but it may not be right away. Just hope that my letters will get to you Darling, so that you will know we are all fine here and our thoughts and prayers and love are with you every day, Darling. I love you so very much.

I made two copies, addressed the handwritten letter to Newk via the North Vietnam Hanoi Post Office, and mailed it. Then I took one copy to the nearest office of the Red Cross. The woman who accepted my letter was kind, but not optimistic.

"We really can't promise anything. At this time, the North Vietnamese are not allowing the Red Cross to check on prisoners. You'll have to contact the Air Force for information about letters going to and from the men who are detained there."

I felt it would be useless to mention that I *had* contacted the Air Force and had not gotten any information whatsoever from them about letters. At least the Red Cross had given me some answers—and insight into their difficulty.

To make matters worse, the harassment from the Sergeant about finances, and whatever I was doing, continued. Finally, I

couldn't stand it any more. I wrote a letter to Captain George
Wehling, the Summary Courts Officer at Newk's squadron, about
this Sergeant's attitude. One of the matters I brought up was that
the Sergeant didn't like it that I made inquiries about our money.
Newk's military pay was allotted three ways: 1) money for me and
the children; 2) money for Newk overseas; and 3) money to our
boat savings fund.

Because of the baby's impending arrival, I needed more money
than was in my allotment. Further I needed to know, I had a right
to know, what the government was doing now with Newk's pay—
all of it. It was months later before I ever got a full accounting of
Newk's finances from the military pay center in Denver.

I dared to ask: "Will the money kept for my husband by the
government be earning interest while he's a captive?" The answer
was "no."

"Then I want that money paid directly to me," I said. "I will put
it in an account where it will at least earn interest."

They were annoyed about that, but I held full power of attorney
from Newk, and I decided that now was the time to use it—for our
family's sake and our needs. That didn't happen easily.
Nevertheless, I persisted, and it was finally agreed that the pay center would send his pay and allowances directly to our bank account
in Fort Sam Houston, Texas.

Fortunately for me, Captain Wehling didn't agree with the
Sergeant's attitude either. I didn't learn until much later that he had
shared my complaints about the problem with Newk's squadron
commander, Lt. Colonel Ray Lowery, who had promptly written a
letter to the Personal Affairs office at Randolph AFB, saying,

> Mrs. Grubb presently has 3 small children and is expecting
> her fourth within the next few months. In her present condi-
> tion, Mrs. Grubb should not be subjected to this inconsider-
> ate treatment, nor should it continue. Request appropriate
> action be taken through command channels to relieve Mrs.
> Grubb of this undue mental harassment, and an investigation
> conducted to determine if tactless situations similar to this
> are occurring elsewhere to unfortunate service families.[13]

Thank you, Ray Lowery! Three cheers. At least he cared about us families—all of us. I wanted to shout those cheers out loud. The Casualty Office assured me that a new Casualty Officer would be assigned to me shortly.

Another month passed, and I couldn't believe I still didn't have a way to write or communicate with Newk. I also hadn't received any mail from him. So I again called Randolph AFB in Texas and inquired how I could establish communication with my "detained" husband. I was told that very little mail was coming to families from the men held prisoner. Okay, that was pretty much what the Red Cross had said. The North Vietnamese weren't releasing the names of prisoners either, I was told. But for whatever reason, they had released Newk's name, and those capture photos, and a tape they claimed he had made! It was very upsetting not to get a satisfactory answer from anyone. No one seemed to know what was going on. We were supposed to be the most powerful nation on earth. Somehow that didn't add up to me. I felt the Air Force was simply ignoring my anxiety, our need for some word about his situation, our right to communicate with him, and that was making me angrier every month.

I learned from one of my neighbors that the Geneva Conventions had established rules about what mail Prisoners of War could receive and send. I immediately went to a library in Washington, D.C., and ordered a copy of the 1949 Geneva Convention rules relative to the Treatment of Prisoners of War. After reading that document, which clearly stated that POWs were allowed to send and receive mail, I resolved to move heaven and earth to reach Newk with a letter and to receive mail from him according to the tenets of the Geneva Conventions.

I think it was at that specific moment that a great resolve, and a well of strength I didn't even know I had were born in me. What my neighbor had told me was very clearly stated in Article 71, Section V of the Geneva Conventions regarding Prisoners of War:

> Prisoners of war shall be allowed to send and receive letters
> and cards . . . the said number shall not be less than two let-
> ters and four cards monthly, exclusive of the capture cards
> provided for in article 70.

And farther down in Article 71 . . . it said:

> Prisoners of war who have been without news for a long period, or who are unable to receive news from their next of kin or to give them news by the ordinary postal route, as well as those who are at a great distance from their homes, shall be permitted to send telegrams, the fees being charged against the prisoners of war's accounts with the Detaining Power or paid in the currency at their disposal . . . .as a general rule, the correspondence of prisoners of war shall be written in their native language.

I made up my mind to find out what a "Detaining Power" was, and where and how in this situation I should go about establishing an account with them for Newk with money in it. Sending packages, something else I had fretted about, was addressed in Article 72:

> Prisoners of War shall be allowed to receive by post or by any other means, individual parcels or collective shipments containing, in particular, foodstuffs, clothing, medical supplies, and articles of a religious, educational or recreational character which may meet their needs . . .[14]

You can imagine how upset I became, reading that. Newk had been a captive nearly three months, and I hadn't gotten any information at all from the Air Force about letters *or* packages! Was Newk the *only* prisoner of war over there not getting mail from his family? It made me sick at heart to even think about that.

I was naïve enough then to believe that the Geneva Conventions regarding Prisoners of War governed these matters. After all, it was an international legal document of great importance. North Vietnam had signed the Conventions. The United States also was a signatory. The other signatory nations were obliged by the Conventions to ascertain through the Protecting Power that countries in conflict carried out the provisions of the Conventions. Was that the same as the Detaining Power, I wondered? Probably not. Did we have a Protecting Power? From my experience so far, that didn't seem to be general information either. I had not been told about any country being designated the Protecting Power. That there should be one was very clear in the Geneva Conventions, but no one seemed to be reading them!

Not knowing exactly where we stood created even more anxiety in me. Meanwhile, time slid by with silence from Newk, and nothing that resolved this dilemma about the Geneva Conventions was explained to me by the Air Force, either.

I was at first bewildered, then fearful. I became more impatient as each week passed. Finally, above all else, I was angry—deeply, truly angry. But I had no way to use that anger effectively to achieve results. So it just roiled around inside me and built steam. There were no other POW wives I could consult, or compare notes with. There was no POW Wives organization that I knew of, and we were not given names or addresses of where the other women were.

I was assigned a new Casualty Officer. Fortunately, this time it was a knowledgeable and caring Air Force captain, who brought his wife along to comfort and help me. They did everything possible to make my situation more tolerable. That was wonderful, and I got along very well with both of them.

Newk's squadron Summary Courts Officer returned Newk's personal belongings to me. That was a dreadful day. Seeing his clothes, especially his dress uniform hat, really did me in. I held it, hugged it, then turned it over and over in my hands. Newk, and Newk's face, weren't under that hat. Would he ever be home to wear it again? The thought that he might not come home again just chilled me to the bone.

I never considered shielding our children from either the hurt or the "yo-yo" of hope and despair that I was experiencing. It was a part of all our lives. Far better for them to know what was happening and what bothered me, than to wonder later why I was behaving differently from before. The younger boys were still too young to have a good concept of time or distance. I was their barometer for emotions about their Daddy. They knew he was a prisoner of war in North Vietnam, but likely didn't even comprehend what that meant. I didn't comprehend it. How could they?

That April, I received a bouquet of roses for our thirteenth wedding anniversary from Newk's squadron with a card that said, "Since Newt is unable, please allow us in his behalf. The 20th TRS (Tactical Reconnaissance Squadron)."

I went into the bedroom, laid down on our bed and cried hard. I felt enormously grateful to the squadron for doing that. It was a wonderful, touching gesture, and one I needed so much to buoy me at that time. When the boys asked, I explained,

"No, the roses didn't exactly come from Daddy himself, because he isn't where they have a florist shop to buy roses, but his squadron friends bought them, because they know Daddy loves us, and would want us to have them."

Later I heard Roke in the living room, where I'd put the roses, telling his friend,

"These are from my Daddy . . . for Mom and us. Well, he didn't exactly buy them himself. He's a prisoner. But his friends sent them so he could tell us he loves Mommy and us."

"Is he in a real jail?" the other child wanted to know.

"I don't think so. Mom says he's in a little room like our bathroom, and he eats stuff like pumpkin soup, and he can't talk to the people there 'cause they don't talk like we do."

"Boy, he must have done something really bad to be locked up in a place like that. Pumpkin soup? Yuck!"

"No, he didn't do anything bad. He's in the Air Force. He wants to come home and be with us, but he can't because of the Vietnam War. That's where he is, in Vietnam."

"Where is Vietnam?"

"It's real far away. Here, I'll show you. Daddy has a globe of the world on his desk."

I heard the globe spinning and spinning and finally realized they were no longer "showing" but just fooling around. That globe was expensive. I went in and suggested another game to distract them, and they raced off to play outdoors.

Weeks slowly passed. I gestated. I heard absolutely nothing from Newk or the Air Force. Silence and worry were my daily rations. To keep myself from falling into depression, I tried to keep busy. I took the children to church every Sunday. I dressed up for Mother's Day. Mother and I took photos to send to Newk and for the new baby to see later.

I played bridge. I did research about prisoners of war and the Geneva Conventions. I felt like I was simply hanging in mental agony. Each day was worse than the last. What must it be like for Newk? Finally I learned from letters from friends and via the ubiquitous Air Force grapevine that most wives and families of POWs

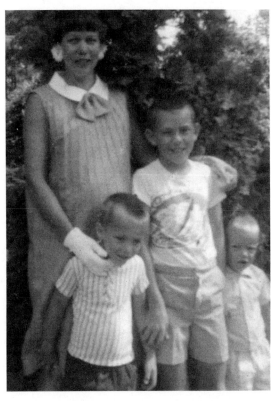

Evelyn, seven months
pregnant, with sons Van,
Jeff, Roke, May 1966.

held by the North Vietnamese weren't getting any mail from their
men either. In fact, there was no assurance that POWs were getting
the mail sent from the families. How did those families know where
to send mail? My mind was full of questions, but I got no answers
from the Air Force. Also, I didn't know any POW wives in my area
I could talk to about this.

What was wrong with our country, I wondered, that we could-
n't make a much smaller country like North Vietnam, smaller than
most of our states, obey a legal treaty they had signed? What good
is a treaty if it isn't enforced? Why *couldn't* our men write home?
Why *couldn't* we ascertain that they received our letters? The whole
situation seemed insane, and was against the international agreements of the Geneva Convention.

Had anyone in our government actually read the Geneva
Conventions? Did anyone in the Air Force read them? Mr.
President, Mr. Chairman of the Joint Chiefs of Staff, do you even
care about our men—or their anguished families?

The answer to that question became clearer in my mind with each passing month. It was NO—no one really cared all that much. The big corporations, the government officials and the American people were going on with their regular daily lives and their commerce. What I saw and heard in downtown Petersburg, and in other places I visited, was that we weren't a country united for a war we needed to win. The public didn't know much about Vietnam, our captured husbands, or the plight of the captives' families. What had happened to patriotism and getting behind your military in a war? I tossed and turned every night but no answers came. I prayed. I made promises to God, if I could only have a letter from Newk.

In May 1966, Newk had been a captive four months, and I was seven months along in my pregnancy. I knew we'd soon need a bigger and more reliable car, to transport the new baby and three growing boys. After test-driving numerous brands, I decided to buy a Volkswagen station wagon. It seemed to be the best value for the money. It was roomy, with enough space for me, the four kids, and Heidi the dog. When he got home, it would handle Newk too, and all our fishing and travel gear. It also would offer safe driving and riding comfort. I knew Newk would love it. We had lived in Germany, and we knew they made good, reliable vehicles.

"I'll take this one," I told the salesman after test-driving it one more time.

"Where is your husband to approve the purchase?"

I was annoyed about that but said firmly,

"My husband is overseas and unavailable. I have the legal right to purchase this car. I'd like to buy it now."

"How do I know that?"

"You'll have to trust that I have the necessary papers, which I can produce for you when we agree on a price and you write the sale up. If you can't, or won't, sell it to me, I'll go elsewhere. But please know I'll continue to do that until I find someone who understands that I'm an adult woman, ready and able to make decisions like this one. I do believe I'll find someone, somewhere, who will sell me this model Volkswagen station wagon."

Looking skeptical, he went away to consult his superiors. I duly produced my power of attorney for them. They sold me the car. I drove away in it. It was a small victory of sorts—winning one major skirmish in what had become a long, dreary war of my own. Thanks to the Power of Attorney, I'd won this round. The discouraging part was how many rounds I had already gone in just a few months, and how many more I might have to face before Newk was freed and came home.

As the baby came closer to term, I began to have an irrational fear that I would not survive the birth. I felt I simply couldn't birth this baby without Newk there to comfort me and watch the boys. I talked to him in my mind, and sometimes even out loud when I was alone.

"This time, I really need you, Newk. Managing four and everything else by myself is just too hard right now. Please . . . .please . . . just write us, let us know how you are. Please?"

Nothing changed except my size. I was weighed down with baby and feeling so tired and alone. If Mother hadn't been there for me, I simply couldn't have done it. July, my ninth month, was fiercely hot. The television news broadcast a horrifying film of U.S. Prisoners of War being paraded through the streets of Hanoi in North Vietnam. The men were wearing some kind of prison pajama like uniforms, and were shackled together in twos, shuffling along, looking haggard, like criminals from an awful foreign jail. Hundreds of angry, shouting Vietnamese jostled the guards, trying to get at our men. They all looked worn, dreadful. Seeing that film upset me terribly but I tried to steel myself and make a conscious effort to blank out my emotions as much as possible so that tears wouldn't cloud my vision as I searched among them for Newk.[15]

My eyes darted from one POW to the next, concentrating on their grim, tired faces. I was desperate for even a glimpse of Newk, but he wasn't among the POWs in that film. I felt both relief and the heartache of disappointment.[16]

On July 27, 1966, almost six months to the day after Newk was shot down and taken prisoner, Roy Fowler Grubb, our fourth son, was born at the Army hospital in Fort Lee, Virginia. Roy's arrival gave me a reason to go on living. He was a healthy baby at six pounds, twelve-and-a-half ounces. I couldn't wait to let Newk know about his new son. I wanted to tell him he'd have his own baseball team if we kept this up! Roy was Daddy's wonderful gift to us all. We loved him on sight.

However, the day after Roy's birth my elation faded. Fear of dying intruded into my consciousness . . . and remained. Maybe it was the loss of our infant daughter. I don't know, I just had this terrible fear for little Roy and myself and I couldn't shake it.

My obstetrician noticed that I was dejected and asked what was bothering me. When I told him about my death fears, he called in a psychiatrist, who explained that what I felt was very common among expectant mothers whose husbands had died or who had lost a previous child. He said he would help me work through these fears to avoid post-partum depression. I stayed in the hospital three more days, sleeping a lot, talking with the psychiatrist there. That respite and his care helped me regain my optimistic nature, I felt I could face going home to take up the care of four boys without Newk. At least I'd have help. Jeff could hardly wait to see his new brother, and Mother would be there. Newk's parents came from Philadelphia right away to see their newest grandson. The neighbors also came to help out by taking the older boys home to play with their kids.

Phone calls and congratulations poured in from all directions. That cheered me up immensely. My overwhelming need and first priority was to figure out how to get news about the baby's birth to Newk in North Vietnam. With help from some influential friends, we were able to get a message sent through our State Department channels. The British embassy contacted their representative in Hanoi, and the North Vietnamese agreed, "for this one occasion," to permit the British representative to transmit the message directly to the North Vietnamese Red Cross. That message read,

> Special birthday gift—number four son, Roy Fowler. Love and prayers are with you. All OK here. Signed: Evelyn and the boys.[16]

I was told through diplomatic channels that the North Vietnamese Red Cross had received the message, and I believed they would quickly get it to Newk.

Now he knows we have little Roy, he knows we are okay here, he knows we love him and that we know he's a prisoner of war, since the message will come to him via the North Vietnamese Red Cross.

I held imaginary conversations with Newk in my head as I

nursed our baby, and I truly believed our correspondence back and forth would start soon. It should now that the message about Roy's birth had been directly transmitted. That is the nature of "where there is life, there is hope." I believed deeply in my country, in the Geneva Conventions, in our innate goodness as human beings. Holding and rocking baby Roy, talking to my husband out loud as if he were there, I had hope, and I kept it alive in my heart.

Hope was the only magic Newk and I had going for us. Nothing else in this POW/MIA situation was going right. I vowed that very soon I would ask our government officials a simple question: *Why aren't the North Vietnamese abiding by the Geneva Conventions for treatment of Prisoners of War, Conventions to which they are signatories?*[17]

But I never dreamed how high up I would have to go, or how long it would take, to get an answer.

4 Invisible Shackles

TIMELINE . . . 1967-1968 . . . <u>WORLD</u> . . . ISRAEL WINS 6 DAY WAR WITH EGYPT . . . FIRST SUCCESSFUL HUMAN HEART TRANSPLANT . . . NORTH KOREA SEIZES USS *PUEBLO* . . . <u>VIETNAM</u> . . . TET OFFENSIVE . . . PEACE TALKS BEGIN IN PARIS . . . <u>USA</u> . . . ROBERT KENNEDY, MARTIN LUTHER KING JR., MALCOLM X ASSASSINATED . . . RICHARD NIXON ELECTED PRESIDENT . . . GREEN BAY PACKERS DEFEAT KANSAS CITY CHIEFS IN FIRST SUPERBOWL(1967)

They are slaves who fear to speak
For the fallen and the weak.
—James Russell Lowell

In 1967 we learned that life was very rough for all of our Prisoners of War in Vietnam, both those held by the Viet Cong in the south, and the Democratic Republic of Vietnam (DRV) in the north. Even so, never in my wildest dreams could I have imagined the extent of the horrific truth of what "very rough" might mean for the victims of Vietnamese torturers. Those truths didn't come to light until later. However, our government certainly had indications that the DRV and rebels were neither being humane, nor were they following the tenets of the Geneva Conventions their government had signed. What we weren't given was any assurance that our government had any specific plans to help those men, or to get them released soon.[1]

In April of 1967, *Life* magazine published still photos of a few of our POWs taken by an East German photographer. The men, dressed in something like pajamas, looked very strange. Their eyes seemed blank, devoid of any emotion or life. We also saw a film clip on television of the interview at which the photos were taken. In the film, one of the POWs, Navy Commander Richard Stratton, came out and bowed like a robot to the north, south, east, and west. That in itself was weird. But when he didn't speak— not one word, this really terrified the POW families and elicited a "stern warning" from our government to the Vietnamese about humane treatment of POWs. The war in Vietnam escalated a lot during those years, and the American Prisoner of War list increased with it. A news announcer said, "We're informed there are approximately 650 American military personnel classed as POWs or MIAs (missing) in North and South Vietnam. The U.S. believes that approximately 200 of these men are being held as Prisoners of War."[2]

The mail situation continued to frustrate me. In January of 1967, a year after Newk's capture, a close CIA friend and confidant of ours told me that if Newk was being held in the Hanoi prisons, he believed I should have his camp number or camp address. But I never received any camp number or camp address.

On February 7, in a letter from Lt. Col. Luther, Chief of the Casualty Division in the Air Force Personnel Center at Randolph Air Force Base, I learned only that:

> ... there has been a slight increase in correspondence from American prisoners in North Vietnam ... we sincerely hope that in the future you will hear from your husband ... Upon receipt of mail from your loved one, you may then write him at the return address furnished in his letter ...[3]

Since I hadn't received any mail at all "from my loved one," the only address I had for Newk was through the International Committee for the Red Cross (ICRC). Since the North Vietnamese were not even letting the ICRC into the country, I doubted any mail was reaching Newk or the other American POWs through them. Nor could the Red Cross confirm anything about mail, one way or another. It was the most anxiety ridden, helpless situation imaginable for a family.

Newk's promotion to Major was official in March of 1967. Although he was already almost 8 months old, I continued to mention the birth of our son Roy in every letter I wrote to him. Now I added the information about his promotion in all letters.

Time passed without any improvement or significant results, except that more and more men were being taken prisoner as the war continued. The mental torment was hideous and ceaseless. All kinds of frightening possibilities assailed my mind. Hundreds of questions I had went unanswered.

Maybe Newk is refusing to write. Maybe he is sick or injured and can't write. Maybe the North Vietnamese aren't letting him write. That would be an egregious violation of one of the most fundamental prisoner of war rights in the Geneva Conventions.

Why should the prisoners and their families have to endure this total lack of communication? Why aren't we doing something about that through international channels? Why aren't the United Nations and the countries who were signatories to the Geneva Conventions doing their duty to protest the North Vietnamese behavior? Why isn't anyone helping us?

Meanwhile, there were other pressing needs. For one thing, we needed to move. We had outgrown the tiny house we'd rented, thinking Newk would be gone 6 months to a year at most, and not figuring on another baby. I found and moved us into a larger rental house in Petersburg. It was newer and the rent was within our budget. Also, it had plenty of space for four boys, the dog, and all our furniture and belongings. Mother was only 3 miles away from us.

We were barely settled in mid-April of 1967 when I received another official letter from Lt. Col. Luther at the Casualty Office that confirmed my CIA friend's suspicions about mailing address-

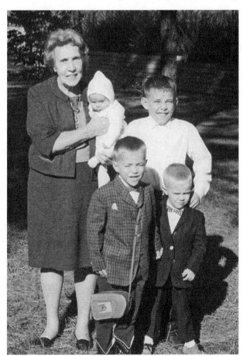

Evie's Mom, Florence Fowler, holding two-month-old Roy Fowler Grubb with grandsons Jeff, Roke, and Van. September 1966.

es. This one sent me into a towering rage, the worst anger I think I've ever experienced in my life. I was so upset that my heart pounded as if I had run miles. I could feel my blood pulsing like a drum in my ears.

The letter began, "This is to advise you of an alternate address you may use in attempting to correspond with your husband." At that, I was elated. Then, as I read further, my fury bloomed and grew like an atomic mushroom cloud. The address they enclosed appeared to be the main address that had to be used for mail going to the North Vietnamese prison camps! The military had known about this POW mailing address for more than a year but as the letter stated: "The use of this address has been previously limited to those next of kin who have been specifically advised to use it by their husbands or sons being held captive in North Vietnam."[4]

Despite the photos of him that had been distributed and published everywhere, photos proving my husband was alive and in captivity somewhere in North Vietnam, but because he had not *personally* written to me, *I was never given the right address by my own government* to send him letters! I simply could not believe what I was reading! As I stared at that sentence I became dizzy. A wave of nausea swept over me. I felt like I would faint, and had to sit and put my head down for a few moments. What if Newk was sick, or had a broken hand, or was injured in some way and couldn't write to me first? We had at that point endured more than a year of total silence and jumped through countless bureaucratic hoops in our desperate attempts to contact him. We'd tried every possible avenue to reach him with mail. We'd even gone through the State Department and the British Embassy.

Now this letter casually and coldly informed me that there *was and had been* another address to which I might have written Newk from the very beginning of his captivity, but at their discretion, the Defense Department and the Air Force Command Headquarters had simply *withheld* it from me and all the other wives and family members who hadn't yet heard from their captured husbands, sons or brothers! It not only blew my mind, it blew their credibility with me to hell and gone, and I'm sure it did the same with many other POW and MIA wives and families, too. What horrible mental torment they had deliberately inflicted on those of us who were the most vulnerable, the most anxious, the frightened ones yearning and wondering and not getting any mail! The letter continued,

> Defense and Air Force have recently decided that it would be in the best interests of all concerned if the address was made available to the next of kin of all personnel missing in action or captured in that country.

How magnanimous of them! The letter then laid out a whole set of rules and regulations about sending mail that the Defense Department and the Air Force had known about, but had never communicated to many of us families. The cruelty of it made me ill. Now we had even more pain to contend with:

> Only one envelope of 20 grams (2/3 ounce) maximum weight may be sent per month to each captured Air Force member; therefore, members of the immediate family must make arrangements to include all their letters, cards and photos in that one envelope. I truly hope that this new address may facilitate an exchange of mail.

How much was not delivered to our men because it weighed too much or wasn't exactly according to North Vietnam's stated rules and regulations for writing to POWs? I recalled Newk's anxiety and frustration in his few letters to me from Saigon, about how upset they were when they didn't get mail, or it was delayed for some unexplained reason.

The comment from our CIA friend about a camp number flashed through my mind. I studied the official address in the letter. It was simply, "Camp of Detention of U.S. Pilots Captured in the D.R.V," but there was no specific camp number. That worried me but I knew without a doubt now that our friend had known there was an address I could use, that I didn't have.

As soon as I calmed down, I sat down at my desk and wrote Newk at the new address. I was careful to keep the envelope to the required weight. Only one letter of 20 grams (2/3 of an ounce, including the envelope!) was a real blow to everyone in our family, and I'm sure in the other families too!

"It looks like I'll have to try to incorporate news about the entire family into my one 'allowed' letter to him each month for the time being," I reported .

What all these regulations, and the current change to "next of kin, one letter per month," would do to the mental and physical health of dear Mother and Dad Grubb, Newk's parents, I couldn't even contemplate. I could see the strain of not knowing about their son etching itself into their faces whenever they visited us. They tried to conceal it from the children. Newk was their only son. Their daughter Beverly was far away in Alaska. They were alone, getting older, were worried and frightened over Newk's silence, and terribly concerned about me and the boys.

The Air Force concluded the new mailing regulations letter by saying we could also try to continue sending mail through the International Red Cross "if you so desire, or use both addresses." I knew the ICRC would be useless. I'd already tried that a number of times with no success.

I was certain that, now that I had received the correct address, had followed all the rules the North Vietnamese laid down, and had written to Newk exactly within the confines of those rules, I'd be getting a letter back from him shortly, and he would tell me if he'd gotten any earlier letters. I went to the post office to assure they still had the forwarding address from our former residence on open file so that any mail from Newk would be forwarded to our new address.

"Don't worry, Mrs. Grubb, the clerk assured me. We're all as anxious as you are for a letter from your husband to come to you and your family. We'll be watching for it and get it to you right away, never fear." That lifted my spirits a lot. People *did* care.

The months continued to tick by, one after another, with no mail for us from "The Camp of Detention" in North Vietnam. Meanwhile, my life as the lone parent of four growing, rambunctious boys continued, and so did the family demands.

The boys were prone to the kind of mischief kids their ages got into. Mother was there for me as always, but I could see that the physical demands of helping me with four active boys, and the mental worry she had about Newk and me, were taking a toll on her, too. We were all trapped in a steel box, with no way out.

The boys were just getting out of school for the summer when I received an unusually long official letter, dated June 16, 1967, from Air Force Headquarters in Washington, D.C., through Lt.

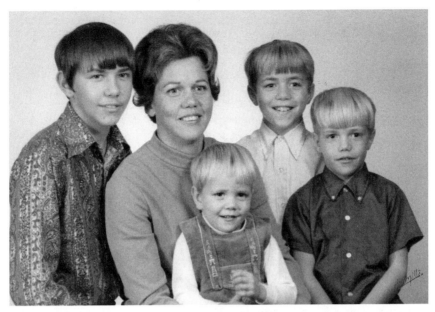

Evelyn Grubb with Roy on her lap. Standing behind are Jeff, Van, Roke. 1968.

Colonel Luther at Randolph Air Force Base. It contained a sobering description of what our government suspected might be going on with the U.S. Prisoners of War held by the North Vietnamese and Pathet Lao.

> Our government is deeply concerned about recent indications that North Vietnam may be mistreating American pilots in order to obtain propaganda statements or 'confessions' critical of United States policy in Vietnam . . .[5]

That foreboding opening was followed by two pages listing incidents that had been verified by our government officials as constituting what we considered humiliation and abuse of the Prisoners of War in North Vietnam, and confirmed that they "continue to received little or no information" about prisoners in South Vietnam, nor had they succeeded in getting anything but "total frustration" from the Pathet Lao about prisoners in Laos. The letter reiterated that our government" had sent a strong protest in March, and Ambassador Averell Harriman had issued a public statement printed in the April 7, 1967, issue of *Life* Magazine regarding the bizarre exploitation of Lt. Commander Richard Stratton in March. The letter said, in part:

> . . . we sent a strong protest to the North Vietnamese gov-
> ernment through the International Committee of the Red
> Cross, (ICRC). As a further measure, the United States
> Government called upon leaders of friendly, neutral nations
> to renew their efforts to bring influence upon North
> Vietnam to carry out its obligations under the Geneva
> Convention.[6]

Well, finally! I doubted that sending the official U.S. government protest via the ICRC would ever get it into Vietnam to their
government. I hoped that with help from our allies, the Vietnamese
would be forced to start invoking the Geneva Conventions regarding prisoners of war.[7] But very few "friendly, neutral nations" supported us in this divisive war.

I had heard from various "military grapevine" sources that many
other POW families, including Al Brunstrom's wife Helen, were
not receiving any mail either. Newk's wingman Al had sent me the
tape he made about Newk's bailout, following Newk's capture by
the North Vietnamese. Then, three months later, in April of 1966,
Al had been shot down over North Vietnam and captured. He had-
n't been heard from since then either. Helen had gone to live in
Florida with their young daughter, and we stayed in touch. We
hoped that somehow Newk and Al had found one another in the
prison camp, and were together. Now, receiving this official letter
about "mistreatment" there, our fear for our husbands escalated.

There were also concerns at home to deal with that demanded
most of my attention. I was worried about Roke's lack of progress
at school. As soon as school was out, I had Roke examined by a
doctor and tested for his school problems with reading. The medical diagnosis was that Roke was "immature for his age." As for
reading, his eyes weren't focusing properly yet and he was "dyslex-
ic"—a new word to us in 1967. Fortunately, one of my fellow
WOOS (Wives of Overseas Officers) friends, Judy Falkenrath, was
a teacher who had taken a year off to have a baby. When I told Judy
about Roke's difficulties, she offered to teach him to read in her
spare time, using phonics, sand writing, and other techniques she

had studied. Roke learned quickly from her in those one-on-one teaching sessions. However, it wasn't until he reached fourth grade that his mind and body kicked into synch and he became a very good and avid reader.

It was a real struggle and learning experience for me to manage everything alone. Worrying constantly about Newk also wore me down. I was often close to losing my grip over small stuff, and I was grateful to have Mother as a stabilizing force in my surreal life as time marched on with no relief or release. In August 1967, I wrote in my journal:

> Waiting—somehow I cannot wait with patience—it seems that when I must wait for little things I become more upset about them than with any other 'emergency.' Perhaps it's because life itself for me is waiting now, waiting and hoping for news from Newk.

There weren't any behavior or coping rules for POW or MIA wives to follow. There were no "how to" books to give us direction. We had no information, no other role models we knew to emulate. I wasn't big on introspection. Who had time? Besides, I had always been an action person. As time wore on with no relief or change in sight, I was becoming more discouraged. My attitude was negative and fatalistic. I also found myself becoming much more introspective.

I wondered about other POW wives, who they were, where they were, and how they were managing. Were they doing better than I was? Except for Helen Brunstrom, I didn't know any other POW wives. Helen had only one daughter to cope with. I knew she and her daughter missed and worried about Al just as much as the boys and I missed Newk. The services didn't encourage or do anything to help the families of POWs to get together. I had the WOOS wives for company, but the active duty Officers Wives Clubs didn't really reach out to us. We had to scramble on our own for footing, and each create her own way to handle the horrible stress and anxiety, learn how to deal with it, and survive it. There was no organization of POW or MIA wives, and I knew that we sure needed one!

You'd think that as time passed, it would get easier, but it did not. It got worse, like a cancer being ignored and not treated. Each month of uncertainty was harder than the last. Patience and nerves stretched thinner and became taut. In late August 1967, Newk had been captive and silent for eighteen months, and it finally began taking a huge toll on me, physically and mentally. I yelled at the boys. I spanked when they were naughty. They began to avoid me, and my temper outbursts. I felt guilty, inadequate. I hated myself, the world, this war, everyone. I was thoroughly disgusted with the North Vietnamese government, furious at our own wimpy, helpless government, and tired of getting mired-in-bureaucratic-claptrap and runaround from the Air Force and Department of Defense. I felt that the U.S. government, and the Defense Department, were making little or no effort to win, shorten, or settle this war. Nor did they seem to have any chops when it came to protesting about the POWs. We just kept throwing more troops into the fray, like dumping more wood on an out of control forest fire.

The students and young people, who were most affected by the draft, had begun staging riots and sit-ins. The general American public, heretofore indifferent to the war (in truth, most Americans still didn't even know, or care, where Vietnam was) suddenly woke up, and they began showing outward restiveness and anger about the ongoing war. It was into its sixth active year, since the late President Kennedy's inauguration in 1961, but actually into its thirteenth since Eisenhower first sent military advisers to South Vietnam in 1955.[8]

At the end of August I received another letter from Air Force Headquarters about the newly formed DOD Prisoner of War Policy Committee. I read it with great hope and interest. Under point 3, the letter said,

> Accordingly, Secretary of Defense McNamara has directed the formation of a Department of Defense Prisoner of War Policy Committee to take cognizance of all matters in the DOD concerning U. S. Military Personnel held captive . . . Assistant Secretary of Defense for International Security Affairs, Mr. Paul C. Warnke, has been designated Chairman.[9]

Not long after that I received a six page newsletter type publication entitled "Viet-Nam Information Notes" (Vietnam was often written Viet-Nam) published by the Office of Media Services of the U.S. State Department (#9, August 1967). In part, it said,

> On June 11 1965, M. Jacques Freymond, Vice President of the ICRC, wrote to the United States Government, the Government of South Vietnam, the government of North Vietnam and the National Liberation Front, reminding each of them of their obligation to apply the Geneva Convention in Vietnam. On August 10, 1965, Secretary of State Dean Rusk wrote to the ICRC, stating "The United States Government has always abided by the humanitarian principles enunciated in the Geneva Conventions and will continue to do so . . . " South Viet-Nam made a similar reply to the ICRC on August 11, 1965 . . . North Viet-Nam and the Viet Cong, on the other hand, have refused on various grounds to apply the Geneva Conventions for the benefit of prisoners of war held by them.*

While frightening to contemplate the stance North Vietnam had taken, it wasn't news to me. We all knew that North Vietnam was not abiding by the Geneva Conventions. What disturbed me was that our country and our military services were complaining about it but *doing nothing specific* to resolve the problem. And meanwhile, the long, dreary wait, the war, and our lives were marching on. On September 5, 1967, Roy took his first steps. I noted it down in my 1967 engagement calendar, so I'd be able to show the date to Newk when he came home.

Then in mid-October 1967, Mary Crow of Virginia Beach, a woman I didn't know, telephoned me to tell me about a POW/MIA wives' meeting that had recently been held in Newport News, Virginia, about 50 miles from Petersburg. That call was an emotional catalyst. First of all, it showed me that I was not alone

---

*Various references are made to Geneva Convention and Geneva Conventions. Geneva Convention usually refers to the meeting itself in 1949; Geneva Conventions to the set of rules promulgated at that meeting. However, in common parlance the two are often used interchangeably to indicate one or both.

with my fears, frustration and anger. Mary assured me that other wives were in the same agony, and most of them had not gotten any mail from their husbands either. What a relief it was to learn I was not alone in this, nor was Helen.

These wives were just beginning to find one another, meet, and talk about their pain. I almost cheered, and promptly gave her my contact information and that of the few other Air Force POW/MIA wives I knew. The call ended with me pleading, "Please . . . please call me again! I want to attend all your meetings."

I didn't know then how critical that phone call would be in changing me as a person and in shaping my life for the near term. At about that same time, pictures of more POWs from Hanoi were shown on the *Huntley-Brinkley Report*. Again, Newk wasn't among them. *Where could he be,* I wondered? *Why doesn't he write to me?*

About then, a second divine intervention came, with a call from a wonderful and generous local lady named Peggy Manley. She had heard about me, had imagined what I was enduring, and wanted to help the POW families any way she could.

"I want to meet you, and please know I pledge my support for any project that you might champion," she offered. I couldn't wait to meet her! Older than I was, Peggy was a thin, serious-faced woman with a source of energy and enthusiasm that transformed her into my angel of mercy.

October 23, 1967, was a red-letter day for me. I attended my first POW/MIA wives' meeting at Navy wife Louise Mulligan's home in Newport News, Virginia. Mary Crow was there to greet me. That day I also met another stalwart and wonderful woman, Phyllis Galanti, from Richmond, Virginia. Her husband, Navy Lieutenant Paul Galanti, had been captured five months after Newk, in June 1966. All this time I'd been feeling so alone and lost, as had Phyllis, and we were living only 30 miles apart! Phyllis had encountered two other volunteers willing to help us. Both were pilots in the Air Force Reserves: Jim Zga and attorney William "Whitey" Park Lemmond. Both men were full of good ideas and had the ability to act on them. We welcomed them. Whitey became my longtime friend and a staunch supporter of the POW wives and families.

The Air Force initially expressed concern when they learned

about our meeting, but the Navy got fully behind us. I called the Air Force Casualty Office at Randolph, and said that I felt the Navy was being much better and more active than the Air Force in keeping the POW and MIA wives informed. I informed them I had just learned from the Navy POW and MIA wives that the Navy issued frequent informative newsletters, and maintained more personal contact with their POW/MIA families. I said we felt that since we had the majority of POWS in North Vietnam, the Air Force could at least do as much as the Navy for our POW/MIA families.

"When we have information, we pass it on to the families," the Air Force representative at Randolph informed me rather coldly. They didn't accept criticism well. I tried another tack. "The Air Force families have more POWs than any another service, yet we get precious little information from Air Force sources to help or comfort us. The Navy is much nicer and more sympathetic to their POW and MIA wives. Why is that? Do you know?" He referred me to another person, who referred me to another person, Lt. Col. Harris. I repeated my comments to each one. Lt. Col. Harris was the only Air Force officer who took my complaints about the lack of support from the Air Force seriously. He went to Major General Wilson, at the Pentagon, and relayed the information I'd passed on. The ensuing hornets nest came back down to a Major Gratch in Texas, who had to reply to General Wilson's questions. Major Gratch contacted me. I was equally frank with him. I said,

"We believe that in geographic areas where there are reasonable numbers of POW/MIA families, we should be helped by the services to get in touch with one another. The wives in my area met recently, and we believe that a single agency should be created to support all the Army, Navy, Air Force and Marine families of POWs or MIAs in each large geographic area of the United States, to keep us updated and informed about our missing and imprisoned men."

Major Gratch was very nice about it but said they had no authority to create such an agency. I said "Well perhaps there is something else the Air Force can do to help us join together as a group . . . .give us an advisor, or other help. Can't you at least look into that, please? We are suffering, our husbands are suffering, and no one is helping us."

I felt good knowing I was not the only POW/MIA wife who would make these suggestions and phone calls. We had decided to be united in this new effort. What was really important about all our calls was that *the services got the message.* The POW/MIA wives were getting together and speaking out. We put the services on notice that we weren't going to sit still any more and simply wait, as we'd been told to do. We had done that for years, with zero results. Now we wanted action instead of reams of empty words. We were a grass roots organization of women. We were inexperienced at charting this kind of action, but we were very determined to do it.

At the end of October 1967, I received another letter from the Air Force. It informed me that I would be allowed to send a Christmas package to my POW in North Vietnam that year. They underscored that the packages would be sent in two increments— first, to the POWs "whom North Vietnam has specifically acknowledged." They then listed the various ways acknowledgement might have occurred, putting Newk in that group. They claimed, "Our rationale is, we honestly feel that packages intended for personnel whom Hanoi has said are in fact prisoners, stand a slightly better chance of being delivered . . ." We were cautioned to "closely adhere to the following instructions . . ." which designated "one package from the next of kin, not more than 3 pounds, content limited to recreational items, tobacco items, hard candy, small gifts made by children, and the like." I sighed. Rules and more rules, restrictions and more restrictions. I just wished we'd get the upper hand with this war. Vietnam was smaller than a lot of our States. Why were we so helpless?

Not long afterward, a second letter came from Air Force Headquarters that changed the instructions of the first letter. That second letter, dated 27 November, with less than a month left until Christmas, informed us, in part:

> . . . unfortunately, there has been an unforeseen change in
> procedures over which we had no control and of which I
> must immediately inform you. In the event you have already
> mailed your package, it will be returned to you by your local
> post office, so I advise you to contact your postal officials

without delay.

Then, they said, we could rewrap the whole package and try again. I wondered if anything would ever go sanely for us in this whole process. The North Vietnamese certainly had us jumping around like puppets with them jerking our strings every which way at will. I read on:

> The package, after you have re-wrapped it in the inner wrapper, must be taken to the post office. Postal officials will then affix the proper postage, at no cost to you, for forwarding from Jamaica (Long Island) to North Vietnam, and the necessary cancellation stamps. You must then wrap the package in an outer wrapper and address it as follows: PERSONAL Mr. Edwin H. Essig, Postmaster, Jamaica, Long Island, NY 11431. You will be required to pay the postage from your postal area to Jamaica, Long Island.[10]

I decided to follow the example of the other wives and make a list of everything I packed and sent to Newk. I still have that 1967 list:

- Family Christmas cards and notes to Daddy from the kids.
- A booklet of photos showing all the family.
- A cribbage board with cards, pegs, instructions for playing.
- A slide rule.
- A harmonica.
- Dice.
- A tablet and 3 pencils, with a sharpener.
- A ballpoint pen.
- 2 pairs of thermal socks.

I was foolish enough to presume that bare essentials, the basic survival supplies, were being provided to the POWs by the North Vietnamese, since they had boasted internationally and in newspapers around the world, that they were providing "humane and lenient treatment" to our POWs. So I figured Newk would want family photographs, writing materials, and other distractions to help him pass the time. Socks were a basic, but I knew our guys' feet were probably bigger than the average Vietnamese's feet, and socks wore out quickly, so I sent those. I was actually feeling almost cheerful as I packed up the holiday box. At last I'd found some other POW wives to talk with about these things.

During this package mix-up exercise, I received an invitation to go to Langley Air Force Base in Virginia on October 31 1967. Mother came over to be with the boys when they got home from school. At that meeting, I encountered a much larger group of Air Force POW/MIA wives, and we were excited to meet each other. Also, we were very encouraged by the fact that this was an official Air Force function, not a Navy event, which meant that our new activism with the Air Force staff in charge of POW matters, had scored a point in our favor.

The Air Force representatives there showed us a film of a North Vietnam Prison camp they had procured. They wouldn't tell us where, how or when they'd gotten it. It showed some of our POWs sweeping the yard in one of the prison camps in Hanoi. We were stunned to learn they actually had such a film. I sat forward and studied it very closely, but Newk was not among these men at this particular camp, nor was Al Brunstrom in it.

Although only a few men were visible in the film, Betty Vogel spotted her husband, Richard D. Vogel, who had been shot down five months ago, in May 1967.[13] After she got over the emotion that brought, they rewound and played it again for her. At one point, she asked them to stop and replay the last segment. Then she said, "My husband isn't left-handed, but he's sweeping left-handed. Do you think he is injured?"

The Air Force group rewound and replayed it once more, and after studying it closely, they realized that most of the men in it were sweeping left-handed. They surmised the film probably had been developed or printed in reverse. We all congratulated Betty for being so sharp. If they were using the film to plot a layout of the prison camp for a rescue or an air drop, their layout would have been the reverse of the real camp. I think they appreciated Betty being quick on the uptake on that. Maybe they even realized for the first time that perhaps the POW wives might be of some help to them on certain matters.

December brought our second Christmas without Newk. The first Christmas he'd been gone had not been as bad as this one. Newk was in Saigon in December of 1966 and still in contact with us, able to send tapes and gifts. This Christmas was a sad one.

Daddy was not there, we'd heard nothing from him, and we didn't know his whereabouts or his physical condition.

Jeff was old enough to help me with the Santa gifts for his little brothers. Roke sang in the church choir. Newk's parents could not come because of heavy snows, so it was just Mother and the five of us. I wrote in my calendar,

> How I miss feeling—the feeling of loving a husband—the joy of having him home, in his favorite chair. The sensations of being loved.

That second year of Newk's captivity, I was close to a breakdown from lack of respite from continuous anxiety. Unrelenting fear and dread for my husband, and what he might be enduring, was with me constantly. I found myself becoming mentally scattered. Activity kept my mind and body occupied, but was not helping me all that much. I kept at it because it was an outlet for built up sexual and emotional energy, and also a diversion from the anger and frustration of my situation. I was neither wife, nor widow. The evenings and nights were so lonely! Sometimes I had to completely exhaust myself, just to deal with my loneliness, and not knowing if Newk was alive or dead, sick, in pain, or what. *Was he not writing because he thought we weren't trying to write him?* That was the worst possible nightmare. I knew that nights were just as awful or probably worse for Newk, wherever he was.

Some nights when I was feeling more positive, I would lie in bed and reflect on what our future might be like. We were young, vital, only in our mid-thirties. We had a lot of living to do with a family of active young boys to raise. I loved and missed Newk desperately. I'd plead with God to help us. "We want to be a family again! That's why we married, and had children. Is it unreasonable to want him here with me again? As a husband and lover, a father to his four little sons, and the chance to try again to have a daughter? Please . . . I want both our lives back! I'm a prisoner in this terrible web, too. We're both chained in different awful prisons by people and circumstances we can't see, can't fight, and can't overcome." I wondered if, after all this was over with, we'd even be able to be a married couple again. Would there be so much regret and anger we wouldn't understand each other any more? Would Newk be physically and mentally okay after his ordeal? Would I? Who knew?

Some of my nights were spent in silent, angry discourse and futile reasoning with phantom officials. Why can't we just go there and tear that place up and bring them back, from a country as small as North Vietnam? Why can't we make North Vietnam follow the Geneva Conventions? We are the most powerful country on earth! This is ridiculous! I want my husband back while I'm still young, so we can watch our children grow together.

Given all that, 1967 had been pretty hideous. Finally, mercifully, it passed. I tried to buoy myself to face 1968 by listening again to the words on Newk's last tape, which I played for the hundredth time, on New Year's Day.

"We'll get together again, one of these days soon . . ."

I had no idea when "one of these days soon" might come. I could only hope it would be "soon."

At five years of age, Van was busy and into everything. He kept the baby and the rest of us entertained. One day during a storm, he earnestly tried to explain lightning to his little friend.

"It's light in a line, with a lot of louds at the end," he said.

And when the television picture went out one night and the announcer said, "We are experiencing some difficulty, please stand by," Van jumped up and stood by the television set, looking very serious. It was a good thing the kids occasionally offered some laughs, because there sure wasn't much else to laugh about in our lives.

It was at that point that I learned I'd have to appeal to Congress to obtain Newk's full pay and be able to deposit it in a savings account that had just been established. I put out my request, and was ordered to attend a "hearing." At that dreadful confrontation, one Congressman, completely ignorant of what we as a family were enduring, snapped at me, "Why should we pay the wives? What did YOU do to earn his pay?"[12]

That simply took my breath away. What indeed? He had not the first clue of what we had gone through during the past two years, and were still going through. What had he done to become my master and judge?

Instead of, "What can we, your representatives of a grateful nation, do to help you and your children endure this agony and survive financially until your husband is repatriated?" He was asking me *what was I worth to my country?* Obviously, in his opinion, I was worth nothing. Or less. The cold reality of what these men we'd elected to represent us really thought about us, the wives and families of the men who were serving their country, was a blow like a face slap to my personal esteem that would remain with me from that day forward. I saw how stunned the other Congressmen looked and fortunately one intervened and shut him up. He didn't ask me any more questions. Nevertheless, a cruel shock like that served to strengthen my inner resolve, and that would turn me in a new direction.

When I got home from that session, I sat and went through my 1966 and 1967 engagement calendars, looking for memories— things I'd done, or the boys and I had done, that I would be proud to share with Newk when he came home. Aside from Roy's birth, that we'd moved, the children's school progress, and my bridge group, there wasn't a whole lot. Okay . . . what was I doing to earn Newk's pay every month? Our families helped and buoyed me in every way they could, and Newk's father did his best to fill in for Newk with the boys, but what was I doing to better our situation? Little or nothing except being anxious, frightened, angry, and feeling sorry for myself. An arrow in my soul was that so many young, stalwart, intelligent husbands and fathers were being killed, wounded, or captured in this war. Many more had been, and were being, shot down somewhere in remote Southeast Asia, and remained MIA, missing in action.

I realized then that there was no "end game" toward which our government was moving, at least not in regard to the MIAs and POWs. That meant that my situation, and poor Newk's, and those other haggard men I'd seen on TV (some of them had been there in prison months or years longer than Newk) would likely continue for the foreseeable future. So I'd need a plan—an end game of my own—for continuing to live my life just as it was now, for who knew how long, until Newk came back to us. When he did, he'd discover to his surprise that I was a different woman.

There were anti-Vietnam protesters massing in cities and on college campuses. Students chanted the rallying cry, "Hell no we won't go!" everywhere. At first, I didn't pay a lot of attention to them. But as time went on, their anti-war chants became louder, and more profane. There was also more violence in their protests. I knew firsthand about the fear and frustration that fueled such depths of fury with our government. I was living it every single day. People fought not to go to Vietnam, not to be drafted, not to become part of the situation in which we were hopelessly trapped. But no one tried to help get us un-trapped. Our men had been prisoners, in the hands of the enemy, for *years*.

As for me, I still was not adjusted to the most painful aspect of my daily routine: waiting for the mail delivery, hoping for a miracle and some word from Newk. The sinking feeling of deep disappointment when it wasn't there. I had to do something to get myself away from the mailbox torture.

In January 1968, on the second anniversary of Newk's capture, I wrote another of the letters to Newk that flowed out of our house like a small river, only to reach a dam somewhere that blocked his receiving them, or blocked his correspondence back to us. This was the first written in the jaunty, cheerful turquoise blue ink I had chosen for 1968. I'd used a different color ink on my letters each year, hoping that might give Newk a little lift and make him smile when he received them. He would be able to look through them and find incidents of a particular year by its ink color. But then, as I got into writing this first turquoise letter, I felt my despair, anguish and yearning must be reflected in my words, cheerful ink or not . . . so much so that I simply couldn't finish it, and never did mail it to him. Reading it again always brings back painful, long-buried memories.

> January 28, 1968
>
> Darling, oh Darling, it's been the longest weekend I've ever spent. Friday it was two years since you were shot down. Two, long, awful, lonely, desolate years without you—the part of me that is most worth existing is fading into awful nothingness without you. When we are together, my life is whole—and without you I simply exist.
>
> The news reported that 3 pilots would be released to 'honor' the Tet holiday on Saturday. My heart stopped when I heard the news—then beat faster, as I thought

maybe—oh, dear God in His infinite wisdom would choose you. It has been both a joyous and fearful waiting time—if only you'd come home, if only you are alive, well, and able to come home—how wonderfully happy, how glorious it would be. I've been short with the children, but last night my dreams were happy dreams. I was able to see you, to touch you in my dreams for the first time in months. Can you imagine my dreams? Have you had them too? Where you were there, but beyond my touch, beyond my call, so near and yet frustrating beyond the point of tears & screaming, just hopeless . . . yearning for you . . . always hoping.

Now the names are released, and it is not your turn to come home. The waiting begins again, hoping for a letter, hoping for some word or sign that you are still alive. Oh, Newk, can this go on and on and on? We are both prisoners—and it's worse being a captive inside your own skull, as I am—afraid to feel, to think about anything, for fear it is the discovery that I'm waiting for nothing. For no one. Even if you return, will you still love and honor our relationship of so long ago? I'm OLD now, ancient in the knowledge of tragic reality, where we appear as mere fly specks on the window of time, to be washed away in the passing showers and forgotten as though we never existed at all. It's awful to feel this OLD at 36—will there be a life for us again? God alone knows, and He is amusing Himself with our frailties—my whole life is a prayer, my body a church. No day passes without a re-dedication to love and peace, and yet for all these endless days it has been for nothing—or is there yet an answer? Is God just waiting to make our reunion a really sacred thing? Oh, Newk, stay alive—I need you so much, and prayer is my only contact with you. Must I have doubts now, when perhaps I should feel stronger than ever that we are important, that SOMEDAY, oh, God, PLEASE—someday soon we will be together here on earth again. I love you Newk, I love you. . . .

Weeping, I threw down the pen, wiped my eyes, and ran out of the room. The letter remained unfinished. The boys had grown so much, and Newk was missing their childhood. It was something neither he nor they could ever recover, and I grieved over that. Jeff was now a sturdy 12 year old, just beginning to leave boyhood and stretch up to adolescence. He and Roke, who had turned 7, watched television news and listened to the radio reports about the war and the rising concern over the North Vietnamese treatment of the American prisoners. Van at 5 was a kindergartner. Soon he'd be reading, too, and watching the news instead of cartoons. He no longer remembered his Daddy, although I played Newk's tapes for them over and over so they'd hear his voice. And Roy was toddling everywhere and climbing on things, starting to talk.

I tried desperately to keep Newk alive in our minds and in our hearts. But a picture wasn't a hug, and an old, often repeated tape wasn't Daddy rolling around on the floor or tickling them or going fishing with them. Our sons had endured so much, and gotten so little in return! I became more active in WOOS—the Wives of Overseas Officers, most of whom were Army wives. The army maintained a formidable presence in Korea, where wives and families weren't allowed, in addition to the escalating deployments to Vietnam. Army wives and children waited in the states while their husbands were sent overseas for periods of a year to 18 months or more. It was accepted as part of being in the service. They had a better attitude about long military separations than I did, and I tried to learn from them.

I had to admit to myself, in the dark of my lonely nights, that I really didn't know who, or what, I was any more. How long could this last, I wondered, before I cracked apart and shattered? To distract myself, I agreed to play bridge with the WOOS wives once a week. And on Saturday nights we had parties with the kids at each others' homes, or went to the movies together as a group. Once in awhile, we got sitters for the kids and went to the Officers' Club for an adults-only dinner in the evening. It was one of those evenings we were at the O-Club, as we called it, when an older woman approached me, her eyes narrow, her lips pursed.

"Are you the woman with a POW husband?" she demanded.

"Yes, I'm Evelyn Grubb. Do I know you?"

"No, but I want to know how you can come here and laugh and be happy, while your husband survives in squalor and torment over there in Vietnam. You should be ashamed! Don't you know how you make others feel? You don't belong here. You should go home and stay there, where you belong."

Again, like with the Congressman's unexpected vitriolic attack on POW wives, I was too stunned to respond. But Judy jumped up, threw her napkin down and spoke up, not quietly.

"She's our guest and we're delighted she's here. Why don't you just go back to your own table and leave us alone?" Another friend grabbed Judy's arm to defuse the confrontation. "Ignore her. She's just ignorant."

At that, the woman huffed and stalked off. We tried to continue to enjoy our evening out, but couldn't get the mood back. Later, home in bed, I thought about it again.

I was still a U.S. military officer's wife, maybe even his widow, for all I knew. Did she even comprehend my life, my fears? Did she think that staying home, having a horrible, weeping time for years on end until I went quietly insane, would somehow help my husband in that "camp of detention" over in North Vietnam?

Once again, an uninvited tirade against me and whatever I was seen as doing wrong had hurt and affected me deeply. I tried not to let myself dwell on it. Mother consoled me when I shared it with her. "I'm sorry that had to happen, Evie. Some people just don't think before they say things they shouldn't. Try to forget it. It really doesn't mean anything, so don't you let it."

In February of 1968, the Viet Cong opened the "Tet offensive." The reporting of it, and the spike in loss of life it engendered, had a substantial negative impact on American public opinion: 2,197 American troops were killed in action in February 1968, the highest number in any month since the war began. As a result, Lyndon Johnson's ratings dropped significantly, and after Tet, he stopped the escalation of the war.[13] I was concerned about the poor leadership we seemed to have where this war was concerned.

On February 26, Major Carleton called from Randolph Air Force Base, and left word with Mother that Newk's name had been brought back by three recently released prisoners. My heart was pounding when I called Major Carleton back, certain that I'd get some real time news about Newk. But Major Carleton said that the released POWs had not actually seen or spoken with Newk themselves. They had learned his name from others and had committed

"Will Grubb's" name, along with hundreds of others, to memory. The three prisoners also said that they had no personal knowledge of anyone dying as a captive.[14] That was a relief, but it didn't answer why I wasn't hearing from Newk.

My sister-in-law Norma called one of the returned prisoners, Lt. Matheny, to try to talk with him briefly. Someone who identified himself as An Air Force representative, but didn't give his name, promptly called me to reprimand me.

"We would prefer that you and your family not pressure us or Lt. Matheny for further information."

"Well tell me who *should* I pressure for further information about my husband? Please . . . just tell me, and I'll contact that person immediately."

There was always a patient silence, inevitably followed by the stock answer: "I'm sorry Mrs. Grubb, I wish I could help you, but we have no further information."

As a country, we certainly weren't putting any pressure on the North Vietnamese on behalf of these men. The North Vietnamese were still openly violating every single article of the Geneva Conventions on Prisoners of War, and had been doing that since the French-Indochina war. President Eisenhower had been right when he wrote in 1954 that he was "bitterly opposed" to ever getting the United States involved in that region.

The Christmas package I had mailed to Newk in November 1967 came back to me. No note accompanied it, nor any explanation. It would have normally sent me into a tailspin, had I not already heard from the Navy wives that many, many POW/MIA packages were being returned with no explanation, even though we were told it was okay to send packages and went through their whole rigamarole.

Vice Admiral B. J. Semmes, Chief of Naval Personnel, sent a sympathetic letter to the Navy wives and families, acknowledging this latest cruel blow to the families. When my Navy friends heard that my package to Newk had come back too, they provided me with a copy of Admiral Semmes' letter, which was a great comfort to me at that difficult time, believe me.

> Most of you who sent packages before Christmas have had
> them returned, and many of you asked whether we've had

any success at all. I don't believe that we have. The whole-sale rejection of the packages clearly indicates Hanoi's pol-icy. The Deputy Secretary of Defense has asked for a status report on the package project. We anticipate that the report will occasion a public statement. I regret that this effort did not succeed, but believe it was worth a try.

Then he elaborated on several other questions we'd raised about finances, and about getting some publicity for our cause, conclud-ing,

Our major purpose has been to avoid exposing you to harassment by 'anti-Vietnam Policy' agitators, and to avoid invasions of privacy by well-meaning news media . . . it is not our intention to inhibit your communication or associ-ation. I realize that our efforts are a poor substitute for some concrete progress toward bringing your men home. All of us have that as our first and foremost consideration . . . I join you in the fervent hope that this year will see your men home. For my part I will leave nothing undone that can contribute in any way to bringing the day of return nearer.[15]

I think I appreciated more than anything his acknowledgment that they had no intention to inhibit our communication or associ-ation, and understood that their efforts were bringing at best puny results. That was human and understanding.

Mary Crow and I decided that maybe if we made some sugges-tions to the Air Force about our needs, it would have a positive effect. So we wrote letters to Air Force Lt. Colonel Luther and Major Gratch with a list of questions we wanted the Military Services and the U.S. government to answer for the wives and fam-ilies. We cited the lack of application of the Geneva Conventions in general and in particular we noted my lack of any letters or information from my husband which was a violation of Section V, Article 70 of the Geneva Conventions regarding POWs, which stated (and I quoted):

Immediately upon capture, or not more than one week after arrival at a camp, even if it is a transit camp, likewise in case of sickness or transfer to hospital or to another camp, every

> prisoner of war shall be enabled to write direct to his fami-
> ly . . . informing his relatives of his capture, address, and
> state of health. The said cards shall be forwarded as rapidly
> as possible and may not be delayed in any manner.[16]

That was clear enough. In addition, we suggested the following actions for the Services:

- We would appreciate a monthly newsletter to cover matters like explaining our Savings Deposit Program, Income Tax and Social Security, legal affairs and other problems the wives and families of POWs and MIAs are experiencing
- We would appreciate a combined services/State Department briefing on a regularly scheduled basis, to give us updates on military and State Dept. information on MIA and POW affairs.
- We request that at those briefings, all photos and films be shared with us for viewing and identification purposes.
- We ask for updates and information on the newly formed Warnke Committee formed by Congress to oversee Prisoner of War matters.
- We request that more knowledgeable and higher ranking casualty offi- cers be assigned to us, who would understand the legalities and intrica- cies of our problems.

We concluded our letters with these remarks:

> Most of us are intelligent, educated women vitally con-
> cerned with every facet of the Missing in Action and
> Prisoner of War problems; as well as striving to maintain a
> stable home life under the stress of so many uncertain con-
> ditions. Yet we feel that those of us who care the most are
> the least informed. It is becoming increasingly clear that
> more information could, indeed should, be provided to us.
> Perhaps these suggestions will promote the action necessary
> to accomplish our requests in a satisfactory way to both the
> families and the Air Force.

In reply, Mary and I both received a gracious and thoughtful letter from Colonel Luther, dated March 21, 1968. Colonel Luther told us in his letter that a newsletter might be beneficial and he planned to publish one regularly for all POW/MIA wives and fam- ilies.

The first will be based upon the debriefing of three recently released prisoners. We estimate that this letter will be
published by 15 April, 1968. We plan to include . . . information on living conditions and daily routines of prisoners,
plus other items of interest you have suggested.[17]

He went on to say that he felt our suggestion about a combined
services briefing had merit, and he would take that suggestion forward to the Warnke Committee.[18] He hoped to have an announcement of progress, as well as answers about disseminating more
information to the next of kin, in the first newsletter.

Most of the pilots who were shot down over North Vietnam
and taken prisoner were officers. Colonel Luther wouldn't commit
to assigning a stateside officer to each next of kin as "casualty officers," because of the large number of officers that would be
required. While there had not yet been an accurate accounting of
POW/MIAs or a reliable list of names from Hanoi, I gathered that
there must be many more pilots and officers MIA or POW than we
knew about. Colonel Luther did assure us that "an officer is always
available to the next of kin, should they require the personal assistance of one."

We never received the promised newsletter in April or follow-
up on any of the matters we addressed to Colonel Luther. I did
receive a letter dated March 7 1968, from Major Gratch that
addressed our concerns about treatment of POWs under the terms
of the Geneva Conventions. It said,

> Dear Mrs. Grubb:
>
> Thank you for your letter of 1 March 1968 pertain-
> ing to your husband, Major Wilmer N. Grubb, and in which
> you enclosed a list of questions concerning living conditions
> of personnel who are prisoners of the North Vietnamese.
>
> Reference is made to the telephone conversation on
> 27 February 1968 with Major Carleton advising you of the
> action to be taken after the debriefing of the three recently
> released officers. The debriefing is in its final stages and,
> upon completion, information that is obtained about the
> treatment, living conditions and related topics will be com-
> piled in a letter and forwarded to the next of kin of our

missing and captured personnel. In their preliminary debriefing, the officers stated that they had been treated reasonably well, by Oriental standards.

Enclosed please find a photograph, just received through our intelligence sources, alleged to be of your husband. Any comments you have regarding it will be appreciated. A self-addressed envelope is also enclosed for your convenience in replying.[19]

Major Gratch later wrote that they believed this was the first photo in a strip of photographs, all taken at the same time as the ones I'd already seen, right after Newk's capture. In this one, Newk was up and walking, followed by armed Vietnamese guards. In the foreground was a water buffalo.

I studied the picture carefully. It was dark in some areas, so I couldn't tell whether the knees of Newk's flight suit were torn. He seemed to have several days' growth of beard, and was apparently shackled at the elbows and shins. The sun created contrasts and appeared to be shining brightly, which made me think it was taken later in the day, or maybe in a different season.

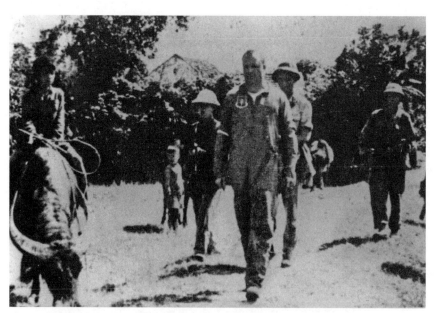

Capt. Grubb following his capture by the North Vietnamese on January 26, 1966, standing up straight, walking, no sign of serious injury.

I wrote and asked whether a closer view, enlarged, might show his flight suit better, so that we could see if the knees were torn the same way as in the other pictures where the young woman was treating his wounds. I closed my letter with,

"I'd appreciate any comments *you* may have regarding the picture, please."

Major Gratch replied promptly, telling me that there were no rips in the knees of Newk's flight suit in the picture when they enlarged it, therefore it must have been taken before the one with the girl treating him, possibly on a previous, sunnier day. He added, "The wounds shown in the (other) color shots, if they were actual wounds, do not appear to be serious enough to have interfered with your husband's ability to walk."

He clarified the phrase "treated well by Oriental standards" with the comment, "Water buffalo are prized possessions of families in Southeast Asia and are given more and better attention than humans in most instances."

Our CIA friend consulted a physician who carefully analyzed the initial photo of Newk being treated by the Vietnamese girl with what looked like a lone gunman right behind him, and another bayonet tip protruding into the photo on the right side. He sent me the doctor's evaluation:

1. I think he'll be bald when you see him again.
2. He has apparently no bruises on his head
3. He seems to be able to focus both eyes on a specific area.
4. He does not seem "cringing" but seems unafraid & able to take care of himself.
5. Right arm OK, leaning on it.
6. Both arms bound behind back.
7. No neck injury—bent in forward position. No swelling noted.
8. Left hand MAY be slightly swollen from poor circulation due to rope. No fractures noted.
9. Would say he was pulled by chute on both knees. Pants seem to indicate that.
10. Left ankle and foot normal flexion.
11. Would guess: Severe contusion (bruise) left knee with abrasions—swelling due to bruise. Prognosis: Very sore,

then to black and blue, then to gradual absorption of fluid, sore at most for 2 weeks.

12. Both legs not fractured. Face does not show evidence of any acute pain.

Conclusion: Think he looks 'GREAT.' Believe he just has contusions and abrasion on left knee. At worst, fracture of the kneecap, but almost completely rule that out, seeing how he's holding his leg. She's cutting his pants back to get better working area. Looks like she has Merthiolate and gauze with her. I'm sure this picture will give you a good deal of 'comfort.' I'm really impressed how good he looks! Those abrasions are very superficial. Just as if you rubbed sandpaper over his knee. No sutures required . . . they won't bother him, only the bruise will be sore."

That helped me a lot. I was beginning to cope better with my situation, especially since the occasional meetings with the group of POW/MIA wives in our area were taking place at Louise Mulligan's. At least I had found other women in similar circumstances to talk to on a regular basis, and could exchange concerns with them. This helped keep the feeling that I was all alone in this at bay. Also, my reaction to that Congressman's taunt had caused me to work hard to change my thinking and attitude. But sometimes it still threatened to overwhelm me. And there was always a family crisis lately, it seemed.

One afternoon during the summer of 1968, I put a rolled and stuffed flank steak into my pressure cooker for dinner. Jeff, Roland, and a couple of neighborhood kids decided they'd put Roy into his stroller and take him for a walk. They had been gone for awhile, when Van came in to the kitchen and asked,

"When are those guys coming back, Mom? Why couldn't I go with them?"

I looked at the clock. They'd been gone more than an hour.

"They should have been back by now," I said. "Go outside and watch for them."

Annoyed, but not alarmed, since Jeff was with them, I decided I'd better go find them. Van was home because he'd been sick. When I got outside I told Van, "You stay there on the front stoop and watch for them in case they come back, okay? I'll drive around the block. If they come back, tell them I've gone to look for them, and to stay right here until I get back."

I jumped in the car and drove around the block. No sign of them. I was even more annoyed then because it meant I would have to go search at the Mall or 7-Eleven, which were off limits to them without my prior permission. I drove back home to get Van. He wasn't outside or at the front window. He was standing in the front doorway, against the closed door, looking scared.

"Everything okay?" I called out, as I got out of the car.

Van called back, "Yeah . . . but the smoke is down to here." He put his hand to the top of his head.

Omigod, the flank steak! I ran to the house, yelling at Van to "*get outside!*"

The house was filled with acrid black smoke, and I could smell burning meat. I dashed to the kitchen, grabbed a potholder, and without thinking I yanked the pressure cooker off the burner. Black smoke hissed out the top. I hurried to the back door with it, face averted, praying it wouldn't explode. Setting it down on the cement patio, I backed away to watch it as it rocked and hissed smoke. When I felt sure the pot wouldn't explode, I left it there and went back in and through the house, throwing windows open to let in fresh air, fanning the smoke away with a folded newspaper. What a mess! My eyes were smarting and burning. There was going to be soot on everything. Dinner and the pressure cooker would end up in the garbage. The whole emergency had taken only three minutes, but as any mother can imagine, they were a very frightening three minutes. Then Van called,

"Here they come, Mom! They're here!"

That night, we sat down to a silent meal of peanut butter and jelly sandwiches in a house that smelled of burnt steak. They all went to bed early without protest. They were glad to be somewhere out of reach. I decided to ignore the house, and pack another package to mail to Newk.

I think Mother realized how close I was to coming apart at the seams, because a few weeks later, she suggested that she and a friend stay with the boys, while I flew down to Miami to visit Helen Brunstrom. Al was listed as a "probable POW." Helen was concerned because she hadn't gotten any mail from Al yet either. Two years had passed, and we both still prayed they were alive, and together in a prison camp somewhere in North Vietnam.

While I was there in Florida, comparing notes and swapping information with Helen, we met with another POW wife, a friend of Helen's, Anneliese Young. We talked about how we felt alienated and cut off from our former military lives and contacts.

"I have some good news to give you," I said. "The Navy and Air Force wives have been getting together up in Virginia near where I live. We hope to start a national organization to speak out in a united voice in support of our POW/MIA husbands."

Helen and Annaliese were thrilled to hear that bit of news. I told them everything we'd been doing and showed them the correspondence with Major Gratch and Lt. Colonel Luther. They agreed to become more active in Florida on the POW/MIA issues. They said they'd try to get the wives there organized into a cohesive group, too.

In the weeks that followed, more POW/MIA wives and families reached out, found one another and we began to communicate. Not just within our own groups, but to other groups everywhere. We compared notes and wrote letters. We gave interviews in our local areas to newspapers and radio stations to raise awareness of the POWs and MIAs in Southeast Asia. We raised our voices to our respective services, and we began to get results. We were starting to coalesce into a strong group.

In March, some of us went to Oceana Naval Air Station where they showed us a film the North Vietnamese had sent via their U.S. sympathizers, who were frequently trekking to Hanoi. The film showed a Christmas party of sorts and some (a very few) of our POWs receiving communion from a priest. Newk and Al Brunstrom were not in that film either. We were told that film was very likely staged propaganda, but it looked like at least a few of them were getting something decent to eat and some religious comfort, even if the film was a fake and staged. We hoped they got to eat the food.[20]

A month later, we went back to Oceana again, this time to finally hear Lt. Matheny in person. Matheny, one of the POWs who had been recently released, came out of the prison camp with the names of many POWs, including Newk's. We were very anxious to hear his POW camp experiences from his own lips. Lt. Matheny confirmed to me that he had *no personal* knowledge of Newk and did not know where Newk was being held in the Hanoi prison camp system. Newk's was just one of the names he had been given by other POWs. Hearing it directly from him, though, and not from someone at the Air Force Personnel Center in Texas, was very important to me, because he'd been there. It also was a measure of just how much I had come to mistrust what I heard via the "official pipeline."

Following that visit to Oceana, I arranged for a short meeting with Congressman L. Mendall Rivers at Fort Lee, Virginia, to talk about the savings program for missing and captured service members and to discuss general concerns about treatment in North Vietnamese prison camps. That went well. He was very receptive and kind. Not long after that meeting, Helen Brunstrom got an appointment to see her Senator. She wrote and asked for suggestions from me. I replied,

> One far-out suggestion is that Congress allow a delegation
> of us POW/MIA wives to go to Hanoi on a peace mission.
> If so many odd-ball Americans who are Communist sym-
> pathizers get to go there, why shouldn't we POW/MIA
> wives be allowed to go?

Of course, hell might freeze over before that delegation would happen, but it was worth a try. The commitment of U.S. forces to the Vietnam War continued to increase. In 1960, the United States had had fewer than 1000 troops in Vietnam, and most of those were Embassy attachés and guards, or advisors to the South Vietnamese army. When Newk was shot down during his reconnaissance mission over North Vietnam in January 1966, barely six years later, that number had increased to close to 200,000 American fighting men in Vietnam. Now there were more than half a million.

December of 1968 arrived, and a rumor was circulating that all our POWs would return by Christmas. I called Major Gratch to see what the official word was. He said he had no news of any imminent or future release of prisoners. That dashed my hopes again. I asked him: "How many POWs and MIAs are there now?"

He replied that the latest count was 336 known to have been captured. He said that they felt there were more men who were prisoners, but our government didn't have an accurate list of names. He didn't have the latest count of Missing in Action, either.

"Well, why aren't we forcing them to adhere to the Geneva Conventions? They're supposed to give us a full and accurate list, and release the sick and wounded men!"

For probably the hundredth time, he made no answer. It had gotten to be a routine with us. A few days later, two Air Force representatives came to my house with a thin album of POW photos. One photo showed a man totally wrapped in bandages. Newk wasn't in any of those photos. Of course, I wondered who the bandaged man might be, and my heart ached for his family. Deep down, I wondered if they'd brought that because they thought maybe the bandaged guy was Newk. At first, I wondered too. But then somehow I knew instinctively it wasn't Newk.

Mother and Dad Grubb came down by train on December 23 to spend our third Christmas without Newk with us. As we opened our gifts and watched the children enjoy theirs, we all thought of Newk and wondered aloud how long could he survive so much time alone, in desolate or even horrific conditions, isolated far from home and family? Despite sorrow-filled hearts, we were determined to carry out the family holiday traditions for the children, and in remembrance of Newk when he was home. He loved everything about the holidays, especially the opening of gifts on Christmas morning.

As I watched my four growing boys open their gifts and play, I couldn't comprehend how or why on earth we would send more than half a million young Americans to fight in a country of less than 130,000 square miles. The way we were fighting it, this war did not make sense, not to me, not to Mother and the Grubbs, not to anyone else I talked with. The Grubbs had lived through the much greater challenge of World War II when, united in spirit and purpose and fully behind our military, we had rallied with our allies and defeated the Axis powers of both Germany and Japan in two distant spheres, all in less time than we'd now spent warring in one tiny peninsular country—Vietnam. What had happened to us? It was frightening and disheartening. Where, how, and when would it all end? No one knew the answer, not even the President of the United States. If he knew, he wasn't telling.

5 The League of Families Is Born

TIMELINE . . . 1969-70 . . . WORLD . . . DEGAULLE RESIGNS AS FRENCH PRESIDENT . . . VIETNAM . . . PARIS PEACE TALKS STALL . . . HO CHI MINH DIES . . . 3 MORE POWS RELEASED FROM N. VIETNAM . . . 55 AMERICANS BECOME POWs . . . USA . . . SUC-CESSFUL APOLLO 11 MOON LANDING . . . CHARLES MANSON CONVICTED OF MURDER OF ACTRESS SHARON TATE . . . JOHN WAYNE WINS OSCAR FOR TRUE GRIT . . . NY JETS BEAT COLTS IN SUPERBOWL . . .

Shake your chains to earth like dew
Which in sleep had fallen on you—
Ye are many—they are few.
—Percy Bysshe Shelley

When 1969 rolled around, the American public was openly expressing outrage over the war. President Johnson had turned the bombing of North Vietnam on and off like a water spigot, for whatever political purposes he felt were expedient. To my thinking, that was no way to wage or win a war.

Military representatives cautioned us not to jeopardize our husbands by saying or doing anything that could be used against them.[1] What did it matter? In 1968, our POWs were all but forgotten by Washington, D.C., and their fellow Americans. Their Vietnamese jailers savagely abused our men, knowing that Americans' interest was focused elsewhere. The Vietnam War dragged on without visible progress on our part. It divided us as a nation—politically, emotionally and financially. It had defeated Democratic President Lyndon Johnson, who declined to run again. Republican Richard M. Nixon won the 1968 presidential election. Americans obviously hoped that a change of administration would bring a corresponding change in thinking and end this War.[2]

While I was eager to hear about government policy changes, equally important to me was the wonderful news I received on January 10, 1969, that the League of Wives of American Prisoners of War in North Vietnam was launched, with POW wife Sybil Stockdale in California at the helm. Her husband, Navy Commander James Bond Stockdale, had been a POW in Hanoi since September 1965. There were other wives to consider, too—the wives of the Missing in Action, the MIAs, some of whom may have been captured and be POWs without their family knowing that. We welcomed those wives into our League of Wives, too.

"This is the beginning, Helen," I wrote on January 12, 1969, to Helen Brunstrom. She had not heard a word from, or about, her husband Al either, and was enduring the same long, silent vigil I was. Newk's wingman, Al was shot down over North Vietnam in April of 1966, three months after Newk. He was classed as MIA. We hoped and prayed he was alive, perhaps a POW. I continued, "It would help if you can get anyone and everyone you know to write or wire the President, Ambassador [Henry Cabot] Lodge, or William Rogers, who will be Nixon's Secretary of State, about helping the POW/MIA situation."

President Nixon had vowed during his campaign that he would end the war, bring our POWs home with honor, and restore solvency to our dismal economy. I knew those were three pretty lofty promises. But like kids at Christmas, we hoped that the new President, like Santa Claus, would deliver the campaign goodies as promised, although no one knew exactly how he was going to accomplish it. The Paris peace talks were not working. The United Nations had not brought peace. World diplomacy was not bringing peace.[3]

In the United States, our whole society was changing fast. From fashions to families, everything seemed to have gone topsy-turvy. What was termed the "New Morality" was spreading throughout the country. Clothing trends had become bizarre. They were much too revealing to those of us accustomed to more conservative clothing and behavior. The national divorce rate continued climbing. Worse, the mood of the general American public turned uglier with each passing month the war continued.

We POW/MIA wives shared our feelings more openly with one another now, too. We talked frankly about our plight. We realized that if we were ever going to see our husbands again, if our children were ever to have their fathers home, we had to organize, stand together, and get the American public behind our cause. We had enormous obstacles to overcome. We'd have to reverse U.S. and foreign policy and public opinion about our fighting men. How to do that was the big question.

It was difficult for us POW/MIA families just to get up in the morning and keep going, day after day, year after year. Newk had been totally silent for three years. In that same letter to Helen on January 12, I wrote,

> I'm in a horrible mood! . . . we need to tell them [our leaders] . . . how we've waited for years in the vain hope that our Government would get some action on the prisoner situation, but feel that by being so trusting and silent we may be doing our husbands a grave injustice—men die from loneliness and neglect as well as from torture and injuries—and God alone knows how lonely three or four years of confinement can be . . . but if I began writing about how I feel our country has neglected the POWs, it would take up another 5 pages . . . What I want to do, (and you should too, Helen), is write down just how I feel, and what I think should be done, so when the Air Force calls to berate us and asks 'what the hell are you doing?' we better be prepared with an answer. But for over three years I have done NOTHING, and have gained NOTHING, so whatever happens from now on I think is fully justified—let the Air Force defend its inaction for once . . .

The POW/MIA wives in my area of Norfolk-Newport News, Virginia, were fed up, too. Together, we vowed that 1969 would bring more positive results. And, that we would do whatever it took to make those results happen. We faced the chaotic, rebellious national mood with resolve and determination. We would stop moping and staying home. We would instead stand up, speak out, and bring world attention to the plight of our men, the forgotten POWs and MIAs, in every way we could.

After I wrote to Helen, I called Louise Mulligan, the leader of the POW/MIA wives in my area. She told me that groups of POW and MIA wives from all over the country were now gathering under an umbrella Sybil had opened, welcoming not just the wives, but the families of the POWs and MIAs. We would now be known as The League of Families of American Prisoners of War and Missing. That news raised my hopes, and my spirits. The first task of the newly expanded League, she said, would be threefold:

> 1. To pressure the Air Force and other services, through every known source, to provide us with more information about the POW/MIA situation in Southeast Asia.
>
> 2. To bombard officials in Washington, and the news media, with letters expressing concern about the treatment and return of our POWs, and demanding accounting for all POWs and MIAs.
>
> 3. To encourage the wives and families of POWs and MIAs to schedule newspaper, radio and magazine interviews, to provide information to educate the American public in more detail about the plight of the American POWs in Vietnam and what was happening to their families here at home.[4]

That was all I needed to hear. I had been a banner-carrying member of the League from its inception, and I was ready for action. The day after Louise's phone call, I contacted the local

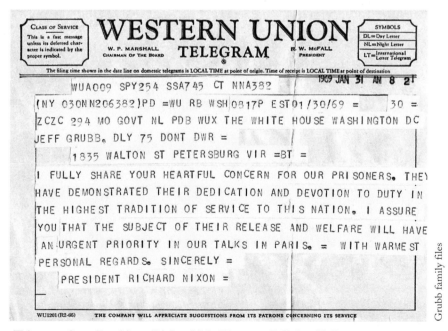

Telegram from President Richard M. Nixon to Jeff Grubb January 30, 1969.

Petersburg Progress Index newspaper and gave my first interview about the POW-MIA situation.[5] I wasn't the only one. Interviews with many different POW-MIA wives and family members cropped up in newspapers across the nation.

On President Nixon's inauguration day that January, Jeff and I sent congratulatory telegrams to President Nixon and his Secretary of State, William P. Rogers. We told them that this month was the third anniversary of the day Newk was shot down. We said that we were concerned about not hearing a word from Newk, even though photographs of him as a captive were still being distributed by the North Vietnamese for propaganda purposes.

"We are counting on you to do something to straighten this situation out over there, Mr. President," Jeff's telegram concluded. Jeff received a very nice telegram in response from President Nixon.

> The White House
> Washington DC
>
> January 30, 1969
>
> Jeff Grubb
>
>   I fully share your concern for our prisoners. They have demonstrated their dedication and devotion to duty in the highest tradition of service to this nation. I assure you that the subject of their release and welfare will have an urgent priority in our talks in Paris.
> With warmest personal regards.
>
> Sincerely,
> President Richard Nixon[6]

That was encouraging. Jeff was very impressed to get a personal telegram from the President of the United States. I later learned that other wives and families also received telegrams like Jeff's from President Nixon. They were the first "official" attention we'd ever gotten from the White House, and the first word directly from our men's Commander-in-Chief, advising us that he was personally aware of our men's plight, and ours, and it would have urgent priority at the peace talks. It was something to hang onto, and we desperately needed even a thread we could grasp.

In March 1969, I attended another meeting of the Navy

POW/MIA wives at Louise Mulligan's. I learned there that some wives and families who hadn't been getting any mail from their POW husbands reported receiving a few letters since Nixon's election. I was happy for them, but forlorn that Helen and I were still without mail or news of any kind. I knew from the photos that Newk had made it down okay, but we didn't know anything about Al Brunstrom's fate. No one could say for sure whether he'd been captured or even if he'd survived. Helen remained as anxious, fearful, and frustrated as I was.

President Nixon soon changed direction in our deep involvement in Vietnam by introducing "Vietnamization." He intended this policy to create what we had sought in the first place—a strong South Vietnamese military force that could defend its own territory. Vietnamization was the first clue that President Nixon intended to get us out of there, and bring our American soldiers home. In that, we would be a helpful force for him. As the publicity coordinated by the League of Families mounted, Nixon's Administration piggy-backed on it with a "Go Public" campaign, openly challenging Hanoi's blatant flouting of the Geneva Conventions and horrible treatment of our POWs. This was the first time an American president had made that public challenge to the North Vietnamese. We were thrilled to hear it.

Our media interviews, and the new President's more open direction regarding the POWs, woke up the military. We POW/MIA wives were suddenly being invited to military briefings at local bases on a fairly regular basis, and we were getting more attention from the military hierarchy. They didn't have much to tell us, but from the top down they assured us that the government was paying attention to us and working for the release of the U.S. Prisoners of War.[7]

By then I'd gleaned enough bad news about the living conditions of our prisoners that I bought medicines, not games, for Newk's next package. I packed aspirin, athlete's foot powder, and vitamins. I included bouillon cubes and drink concentrate cubes. What little I'd learned about the rotten conditions in the prison camps in North and South Vietnam upset me terribly, so much so that on June 10th, 1969, I decided to write a letter to Ho Chi Minh, the President of North Vietnam. Why not? Nothing else was working. I'd try anything, if it would help me find out something about Newk!

> Dear President Ho Chi Minh:
>
> It is with great respect that I write this letter to you. I appeal to you for some positive information on the present health of my beloved husband, American pilot Wilmer N. Grubb, FV2211784, captured January 26, 1966 in the Quang Binh Province. Soon after his capture, a photograph of him was published in the American newspapers showing him being treated for injuries. Since that time, I have heard nothing from him. My anxiety, after 3 1/2 years, surpasses all imagination. I fervently hope that my personal request for your help and assistance will bring a favorable response from you soon.
> Very Sincerely,
> Mrs. Wilmer N. Grubb

I kept a copy and mailed the letter to Hanoi using regular international airmail. I hoped that my letter would reach him, and move the North Vietnamese President to send me information about Newk. Apparently it didn't, because I never got a response from him or anyone else in his government.

In July 1969, we celebrated Roy's third birthday. He was very independent and a great talker. It tore my soul that Newk had never seen him and now I couldn't prevent the thought from creeping into my head: *Maybe he never will.*

In keeping with our new League and its determination to raise public and official awareness, I called and made an appointment to speak at the Virginia State Capitol. In August 1969, Jeff and I went to Richmond to the Capitol building where Jeff also made his first public speech about his Dad. The people there were so friendly and caring that it was difficult for me not to break down and cry. Following our speeches, they helped me get an appointment to see Senator Robert Byrd of West Virginia, scheduled on August 8 in the Senate Chambers in Washington.

Louise and our group of POW/MIA wives and families were excited and positive when I told them what I'd done. I was nervous when I got to Byrd's Washington office, but Senator Byrd, a short, dapper man, was a true gentleman charmer and put me right at

ease. His staff made it quite a day for me indeed. Besides Senator
Byrd, I also was able to meet briefly that day with Senator George
McGovern (D-South Dakota), Senator Richard Schweiker (R-
Pennsylvania) and Steve Blakely, an aide in Representative L.
Mendel Rivers' (D-South Carolina) office. I also had the opportu-
nity to speak at length with Mrs. Neta Stockstill, secretary to the
House Armed Services Committee.

For those distinguished congressmen and Mrs. Stockstill, I
went over the basic grievances: that despite the photos proving he
was alive and a POW, I'd had no communication from Newk for
three years, and we weren't the only family without mail for long
periods. They were shocked to learn that, and openly expressed
their combined sympathy to me. I stressed that not only was it terrible hardship for the families, but also this lack of information and
communication was a flagrant violation of the Geneva
Conventions, which North Vietnam had signed, as had the United
States.

"I don't think you can imagine what this silence has done, and
is doing, to our family. *All* the wives and families of POWs and
MIAs are worried about their husbands and the terrible conditions
of their imprisonment in Hanoi. We are concerned that the
Congress and the American people do not know or care about their
situation."

I was immediately reassured by each of these distinguished legislators and Representative Rivers' aide, that the Congress and the
American people indeed knew and cared about us.

"I am here to beg you to please bring up the issue of the plight
of the POWs and their families on the floor of the House. I ask that
you demand that Hanoi make a full accounting of our prisoners
and, at the very least, allow them to communicate with their families. We are desperate, Sir."

All were most gracious. Each assured me he or she would help
the families' efforts to bring recognition to the plight of the POWs,
and the concerns of their families. I was elated when not long after
I returned home, I received a call from Neta Stockstill's husband,
Louis, who, with Neta, became lifelong friends of mine. Lou told
me he was writing two articles, one to be published in *The Air Force
and Space Digest* in the October 1969 issue, and the other would be

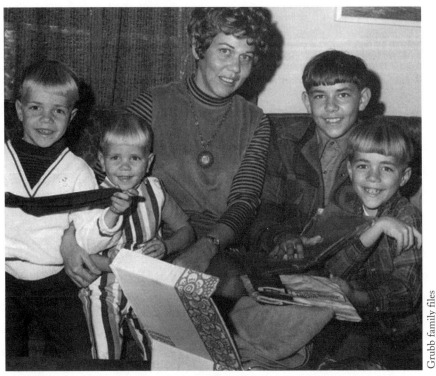

Grubb family files

Evelyn and sons Roke, Roy, Jeff, and Van prepare a Christmas package for Newk.

a condensed version of the same story, slated for the huge circulation of *Reader's Digest*. I was thrilled to hear that, and so were the other wives in my League group.

"Congress definitely heard your pleas, Mrs. Grubb," said Lou. "Through the articles, both publications will tell the American public the truth about the treatment of our POW/MIAs, and what they can do to help the POW/MIA cause."

We were soon on a first name basis. Shortly thereafter, Lou and I had a long telephone interview and he asked me to send him pictures of Newk and our family. They ultimately published the one of us packing that year's holiday package for Newk.

About the same time, Phyllis Galanti from our area League group in Virginia had a radio interview with Bob Bauder on WTVR in Richmond. A week later, Bauder called me.

"Mrs. Grubb, I'd like you to come to Richmond for an appearance on my television show. We'd like you to share with our audience your visit to Washington and meeting with the U.S. Senators." I accepted with pleasure. Phyllis had paved the way for that follow-up. It allowed me to expand our message, and also give the Senators by name some "attaboy" radio coverage for their kindness and personal attention to our plight.

It was on a Sunday not long after those interviews that I felt especially close to Newk during church services. It was like God opened a window for me and I could see Newk, sitting alone somewhere. How awful for him! He looked so lonely. He had no one—no family, no busy, active and wonderful children around him like I did. Tears came to my eyes, my throat ached, and I wanted so badly to gather him close, to hold and console him. Then Newk turned and looked straight at me. "Evelyn, don't worry about me. I'm fine where I am," he said. But I couldn't see where he was. Nonetheless, that vision of Newk was a comforting and spiritual experience. I could not explain it then, nor can I today, as I recall it. Afterward, for whatever reason, I felt myself growing calmer. I was more at peace and better able to cope with the stresses of daily life.

On Tuesday September 16, 1969, I went to Oceana Naval Station to hear two recently released POWs, Seaman Douglas B. Hegdahl and Navy Lt. Robert F. Frishman. They were visiting military bases to speak to the POW/MIA families.

When they first arrived home a month previously, according to eyewitnesses who had seen and interviewed them, the two men had looked terrible. They were gaunt, hollow-eyed and malnourished and Frishman's elbow, injured on bailout, hung wasted at his side. A third released POW, Air Force Captain Wesley Rumble, was so "ill, stooped and pale" he'd been rushed to a waiting medical evacuation plane as soon as he'd landed in New York.[8]

Hegdahl and Frishman had both been captured in 1967, and Rumble had been a prisoner since 1968. In the month since their repatriation, the medical staff at Bethesda Naval Hospital had done everything possible to improve the health and appearance of the men before we saw them. Even so, it shocked us. They had regained some of their lost weight. Frishman had dropped 45 pounds during captivity, Hegdahl 60 pounds. But their sunken pallor remained, and what they told us about the awful treatment our POWs in Hanoi were receiving made my hair stand on end.

After his capture, despite his serious injuries, Frishman had been trucked around North Vietnam, where frequently he was abused and stoned by villagers! Was Newk also subjected to that on his way to Hanoi? I wondered. Frishman related that, instead of being treated at a North Vietnamese hospital for his injuries, he was taken to prison in Hanoi. Instead of receiving any medical or humane treatment there he was tightly tied up with ropes that were then pulled by his jailers, nearly forcing his arms from the sockets, while they badgered him to talk about military information until he passed out from the excruciating pain. We gasped in shock at that horrific description of torturing an injured man. He said that although Vietnamese doctors eventually operated on his arm, they did not remove the missile fragments in it. The wound soon infected and remained infected, draining pus for the entire period of his captivity. He received no further medical treatment from his captors after that one operation. Imagine our shock and horror and our fear for our men still there, upon hearing that. Hegdahl, a young Navy man, told us he was kept in solitary confinement for more than a year. I had heard rumors of solitary confinement, but we were stunned to learn from him that most prisoners were isolated that way, kept alone in single man cells.

We expressed our concerns about what might happen to the remaining men because Frishman and Hegdahl revealed those conditions in the prisons. The ex-prisoners assured us they didn't intend it to frighten us, but that the POW commanders had assured them that those imprisoned there had told them they *wanted* them to tell the American people the truth when they got here. The prisoners wanted the facts revealed about their hideous situation. They wanted the world to know about the torture they were enduring. Frishman said a fellow prisoner had told him, "Don't worry about telling . . . if it means more torture, at least we'll know why we're being tortured. It will be worth the sacrifice just to know the folks back home know what's going on here."

Afterward, I was sick with outrage and fear, as I'm sure the other families were too. I kept thinking that Newk and many others had been prisoners much longer than the two we had just seen. What might their physical condition be? The League just had to get busier and demand that those prisoners receive better treatment. Actually we needed to get them out of there before they died of torture, starvation, and disease. Armed with that horrifying information, the League of Families members nationwide stormed Congress with letters. The legislators became as incensed as we were. They issued a strong statement condemning North Vietnam for its cruel treatment of our prisoners.

The unsatisfactory results in Vietnam and the alienation of the American people, underscored by riots, draft card burnings, and other demonstrations of their feelings pressured America's national leaders to reconsider things from a strategic standpoint. Our publicity about what was happening in the prison camps also forced our leaders to think differently about the POWS, as well. Everything the League did to get the word out had further galvanized Nixon's "Go Public" campaign. The public was listening and learning, and they didn't like what they were hearing any more than we did.

As promised, Louis Stockstill's article, "Prisoners of War: The Forgotten Americans of the Vietnam War," appeared in the *Air Force/Space Digest* in October. The editors called it "one of the most important articles ever published in this magazine."[9] Immediately afterward, in November 1969, the POWs and their terrible plight received enormous worldwide publicity when his condensation was featured in *Reader's Digest*. Entitled "What You Can Do for American Prisoners in Vietnam," its lead caption read, "Nothing less than a worldwide cry of outrage is likely to bring a halt to the grossly inhuman treatment our men are receiving in the enemy's prison camps."

Stockstill's article starkly illuminated the plight of the prisoners and the anguish of their families. It began,

> Once a month from her apartment in Arlington, Va., Gloria Netherland walks down a long hallway to the mail chute and deposits a letter. She watches it drop from sight on the first leg of a long journey . . . The letter begins 'Dear Dutch.' Whether Dutch [Captain Roger M. Netherland, missing in action] will receive it is impossible to say.[10] Gloria and Dutch have been married 18 years, but she doesn't know whether he is alive or dead. For more than two years she has written the monthly letters—six lines each, according to current communist rules. None is answered; none is returned. But

in the pattern of 'dreadful uncertainty' that characterizes her life, she never fails to write . . .

Gloria Netherland is but one of hundreds of American wives and parents whose husbands and sons are the forgotten men of the Vietnam War. Approximately 1400 men are captured or missing and possibly in enemy hands. Most of the known captives are imprisoned in North Vietnam. Others are held by the Vietcong in the South. A few are interned in Laos and Red China.

Stockstill then pointed out that despite being one of the signers of the Geneva Conventions in 1957, "In blatant disregard of international rules, Hanoi refuses even to identify the prisoners it holds, to release the sick and wounded, or to allow proper flow of letters and packages . . . " Then he went on to reveal my situation.

Evelyn Grubb's only knowledge of her husband, for example, has come from a Hanoi propaganda gesture. An unarmed reconnaissance aircraft, piloted by Maj. Wilmer 'Newk' Grubb, was shot down in January 1966. Hanoi gloatingly publicized his capture. Each time Evelyn writes, she sends photographs of their four sons—stapled to the letter so that Newk will know if they have been removed.

She doesn't know whether he has received a single photograph or letter. In almost four years, she has received no further official word of her husband. Until recently, the American public has been provided scant information about American POWs in Vietnam . . .

At last, I thought, *the truth has gotten to the millions who read* Reader's Digest! *Maybe now, world pressure would be brought against North Vietnam to force them to release the POWs and account for the MIAs.*

Stockstill concluded the article by embracing our League's desire for a "vigorous letter writing campaign," telling the readers to write to:

- representatives of foreign nations and the press of those nations
- your Congressmen
- Xuan Thuy, chief North Vietnam negotiator at the peace talks

in Paris.[11]

The *Reader's Digest* offered to forward the addresses of ambassadors and foreign newspapers to anyone interested in writing to them and included an address for Xuan Thuy in care of the Paris Peace Talks.

It would be impossible to describe how excited and happy I was when that article appeared. It was the impetus I so desperately needed. I was convinced it would awaken America and the world to the inhumane treatment of our men. I was partly right. It woke up the American public and the League's national letter- writing campaign took off like a rocket. But it didn't budge the North Vietnamese.

I sent my next letter to Paris, on November 3, 1969, to Xuan Oanh, Delegation of the Democratic Republic of Vietnam at the Paris Peace Talks. I gave him the details about Newk's capture, and said, "I have never received a letter from him and am deeply worried about his well-being. Is he in need of any special medication that I could send to him?"

I never asked for Newk's release in my letters, knowing that would be futile, since our delegates were getting nowhere negotiating those terms at the Paris talks. I asked for them to "please give me some information, any information, through official channels, about my husband." As usual, I received no acknowledgment of any kind.

President Nixon had proclaimed November 8, 1969 a "Day of Prayer and Concern" for Americans being held prisoner in North Vietnam. As residents of Virginia and recognized members of the Virginia area Chapter of the League of Families of POW/MIA, Phyllis Galanti and I were invited for a visit with Virginia governor Mills Godwin. He called upon everyone in the state of Virginia to join "in this united evidence of concern this Sunday." The press coverage in the Virginia papers carried information about Newk and my own plea for the American public to join me in "informing the world how badly the North Vietnamese are treating these prisoners and then Hanoi will react to world opinion."[12]

Sweden was the first Western country to formally recognize the government of North Vietnam and therefore had diplomatic relations with them. So I wrote to Swedish Ambassador Olander, explaining that only 100 families out of 1300 prisoners had heard from their captive men. I asked for Sweden's help in pressuring North Vietnam to "change its policy about the prisoners of war." I hoped Sweden would volunteer to act as the Protecting Power cited in the Geneva Conventions to handle repatriation of prisoners and receive lists of prisoners. I closed my letter to the Ambassador, "please, please, in the name of humanity, try to help us."

Meanwhile, I'd been in touch with the American Friends Service Committee, Inc. from Philadelphia. One of their members, Dr. Joseph Elder, a professor of Sociology and Indian Studies at the University of Wisconsin and a Quaker, had traveled to Hanoi twice on humanitarian missions—once to deliver some needed heart surgical equipment just as he had previously done to the South Vietnamese. The wives of two POW pilots, Richard Walsh and David Winn, had spoken with Dr. Elder and invited him to address the League's local meeting at Louise's. He told our group that in a visit to Hanoi in June, he had met with a Mr. Houang Bac and asked him if he might visit a POW camp, talk with American POWs, or take POW mail back to the United States. He also asked if he could obtain a list of prisoners in order to notify their relatives. According to Dr. Elder, Mr. Bac replied that he did not have access to military authorities, that many prisoners were a long way from Hanoi, and that perhaps a list of prisoners would be ready for him when Dr. Elder returned to Hanoi on his next visit.

Leaving Hanoi, Dr. Elder had met with U.S. Ambassador Ellsworth Bunker in Saigon and visited some prisoners being held in South Vietnam. Upon his return to the United States, Elder met in Washington with Dr. Henry Kissinger to relate the events of his trip.[13]

After I heard Dr. Elder speak, I forwarded to his care a letter for Newk. I received a letter back from Dr. Elder written on October 6 from the Hotel Monorom in Phnom Penh, Cambodia, saying,

> This is just to assure you that your letter to your
> husband did reach me in time, and I am including it with
> other mail to prisoners that I am taking with me to Hanoi.
> I am not optimistic about my chances to visit any of the

prisoners. However, if I don't get to see them myself, I plan
to turn over the letters to the most responsible authorities I
can. Please accept my sincere concern for the hardships you
have undergone these past three, nearly four, years. One of
the tragedies of this war is that so many people like yourself
are suffering so much . . . on all sides.[14]

On Sunday, October 12, 1969, Dr. Elder was in Hanoi and
turned over to a Mr. Toan the POW mail he had brought including my letter. He then visited a province about 5 hours south of
Hanoi. Upon his return, he inquired of Mr. Toan about the letters
and was told they had been delivered to prison camp authorities.
The North Vietnamese then lectured Elder about their prisoner
policy, claiming they offered "humane" treatment, adequate medical
care, and adequate diet, even for the pilots, who were "aggressors"
and not "victims of aggression."[15] They refused to allow Dr. Elder
into the camps. He received a verbal wrist slap from the
Vietnamese about the letters he delivered. They told him, "Your
government is using the families of the missing men and POWs for
propaganda purposes."[16]

Dr. Elder responded that their policy of refusing to release the
names of all prisoners hurt the families of the men. They didn't
budge. Dr. Elder returned home without any names and without
information about any of the prisoners. Nevertheless, I was grateful
to know that he had delivered our letters directly to the prison camp
authorities.

"The North Vietnamese administration is bureaucratic and
pursues details, so they must keep an accurate listing and accounting of all the men they are holding. However, they do not release
that list to anyone," Dr. Elder informed us.[17]

In early December 1969, I wrote a letter of thanks to Dr. Elder
and the American Friends for trying to help me and for taking my
letter to Hanoi. Then I turned my attention toward making preparations for our fifth Christmas and New Year without Newk, our
fourth without a single word from him.

At about that time actress Jane Fonda was drawing attention to
herself as a dissenter and an anti-war activist. I was stunned to see
how far she would go in slamming her own country. "I would think
if you understood what communism was you would hope, you

would pray on your knees, that we [the U.S.] would some day become communists," she was quoted as saying.[18]

Time seemed to be going by faster, probably because I had something positive to do besides being lonely, angry, and frustrated. I felt organized, involved and positive as I worked with the League of Families to improve my husband's POW/MIA situation. We were pleased when Texas businessman H. Ross Perot, who had tried to fly Christmas meals to our POWs but had been rebuffed by North Vietnam, joined our crusade.[19]

Perot quickly became an influential and driving force in our League of Families get-the-word-out and letter-writing campaigns. We were grateful for his participation in our cause, and even more grateful for his influence with Washington on our behalf.

The local groups affiliated with the League began a letter writing campaign to apprise our politicians about the POW situation. Mr. Perot is the one who suggested that we expand it to involve *all* Americans in writing "Letters to Hanoi." We were more than happy to do that. League wives and family members in all areas of the country proceeded to give speeches everywhere they could-at schools, clubs, civic and military organizations—encouraging the American public to write letters to Hanoi and ask for improved treatment for our POWs and a full accounting of all the POWs they held.

It was primarily from that letter-writing campaign under the auspices of the League of Families that the American public finally truly connected with the POWs and MIAs. Americans were shocked to hear the truth from the mouths of the families of these men. To our joy, they got very worked up over the mistreatment of our incarcerated fighting men. It was exactly what we had been hoping would happen for so long, and it did happen. We had counted so much on the American citizens, a formidable force when they got really angry about something, to back us and our cause. We were not disappointed.

I speak for myself here, but I believe I speak for all the POW/MIA families of the Vietnam War, when I say we will be forever grateful to those American people who wrote, and for their splendid letters. We're also grateful to Ross Perot for his faith, his help, and his outreach with a strong hand and for putting his money where his mouth was! To us, in those dark and trying days, Ross Perot exemplified the American citizen and patriot in the truest sense of the word.

Another lonely Christmas came and went, and it was 1970, the start of a new decade. *Time passing should make things easier now, but it doesn't,* I thought when I woke on that New Year's morning. In three weeks, it would be four years since Newk had been shot down. That meant more than a thousand days of a mailbox without any word from him. It would mean hundreds of letters written and mailed by me . . . in hope, in pleading, in begging for information from someone, anyone . . . all unanswered. And here I was, with another year starting, and no way out of my predicament. Nor did Newk have any way out of his. We were trapped . . . like rats in a box with no exit . . . and for what gain?

No sense lying there. It wasn't going to be solved by my staying in bed. I got up, put on my robe, and peered at myself in the bathroom mirror. The woman who stared back at me looked neither young nor happy. I was 38 years old, not even 40 yet, and already felt like an old, worn-out woman. I spoke aloud to myself in the mirror.

"I've completely lost all my femininity. I'm a robot. Does anyone even see me as a woman any more? Am I just a cranky, complaining female animal, fighting against the world? Probably so . . . but what other choices do I have right now?"

I stuck my tongue out at myself in the mirror. Checked my teeth. Wrinkled my nose. Waggled my unplucked eyebrows. Finally, I broke out and laughed at myself and my reflection in the mirror. Some "glamour puss" I was! I was shocked to see my eyes fill with tears that started to spill over . . .

"Let it be," I ordered myself and wiped my eyes. "No self-pity today." I brushed my hair, added some lipstick, and went downstairs to make breakfast for the boys. I needed an attitude adjustment, and I vowed to make one this year. My New Year's Resolution Number One: Try to be happier, more pleasant, and accepting of my situation. But who in their right mind could do that? Two minutes later, as I poured my coffee, alone again with nothing facing me except the same weary fight every day, the thought came: *Who am I kidding? There isn't anything happy or pleasant about this!* Somehow, just accepting how it was, and thinking that, made me feel a lot better.

Once the boys were fed and off to school, I made a list of medicines to buy for Newk's next package. I picked up the letter and information sheet I had just received from Dave Dellinger and Cora Weiss' "Committee of Liaison with Families of Servicemen Detained in North Vietnam." I had written them in 1968 about my husband, hoping they might be able to get some information about Newk on their frequent trips to North Vietnam, but they had never replied to my letter. There were many groups of varying sizes and memberships that had formed in the United States, with various agendas and purposes that were linked in one way or another to the Vietnam War. Some were quite radical in their thinking and behavior, what we'd call out of the mainstream.

Cora Weiss' Committee of Liaison considered itself a "peace movement only" standing firmly against the war in Vietnam. It was active with a variety of other organizations. Some I truly appreciated, like the American Friends. Others I knew little or nothing about, nor was I particularly eager to know, like the New Mobilization Committee to End the War in Vietnam; Clergy and Laymen Concerned About Vietnam; Women Strike for Peace; The Conspiracy; and (this one made me smile) Women Against Daddy Warbucks. In the clarification section of the information sheet on Weiss' Committee of Liaison, I read "The Committee will be dealing solely with the government of North Vietnam, and will not have any information on men held in South Vietnam by the Provisional Revolutionary Government. Nor will we be able to provide information at this time concerning men held in Laos or any other Southeast Asian country where U.S. Troops and aircraft are presently involved in combat missions."

I wondered how she'd gotten the authority to "deal solely with the government of North Vietnam" and felt little trust in what the information sheet implied. However, I cared that the Committee without a doubt had contacts with the North Vietnamese officials. They had gone to Hanoi, and they had returned with released prisoners.[20] Granted, they were not the POWs held the longest or the injured POWs, as required by the Geneva Conventions, but nevertheless, they were American POWs who had brought back names and first-hand information about conditions in the prison camps.

That was more than our government had accomplished in all the years since the first American was captured. The letter invited me to contact them again and intimated that it was the North Vietnamese who were encouraging such contact.[21] I didn't believe that and tossed the letter back into the box on my desk. A few days later, I received a copy of a letter, undated, sent to me by Pat Mearns, wife of MIA Major Arthur Mearns U.S. Air Force, who had been shot down November 11, 1966 and hadn't been heard from since. Pat wrote:

> Cora Weiss and a Mrs. Vincent Duckles (someone I'd never heard of) have just returned from Hanoi, and were saying that my husband and four other men either missing in action or Prisoners of War were 'known dead.' The Air Force did not change my husband's status and stated that 'it is impossible to check the story.' This word added further to my three years of torture and caused a very unhappy Christmas for two small girls who believe that their Daddy is still alive. . . . She [Mrs. Duckles] said that North Vietnamese prison officials through her North Vietnamese hostesses told her this . . . and she said 'the North Vietnamese wouldn't say such a thing unless it was true. She [Mrs. Duckles] had no further proof that what they said was true.[22]

I shook my head in disbelief. After reading her letter twice and feeling sick for Pat and her daughters at this new torment, I filed the letter on my desk with the one from Cora Weiss' Committee of Liaison. At the end of her letter, Pat had informed the League that she was leaving (actually had already left) on January 3 with three MIA wives on a trip around the world "to uncommitted and Communist countries. We will seek information and humane treatment for the POWs and their families. We feel that public opinion is one way to get Hanoi to change its attitude on the fate of our loved ones."[23]

Several weeks passed. On January 26, 1970, just after the fourth anniversary of Newk's capture in North Vietnam, I took that letter from Pat Mearns out and read it again.

I decided to write Cora Weiss and her Committee of Liaison,

giving them all the personal information about Newk, including the photo showing him after his capture. I concluded my letter with, "I do know he was captured and presume he is still alive. But you can imagine how terribly anxious I am for some information from him or about him. I do hope you are successful, and appreciate your efforts to help us—for we need help so desperately."

On February 7, I received a reply from the Committee's Barbara Webster. She informed me that they had written to the North Vietnamese about Newk and enclosed my latest letter to him. They did not forward the photo I had sent as evidence, saying it was not needed. "I do hope we will have word for you soon. In the meantime, I am enclosing an air letter form which you may wish to use the next time you write to your husband."

The form letter enclosed was new to me. The Committee also included instructions on how to send mail to the POWs. The air letter form, about the size of a postcard, allowed the family only six short lines of correspondence and appeared that they were letting me know this was the North Vietnamese regulation form for corresponding with POWs in Hanoi. It would be difficult for anyone else to comprehend the frustration we endured about not getting proper information about just how to contact our prisoner husbands and sons. Yet again, I wondered if any of my previous letters had ever reached Newk because all of them had been longer than what apparently was a limit of six lines, and none of them had been on this form. That gave rise to a whole new horizon of fears. Maybe that's why we've heard nothing back from him! Not ever knowing whether what I was doing was the right thing to get to Newk kept me in a terrible state of heightened anxiety. Again I worried: What if he hasn't written because he thinks we haven't cared enough to write or send him anything?

I decided then and there that we had to stop living in this temporary day-by-day manner and attitude. I was living in fear and anxiety every minute of every day. We needed a real home, a more settled life, while we waited for news or anything to come to us regarding Newk. I knew I simply could not go on much longer in this "circling the airport waiting for landing instructions" way any more. I was almost out of gas, and the children were suffering because I was kept in such an anxiety-ridden emotional state all the time. I was like a volcano, building, building, and about to blow any second.

A few weeks later at church, I was talking with Glen Hastings, a builder from our area. I shared with him that I was considering changing my living situation and thought I might buy a home. I figured it would be a wise investment, and we could sell or rent it when Newk got back and we learned where our next base would be.

Glen agreed with me and suggested I look at Colonial Heights where he and his family lived. I did. It was a wonderful community, so I selected a lot with plenty of trees and chose a modern, split-level house plan from the drawings Glen gave me. Buying that lot was a tremendous morale lift for all of us. Mother was thrilled, and so was I. It gave me a sense of finally being someone myself, of belonging to a community. As soon as we could, we broke ground and began building.

Meanwhile, I continued to travel around Virginia, sometimes with Mother and the boys, sometimes with Jeff, or Peggy Manley, sometimes with other POW/MIA wives. I made speeches and collected letters written to Hanoi. I was making a difference through the League of Families, and that was gratifying, too. More and more Americans were concerned about the POW/MIA situation, and Congress was beginning to mirror their concern. But nothing moved North Vietnam so much as an inch, and that was a huge disappointment for all of us. We were working so hard to change things over there, but we were having no noticeable effect on them. I began to see what our country really was up against with the North Vietnamese; what Presidents DeGaulle and Eisenhower had meant about staying the heck out of that internal mess. What had happened to the French was a lesson we totally ignored, thinking we were more powerful. Hah! Look where that had gotten us. While we hadn't budged the DRV, there were some encouraging advances on the home front in Washington.

Representative William J. Scherle (R-Iowa) took a bold step and inserted this quotation into the Congressional Record to run every day, beginning on January 26, 1970. He vowed to continue it daily until all American POWs were released:

A child asks: Where is my daddy? A mother asks, How is

my son? A wife asks, Is my husband alive or dead? Communist North Vietnam is sadistically practicing spiritual and mental genocide on over 1500 American prisoners of war and their families. How long?[24]

Representative Scherle claimed that he and other members of Congress were determined to keep up the pressure until the United States received an accurate and complete accounting of the men they were holding prisoner and were assured of their humane treatment. I nearly cheered out loud when I heard that.

In March, I went to Fort Lee, Virginia, to obtain the commander's permission to ask military families and servicemen to write letters for the League's "Letters to Hanoi" campaign. As always, each individual could choose whether or not to write a letter. The commanding officer there turned me down flat, saying that if he said yes, he would be condoning solicitation on a military post. I decided to elevate his decision, and addressed the issue in a letter to the Legislative Affairs officer at the Department of the Air Force. On March 10, I received a very welcome response. The letter said in part,

> I am sure that it is obvious by the statements made by the President, Secretary of State, and Secretary of Defense that the present policy of the government is to bring to bear on Hanoi the pressure of world opinion . . . anything that anyone could do to focus world opinion on Hanoi is useful. We measure by two criteria. First of all any program should not be harmful to the men or to their families. Secondly, it must not violate the U.S Code. The enclosed item, relative to letters by active duty personnel, testifies to the fact that we believe that letter campaigns directed to the humane aspects are not in violation of the Code. I am sure you will understand, but again I will repeat that we are pleased to see these programs are taking place. I think they will continue to further our efforts. With best wishes,
> (signed) Milton K. Kegley, Colonel,
> USAF, Special Assistant, Legislative Affairs[25]

When I took that letter to Fort Lee, the commander not only

allowed the "Letters to Hanoi" campaign to begin on his base, he pledged his full support to help my family in every way he could.

May of 1970 brought another defining moment, and a great opportunity that raised the League's ability to raise worldwide and national POW-MIA consciousness. The fledgling League of Wives of Prisoners begun by Sybil Stockdale in 1969 was growing fast, and changing with that growth. First we had morphed into the League of Families, welcoming all members of a POW or MIA family to join us in our work, and now we became officially The National League of Families of American Prisoners and Missing in Southeast Asia! The League had been incorporated as a non-profit, non-partisan organization, to be financed by the families of POW/MIA and contributions from concerned individuals and organizations. The various chapters of the League of Families in regions all across the United States were now gathering together under that important national umbrella.

On May 1, we held our first Appeal for International Justice

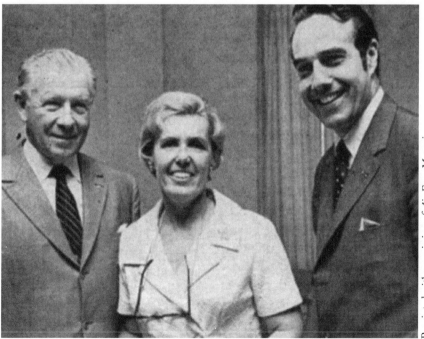

Sybil Stockdale, Senators Bob Dole and George Murphy at first Mayday Conference of the League of Families, Washington D.C., May 1, 1970.

Reprinted with permission of *Air Force Magazine*

Conference in the Daughters of the American Revolution Constitution Hall in Washington, D.C. We called it the "Mayday" Conference, not just because of the date, but because Louise Mulligan opened the conference by shouting "Mayday!" Mayday!" the international distress call, into the microphone.[26] We were all so proud of her! The families and our POWs and MIAs were in great distress. We needed help, and we wanted the world to know it.

Thanks to Sybil and her contacts, that first Mayday Conference was a star-studded Washington political event. President Nixon wrote the foreword for the official program booklet. Senator Bob Dole (R-Kansas), the chairman of the Senate-House Appeal for International Justice Committee, kindly acted as master of ceremonies; singer Jack Jones sang "To Dream the Impossible Dream" from *Man of La Mancha;* H. Ross Perot introduced "United We Stand" in a speech.[27] Senator Barry Goldwater (R-Arizona) introduced astronaut James Lovell, the *Apollo 13* Command Pilot, as the

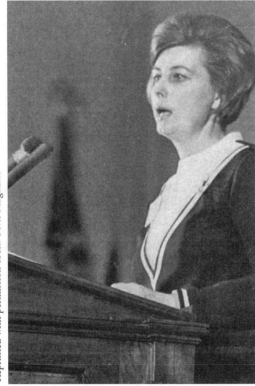

Navy POW wife Louise Mulligan shouts "Mayday!" to open the first League of Families Mayday Conference.

featured speaker. Lovell spoke about the POW/MIA situation being a challenge to America.

Recently released POWs Robert Frishman and Doug Hegdahl were introduced to the Mayday gathering and received a great ovation.

Mrs. Iris Powers, whose son Lowell was MIA, served as the interim National Coordinator (President) of the National League of Families of American POW/MIA in Southeast Asia, until elections could be held at the League's first National Convention, slated for October of 1970.

Since the League's official name was a mouthful to say or type, we called it variously the League of Families, or simply the League. Sybil, along with Mrs. Bruce G. Johnson, an MIA wife from Salina, Kansas, and Mrs. Jerry A. Singleton, a POW wife from Dallas, Texas, made touching appeals for international justice for our men. When they finished, the Convention drafted two important resolutions regarding justice and humane treatment for the POWs and demanded that the North Vietnamese government provide an accounting for all prisoners and those missing in action. Copies were presented to a representative group of POW/MIA wives and mothers, including Louise Mulligan, who took the resolutions to Congress for their sponsorship. The resulting Senate-House Joint Congressional Resolution called upon, "Men of compassion and good will throughout the world . . . to search all peaceful avenues available to insure that these men be treated humanely and fairly, in accord with . . . the Geneva Conventions;" and "that every possible effort be made to secure their early release from captivity." It further required that "copies of this resolution be delivered by the appropriate representatives of the United States Government to the appropriate representatives of every nation of the world."

We League of Families members were elated. The U.S. Congress had finally added its considerable weight to our cause! We also were grateful for the help and presence of the astronauts like James Lovell, Frank Borman, and Alan Shepard, who lent so much prestige to our cause. Americans looked up to their astronauts and would back a cause they supported. Lovell's friend and fellow Gemini VII astronaut, Air Force Colonel Frank Borman, even made a worldwide tour as a Special Presidential Ambassador to seek support for the release of the American POWs held by North Vietnam. The League was deeply indebted to him for trying to get our POWs released and brought home.

On May 10, 1970, Helen Brunstrom called me, breathless. She was beyond excited and happy. She had received a letter from Al, her very first word from him, after four long years of total silence! That threw my system into high gear. Elated for her, I rushed out to the mailbox every day after that, expecting to find one from Newk. I was truly thrilled for Helen, but as the days continued with the hollow emptiness of the mailbox as to Newk, I became even more distressed and depressed about my own situation.

"Somehow Helen's good fortune in getting a letter from Al makes my own vigil seem so lonely," I wrote in my journal. I still had hope that one day I'd receive a letter from Newk out of the blue, just the way Al's letter had suddenly dropped out of the sky into Helen's mailbox.

In early June, I wrote to Newk about our new house. I abbreviated as much as possible to get everything into the short, six-line space we were allotted by the North Vietnamese:

> June 2nd '70
> My dearest Newk,
>   I love you. School will soon be out . . . We are bldg. a house Darling, & I have tried to choose things you would like in it. Our address will be 307 Norwood Dr., Col. Hts. VA. It will be finished in Aug. I will send pictures in the pkg. to you. Jeff, Roke, Van, Roy & I miss you and need you. I hold and comfort you in my dreams Newk. Our families are all fine.
> Always yours,
> Evelyn

Off it went, and with it my hopes and dreams for our future together as a family.

The recently released statistics regarding the flow of letters from the Vietnamese prison camps to the POWs' families only underscored our frustrations. It remained very disheartening. At the end of 1965, just before Newk was captured, there were an estimated 173 American servicemen classified as POW or MIA in the Vietnam War. Of these, only 19 wrote a total of 35 letters during that entire year.[28] That was fewer than two letters per writer, per year, counting only the 19 that wrote! What about the others, who didn't write? Were they alive or dead? How did their families handle it? The same way I did—with fear, anger, deep distress and frustration. However, those terrible statistics reminded me again that I was not alone, that there were many, many other wives in the same no-communication-whatsoever predicament I was trapped in. We might one day be like Helen, and unexpectedly there would be a letter. From the depths to the heights. What an awful way to live.

By 1968, the number of prisoners and missing had risen considerably.[29] Yet only 246 letters were received by the families of about 110 prisoners that year.[30] Again, barely two letters per year, per *writing* prisoner, who were far fewer than the total number of prisoners! What about the other POWs or any we called MIAs who were prisoners, who didn't (or couldn't or weren't permitted to) write anything at all to their families? That was the kind of reality the POW families lived with every day. No acknowledgment and complete silence were the cruelest blows and mental torture imaginable to the families, especially when it continued for years, as it did for so many of us. In our internal statistical studies, one of the prisoner categories was "silent for reasons unknown." Newk was a member of that category. My Newk, who always wrote me love notes and long, chatty letters when he was away on assignment. Our Newk, who smiled and laughed and chatted with us. Newk Grubb, who loved his family, and whose family loved him. *That* Newk's family had not received a single letter, nor had anyone reported seeing him, since January 1966.

It was now July 1970. Four and a half years had passed in complete dark silence. Did that mean he was alive or dead? Who knew? In truth, my situation was not much different from that of the MIA wives. Their wait was equally as agonizing as mine. Most didn't know if their husbands had been killed, perished after going missing, or were captured and not writing for reasons unknown. At least I had that one scrap of knowledge, that photographic proof from North Vietnam that Newk had been captured and was in North Vietnam's "humane" custody.

The Geneva Convention specified that a prisoner of war must be allowed to write no fewer than six letters and cards per month to family.[31] By now, I should have received more than 300 letters—as many from Newk alone as were actually received from *all* the prisoners during that time. The deepest, worst black hole imaginable had opened between POW/MIA families and their husbands, fathers and sons. It was beyond cruel. It was beastly, uncivilized, and downright sadistic.

As for coping with Newk's silence—I desperately struggled to hold together the thinning shreds of what once had been our solid life together. I had once been ready to divorce him because I couldn't imagine spending two or three years without him, and didn't believe our family could survive that. Now, I had been alone for four years—frightened, angry years spent without so much as a word from the man of my life. And what about our children? If anything, my love and longing for Newk was stronger, I missed him more than anyone could possibly imagine. The children? That was a different kettle of fish, as the saying went.

Fortunately, Jeff still remembered Newk, and Roland occasionally recalled times with Daddy. In the night, tossing restlessly, I pondered how we would ever put our lives back together again. I didn't know, and could not imagine how. I just hoped that God would help and he would come back to us. Only when that happened would I have the opportunity to re-fashion some kind of family fabric for us. Only then.

Barely a month after our Mayday Conference in June 1970, The League of Families marked another major milestone: We opened a national headquarters office at One Constitution Avenue NE, in the Air Force Association building in downtown Washington, D.C.[32] How our founder, Sybil Stockdale, had managed to organize us into area groups and then coordinate us into a national organization with a headquarters in the nation's capital was mind-boggling to me. Sybil was just an amazing woman. It was her single-minded perseverance that got us joined together. The boys and I were proud to attend the opening day ceremonies that marked the League's new national office.

In her opening remarks as Chairman of the Board of the League, Sybil declared that the POW/MIA families had worked too long out of their living rooms and kitchens. She was right. Having an office in the nation's capital would not only focus more attention on the POW/MIA issue, it would also give the League of Families a prestigious base in our national capital, a central point from which the League could coordinate activities and contacts. It would permit broader communications between POW/MIA wives and family members and members of the Federal government. It would promote improved press and public awareness. A Washington, D.C., address on our letterhead from which to operate would also give us the patina of official status and would likely bring greater world pressure to bear upon North Vietnam. That was the icing on the cake for us. For my part, I encouraged the League Board and members to focus world attention on North Vietnam's sins of omission—by pointing up their failure to adhere to any of the provisions of the Geneva Conventions. I wanted us to be relentless about that.

Thereafter, the League concentrated heavily on the POW "Discrepancies:" the men like Newk, who had been photographed or taped by the North Vietnamese following capture, and whose photographs and/or tapes had been used by the North Vietnamese for propaganda purposes in clear violation of the Geneva Conventions. The names of many of these men like Newk's had been omitted from the first list of prisoners the Vietnamese had recently given to the Committee of Liaison, Cora Weiss and David Dellinger's group.

The League ensured that these discrepancies were highlighted in the press, underscored with the photos like Newk's that the North Vietnamese had used, or released to the press. Admittedly, the League's maneuvers were small triumphs, but to the families, in our desperation and hunger for any news of loved ones after years of silence, every small triumph was a bold step forward in what had been an agonizing stalemate for years. Sybil had showed us all how quickly "small and insignificant" could sprout and become "big and bold."

That boldness was both a relief to me in my present situation and a worry for the future. I was now the one who made all the family decisions at home. I was the person to whom the boys automatically turned for answers. I had raised the kids my way, and now

I was becoming an outspoken public activist on national and military matters. What would Newk think of that? I knew I was definitely no longer the woman Newk had left at home in Petersburg in late 1965. Neither would he be the same Newk when he returned to us. What would he be like, I wondered? Balding, the doctor had predicted. Would he be physically and/or mentally okay? Would he, could he, still love me . . . and our four kids? How would Roy react to him? Would Newk even like us the way we are now? Would I be able to just hand it all over to him again when he came back? What would life be like for us, after this terrible ordeal he'd been through for so many years? There were so many questions burning holes in my mind . . . but as always, no answers for any of them.

It had long been rumored that the North Vietnamese were ignoring us as a threat at the Paris Peace Talks, and treated our prisoners as sadistically as they pleased, because they didn't believe the American people cared anything about the small handful of men they held.[33] The League knew that we had to convince them beyond a shadow of a doubt that the American people did care. There might be comparatively few POWs in the overall scope of population of the United States, but their families, the League, and millions of Americans cared a whole lot about those few, and were starting to show the world that we cared. This realization was very gratifying to us in our desperation to get those men better treatment.

In 1969, Sybil had outlined the League's mission in a bulletin that announced the formation of the League. She had said in part,

> Our aims are to inform Fellow Americans and World Citizens of the codes for treatment of Combatant Prisoners as established by the Geneva Convention for the dignity and protection of Mankind . . . Ours is an effort to supplement that which our government is doing to ensure humane treatment for our men . . . We believe that the cumulative voices of indignation from people all over the world will have a profound influence on the North Vietnamese government if they want to be recognized as a respectable government in the world community.[34]

I would be right there with them, but I wasn't going to neglect my family either. I was head of the Grubb household now. Everything rested on my shoulders, including matters regarding Newk. I'd just have to solve each problem as it arose.

By July 1, 1970, our new house in Colonial Heights was almost finished. In keeping with my resolve to maintain our normal family life, I left with the boys, my mother, and my brother's family, for a week of carefree summer vacation in Southern Shores, North Carolina. It was wonderful being together with other regular summer vacation friends and their kids, too. At one point, the boys got me out on a five-man raft. Off balance and laughing, I upset the raft three times. After the final time, they deposited me unceremoniously on the beach. There was lots of fun and laughter; the sadness that Newk wasn't there to share that fun and laughter with us caught me like a sudden lancing pain from time to time, as it always did when wonderful family moments like this happened without him. Following our great week at the beach, the four boys went to a friend's cottage in Pennsylvania for another week, while Mother and I returned home. Together we moved things into the new house. Mother was such a stalwart companion to me, and I loved her so much, but I could see what worrying about us, and about Newk was doing to her. She was aging fast.

We had just completed our move and were settling in at the new house, when in August 1970, a photo of Jeff and me appeared in *Air Force Magazine* with an article about the opening of the League's new Washington, D.C., office.

When the boys arrived back home from Pennsylvania, I took them to register at their new schools. Jeff would be attending Colonial Heights High School. I knew that changing schools wasn't easy for him. I couldn't believe he was in high school. He was growing up fast and was a big help to me. Barely a week later, tragedy struck. We lost our beloved hound Heidi. It was in a tragic accident, and we grieved deeply over it. She was Newk's gift to us when he left for Saigon and had been the living symbol of Daddy to all of us for more than four years. We held a solemn burial ceremony in the back yard under a tree. The boys were inconsolable. Afterward, Van sobbed and begged me to dig poor Heidi dog up again, "She'll be okay, Mom." It took a lot for me to distract them to something else.

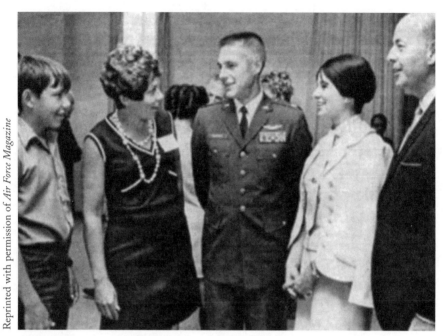

*Evelyn Grubb and son, Jeff Grubb at left, attend the opening of the first
National office of the League, in Washington, D.C., August 1970.*

Not long after that, Mike Wallace and his crew from the television news show, *60 Minutes,* came and spent two days interviewing me and my family. To his deep dismay, I refused to talk on camera against the military, and declined to speak out against the war, and our President. When the show aired on television, my comments had been cut to one sentence, and that sentence had been taken out of context. Mr. Wallace wasn't happy with me as an interview subject, since we had differing views, and agendas.

I was astounded to learn one evening that Mother wasn't happy with me either. She openly expressed her dislike that I was spending so much of my time with the League of Families and our projects to get better treatment for the POWs and accounting for the MIAs.

"You've been at it for more than a year now, Evie, and it hasn't done a bit of good. You've still heard nothing from Newk. Why do you keep on with it? You should stay home with the boys and stop all this."

Mother was sounding a lot like the older woman at the Officers'

Club who had berated me for going out for dinner and smiling. It was impossible to convince Mother, who had very narrow views of a woman's role, and had never worked at a job in her life, that what I was doing for and with the League of Families was important to me, even vital. She didn't want to accept that working with the League was something I wanted to do. It was keeping me focused and active. Most importantly, it kept me sane.

By October of 1970, the League had moved into larger office quarters donated for our use at the American Legion Building on K Street in Washington, and we had many national and local area projects underway simultaneously. Our Virginia Chapter efforts were reported in a newsletter by our Coordinator, Dorothy McDaniel, wife of POW "Red" McDaniel. As a result of the untiring efforts of my friend, Phyllis Galanti (wife of Navy POW, Paul Galanti, who like Newk had been gone since 1966) several statewide banks mailed POW information brochures out with their monthly bank statements. These brochures contained a tear-off sheet with a printed letter ready to be completed, signed and returned to a Richmond post office box for distribution to Hanoi. Jim Gunter and Whitey Lemmond volunteered to distribute the extra brochures with the letter at the American Fighter Pilots' booth at the Virginia State Fair. We were thrilled. The Norfolk-Virginia Beach families launched OPERATION WE CARE in October, 1970, with the goal of sending a delegation of private citizens, accompanied by two mayors, to the Paris peace talks to present petitions to the North Vietnamese delegates.

October also brought our first League of Families Convention, which came and went in a whirlwind blur of activity for me. MIA wife, Joan (she pronounced it Jo-Ann) Vinson, succeeded MIA mother, Iris Powers, as National Coordinator of the League of Families. U.S. Navy MIA wife, Kathy Plowman, became Assistant National Coordinator.[35] Air Force POW wife, Carol North, of Massachusetts succeeded Sybil Stockdale as Chairman of the Board, and Mary Jane McManus, wife of an Air Force POW, was made Secretary-Treasurer.

Before we could catch our breath, the holidays were upon us. Army POW wife, Valerie Kushner, began a LEST WE FORGET campaign in Danville with Christmas cards featuring Pat Mearns'

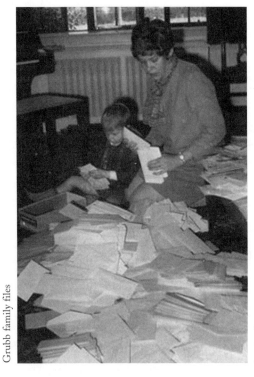

Grubb family files

*Evelyn Grubb and youngest son,
Roy, sort letters to Hanoi from
American citizens.*

two young daughters, and holiday ads about remembering the
POWs during the holiday season.

Dorothy McDaniel and I convinced Virginia Governor
Linwood Holton to again proclaim the week of November 9-15 the
"Concern for Prisoners of War Week."

I attended a League meeting in Washington with the
Richmond group to hear business magnate H. Ross Perot and a
psychiatrist, Dr. Martin Orne of the University of Pennsylvania,
speak. The League began working on how to ship the boxes of
more than 12,000 letters we'd gathered already to the North
Vietnamese officials. At home, Roy helped me sort and box the
thousands of letters we collected.

Although the purpose of the letter campaign was primarily to
raise awareness and get Americans involved in the POW/MIA
cause, the League had those letters and felt they should be delivered. Why not to Hanoi?

One Sunday during that hectic October of 1970, a couple from
our church asked me frankly whether I really believed Newk was

still alive. "It depends on the day," I replied honestly. "Some days I think Newk is alive and okay and just doesn't want to write us for some reason. Other days I think Newk must surely be dead, or we'd have heard from him by now. Other times I think that we haven't heard because he is sick or terribly injured and can't write us. In truth, I don't know *what* I believe any more. My friend Helen Brunstrom got a letter from her husband after 4 years of silence. So there's always hope."

Early in November, Newk's parents flew down for Thanksgiving. Dad Grubb immediately began planting tulip and daffodil bulbs around our new house, hoping that Newk would be there to see them come up and bloom next spring. Mother and the Grubbs looked worn, weary and terribly sad. The toll this situation had taken on them angered me. I knew I didn't look all that good myself. I felt that things couldn't get any worse . . . but they could. The evening of November 12, I returned home from doing my weekly shopping to find Dad Grubb pacing the floor, waiting for me to arrive.

"The boys said you received several calls from Randolph Air Force Base in Texas, Evie. Colonel Gratch wants you to call him back right away. It must be something to do with Newk."

I immediately became concerned and fearful; I could see in Dad's eyes that he was, too. I checked my watch. It would be about 5 p.m. out in Texas. I snatched up the phone and dialed Colonel Gratch. When he answered, his voice was somber.

"We have received some information today from the State Department, Mrs. Grubb. I wanted to inform you right away before you hear it elsewhere. Cora Weiss, of the Committee of Liaison, says she has a list from North Vietnam of six men who have died while in prison camp: three Air Force and three Navy men. I feel we should inform you that a Major Wilmer Grubb was listed as one of those six men."

I stood there, silent, gripping the phone, trying to absorb the impact of his words. Colonel Gratch went on to say that Mrs. Weiss had informed the State Department that she had particulars about each man, and that she would share them with the families tomorrow at her press conference, which was scheduled for 11 a.m.

Dad Grubb knew from the look on my face that it was bad

news, news none of us wanted to hear. I handed him the phone. When Dad hung up from his talk with Colonel Gratch, we hugged each other, and then went to tell Mother, Mrs. Grubb and the children what Cora Weiss had reported. There was no wailing, no sobbing. There was only silence. Tears don't make any noise as they slide down your cheeks.

My anger finally boiled up, and broke the silence and grief. "If Newk is dead, then those North Vietnamese bastards killed him!"

Mother Grubb said, her voice quivering, "They used his picture for five years as an example of the humane treatment given to U.S. pilots?"[36]

No one responded. No one could.

We continued to express our thoughts in short sentences and brief outbursts of memory, of denial, of disbelief. It was comforting that Mother, the Grubbs, and the boys were all there with me to help me bear the brutal pain of that phone call. Once again, we had received dreadful news in an offhand way. After five years of anxiety and fear, we received the ultimate blow from a stranger named Cora Weiss, who had not even had the decency to inform the wives and families of these men before publicly disseminating such life-shattering news. I was to believe a phone call to transmit unsubstantiated information passed to the Air Force and our government by a Communist sympathizer who had no official capacity? It was a nightmare scenario of the worst kind. Should we believe her? I thought back to Pat Mearns' letter almost a year ago and wondered if her husband might be one of the men named on that list of six.

The doorbell sounded. Jeff went to answer it. Captain Robertson of the Casualty Office at Langley Field had arrived to personally convey his regrets. He elaborated some on what Colonel Gratch had told us. According to Cora Weiss, he said, the North Vietnamese claimed that Newk died of injuries related to his bailout.

"What a crock!" I exclaimed. "Newk was up, standing straight, and walking. A doctor has carefully examined all those photos of him and deduced from them that Newk showed no signs of shock, injury, or internal bleeding of the kind that a serious bailout injury might have caused. They're lying."

"I understand how you and your family must feel, Mrs. Grubb.

He glanced around the room at each tear-stained face of our parents and our sons. I saw his face soften. He drew a breath. "I know this is unbearable, but we can't confirm anything at this time. Nor can we stop Mrs. Weiss from speaking out in a press conference. We're simply informing you now what she claims the North Vietnamese told her, and what she'll probably say in her press conference tomorrow. I know it's very difficult to comprehend. We're not saying that her information is true, as we have no official proof that it is. Nor can we keep her from saying it publicly, and we wanted you to know what's coming."

"I appreciate that, but this is all very contradictory to what the photos of Newk after his capture showed. I want better proof."[37]

Robertson was very kind, and quietly sympathetic to us. I didn't envy him his job. "I understand. Mrs.Weiss might have further details to reveal tomorrow at her press conference. We're very sorry this is happening this way, Mrs. Grubb."

I stood up. "Thank you. I appreciate that. Thank you for being here, and for being so kind to us. Right now, I need to go to bed and just be alone. I need to think about all this." With that, I turned and went upstairs to my bed.

6 Reaction and Resolve

TIMELINE . . . 1970 . . . <u>WORLD</u> . . . ROLLS ROYCE DECLARES BANKRUPTCY . . . NIKITA KRUSHCHEV, 77, DIES . . . <u>VIETNAM</u> . . . SOUTH VIETNAMESE TROOPS INVADE LAOS . . . U.S. DECLARES AIR RAIDS AND BOMBINGS WILL CONTINUE UNTIL VIETNAM RELEASES ALL U.S. PRISONERS OF WAR . . . <u>USA</u> . . . 1970 CENSUS RESULTS: 204.8 MILLION IN U.S. . . . WHITE HOUSE ANNOUNCES PRES. NIXON TO VISIT CHINA IN 1972 . . . "ALL IN THE FAMILY" WINS TV EMMY AWARD . . . KC CHIEFS BEAT VIKINGS TO WIN SUPER BOWL . . .

Show me a good and gracious loser
And I'll show you a failure.
—Knute Rockne

I didn't sleep throughout that long, long night. If I accepted Cora Weiss' information, my Newk was gone. I was prepared for this, or so I'd thought. In truth, I felt cheated. I mentally reviewed the symbolic "bargain" I believed I had made with God.

Have I not remained faithful to Newk? Have I not been a good mother to the children in his absence? Why does it have to end with Newk being dead? Why couldn't we have him back with us? Slowly, angry yet subdued by sadness, I began to accept that in all likelihood, Cora Weiss was telling the truth about Newk. Yes, it was truth without proof, without supporting evidence, without legitimacy. My thoughts tumbled over one another. Newk is dead. He will never hold me again. The boys will never see their father again. Okay . . . I've asked for answers, I've prayed for answers, I've begged for answers. Tonight I got an answer: Dead . . . one cryptic word. But whose word? Do I accept that? Can I accept that? And worse, what will it mean for all those other POWs if I do?

It was near dawn when I got up, dressed, and headed downstairs. Mother was already up and sitting at the kitchen table, nursing a cold cup of coffee. She looked absolutely haggard. Obviously, she hadn't slept much either. I knew she was heartsick hearing this about Newk and probably frightened for me and our future. She loved Newk so very much. I couldn't even imagine how Newk's parents, still in bed upstairs, must feel. What a horrific blow this was to them, after all our hopes and prayers.

I poured myself a coffee, glanced surreptitiously at my mother, and was shocked to see her glaring at me, angry as a cornered hornet! I raised an eyebrow, and without preamble, she lashed out.

"So . . . look at you, Evie Grubb. Exhausted. Beaten down. What have you accomplished, with your trips, your speeches, your letters, all those efforts? What good has it done Newk? Or you? Or the children? No good at all! It got you nowhere, gave you nothing. Newk is gone. Dead, if we're to believe that woman."

I tried to stay calm. She was overwrought. This was the terrible last straw. "Oh, dear, I know you're upset . . . as I am, Mother. We all love Newk. This is a dreadful way for all our hopes and prayers to end. We need to think of Newk and his parents and the children today. Tomorrow the rest can be dealt with."

"What rest can be dealt with?" Mother stared at me, aghast. "What can you do about it, Evie? Surely you won't continue this useless fight with those people!"

"I'm afraid I will, Mother. I know you don't want to hear that. But without the official notice or explanation from their government to ours that I'm entitled to receive, of how and why Newk died, according to the Geneva Conventions, which North Vietnam signed, I simply cannot accept this as official. You heard Captain Robertson: they have heard it, but they're not agreeing it's true, or official."

I stopped to draw breath. Mother jumped right in.

"Oh, Evie, let it go! Quit that League. I worry every time you go up to Washington alone. That city is a dangerous place. So much crime and murder, bombings and anti-war demonstrations. You should stay home now, with your children."[1]

I sighed and closed my eyes for a moment. I wanted to avoid tangling with her, but Mother was on the warpath, not to be deterred. I knew her well. I was just like her, in fact. So I might as well speak my mind, and give her more to jump on, which she needed and wanted right now, in order to cope with this latest shock.

"First, Mother, I believe we in the League have indeed accomplished something simply by doing all those things that you don't want me to do any more. Finally, I got *someone* to answer *something* about Newk, didn't I? It isn't the answer we wanted to hear, nor is it the answer we prayed for. It isn't even an answer I can officially accept. But you know . . . I think it's true. So I'm not in denial."

"I think we've all felt that way, Evie, at some point. But . . . what if she's wrong?"

"Who knows? We may *all* be wrong. Is it true . . . or false? We don't know. So no, it's not over, not by a long shot. We owe Newk more than this. Like demanding to know how . . . and why . . . did he die? Like those returned men have told us, he was probably so brutally mistreated he died from it. I believe if he's dead they killed him! I do know that, for his sake and for the sake of the rest of our POWs I cannot meekly accept what Cora Weiss said, whether I believe it or not. Certainly I can't accept it without some more specific official explanation or proof."

"What if Newk *is* gone, as you think he is, Evie? You're the children's only parent now. You have to look out for yourself and for them. Haven't we been through enough already? It's been nearly five years! How much more can we all stand? This can't go on and on forever! It's too hard, too horrible."

"I know. You're right . . . of course it can't continue like this, Mother, and hopefully it won't for much longer. For the moment, though, I must keep on. It's important to the men still in prison over there, and it's important to me and Newk, for many other reasons."

"Why? Help me understand why, Evie, because I don't."

Well, for one, why should I believe *anything* Cora Weiss tells me? It could be just a brutal lie. They *are* brutal, we know that. She is *not* an official of the North Vietnamese government! She is *not* an ambassador. She's *not* a representative of our government. She is an American but doesn't respect us. She comes and goes to North Vietnam at will and they welcome her, so she must be one of them. And we allow it. Okay . . . let's say we believe her on the face of it, and accept that Newk and the others are dead on that list she claims to have. Which means that Hanoi is officially responsible for those deaths. Why aren't *they* notifying me? They know how to write. They're in Paris negotiating. What kind of game are they playing? And why? They could notify me as easily as Cora Weiss can. But they'd have to do it through official channels! And they won't. Why not? Because they want to be free to do to other POWs what they did to Newk? I can't accept this so easily, and let that possibly happen, Mother. I just can't. I'm going to fight back."

"What about the children, Evie? They need you here with them now, not off fighting governments."

"They needed their father too, Mother. And no one gave him all this argument when he went off to fight governments. Of *course* we've had enough! Five months, even five days of this was more than enough. But we've hung in there believing he was alive, for five long, miserable, lonely years, and I'm not going to let them beat me down now. I want justice, that's all. Simple international justice prescribed by law. I won't accept this until both sides, my government and theirs, take the responsibility for the Conventions they signed. If Newk is truly dead, neither side can hurt him anymore and no one can intimidate me anymore, either. So what does it matter if I decide to continue to fight for my rights as a U.S. citizen, a wife, a mother, and a woman who deeply believes in justice?"

My voice had risen almost as high as my mother's eyebrows. We were certainly digging into the depths of it all. I knew I had to calm down. Mother gave me one of her "I don't believe this" looks. "What do you mean, Evie? What can you possibly do now that will help anybody? You've done so much already—enough! Do you really believe Newk is gone?"

"Mother, I know my husband better than anyone. If he were still alive, my Newk would have found some way, somehow, to let us know that. Yes, I believe Newk is dead. Therefore, I can speak out, fight dirty, fight back. I'm not ready to roll over, Mother."

"No one's asking you to, Evelyn! You're distraught, and grief-stricken. You're only one woman. You can't take something this big on all by yourself!"

I'm not alone, Mother. I have the League with me. The POW/MIA families have seen and heard such terrible things about conditions over there in Hanoi and the POW camps, they are afraid that anything they say will be used against their men! The North Vietnamese have gone beyond vicious. Newk died in captivity, while supposedly under the rules and protection of the Geneva Conventions. He died while reportedly receiving their "humane treatment." We don't know how or why he died. So I'm going to fight hard for him, Mother, for myself and all the other POW/MIA wives and families."

"Oh, dear, no! For all our sakes, Evie, give up this endless, impossible fight!"

Mother's voice had now risen to a level that matched mine. I turned away and thought for a minute. My mother had lived through World War II, Korea, and my father's death. Now it was Newk's death she'd have to face with me. She was older, and I needed to be more gentle with her. I kept my voice quiet and level when I turned back to face her.

"I understand what *you* want, Mother. Please understand me, that I can't surrender. If I fail Newk and all the POWs now, what's to stop the North Vietnamese from simply killing *all* the American prisoners over there, one by one, or torturing them to death, just like they probably did Newk and these other five? If we do nothing, they can do that, with impunity. Cora Weiss can come next time and tell us they're all dead. "Too bad, so sad!" Then what do we do, declare war on them? We *are* at war with them! Think about that, Mother."

Mother sighed, got up, and went to get her coat. She came back, buttoning it up, her voice soft and sad now, too.

"I'm so sorry, Evie. Neither of us is in any state to talk about this. I cannot imagine what you must be feeling right now. I love you, and I love the boys. You're the living, you're all we have. I'm going home now to rest. I'll make dinner for everyone tonight. Please come around six. Let's just leave this be for today."

"All right, Mother, I agree. We all need some rest. Thank you for understanding. You're right, there's really nothing more to say." I went over and put my arms around her and we hugged one another tightly. When the door closed after her, I ran upstairs and let the tears for Newk—my dear and wonderful love—and for myself, just pour out. I cried until I was totally exhausted, then fell asleep and slept solidly for two hours. When I awoke, Mother and Dad Grubb were up, sitting in the kitchen. One look at their ashen faces only hardened my resolve. I tried to smile.

"Good morning. We all look the way we feel today, I see—terrible. Where are the boys?"

"Over at the neighbor's," said Dad. "We fixed them breakfast and told them to go on ahead—hope that's okay with you, Evie. We figured you needed your sleep."

"Thanks, Dad . . . I do need some down time. Got lots to think about."

We talked quietly, in broken sentences for a bit, and finally Newk's parents confirmed that like me, they truly believed Newk was dead.

"If he was alive, Newk would have found some way to let us know that." Dad said. "I've suspected for quite awhile that our boy's gone, Evie. Died over there."

"Poor little Roy. He never will know his Daddy," said Mom Grubb, her face crumpling. She began to sob loudly, the tears running down her face.

I looked at their dear, sweet faces and my love for them just overwhelmed me. No one could ever have better in-laws. The Grubbs were rock solid people, always there for me . . . for us . . . their grandsons. I also knew they'd undoubtedly overheard my fierce argument with Mother earlier. After we'd all cried a bit, and settled down again, I ventured,

"I'm not deaf to what my mother is saying either, but I'm very troubled, Dad. The long silences and their cruelty are well known. We need to demand hard, official proof of Newk's death. All the families of POWs who die in captivity should get that at least. I'm just not going to give them the satisfaction of accepting Cora Weiss' word on this."

They nodded, unable to speak, bitter tears still sliding down their cheeks. I got up to get us some tissues. It looked like we'd be needing boxes of them today. They were suffering as deeply as I was. After five years of hoping, it was unbearably painful to accept that all that hope was gone. Now we could at least spill out some of the grief and despair that had been building inside us for years. I sat and wept with them for a few minutes. Then I stood up, took another deep breath, and cleared my throat. We went about our daily routines and comforted one another, and the boys, whenever one of us needed that. Eventually, when we were having some tea after lunch, Dad Grubb looked at me and said, his voice weak and gravelly from grieving, "Evie, Mom and I have talked about this. We'll respect your wishes fully. You need to do whatever will help you and the boys get through and past this. Get on with your lives. Five years of pain is more than enough. No matter what we do, we can't bring Newk back."

"I know that, Dad, and thank you. I want to make his death, and those other POW's deaths, more than just a passing yawn to his jailers, or a statistic to the Vietnamese. Thank you both for being understanding. I need to stay on this path for awhile longer. I don't even know what my status is now. That will all need to be resolved officially too. There's just so much to deal with."

Cora Weiss' press conference revealed nothing we didn't already know. She didn't expand, she didn't give more details. It appeared to me she just wanted publicity and comfort for her cause and for the North Vietnamese over the "accidental" deaths of these men. Well, she could look long and hard, but she wouldn't get it from me. That same afternoon, I began re-reading my copy of the Geneva Conventions, most particularly the section about prisoners who die in captivity. Sure enough, it was covered in detail in Section III, Articles 120 and 121, which stated in part:

> Death certificates, in the form annexed to the present Convention, or lists certified by a responsible officer, of all persons who die as prisoners of war shall be forwarded as rapidly as possible to the Prisoner of War Information Bureau established in accordance with Article 122.
>
> . . . The death certificates or certified lists shall show particulars of identity as set out in the third paragraph of Article 17, and also the date and place of death, the cause of death, the date and place of burial and all particulars necessary to identify the graves . . . the detaining authorities shall ensure that prisoners of war who have died in captivity are honorably buried, if possible according to the rites of the religion to which they belonged, and that their graves are respected, suitably maintained, and marked so as to be found at any time. Whenever possible, deceased prisoners of war who depended on the same Power shall be interred in the same place.

Article 121 covered the subject of death or serious injuries, saying in part,

> Every Death or serious injury of a prisoner of war caused or suspected to have been caused by a sentry, another prisoner of war, or any other person, as well as any death the cause of which is unknown, shall be immediately followed by an official enquiry by the Detaining Power. A communication on this subject shall be sent immediately to the Protecting Power. Statements shall be taken from witnesses, especially from those who are prisoners of war, and a report including such statements shall be forwarded to the Protecting Power. If the enquiry indicates the guilt of one or more persons, the Detaining Power shall take all measures for the prosecution of the person or persons responsible.[2]

Every time I read the Geneva Conventions, I was overcome with admiration and respect for the group that had drafted them. I saw how thorough they were in covering every aspect of war and the prisoners of war, although they had been written decades earlier.

I read again the small booklet that contained the Third Convention relative to the treatment of prisoners of war, and wondered how many people in the United States government knew what the Conventions contained. Everyone talks about them, but I don't believe many people have ever actually read them. Looking over the list of signing nations, I noted that none were paying attention to, or attempting to enforce, the Geneva Conventions, as they had been charged with doing as signatories. And North Vietnam had done nothing that Articles 120 and 121 required them to do. All we'd gotten from Cora Weiss and all the Air Force had gotten, was that Newk Grubb was one of six men listed as "dead."[3]

That night at Mother's house, our attorney friend, Whitey Lemmond, stopped by to visit and offer his condolences. As soon as Whitey appeared, Mother started in again, right where she'd left off that morning.

"Don't get into any more problems, Evelyn. Just give this whole idea up, for the children's sake?" She then turned to Whitey. "Can't you reason with her, Whitey?"

Poor Whitey! He looked stricken. Then he ventured,

"Why do you want to fight them, Evie? Can't you accept it that

Newk is dead?" he asked, not unkindly.

"I believe he's dead," I responded. "How can you even ask me that question, Whitey? You're a lawyer! You should know that if we give in on one more article of the Geneva Conventions — and we've already given in on plenty — we'll soon be sacrificing more men, not just Newk. Don't you see that? Look. If and when I am *officially* notified of Newk's death according to the Geneva Conventions, and North Vietnam provides me with the factual information about his death that I'm entitled to receive, I will accept it, of course. I'd have no other choice. I got no indication from Colonel Gratch that our government or the Air Force is going to accept it, so why should I? Are they going to accept this information from Cora Weiss?"

"I haven't heard anything, but you're right, Evie. I doubt it," Whitey said.

"So until that happens, absent official notification from either government that Newk is dead, nothing changes, officially. But I can and will fight back at the North Vietnamese. To do that I need you, Whitey. I'll need your legal expertise, and your honest perspective. Please don't abandon me now, when I need you the most. This is just another dreadful thing I have to deal with."

Whitey hesitated, glanced quickly at Mother, and then said,

"Well, I see your mind is made up, Evie. Okay, I do understand, and I know what you want to do, and why. I'll help if I can."

"Thanks, Whitey."

He smiled at me. "Glad to do it, Evie, if it will help you deal with this awful news. You knew I'd be hooked by the legal aspects of the dilemma, and you know I'm with you in whatever you want to do for the League of Families."

"I'm glad you understand that this does affect the League and its work. This is something I simply have to do. For Newk, and all the other POWs." Without warning, I broke down in tears again. Before Mother could utter another word, to my astonishment, Jeff stood up and said,

"Okay, enough for today. Let's go, Mom. Your face is white, and you're exhausted. Whitey, will you bring Grandma and Grandpa Grubb home to our place later?"

Whitey nodded, "Sure . . . I'll be happy to do that, Jeff."

Jeff corralled his brothers and got us out of Mother's house and into the car. On the drive home, Jeff and Roke kept patting my shoulder to comfort me. When we got home, Jeff brought me a glass of water and an aspirin. He hugged me and said,

"Listen, Mother, don't let Grandma or anyone else upset you like this anymore. You do whatever your heart tells you to do. Don't worry. We're okay, and we'll get along just fine. Go to sleep now. You need some rest, and we need you."

"Oh, Jeff . . . I'm so proud of you! You boys have been so grown up these past two days. I know it must be awful for you to hear that your Daddy is gone. After all this hoping, waiting, and praying, I wanted so much for him to come back, so we could be a whole family again."

I looked at my boys through tear-blurred eyes. These four sons were a mixture of the best parts of both Newk and me. More fatherless sons and daughters. That was the real legacy of this Vietnam War. The enormity of it, on both sides, staggered the imagination. I knew I was at peace with my decision. I slept soundly that night for the first time in months. I knew with certainty that I was headed in the right direction.

The next day, I formulated some plans. First, I called the Governor of Virginia's secretary and asked her to please schedule a news conference at the Capitol Building in Richmond for me, which she agreed to do. She called me back within the hour, saying it had been arranged for November 19, 1970, and the Governor had approved it.

On November 14, the *New York Times* quoted "a State Department official" as saying about Cora Weiss' list naming the six dead men: "There is grave concern over the news, since no information has been supplied on the dates or circumstances of the men's deaths." As nothing else had to this point, Cora Weiss' reporting the death of these six men with no specific details served the purpose of the League admirably. It finally stirred the American press and the American public to action on behalf of the rest of our POWs. They had seen what I saw, that there was danger ahead if we accepted this without protest. The U.S. government initially was silent on the matter, but not for long. They soon reacted to the ire in the press. I went to work to prepare the statements for my press conference, and on November 19, 1970, I presented it on the steps of the State Capitol. Afterward, Representative John G. Schmitz (R-California) asked that my full statement be included in the *Congressional Record* of December 1, 1970. That record reads:

> Cora Weiss, from the Committee of Liaison, has just returned from Hanoi with the names of six men who have died in captivity. My husband was one of the six. Cora Weiss was to have a press conference with the details of her trip. Only then would she release written information concerning the death of my husband to the State Department, she said. But, as of today, she still has not produced any written evidence, and I am again left dangling at the whim of the enemy. Can you imagine the suspense and horror of the past three days? . . . Hanoi confidently expects that the news will be passed over with a few kinds words—and then—forgotten. Don't let that happen!
>
> Newk, Major Wilmer Newlin Grubb, my husband, was called to Vietnam, thousands of miles away, to fight Communism . . . Now, five years later, I am notified of his death by a highly organized, well-financed Communist organization right here in our own United States! You must comprehend the significance of this ludicrous situation. When other families and I must depend on this Communistic source as the only source of information from and about our captive men, then we too are prisoners of a foreign government. If you and I allow this unofficial death notice to pass unchallenged, we will forsake the sacrifice of every American in the Vietnam conflict.
>
> During the [years of] lonely waiting—and these last tearful days of anguish—I have made a decision. This decision must have your understanding—and your support. This is my decision: I will not accept notification of my husband's death until it is submitted according to the articles of the Geneva Convention. The Geneva Convention was written to protect all captives. Hanoi has never adhered to this Convention. Propaganda photographs portray the fact that my husband was in excellent condition after his capture. If he is dead, then it is my moral—my legal—right to

know all the circumstances of his death. Here is how you can help me. I need lawyers knowledgeable both in national and international law. I need funds to pay the many expenses of possible legal proceedings, but most of all I need your moral support to strengthen me and my family in the coming months. I am determined to put aside my grief, to dry my tears, to turn from bitterness and self-pity, and begin a journey—a mission to force all countries to recognize and adhere to the Geneva Convention, which will ultimately benefit our now 1600 missing men.

Forsake my husband? I will not. Let us instead make this effort a tribute to a gallant hero—my beloved husband. America, I need you, and you are my America. I am depending on you.[4]

The *Richmond News Leader* published the full text of my speech and wrote a strong, vehement editorial that endorsed my position. Their editorial was also published in the *Congressional Record* of December 1, 1970. The final paragraph of the editorial asked:

And what did Major Grubb think about as he lay dying? Did he wonder about the abject weakness of a nation that will not retrieve its prisoners? Did he wonder whether his presence in Vietnam had done any good—any good at all—given the ingratitude of so many in the United States? Indeed, did he wonder whether his imminent death would be but a prelude, a foretaste, of what is in store for his beloved nation? It is too much, too much, the way this good man was treated. Weep for him. And ponder what perhaps were his anguished thoughts as he approached his first glimpse of eternity.[5]

Meanwhile, Secretary of Defense Melvin Laird, in a statement before the Senate Committee on Foreign Relations, regarding the unsuccessful Son Tay prison camp raid, said in part:

At a time when Americans are dying in captivity, some have claimed that this search and rescue attempt might have jeopardized the lives of American prisoners. It is my firm belief that the lives of our American servicemen held captive are in danger every day that Hanoi holds them and

refuses to abide by the humanitarian provisions of the
Geneva Convention. In the absence of inspections by the
International Red Cross or another impartial organization,
we can never be certain of the safety and well being of our
men . . .[6]

Probably because of all the furor her handling of the list of dead
POWs created, The Committee of Liaison's Cora Weiss subsequently published, in the *New York Times,* December 12, 1970, an
article "But It Avoided the Real Facts," disputing the known facts
about ill-treatment and deaths of U.S. POWs in captivity, and
accusing Lt. Frishman, a returned POW, of "tales of highly dubi-
ous credibility." She claimed, "there is no foundation for the charge
that these are deaths in captivity . . ."[7] I wanted to throw up. They
were such straight-faced liars.

Instead, I kept silent and sent a telegram to Ambassador David
Bruce, member of the United States Delegation to the Paris meetings on peace in Vietnam, and informed him of how I'd found out
about my husband's supposed death as a POW. I received a very
nice reply from him dated December 14, 1970. He enclosed a copy
of his opening remarks on the Prisoner of War issue given at a press
conference in Paris on December 1.

In his remarks, he addressed many of my main concerns by asking a series of questions of North Vietnam. I was glad that someone stated a clear U.S. government position on the humane treatment issue, though I noted that Ambassador Bruce didn't indicate
if any action would be taken if North Vietnam continued their
refusal to comply. Ambassador Bruce's remarks on December 1
included:

- What is humane about keeping hundreds of families in
  agonizing doubt by refusing to identify the prisoners they
  hold, and to provide full information on the men they
  know to be dead?
- What is lenient about keeping prisoners incommunicado
  for years, and . . . allowing little or no communication
  between many of them and their families?
- What is humane about refusing to permit impartial
  inspection of prisoner of war facilities?

• What is lenient about failing to release sick and wounded prisoners of war, and those held captive a long time?

. . . It is clear that the other side has deliberately chosen to flout their international legal obligations under the 1949 Geneva Convention, and their moral and humanitarian obligations to the prisoners and their families . . . Here in Paris we have pursued the prisoner question as a matter of the highest urgency . . . in this matter . . . I do not reflect a uniquely American position, but a universal position as set forth in the Geneva Conventions. . . . We will continue to pursue the twin objectives of humane treatment and early release of our men by all means available to us. Our men and their families deserve nothing less.[8]

On December 23, a long article by R.D. Patrick Mahoney, "We Must Free the Prisoners," appeared in *The Review of the News*.[9] This article finally roused the right wing of our government. It certainly strengthened my own resolve to continue. The basic question Mahoney asked about the prisoners in Vietnam was, "What is being done to free them from captivity?" He answered his own query with "Damn little." He then thoroughly castigated the administration and the Congress for doing so little to help our men. Mahoney was not afraid to name names. He liberally quoted the wives of the prisoners, and illustrated the poignant anguish of the families:

For years, these families listened as faceless men in our government double-talked and lied to them. They were boldly told to keep their mouths shut or face reprisals. It was over a year and a half ago that Mrs. James Bond Stockdale, accompanied by relatives of ten other prisoners, moved into Defense Secretary Melvin Laird's office to urge a major campaign to free the prisoners. They were there 'seeking aid and comfort,' according to the July 29, 1969 *New York Times*. But, said the *Times*, they received 'little comfort and even less aid.' That did it! They would fight, and they would fight even their own government if necessary. Within weeks, some three thousand women had banded together to form *The National League of Families of American Prisoners and Missing in Southeast Asia*.

... (Valerie Kushner says), "I have never lost faith in my husband, but at times I wonder if my country has lost faith in him ... I come ... today to tell you that I am tired, I am tired of traveling and I am tired of publicly baring my anguish. And I am *most tired* of Presidential platitudes and Congressional convocations. They no longer reassure me, and they have never brought any relief to the men involved.[10]

Mahoney included most of my story, too, with a few of my quotes from Lou Stockstill's article in the *Air Force and Space Digest*, and commented:

> The courage of Evelyn Grubb has been tested almost beyond endurance, but she is a valiant lady who will not break. It was she who told the *Richmond News Leader* that 'in all the history of warfare, this is the first time that the wives and families have had to work to free their men. Never before has this kind of thing happened. And I am not too sure that it is something that our country can be proud of. To hear nothing from a country that can produce the names of the My Lai massacre civilians in five days and cannot produce a list of prisoners in five years is beyond belief.' The plight of these women is a national disgrace," wrote Mahoney. "Little indignities are repeated and repeated ... Mrs. Galanti being overcharged for repairs to her car; Mrs. Grubb not being able to get a credit card because her husband can't sign the application. These brave ladies can't even buy or sell a home because their powers of attorney have expired. ...

Mahoney went on to excoriate the activities of Cora and Peter Weiss. He told about their Communist activities, and how I'd learned about Newk's death.

> After five years of being separated from her husband, Evelyn Grubb would no longer worry about him. "Newk" Grubb's youngest son, Roy, born while he was in captivity, would never look into the face of his father. Jeffrey, Roland, and Stephen "Van" Grubb would never see their Dad again. Cora Weiss had delivered a Christmas message from the Reds. Her husband [Newk Grubb], it said, was dead—

probably tortured to death in North Vietnam . . . Merry
Christmas Mrs. Grubb and Jeff and Roland and Stephen
and Roy—we have killed your husband and father. Merry
Christmas from Hanoi . . .

He also talked about House Resolution 1378, introduced by
Congressman John G. Schmitz , Republican from California's 35th
district, President Nixon's home territory, that was still bottled up
at that point in the House Foreign Affairs Committee:

This Resolution is written in language the Enemy can
understand. It reads in part: . . . unless within thirty days
following passage of this joint resolution the government of
the Democratic People's Republic of Vietnam indicates a
genuine desire for peace in Southeast Asia by (1) the release
of all United States prisoners of war and also (2) the large
scale withdrawal for its fighting forces back within its own
territorial limits indicating to the satisfaction of the
President of the United States that their aggression is
ended, the state of war that has been thrust upon the United
States ...is hereby formally declared." . . . Call it, if you will,
the Newk Grubb Resolution.

When I read that final phrase, I felt that I had been given a
wonderful Christmas gift! In his conclusion, Mahoney said,

I write, in the days just before Christmas, with the hope
that as President Nixon sits down with his family and his
conscience he can spare a thought for another family whose
father and husband died in captivity in North Vietnam. She
and her four sons, Mr. Nixon, live at 307 Norwood Drive in
Colonial Heights, Virginia. Cora Weiss sent them a
Christmas card this year. Merry Christmas, it said, we have
killed your husband. Unlike you, Mr. Nixon, [Evelyn
Grubb] would not back off. She would not surrender. God
bless her. God bless them, every one.[11]

Accompanying Mahoney's article was a print of artist Maxine
McCaffrey's painting of two sad-faced young girls. It was the 1969
portrait of a very sad Frances and Mary-Ann Mearns, the daughters of Major Arthur Mearns, U.S. Air Force MIA. In the portrait,

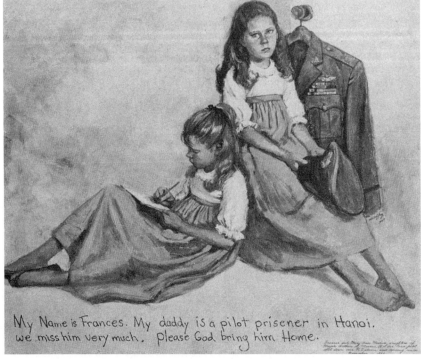

From "Review of the News" Dec. 23, 1970

The National League of Families' 1969 Christmas Card featuring the daughters of USAF MIA Major Arthur Mearns. (Mearns was eventually classed as KIA in North Vietnam, his repatriated remains were buried in Arlington National Cemetery in 1977.)

the girls are sitting in front of their father's empty Air Force uniform jacket. One clutches his empty uniform hat, the other is writing a letter to him. "No one has to ask what these children want for Christmas," the caption reads. At the bottom of the portrait, in childish script, is written: "My name is Frances. My daddy is a pilot prisoner in Hanoi. We miss him very much. Please God, bring him home."[12]

That portrait reflected the kind of sad Christmas holidays we'd all had for many years now. As the calendar turned to January 1971, I was gratified to receive a long letter from President Nixon, that he had written to "all the wives and families of our men held prisoner and missing in Southeast Asia—and also to the many others who care so intensely about them." The President wrote, in part,

The White House
Washington
December 26, 1970

Although I have corresponded with many of you individually, I would like, during this Christmas season, to address this letter openly to each and all of you—to all the wives and families of our men held prisoner and missing in Southeast Asia . . . I would like to tell you about our efforts to solve this problem, what we have achieved so far, and what we plan to do.

The basic obstacle, of course, is the barbaric, inhuman attitude of Hanoi in violation of the Geneva Convention. . . . .Early in 1969, I directed . . . intensive review of the prisoner of war problem. . . . it was time to take new measures, that the enemy's cruel and manifestly illegal policy toward our men should be exposed fully to public attention in the country and around the world.

Hanoi, however, has so far rebuffed every effort to obtain release of our men or to verify the conditions of their treatment. This attitude violates not only the Geneva Convention, which Hanoi had pledged to observe, but all common standards of human decency. It is barbaric. It has been universally and justifiably condemned.

I will not forget the strength, the loyalty and the dignity with which you have borne your burden. I can do no less than pledge to you that we will not rest until every prisoner has returned to his family and the missing have been accounted for.

With every good wish,
 Sincerely,
(Signed)
Richard Nixon[13]

I was grateful to the President for this strong condemnation of the North Vietnamese attitude about our POWs and MIAs. This would help us and my cause, but I realized that the League still had a long way to go. Perhaps generating this sense of public outrage over Newk's fate would be a good start.

I asked Whitey to document and respond to the replies I had received from my recent public appeal for legal assistance. I certainly had a good cause, but now I needed a plan of action. That plan came from John Norton Moore, Professor of Law and Director of the Graduate Program at the University of Virginia in Charlottesville. He shared my interest in securing adherence to the Geneva Conventions of 1949. In his kind and encouraging letter to me on January 15, 1971, he said, "I believe that the effort to develop an international-legal approach and to call attention to the duty of signatory states of the Geneva Convention not only to respect but also 'to ensure respect for the Convention' is a sound approach."[14]

Professor Moore sent me a draft outline of a legal memorandum to help me develop such an approach, and included a copy for Whitey. He said he was "happy to be associated with the effort which you have initiated to utilize international law to promote adherence to the Geneva Conventions," and said he'd look into doing whatever he could in the matter.[15]

The plan to create and present a class action petition to the United Nations began with that letter. That plan lifted my spirits and gave me confidence in what I was doing. My spirits took another jump upward when I learned that the full text of R. Patrick Mahoney's December 23 article, "We Must Free the Prisoners," was read into the Congressional Record on January 2, 1971.[16]

That January, the military also changed the status of one of the men on Cora Weiss' list from Prisoner of War (POW) to Killed in Action (KIA). When I inquired about this unusual move at the Air Force Casualty Office, I was told that additional information had been received that enabled the Government to officially confirm the prisoner's death.

I then wrote a letter to the Department of Defense and asked for clarification on my own legal status. On January 22, Brigadier General Daniel "Chappie" James, Jr., Deputy Assistant Secretary of Defense for Public Affairs, replied to my letter and said in part:

> ... the Secretaries of the Military Departments are charged
> by law with the responsibility for determining the status of
> men assigned to their departments. Changes in status are
> made only after review and evaluation of all available infor-

mation. I want to emphasize that there is no statutory responsibility, which the Service Secretaries and their authorized designees take more seriously than in making such determinations. Please be assured that any additional information we receive about your husband will be passed on to you as quickly as possible.[17]

Well, that meant that for the moment, and until they received further confirmation or information, the military would not change Newk's status. It was January 1971, exactly five years since he'd been shot down and taken prisoner, and although Cora Weiss claimed he was dead, our government, because they had received no official word or proof of his death, still classed Newk as a live POW in North Vietnam. That made me still a POW wife, even if I believed that I was very likely now a widow. I felt like I had just been awarded the lead role in a macabre play.

7 A Plan of Action

TIMELINE . . . 1971, JANUARY TO JULY . . . <u>WORLD</u> . . . U.N. PROCLAIMS EARTH DAY . . .
<u>VIETNAM</u> . . . SECRET PEACE NEGOTIATIONS RUMORED BEING HELD BY KISSINGER . . .
NIXON SAYS US DEPARTURE FROM SOUTH VIETNAM DEPENDS ON PRISONER EXCHANGE
. . . <u>USA</u> . . . ATTICA PRISON RIOTS . . . ASTRONAUT ALAN SHEPARD TEES OFF ON MOON
. . . COLTS BEAT COWBOYS IN SUPER BOWL . . .

> *These unhappy times call for the building of plans . . .*
> *that build from the bottom up and not the top down*
> *and put their faith once more in the forgotten man . . .*
> —Franklin Delano Roosevelt

The American Legion had assigned Mike Schlee, a bright, friend-ly young man, to help us get settled in our new office, make con-tacts, and set up meetings with other military service organizations. The League office was a continual beehive of activity that often bordered on chaos. There was much to accomplish and little time available in which to accomplish it. Our POWs needed help fast, not years from now. So organization never took priority over mov-ing along and *getting things done*. The League was always moving full speed ahead. We were willing and able to make quick decisions.

Joan Vinson's first priority as National Coordinator was to carry out the obligations designated by the League Board. The Board of Directors consisted of 15 members. They met monthly at Bolling Air Force Base in Washington, D.C.

Carole North had succeeded Sybil Stockdale as Chairman of the Board, which responded to the many POW/MIA family mem-bers who had projects and ideas about how to bring national and international attention to the League's American POW/MIA situ-ation. The Board considered, and decided on, which projects the League would sponsor or adopt.

Sybil Stockdale, the acknowledged spokeswoman and leader of the League since its inception in San Diego, was very respected. Many of us revered her. She was a woman who had the John Wayne kind of "true grit." Sybil had traveled to Paris to try to meet with Chinese and North Vietnamese representatives. She walked the halls of Congress and constantly pursued news coverage to publicize the existence of the League of Families. It was she who had done the groundwork to get us a national office, so we weren't operating solely from our "kitchen tables."

As National Coordinator, Joan Vinson also was tasked to stay in contact with the League's state chapters and their activities and direct the all-volunteer staff in the Washington, D.C., national office. Joan was a well-educated, intellectual woman. I always picture her with eyes flashing, and a phone receiver clutched in her hand, talking away. Joan had married Bobby Vinson, a gregarious, athletic West Point graduate from Texas, after his stint in the Korean War. They had four children, two sons and two daughters. Major Bobby Vinson had been listed as MIA since the plane he was piloting, a *Phantom* F4D, had gone down in April of 1968. There had been no word since of Bobby, nor of his copilot, Lt. Woodrow Parker, also listed as MIA.[1]

In January of 1971, Sybil tentatively set up a meeting between the League's Board and President Nixon at the White House. At Sybil's request, I was designated as one of the League's delegation of attendees. That was an honor, and I was very excited about it, as anyone can imagine. However, just before the meeting, the League office was informed that the President had urgent business that would not allow him to attend. Instead, we'd meet with Dr. Henry Kissinger, the President's National Security Advisor.

Although we were all disappointed that the President wouldn't be at the meeting, we were nevertheless delighted to be invited to meet with such a high-ranking member of the Nixon administration as Dr. Kissinger. We were confident that as one of the prime movers at the Paris Peace talks, he would know a great deal about our situation. We all prepared important questions to ask him.

On the appointed day, we were taken by special bus from Bolling Air Force Base to the White House. We were ushered into an impressive, executive style meeting room, where we took our places around a sleek, dark wood conference table. An Army brigadier general and two civilian assistants came in, and went to the head of the table. We all ceased talking and sat up straight.

"Ladies and gentlemen," the General greeted us, his voice sure and strong, "my name is Alexander Haig, and I am here today in Dr. Henry Kissinger's stead. He deeply regrets that he is unable to attend and speak with you today."

At that, audible murmurs of surprise and disappointment could be heard around the table, reflecting our disappointment and from some, overt displeasure. Obviously taken aback somewhat by that tone, General Haig stepped back a few paces, placing himself a bit farther away from the end of the conference table where we were seated. He put one hand in his uniform pants pocket and began nervously jingling some coins. He seemed unaware of both the action and the noise the coins made. A brief silence ensued, as we waited for him to speak. Then he said,

"I . . . will be happy to answer any questions you have."

Hands immediately went up. Soon, we were bombarding General Haig nonstop with the questions we all had brought for Dr. Kissinger to answer. Each of us had an important League agenda issue to present. Scarcely had he answered one question before hands went up to articulate rebuttals or ask another question. We weren't getting much in the way of candid responses from him, and our disappointment with that became obvious. The coins in General Haig's pocket jingled faster as he tried to field our questions. He didn't appreciate our rebuttals of his inadequate responses. It had become apparent to us soon after the meeting began that he hadn't really been briefed or prepared for it. Perhaps we should have given him more breathing room, but this had been a long-anticipated unique opportunity for access to someone who knew what was happening, and now it had been diluted down the line, and was slipping away without any substantive information or resolution of issues that concerned us. Some of us had come from quite a distance. We were in the White House, and that was a memorable occasion, to be sure, but we all had great expectations that didn't come to pass. Nor were we getting answers to any of the questions we fully expected to have answered. On some questions, General Haig looked rather desperately to his two aides, but they had little or nothing to offer in the way of help for him. The situation deteriorated fast. Ultimately, the sound of coins jingling in his pocket could be heard above our disappointed voices. They must have worn a hole in his pocket, because suddenly they were cascading out from the bottom of his pants leg and rolling all over the polished wood floor. The aides were scurrying around grabbing them, trying to retrieve them. General Haig turned bright red, whether in embarrassment or anger, I don't know. He stopped speaking and raised a hand.

"Quiet, if you please, ladies and gentlemen," he requested. We stilled our voices and waited. A moment or so later, when he had regained his composure, he spoke in a strong, sincere voice that revealed he was accustomed to command. General Haig apologized to us, said that he understood our frustration and acknowledged that he realized he wasn't the person we had expected for this meeting, nor did he have the answers we sought. He assured us that Dr. Kissinger's last minute cancellation was due to "matters of great national concern." There had not been time for anyone to adequately brief him as Dr. Kissinger's replacement in advance of the meeting. Therefore, he regretted that he was unable to adequately respond to the complex questions we were asking him. "I'm afraid you'll have to excuse me . . . ladies . . . gentlemen." He gave an apologetic nod, turned and left the room. We sat there in stunned silence for several minutes. Then someone on the Board said, "I believe this meeting has just been adjourned. Should we leave?"

One of the aides came back in to apologize again for the inconvenience to us. He confirmed that General Haig would not be returning to the meeting. The aide asked us to remain where we were, and assured us that shortly we'd be escorted back to where our transportation awaited us.

We heard later through one of our contacts that General Haig had said he would go anywhere or do anything rather than ever again have to meet with the League of Families. I can't say I blame him for that, as we had given him little or no relief that night from the start. But then, we'd had no relief from our nightmare either. Nor had our men gotten any relief . . . not for years, and years. We had gone to the White House for answers. We wanted to hear a plan of action. We weren't disposed to being shuffled around and dismissed any more. General Haig had simply fallen victim to the vise of our frustration. We wanted action, not evasion. He had innocently walked into a barrage.

By February 1971, I felt I had developed a novel idea. I presented it in some detail to Whitey Lemmond and to Charlie Havens, the League's lawyer. They gladly backed me and helped me secure an appointment on February 12 to see U.S. Attorney General John Mitchell at the Department of Justice to present my idea. Whitey and Charlie went with me. Attorney General Mitchell stood to welcome us. He was past middle age, medium height, balding, with pleasant features. He paid close attention as we explained our desire to bring to the attention of the delegates and representatives to the United Nations North Vietnam's failure to comply with the tenets of the Geneva Conventions as they apply to Prisoners of War. I wanted to do that through a formal, legal avenue, perhaps by presenting a Resolution, or a Petition, to the U.N.

Mitchell thought it was a fine idea. When I asked if there was any way he could assist us, he thought a moment, then offered assistance from Charles Gentry, one of the White House Fellowship winners working for him at the Justice Department.[2]

Gentry was a pleasant and solidly built man who had been wounded in Vietnam and was sent home to recover. Following that, he'd excelled at college and law school. He had recently been selected as a White House Fellow, a great honor. Being a Vietnam vet, he seemed delighted with this new assignment to us and our cause. After reading John Norton Moore's outline, Charley was eager to get started on the project. That pleased us immensely. From then on, Whitey, Charlie Havens, and I met with Charley Gentry regularly in his tiny corner office, high in the Justice building. Since the building also housed the executives of the FBI, war protestors frequently picketed outside. On more than one occasion, I had to work my way through a milling crowd to reach the front entrance. *We are struggling at opposite ends of the same war,* I mused, listening to them shout antiwar slogans and chants.

With help and input from Whitey and Charlie Havens, Charles Gentry and I developed what would become a class-action petition, initiated by me on behalf of my husband and all Prisoners of War. I presented my plan to the Board of the League of Families, who voted to fund the cost of developing and publishing the petition.

With a positive and funded plan in motion, we forged ahead. It required a lot of my time, but I was more than willing to devote that time to the League, in order to develop the petition to the United Nations. That in turn focused my attention on new family needs. I learned how much is required of one person to handle being head of a family of four young children when you worked outside the home, too. My first priority was to assure that the boys were cared for after school hours. Roy was five and starting kindergarten. I found a reliable neighbor who agreed to watch the boys after school until I got home. I knew that Mother would also give me some help, even though she still didn't approve of what I was doing. Given her age, it was too much to expect her to handle four rambunctious young boys. Getting extra help during those after school hours I was in Washington was a must. Predictably, Mother grumbled about it, intimating that I didn't trust her with the boys any more. However, she accepted the inevitable with good grace, and probably with some relief she wasn't willing to acknowledge.

By then the League had grown in size and national recognition, and we were gaining plenty of notice in Washington, D.C., as well. Joan and the League staff met weekly with our small group of advisors, who were all excellent, capable and dedicated volunteers. Charlie Havens, our legal advisor, had worked with the Department of Defense, and in that work had met many POW/MIA family members. Paul Wagner, of Wagner and Barooty, a Public Relations firm, was a well-known and liked volunteer. Fletcher Prouty, of Madison National Bank, kept an eye on our financial status, and made certain that we complied with our organization's non-profit status. And always welcome at the office whenever they were in town were Major Nick Rowe of the Army, Lt. Robert Frishman of the Navy, and Col. Norris Overly of the Air Force. All three of these men were former Vietnam POWs. Rowe was nationally known for his escape from brutal captivity in South Vietnam, and was an excellent speaker who brought valuable attention to our cause. The nation's astronauts, particularly Alan Shepard, Frank Borman, and Jim Lovell, were revered Americans whose willingness to speak out on our POW/MIA cause brought it great prestige across the country.

Other members of the League volunteered a good deal of their time too. We had a pressing purpose to fulfill, one for which time was of the essence. Iris Powers, an MIA Mom who had been the League's first National Coordinator, was a gem. Older and more experienced in these matters than Joan and I were, Iris volunteered to address the humanitarian aspects of prisoner treatment during and after their captivity. She also looked after the welfare of the POW/MIA families.

Iris was one of the most dedicated and interesting women I'd ever met. She became a strong influence in my life. A small, slight woman with gray hair and a ready smile, Iris had once been an acrobat and bareback rider in the circus. Then, during World War II, while working as a taxicab driver in New York City, she learned that her husband was missing in action on Okinawa, in the Pacific theater of that war. He was later officially declared dead. (We referred to that in acronym shorthand as OPFD, "official presumptive finding of death," or just PFD, which meant that the government had decided to declare a missing person legally deceased.)

However, in Iris' case, several years after World War II ended, her husband turned up alive. By then Iris, legally a widow since before the end of the war, had remarried. It was a dilemma for her that could not be imagined by any of us in our worst nightmares.

Ultimately, Iris decided to petition for annulment of her second marriage, which was granted. Then she remarried her first husband, who was the father of her two sons. Iris was a bona fide widow now, as that husband had passed away. Unfortunately, she was to become a war statistic again as a mother, this time the Vietnam War. One of her two sons, Lowell Powers, a helicopter pilot, was MIA. To us, that was a cruel *déjà vu* blow to poor Iris. We all prayed her son would be found alive. According to his aircraft commander, who had been rescued, Lowell was alive following the crash of their helicopter. Iris held to constant hope that her son would turn up, but he had not been seen or heard from since the crash. Our hearts went out to this staunch and courageous lady, who never let her spirits flag. Iris Powers inspired us all, every single day. She epitomized the saying, "Of few, much is asked . . . "

Another MIA Mom, Nancy Perisho, frequently traveled to Washington, D. C., from Illinois to help at the League office. Nancy also was trying to cope with the position she was in regarding her missing son, as her daughter-in-law refused to give or share with Nancy any information about him. Given my wonderful Mother, and my in-laws, Newk's parents, and how caring they were to me and my children, I couldn't even imagine such a thing happening. However, sadly it did happen. A kind and generous lady, Nancy was always up for the challenges we faced, and she was a very welcome addition to the national office.

I had by then done enough volunteer work at the League's Washington office that I knew all the staff quite well. I was in Washington often to work with Charles Gentry on drafting and writing the U.N. petition, and therefore often accompanied Joan to meetings and official events to which the National Coordinator had been invited and/or needed to attend. I had also taken on the task of writing a letter to the Ambassador or some other official from every country that had signed the Geneva Conventions, asking for their help to get the North Vietnamese to comply with the 1949 Conventions regarding treatment of Prisoners of War that they had signed. I participated in meetings that were official business of our organization.

One example was getting the free Public Service Announcements the League had qualified for with the Advertising Council (Ad Council) in New York City. They were to air on radio and television. One of the Ad Council's members was to produce audio and video ads for us free of charge, after which the Federal Communications Commission would be asked for their approval. Then the Ad Council would arrange for the ads to be distributed and aired nationally. That kind of extensive public exposure was very important to the League's mission. I went with Joan the afternoon that two men from the advertising firm SSC&B-Lintas, (Sullivan, Stauffer, Colwell and Bayles) of Smokey the Bear fame, came to make their initial presentation of their Public Service Ad to the League.[3] The first issue, they said, was our "brand" (the League name), which was long and unwieldy. So their first suggestion was that we should shorten the official name of the League to letters, like their firm's name. The man at their display board flipped a page, and we saw "NLF" in huge letters. Joan and I stared in disbelief.

"You will be known everywhere now as the NLF!" The ad agency representative announced triumphantly. He looked around with an expression of delight and WOW! on his face, as if waiting for cheers and applause. That expression was short-lived. "Stop right there!" Joan commanded, jumping to her feet. "We will *not* be known as any such thing. If you had done *any* research at all about this situation, gentlemen, you would know that NLF stands for National Liberation Front, which is more popularly known as the Viet Cong, the Communists who are our sworn enemy in Vietnam."

The man's expression went from proud to stunned.

"Please do us the favor of reworking this ad campaign." Joan said.

"I think if you had contacted our office first, you'd have been more certain of who we are and what we're about." With that, she headed for the door. I followed in her wake. We subsequently reported to the Board that the ad campaign had been tabled pending the arrival of new material from SSC&B.

Sometimes nothing went right for us because we were relative amateurs dealing at highly professional levels. But we learned fast from our errors. At another meeting I attended with Joan, a high-level member of the huge AFL-CIO union group was present. Joan described the League's purpose to him, explaining that we desperately needed help. After listening attentively, he asked her kindly, "so . . . just what kind of help would you like from us, Mrs. Vinson?"

I was at the edge of my chair, thinking, *Okay, we've got him on our side. Ask for a donation of a dollar annually from every member, until all the POWs and MIAs are accounted for!* But I had no way of passing her a note. Joan waited for a moment and then said, "You know we would appreciate anything you could do for us and the plight of our prisoners . . . " and left it hanging there, waiting for him to suggest something. He really knew nothing about what we needed, so nothing happened. Without a specific goal or action being offered with which he could then approach his members, he committed nothing concrete to us. The meeting ended, and we left.

The League had missed a huge opportunity there. I made a mental note then to always have a plan or an agenda with a specific suggestion or request *before* meeting with the important people who could help us with our cause.

Not long after that experience, I received a reply to one of my many letters to countries that had signed the Geneva Conventions.

This reply was from Sweden. Foreign Minister Rune Nystrom of the Swedish Royal Ministry of Foreign Affairs wrote,

> It is my sad duty to convey to you the information given to the Swedish Government by the Government of the Democratic Republic of Vietnam, namely that your husband died in North Vietnam on February 4 1966. Please accept my most sincere condolences in your loss.[4]

The North Vietnamese government had now confirmed Newk's death to Sweden. I was confused and stunned about them stating February 4, 1966, as the date Newk had died. That was incredible, since that date was *before* they published the pictures of a captive Newk being treated for minor injuries, and then later, up and walking on his own. February 4 was also before the date of the alleged broadcast they claimed he had made.

It was a quasi-official confirmation of what Cora Weiss had told me, but again, the date was questionable at best, a lie at worst.[5] No specific cause of death or circumstances surrounding his death in North Vietnam was offered by anyone. Sweden had been the first country in Europe to openly recognize the government of North Vietnam, which to my mind put them on North Vietnam's side in this dispute. I was fine with the confirming information, but at odds with the date and sketchy details. Without question, we as a family needed information and closure on this long ordeal. However, absent any details or reliable proof of Newk's death, I wasn't convinced that I could trust their claim. Neither did our government seem inclined to accept it.

That February, the Secretary of the 5,000 member strong Delaware County (Pennsylvania) Federation of Women's Clubs wrote to let me know they'd written letters of protest to Hanoi and to the International Red Cross about the way that they'd sent the news of my husband's death. She also said they were looking into creating a scholarship in Newk's name. She assured me they'd help the League in any other way they could. I was very touched by that letter, and it meant so much to me to know I had the support of those American women.

In March 1971, Representative Paul McCloskey (R-California) suggested that President Nixon should be impeached for his policy of continuing U.S. involvement in Vietnam. That was a national shock. California Governor Ronald Reagan promptly asked McCloskey to resign from the Republican Party. McCloskey refused, declaring that if no other Republican contender came forward to challenge Nixon on his administration's war policies, he would run against Nixon himself. That was an interesting turn of events! The war had turned our country into a nation of turmoil and dissidence.

In an effort to improve his image with the country regarding the war, President Nixon named the week of March 23, 1971, the "National Week of Concern for the American Prisoners of War Being Held by North Vietnam." During that week, local League chapters in most states held meetings and encouraged prayer services. I went to Washington to testify before the House Foreign Affairs Committee to make specific recommendations on how Congress and the American people could help the POW/MIA situation. In my remarks to the Congressmen, I explained my situation and said in part,

> Congress passed the Gulf of Tonkin Resolution, legally sending my husband, along with thousands of other men, to defend South Vietnam. Now the Tonkin Resolution has been revoked. But it's still YOUR war, and you are still responsible for the return of all those men. Those still living, that is, and there are an unknown number of them being held in prison camps all over Southeast Asia. Men who have already sacrificed everything but their lives for this "revoked" war . . . In December 1970, nearly five years after my husband was captured, Newk's name appeared on some Communist lists as "dead." The second list of twenty, with his name as dead, was presented to representatives of Senator Kennedy and Senator Fulbright in Paris, with the addition of a date of death for the twenty men. Once again I waited for my government to respond, and once again waited in disappointment. Was there a demand by our government for more information about the twenty men listed as dead? None that I know of. Was there vocal surprise, or better still—outrage, at Newk's death after being so highly advertised as a prisoner? None. Did anyone question why it

has taken Hanoi up to five years' delay in sending the death notices? None. Was there any information other than a terse report given to the family? None. The government was content to accept the lists without question. But I could not sit back and quietly accept the list. It was decided to take legal action. I have chosen that way to gain recognition of the Geneva Convention Relative to the Treatment of Prisoners of War. This Convention was written to protect all prisoners. It was signed by 135 countries, including North Vietnam . . .

Two proposals were made last year and never acted upon. The first was by H. Ross Perot. He said, 'through our labor unions, through our Congress, we say to our friends around the world who are trading with us and trading with North Vietnam, make a choice. Until we get our men back, if you send anything into North Vietnam, you won't get anything in this country.' I must add in all candor that now people within our own country should also have to 'make a choice,' for they are trading with the enemy, too.

The second proposal was made by Mr. Zablocki. He said, 'We have testimony from the chairman of the House Armed Services Committee that the United States should issue an ultimatum to the North Vietnamese, that they either release our prisoners by a certain date, or we would blockade Haiphong or take other serious action.[6]

In conclusion, I referred again to Newk, and then said,

. . . I stand before you today, like my husband, with my head held high. To all the Congressmen who bear the burden of the fate of all these men I say . . . look closely and listen. Unless we all work together for our prisoners of war, these men could be sacrificed. . . . Let the words of author W. Somerset Maugham burn into your collective conscience: 'If a nation values anything more than freedom, it will lose its freedom, and the irony of it is that if it is comfort or money that it values more, it will lose that, too.'[7]

Following that appearance, I was interviewed in depth by Fulton Lewis for his "Top of the News" radio program. He included my interview verbatim in his weekly publication, the "Top of the News Newsletter," under the bold headline, "1600 MEN—MISS-ING BUT NOT FORGOTTEN."[8] Fulton Lewis was a popular celebrity newscaster. That interview gave the League of Families and our efforts and suggestions considerable visibility—not only in Washington, but throughout the country.

I was gratified to learn later that people understood what I was saying. The proof came when U.S. ambassador to the United Nations, Honorable George H.W. Bush (later to be the first President Bush) spoke to a League delegation from Chatham Borough and Chatham Township, New Jersey.[9] He invited them and some members of the press to his office at the United States Mission to the United Nations in New York City on March 24, 1971, where they presented him with more than 6,000 letters—statements of concern for American Prisoners of War in North Vietnam. Ambassador Bush said, in accepting them,

> These letters represent the work of volunteers . . . in two communities. To me, they symbolize the national concern about the prisoner of war problem. They have asked me to discuss these letters with the Secretary General of the United Nations (U Thant) which I intend to do. And let me simply say that I think it is tremendously important that everyone in this country—but more, in the world—focus on this human problem of prisoners of war, and that we each in our own way do something to end the misery that has been brought about by the treatment of prisoners of war in Southeast Asia.[10]

One of the reporters asked him, "Mr. Ambassador, where does the pressure ultimately have to be put?" Ambassador Bush replied, in part,

> The pressure ultimately has to be felt in Hanoi, or wherev-er these prisoners are held. World opinion, in my opinion, means an awful lot. And it is a human question. It is a ques-tion of the breaking of treaties [Geneva Conventions]. It is not a question of communism, or our way of life. It is some-thing far greater than that, I think, the outpouring of human concern. These ladies symbolize an effective way of

influencing world opinion . . . to me the very fact that there has been public opinion, that Ross Perot is with us today, and he and others have brought opinion to bear, has resulted, we think, in better treatment for the prisoners. Perhaps more pressure, more concern, will bring about the release of some of them, and maybe all of them. And I think it is worthwhile. I think it is important work. I think it is work that the international community should address itself to all of the time, a lot of the time.[11]

The basic text of the letters was:

Dear Mr. Secretary-General:

As a citizen of the United States of America, may I take this opportunity to express my deep concern for the over 1600 men who are held prisoners of war in North Vietnam. As you well know, the Geneva Convention calls for: "immediate release of the sick and the injured; impartial inspection of prison camps; the identification of the men held; and proclaims the right of prisoners to correspond with their families." Since more than 120 countries, including North Vietnam, are signatories to the Geneva Convention, it is my earnest hope that this letter, among others, will be of help to you and/or the United Nations, in persuading North Vietnam to review and fulfill its commitment as outlined above.[12]

Through Bush's kind and generous help, and with that of the rest of the U.S. Mission to the United Nations, Joan Vinson and I secured an appointment to meet with United Nations Secretary-General U Thant on March 25, 1971. The Secretary-General's office was on the top floor of the United Nations building in New York City. His large waiting room was lined with windows that afforded a breathtaking, panoramic view of the Hudson River and the bustling Port of New York. Joan and I couldn't help expressing admiration for the view. As we stepped closer to the windows to see better, one of the gentleman from the U.S. Mission escorting us exclaimed, "Oh my . . . look at that!"

He pointed to an area of the river—where a barge was anchored in place, displaying a huge banner that proclaimed:

THERE ARE NO U.S. POWs IN HANOI.

"Surely that's not being done to protest our presence here!" I said.

"No, I'd think it's probably more permanent than just there today," he responded. "It's probably being kept there long-term, for the U.N. delegates to ponder."

Shortly after that, Secretary General U Thant entered. I was awed just to be in the same room with him. He was small, very dignified in appearance, with a formal, polite manner. He spoke softly. He frankly informed us that our appeal to the United Nations for help likely would have no impact because there were so many obstacles and diverse opinions at the U.N. about the Vietnam conflict. Therefore, he sincerely regretted that there was little he could do to assist us. Our disappointment was obvious, but we pressed on, asking other questions. The Secretary General acknowledged that a class action petition such as the one we were developing *might* get some attention from the delegates. However, in sum he remained noncommittal on helping us get it to the delegates. After about ten minutes, we were politely ushered to the elevator door by Mr. Thant's assistant.

"Do you know anything about who owns or leases that barge out there with the banner on it?" I asked the assistant.

He shrugged. "No, Madame. We know nothing about that."

The Secretary General's remarks had effectively dashed our hopes for any help from the United Nations. Our gloomy mood matched the grey skies of New York. Then Joan pointed out, "Well, all is not lost. We've made the Secretary General aware that we are creating a human rights petition, and we intend to present it to the United Nations. What more could we really expect from him?"

"Well, in my opinion, he could have been more openly supportive. He could have said he would help us insist on humane treatment of our POWs," I grumbled. To me, the United Nations was little more than a gigantic Tower of Babel on Manhattan Island, filled with people who got nothing much done and took money from Americans' pockets, but openly showed their disdain for us, even as they demanded our help and spent our money. It made me angry as an American taxpayer. My personal respect for the United Nations fell to rock bottom that day. Nevertheless, I returned home more determined than ever to complete and present my petition to that international body.

More and more POW/MIA wives and families were being created by the continuing Vietnam War, and the families were becoming increasingly active. They energetically joined in the League's activities. That strengthened our visibility and power as a group, and increased our sphere of citizen influence. Congress noted our activities, as did the military services. On March 5, 1971, Iris Powers was sworn in as "Consultant to the Army in POW/MIA Next of Kin Affairs." In that capacity, she would serve as liaison between POW/MIA families and the Army. At about that same time, Phyllis Galanti, along with other League members and friends from the Richmond, Virginia, area, left for Sweden with 750,000 POW/MIA letters from Virginians. They had appointments with Foreign Minister Nystrom (the official who had written me regarding Newk's death), U.S. Ambassador Jerome Holland, and with the President of the Swedish Red Cross.

With so much going on at the League, 1971 seemed like it was flying by. I had a nagging concern about my recent decision to continue the fight to force North Vietnam to officially confirm Newk's death to me, and to our government, according to the terms of the Geneva Convention. I feared it might be misinterpreted at home as a selfish desire to retain my status as a wife, rather than accept that I was very likely a widow. I'd heard some gossip to that effect, and that upset me, as that was not the case at all. I felt that passive acceptance of these things on our part gave North Vietnam too much leeway regarding their treatment of all of our POWs. I decided to write a letter to the Defense Department, informing them that I wouldn't object if they decided to change *my* status and eliminate my financial benefits as a wife. However, I asked that they not change Newk's status without some kind of official proof from the North Vietnamese Government. They could work out the financial details of that, and I would accept their decision.

Very soon thereafter, I received an official letter from General Daniel "Chappie" James about the military position on the allegations that POWs had died in captivity, and a very nice note from Senator Bob Dole (R-Kansas), who enclosed a copy of a letter from Armistead Selden, Jr., the Assistant Secretary of Defense, regard-

ing the status of the men, now numbering about twenty, reported
by Cora Weiss or others to have died in captivity. Newk was one of
those twenty. It looked like it was the original document from
which General Chappie James excerpted the paragraph he had
included in his letter to me.[13] Senator Dole, a wounded World War
II veteran, had apparently seen or been apprised of the letter I wrote
to the Department of Defense (DOD) concerning my status versus
Newk's.

On May 10, 1971, I was invited to meet with Dr. Roger Shields
and Vince de Mauro. Dr. Shields was the person working most
closely within the DOD on the POW situation. When we met, he
asked me why I had written that letter to the DOD. I answered, "I
wrote it because I am fighting for the Geneva Conventions to be
followed, not to keep my income and benefits, as some people
appear to be intimating I'm doing. I am not refusing to accept reality about Newk's reported death. I just don't want my acceptance of
his death to trigger deadly actions against other prisoners. I am
afraid that if they get away with killing Newk and these others, and
we accept it without question, as we seem to be doing, they might
then take similar action with other prisoners. Why not? Therefore,
I am amenable to accepting a change in my status, if that will make
the situation easier for everyone, but I am adamant that Newk's status not be changed."

Dr. Shields nodded. He was obviously thinking about what I'd
said. Then he smiled at me and said, "Officially, Mrs. Grubb, I must
tell you that your letter upset us. Unofficially, it was a very good
thing to do."[14] He further assured me that no one in the military or
the government suspected, or spoke of me, as having ulterior
motives in not accepting Cora Weiss' word at face value. He also
assured me that the Defense Department fully supported my efforts
in the class action petition I was preparing to present to the United
Nations. He also reiterated that, without further, more specific
information, the DOD was not contemplating any change in status
for Newk or me.[15]

Following that meeting, I continued working with Charles
Gentry and the legal group on the U.N. Petition. In those pre-com-
puter days, everything had to be laboriously typed, and retyped,
with carbons for copies. Every major change or correction meant

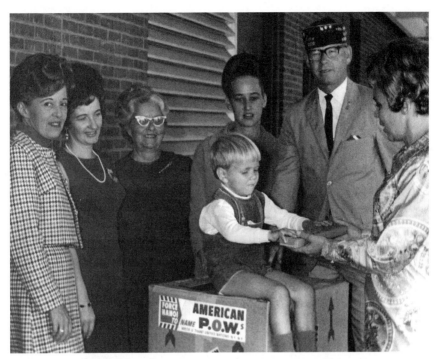

As League of Families activists and an American Legion official look on, Roy Grubb, age 4, and his mother, Evelyn, mail a package to his father, Newk Grubb, a POW in Hanoi.

that pages and pages were retyped and renumbered. It was like writing a doctoral dissertation – it had to be perfect in every way. Meanwhile, I continued with my schedule of interviews and speeches on the POW/MIA situation, and participated actively in our international letter-writing campaign efforts.

At home, in the evenings and on weekends, I devoted myself to the boys, their needs, and their school activities. They were becoming more understanding of what I was doing and what it meant to me. Also, my positive activity for the POW/MIA cause kept me energized, and that period became a very productive time in my life. My days were filled with worthwhile efforts and actions that kept me far too busy to dwell endlessly on painful thoughts of Newk's and my unresolved situation and being in limbo for years on end. It also helped me to work through, in a positive way, the deep grief and hostility I had felt for so long.

Of course, certain events and setbacks occasionally brought

anger and frustration boiling back up to the surface, but it happened less often than in previous years. I was part of a group that
was suffering the same pain, and making things happen, and that
helped me immensely to cope. Perhaps the League of Families
engendered the birth of the "support group" concept, who knows?

The boys also thrived on our new routine. They had a more
cheerful Mom to be with, for one thing. Another big plus was that
Jeff was taking a great interest in the work I was doing with the
League. He helped me edit speeches and was full of creative ideas.
He gave his own speeches, too, and wrote letters on behalf of his
Dad. It was a tough situation for him as a teenager—especially
given the anti-war, anti-military political climate. He really needed
his Dad to help guide him as he grew into male adulthood. Often
he was surrounded by shouting "peaceniks" who considered our
military men in Vietnam little more than traitors. Jeff fearlessly
faced audiences that were far more hostile than any I ever faced. I
was very proud of his courage and determination.

At the end of May, Joan Vinson escorted a group of more than
140 League of Families members to Geneva, Switzerland, to meet
with the International Committee of the Red Cross. Then some
went on to visit other capitals in Europe, while Joan, her sons
Charles and Robert, and Betty Burford went to Paris, where they
were unable to meet with the North Vietnamese, but got a lot of
publicity for the League's efforts. I had volunteered to stay behind,
to cover the League office during Joan's absence.

It was at about that time that "Little Joe" McCain, the younger
brother of Navy POW Lieutenant John McCain, came in and volunteered to work in the League's Washington office. He was an
enthusiastic helper and morale builder, and we soon became good
friends as well as POW/MIA colleagues. Joe was immediately
interested in our Discrepancies Report, the list of men who had
been seen alive and/or captured, but were not on any of the lists
we'd gotten so far from the Vietnamese government. He soon
assumed responsibility for maintenance of the Discrepancies
Report and its accompanying exhibit boards, which contained photos or other evidence of men who were seen alive following the loss
of their aircraft, but not acknowledged by the North Vietnamese or
heard from since. Joe did a great job with it from the very beginning.

One day, I asked the Air Force personnel office at the Pentagon if I could review Newk's records that were kept on file there with those of other POWs and MIAs. I wanted to be certain that I had everything I needed to include with the petition to the U.N. At first, the Air Force personnel office refused my request, informing me that Newk's personnel records "are classified."

I couldn't understand why they would be classified, and contacted General Don Hughes, the League's White House liaison, who succeeded in getting me an appointment to see Newk's file at the Pentagon. Gil Calhoun, my steadfast friend, who was an intelligence specialist in Asian affairs with excellent security clearances, accompanied me.

We were ushered into a small room with a table and two chairs. Newk's file was lying on the table. When we opened it, we found a jumbled pile of papers and photos in no coherent or chronological order. There also were photographs of Newk as a captive that I had never seen. To me, the file was a mute testament to how little attention the files received, stuff was just jammed in there. Those men were missing or suffering God knows what in brutal prison camps in Southeast Asia, and no one at the Pentagon could bother to even keep their personnel files in decent order?

That to me underscored how little anyone in the bureaucracy of the military cared about what was happening to the MIAs or POWs. Stuck in among Newk's papers were some documents pertaining to Peter Grubb. Peter was MIA, and was no relation to Newk. I went to the administrative desk with Newk's file.

"We would like to see Peter Grubb's file too, please."

The airman on duty replied, "I'm sorry, Ma'am. You can't see his file. Why do you need to? Are you related to him?"

"No, but some of his papers are filed in my husband *Newlin* Grubb's file, and since no one appears to be maintaining any order in these files, I'd like to check to see if Peter's file has papers in it that should be in Newlin Grubb's file."

"I'm sorry. We'll look into that for you, Ma'am," he said.

"Please do. These files are a real mess. Someone needs to straighten them out. You should be ashamed to have anyone review them in this condition. I would like copies of these photographs, please." I handed him the photos.

"I'm sorry you're unhappy about the files, Ma'am. I'll get these photos copied for you right away." Although I got the impression he really didn't care what I thought, he did have the photos copied and they were ready for me later when I left.

Later, at the League office, I called General Hughes at the White House.

"Thank you for getting me in to see my husband's file, General Hughes. I reviewed it today." When he asked if I'd found what I needed, I replied, "Well . . . I'm sorry to tell you that the personnel files of our POWs and MIAs at the Pentagon are in disgraceful order."

He was surprised at that, and asked me what I meant. I explained about the general disorder of Newks' file, the misfiling of Peter Grubb's papers in Newk's dossier, and the photos I'd found in there of Newk that we, his family, had not even seen. "I'm planning to address this deplorable situation in the next issue of the League of Families newsletter. Perhaps the League members can field a volunteer committee of family members to review these files of our men who are in prison or missing, and give them the attention required to at least straighten them out. (I could imagine General Hughes' horror at the mere thought of that.)

"I'm sure that won't be necessary, Mrs. Grubb. I'm very surprised to learn of this situation."

"Thank you, sir. And I'm sorry to bother you with it, or be so insistent, but I believe that the files of these missing men and POWs, who have sacrificed so much for their country, should at least be maintained in some semblance of decent order . . . lest we be led to believe that our husbands and fathers and brothers have been overlooked and forgotten by their own military buddies, don't you agree?"

The General strongly agreed. "I'm very sorry you had to experience this situation, Mrs. Grubb. I assure you I'll see to it that those files are reviewed and straightened out immediately." I knew he would do that, and I thanked him for relieving the League of Families of concern that the services weren't keeping proper personnel records of our men up to date.

By the end of the month, the human rights petition to the United Nations was finished. On Monday June 7, 1971, I traveled to New York with Charlie Havens and Paul Wagner to present it to the United Nations. It was a big moment for me, for all of us, and I was nervous but excited to be doing this.

Present to welcome us were Ambassador Arthur Stillman, Advisor on U.S. Economic and Social Affairs to the United States Mission to the United Nations,[16] and Mr. Roussel, a press advisor for the U.S. Mission. We proceeded to an office where we formally presented the Petition to Mr. Lawson of the United Nations Commission on Human Rights in the U.N. building. He read the cover aloud:

> PETITION TO THE HONORABLE U THANT
> SECRETARY GENERAL OF THE UNITED NATIONS
>
> Violation of Fundamental Human Rights of Mrs. Wilmer Newlin Grubb, Her Children, and All Similarly Situated Families of Servicemen Held Captive by the Democratic Republic of Vietnam and Its Allies in Indo-China
> June 7, 1971[17]

After the Petition introduced me as a United States citizen, and gave my status as the wife of Major Wilmer Newlin Grubb of the U.S. Air Force, and the names of each of our children, the body of the Petition stated:

> It is my understanding that under the United Nations Charter and the Universal Declaration of Human Rights any person on earth, and particularly a citizen of a nation subscribing to the United Nations Charter, has the right, either individually or in association with others, to petition (or by other process communicate with) the authorities of the United Nations to remedy a wrong committed by another nation that violates a fundamental human right.
>
> Therefore, Your Excellency, I respectfully request and humbly implore you to receive and earnestly consider this document as an informal petition, on behalf of my children and me and on behalf of all persons similarly situated, for the General Assembly, on the basis of facts which I will fully present, to recognize a violation of fundamental human rights and take action to redress that violation.[18]

It went on to expand and explain our contention that we had the fundamental human right to know whether my husband, the children's father, was dead or still alive, and if dead, the circumstances and details surrounding his death. The Petition was ten typed pages in length, single spaced. We had also attached three pages of the North Vietnamese photos of Newk that had been published in various newspapers and books that showed him standing up and apparently walking with no sign of serious injury or disability. We included a transcript of the tape Newk had allegedly made *after* his capture which had been broadcast by Voice of Vietnam *after* the date he was supposed to have died. We offered them as proof that North Vietnam had used the pictures and tape of Newk extensively and solely for propaganda purposes and that use alone was a violation of the Geneva Conventions.

We felt that the presentation went very well. Nonetheless, Mr. Lawson hastened to caution us that the Petition had little hope of ever gaining answers through the Commission on Human Rights. When we questioned that, he gave us several specific reasons. First, the Petition had to be forwarded to the country involved for an appropriate response, and he felt that since the Democratic Republic of Vietnam was not a member of the United Nations (although they were a signatory to the Geneva Conventions) the Petition could not be submitted to them except by a U. N. member nation. Second, any action by the Commission would depend upon the Democratic Republic of Vietnam *responding* to the petition, through a member nation. Even if the DRV responded, Commission action would be extremely slow because they received more than 15,000 Human Rights petitions a year. I was stunned at that number, and my hope for any resulting consideration began to fade. The barriers were enormous, and overcoming them would take years. Third, he informed us, the Human Rights Commission actually preferred "group" or "class" petitions, rather than single person or family petitions (U.N. officials had advised us exactly the opposite when we first conceived the project.)

Noting my obvious distress at his response, Mr. Lawson further informed us that another committee was being formed to "study" the problems involving the negligence of Human Rights by non-U.N. members that affected the countries who belonged to the

U.N. However, he acknowledged this would take a great deal of time to achieve any results. Mr. Lawson then offered us some alternatives, the first being that I present my petition to individual countries that were in a position to contact Hanoi and present it to the DRV. Or, I might consider reworking and then re-submitting the petition as a class petition from the League of Families on behalf of *all* the POWs, MIAs, and their families. He also suggested that I appeal to the International Committee of the Red Cross. I assured him we'd already done that countless times both individually and as groups without measurable success. I again stated that "the North Vietnamese have taken a hard and immovable position that is completely contrary to the Geneva Conventions, which they have signed."

He made no response to that, and said that to his knowledge, the only other avenue available to us would be to ask the American delegation to press for direct United Nations action on the U.S. POW/MIA problem. That action had not ever been taken before by the United States, he admitted, although the U.S. had recently presented a resolution supporting the Geneva Convention on POWs that the General Assembly had passed in December 9, 1970. I knew about that, since it had been confirmed to us by President Nixon in his December 1970 letter to all the POW/MIA families.[19]

In sum, although ultimately a huge disappointment to us as far as getting action on the Petition was concerned, I felt that the meeting had gone as well as could be expected from the United Nations, which was noted for endless delay, haggling, and inaction. We made plans to pursue those of Mr. Lawson's suggestions which were more specific and might help our cause. Ambassador Stillman was very kind to us, and he also took careful note of Mr. Lawson's suggestions. Stillman personally assumed the obligation to do something on our behalf at the United Nations. I told him I sincerely hoped he would succeed.

On June 21 1971, Charlie Havens received a rough draft outline of a proposed paper on "The Geneva Conventions and the Obligation of Signatory States to Promote and Assure the Humanitarian Treatment of Prisoners of War" from professor John Moore of the University of Virginia School of Law. As promised, he was collaborating with Peter D. Trooboff, of the District of Columbia Bar, on behalf of the prisoners *vis-à-vis* the Geneva Convention.[20]

Moore said in his cover letter that they hoped to form an ad hoc committee of international legal scholars concerned with initiatives for the humanitarian protection for victims of armed conflict. When it was finally drafted and completed, the Committee planned to send the statement to all of the signatories of the Geneva Convention. Professor Moore invited my review and input to this outline, and included a list of the professors who had agreed to participate in the review of the completed Statement. The list was impressive and included professors from the Schools of Law at Yale, Columbia, University of California at Berkeley, State University of New York at Buffalo, St. Louis University, Southern Methodist University, and others. The enclosed outline was very comprehensive. I was grateful to Professor Moore, and we carefully reviewed the document he'd sent us. My few scribbled marginal notes back to Professor Moore suggested adding something about "the humanitarian and legal rights of prisoners of war who die during captivity," which I penciled in as *Section H under IV: Specific Obligations Under the Convention and Their Application to Military Personnel Held in Indo-China*. Under another section that addressed Convention requirements, I suggested inserting something about "initial status and treatment as a Prisoner of War."[21]

Charlie Havens also contacted Peter Trooboff to commend the draft outline and encourage him and Professor Moore to organize their committee to address legal initiatives to get humanitarian protection for victims of armed conflicts.

Also, following Mr. Lawson's suggestion, with our League lawyers, we began work on a class action petition from the League on behalf of *all* the American POW/MIA families.

Barely two weeks later, on June 23, 1971, I was back at the United Nations, this time accompanied by Mr. Murphy Martin from Ross Perot's United We Stand organization.[22] Our recent visit and our initial Petition had apparently made quite an impression on the U.S. delegates. I was given a two-day agenda of appointments that had been set up by Ambassador Stillman, allowing me to make formal calls on delegates from seven individual U.N. member countries: Romania, Algeria, Yugoslavia, France, the United Kingdom, Sweden, and Norway, to give them our Petition.

I made the appointed rounds. Each country's delegates were very cordial and most were interested in my petition and expressed sympathy about my very difficult personal situation. The delegates from each country promised to do everything in their power to get my petition submitted directly to the Democratic Republic of Vietnam, and to attempt to gain all possible information about POWs and MIAs from the government of North Vietnam. I was very pleased that the mission delegates from these countries demonstrated such a sincere interest and concern for Newk and all our other missing and detained men. I was impressed that they had become well-informed on these issues.

My visit brought The League of Families to their attention. The League was already fairly well-known in the United States, but through this interaction with the United Nations, and some trips abroad by League members, we were becoming better known internationally as well. I was learning what a formidable task it would be to exert influence on world opinion, but we were not deterred by the word "formidable" in the League. We dealt in "formidable" situations every day! We simply kept going, kept chipping away at international opinion, nation by nation. This round of meetings would help that effort enormously. I had emphasized to the international delegates that time was passing for our men and for their families. Their children were growing up without fathers. "We are desperate for resolution," I implored them.

One example the League used in these discussions was Navy Lt. Everett Alvarez, Jr. Lieutenant Alvarez had been shot down and taken prisoner by North Vietnam on August 5, 1964. At age 26, he was the first American prisoner in North Vietnam. Seven years later, in the summer of 1971, he was 33 years old and still a POW in North Vietnam. Hopefully, he was still alive.[23] In the interim, more than 1600 of his fellow Americans had become POW or were MIA, and the news from returning POWs about the conditions and treatment there in the camps of Hanoi and South Vietnam was very grim.

I emphasized that to every influential person or national representative I met, and said that we knew with certainty that we could not, would not, leave them there to die abandoned in the prisons of North Vietnam. No matter what it took, the families had to keep up the fight to get them acknowledged, accounted for, better treated, and returned home. We just weren't certain how much longer they could survive. To us, the time clock was running out in this game.

As the League of Families, we shared Knute Rockne's philosophy: we were never going to be good and gracious losers! The League of Families would never give up on these POWs and MIAs.

8 National Coordinator of the League

TIMELINE . . . 1971, JULY to DECEMBER . . . WORLD . . . PEOPLE'S REPUBLIC OF CHINA TAKES U.N. SEAT OF TAIWAN . . . ALEXANDER SOLZHENITSYN RECEIVES NOBEL PRIZE FOR LITERATURE . . . VIETNAM . . . NGUYEN VAN THIEU UNOPPOSED FOR PRESIDENT OF SOUTH VIETNAM . . . PRESIDENT NIXON PLEDGES TO END U.S. INVOLVEMENT IN VIET-NAM . . . USA . . . DANIEL ELLSBERG LEAKS CLASSIFIED PENTAGON PAPERS . . . WALT DIS-NEY WORLD OPENS OCTOBER 1 IN FLORIDA . . . U.S. VOTING AGE DROPS TO 18 . . .

In mighty enterprises, it is enough to have had the determination.
There is something beyond the grave; death does not end all . . .
—Sextus Propertius, Elegies, c. 30 BC

It was sometime in late June 1971 that Joan Vinson asked me on the way back from a meeting, "Evie, you wouldn't want to run for National Coordinator of the League of Families, would you?"

"Well, I haven't really thought about it, Joan. I'm deep into the U.N. Petition project, you know, and that's still going on. Then there's the letter-writing campaign, fighting the legal aspects of my own situation, and all the other League activities, not to mention my family, and the new house."

"My, you're certainly keeping busy! I have the same problem. I hope you'll find some time to help with the League Convention in September. I'd like you and Mary Jane McManus to work with Bob Earle from the Red Cross. He's volunteered to help us. That's wonderful because he has already handled many conventions. Also, I'd like you and Mary Jane to arrange the Armed Services luncheons for me."

"I'll help you as much as I can," I said. I knew that our annual Convention was always a big chore for whoever was Coordinator of the League, and we all pitched in and helped as much as we could.

By July 1, Mary Jane and I had met with Admiral Epps and Colonel Haggard at the Pentagon to arrange for the four military-sponsored luncheons at the League Convention. Each luncheon would represent, and have in attendance at each table, at least one knowledgeable representative from one of the Armed Services (Army, Navy, Air Force or Marines). These representatives would answer questions from the POW/MIA family members seated at that table.

We had also requested military assistance in flying the primary next of kin of each POW or MIA to and from the Convention. That meeting went well, too, so we felt those luncheons and travel arrangements were all set and in very capable hands. Then Joan tasked Mary Jane and me to arrange the formal Speaker's dinner. President Nixon had been invited to be our main speaker, and we were hoping he would accept.

The Board, Joan, her staff, and the other League volunteers handled the business part of the convention. They printed and mailed ballots and counted them as they were returned to the office. They invited the speakers, arranged for panel discussions, and covered many of the myriad tasks associated with a big national convention.

On many evenings that summer, I was simply too tired to drive home, so I stayed nearby at the Army and Navy Club where my father, a disabled vet of World War II, had stayed many times. When the Club members were made aware of my POW/MIA situation, and the League of Families, they invited me, and any guests of mine to use their lovely dining room for business lunches and dinners, and to stay overnight when necessary.

In late July, Mother and I took two weeks off for summer vacation and drove with the boys down to Auburndale, Florida, where my brother, Bill, and I had bought an old Florida-style house. It had an enclosed veranda and huge live oaks draped with Spanish moss in the front yard. The boys loved it. While there, I finally found time to read the captivating but hair-raising book by escaped POW James N. "Nick" Rowe: *Five Years to Freedom,* the story of his years as a captive of the brutal Viet Cong in South Vietnam.[1] It was especially difficult for me to read about what he had gone through. The Viet Cong certainly took "man's inhumanity to man" back to the dawn of civilization. It took awhile for me to finish it because periodically I had to put it down, just to rest my mind for a bit so I could get past the countless horrors he'd had to endure at their hands.

On July 26 1971, the boys and I were at Kennedy Space Center, to watch our first live space shot, *Apollo 15,* headed for the moon with the Lunar Rover vehicle aboard.[2] General Chappie James had arranged for a VIP car pass that allowed us to get fairly close to the launch site. As we watched the rocket ascend toward the heavens with a ground-shaking roar that reverberated through our bodies, trailing that gigantic flaming tail, I screamed, applauded, and exclaimed as it climbed and the roar subsided. "Wow! I've never seen anything like this before!" I yelled. Jeff gave me one of those eyes-rolling-up looks, and in that world-weary voice teenagers use when talking to their parents said, "Mother, none of us have ever seen anything like this before!" We were all happy to learn that they'd reached the moon safely, and the Lunar Rover had been successfully deployed and operated four days later. We were having more success and progress exploring space than we were in negotiating with North Vietnam.

That September I received a letter from Department of the Air Force Headquarters in Washington, D.C., informing me that Newk had been selected for promotion to Lieutenant Colonel. I was told that I'd be informed of the promotion when it became effective, but "his selection will not be released to the news media, nor will his name appear on the list of selectees distributed throughout the Air Force . . . " which made me wonder if they'd gotten information I didn't have.[3] They said that ploy was "to assure that it may not be used to subject him to any additional pressure or stress," which hadn't happened when he was promoted to Major while a captive. I knew then that the Air Force probably believed as I did that Newk was dead. However, Congress had passed H.R. 8656, "to amend titles 37 and 38 USC relating to promotion of members of the Uniformed Services who are in a missing status." That bill provided that promotions of personnel carried as missing "are valid for all purposes, including Federal benefits to survivors, even when the date of death of the missing member is later determined to have occurred prior to the promotion."[4]

The Saturday night before the League Convention opened Iris and Sybil asked me to please join them in their hotel room. "We have something important we need to discuss with you," Sybil said. When I got there, she explained in more detail.

"Evie, Joan Vinson has made it clear to us that she does not want to commit outright to another full term as National Coordinator. We feel that the League desperately needs a full one-year commitment by its elected National Coordinator. Joan is insisting on an initial three-month term, with three optional and tentative three-month extensions, at her discretion, to follow. That isn't solid enough for the League's heavy business agenda this coming year. We don't know if there will be peace accords signed, or if our men will be released, with all that entails for the League. We need an elected Coordinator who will commit to serve the full year from beginning to end. If you'll agree to do that, Evie, we'd like to propose you to the Convention as the nominee for National Coordinator for this next term."

To say I was surprised would be an understatement. I had done enough work at the League at the national level to agree completely with Sybil and Iris' opinion that Joan's piecemeal proposition wouldn't work for the best interests of the League. We needed a full one-year commitment. My qualifications for National Coordinator weren't an issue. In my recent activities with the League, I had learned my way around official Washington and the Pentagon, and I had become familiar with the political machinations of the United Nations. I had met and interacted with many high level civilian and military "players" and had already done a lot of public speaking. I had also managed various League projects. However, I was concerned that Joan hadn't turned down a second term as National Coordinator, but had requested that they change the terms for serving in that position. I understood the Board's dilemma very well. I replied a bit hesitantly, choosing my words carefully.

"I'm very honored that you have the confidence in me to consider me for this nomination. In return, I'll be candid with you. I don't want to upset Joan, or cause a rift in our friendship. That's a major concern. Another is my children. They're all in school, but I know I'd need to be in Washington all during the week, and sometimes on weekends too. I live too far away to commute, so I'd have to find a reliable live-in couple before I could even think of agreeing to this. I know it's a volunteer position with no pay. I'm concerned about the personal outlay of expense involved. We're all on pretty tight budgets at home, as you know. I can barely afford to be a volunteer for the League as it is. Also, although I'm qualified in a lot of areas, I have no background in the administrative details of being Coordinator, like the office procedures, staffing, budgeting, and basically whatever else it takes to coordinate and run the National League of Families' main office."

Iris and Sybil appreciated my candor. "If you'll just say you'll consider it, Evie, we'll do everything possible to resolve those concerns," Iris assured me.

Sybil added, "You are the most appropriate candidate we have, since you already know the ropes in Washington better than anyone else. Also, there is no doubt in anyone's mind about your dedication to the POW/MIA cause and the work of the League. Please tell us you'll let us nominate you, Evie."

They promised to help me find a place to live in Washington, and assured me that the League would reimburse my out-of-pocket expenses for conducting League business and staying over in Washington when necessary. They also assured me they would help in every way they could to make my job easier. With that kind of backing, I felt I could devote a full year to being National Coordinator. I knew Mother would have a fit, but if I could find good help for the boys, we'd do all right. She had adjusted well to this past year, when I'd been at the League's Washington Office a lot, working on our Petition to the United Nations. Finally I said, "Okay, with the promise of your help, I agree to be a candidate for National Coordinator."

They were visibly delighted that I had agreed to be a candidate. I was nominated and on September 28, 1971, I was elected National Coordinator for the League of Families for the 1971-1972 term. It was quite a change for me, but I was proud to be elected to that position. Even more important was the confidence and trust in me it implied.

I learned soon afterward that President Nixon had accepted our invitation to speak. A security team arrived before dinner to make arrangements for the President. We had to scurry to add extra places at a few of the tables for his men and exchange the podium for one that was bullet-proof. But all our weeks of planning paid off handsomely. It was a great honor to have the President there to speak to the families. I was too nervous about being the newly elected National Coordinator to really register all that went on when he arrived to speak, but as anyone can imagine, having the President of the United States appear in person was a very big boost for us and our event.

My term as National Coordinator of the National League of Families of American POW/MIA in Southeast Asia began right after the Convention closed. Carole Hansen was the new Chairman of the Board. We avoided national politics at the League as a policy, but I quickly discovered that office politics were a constant reality. We wrote our job descriptions as we learned them and helped each other when needed. Jan and Cathy Ray, two sisters whose brother was MIA, were there as volunteers, and they handled routine duties, wrote thank-you notes, provided information about the League to visitors, helped the volunteers, made copies, typed press releases, coordinated liaison with various Washington contacts, and accomplished many other administrative duties. Although they worked long hours, they were always cheerful and helpful.

My job description as National Coordinator was to be spokesperson for the League, carry out the mandates of the Board (which meant being very diplomatic), and consider both sides of issues. Luckily, the Board, the office staff, and our advisors often worked as one voice. Without their dedication and support, I would not have been able to accomplish anything.

The boys were very proud of me and my new position, which was quite a change for me. Not surprisingly, Mother was less than thrilled about it, but was also somewhat proud that I'd been elected to an office as important as National Coordinator of the League. What she didn't like was my weekly commute to and from Washington, and that I'd be away from the boys during the week and on some weekends during that year.

"I think you should be staying at home with your sons, but I'll do whatever I can to help you and the boys, Evie, you know that."

With Sybil's recommendation, I found a reliable, pleasant and honest young military couple from nearby Fort Lee, Sharon and Bruce Carlson, who were exactly what I wanted and needed for the boys. They were eager to jump right in, and Mother agreed to oversee them during the early weeks. They were wonderful, and soon became a part of our family. In Washington, I rented a well-used efficiency apartment in Foggy Bottom. My one window looked out on the back of the Howard Johnson Motel, a slice of the Kennedy Center, and the front of the Watergate building.

Getting started in my new job was a bumpy ride. First of all, I was alarmed to find that the turnover review of the League's financial status showed that we were about $7,000 in the red! That was mostly because some members had charged travel expenses and purchases to the League that shouldn't have been charged. During 1970 and 1971, a fund-raising organization with a mailing list of "Caring Americans" had collected a lot of money for the League and we had counted on that income to cover those expenses and put us in the black. Too late, we learned that the organization intended to keep 60 percent of what they collected on our behalf, *plus* expenses! We only got what little was left. I resented that this organization had used the League to make more money for themselves than for us. I raised that issue at the next meeting and the League Board decided that fundraisers like that were *not* a good way to raise the funds we needed.

I then turned to two of our sage League Advisors, Fletcher Prouty and Paul Wagner, who suggested we find and initiate new ways to raise funds. Initially, to cover our present emergency, League members appealed to their own family members, local churches, military chaplains, military officers' and officers' wives clubs, and other military service organizations. That appeal helped reduce our debt for the near-term.

Senator Barry Goldwater (R-Arizona) heard about our dire financial straits and kindly offered us his mailing list to solicit donations. Other Congressmen followed suit. It became a very patriotic thing to do at a time when patriotism wasn't all that popular in our country. Next, we applied for grants from various sources, which yielded a good sum. Finding alternate fund-raising projects was not without problems—and yielded a few laughs, which in our circumstance were welcome.

One of our Board members was adamantly against the League's acceptance of any donations from the military. He called me almost every day to ask about our financial status and always ended the call with a caution against accepting money from military contributors.

Before long, with our new efforts, we were in the black again, instead of the red. I was thrilled and excited to report at out next Board meeting that we had received a large grant from General Mills.

"Dammit, Evie, I said *no* military money!" shouted my ever vigilant watchdog.

"Wait," I said. It isn't *a* General Mills, it's *the* General Mills. The company that shoots cereal, not bullets."

"Oh, that General Mills." He reddened in embarrassment and his anger diminished. The Board enjoyed a good laugh about it, and he actually joined in.

Another complication during my first week involved the organization called Voices In Vital America, known as VIVA, purportedly a student organization that sold the very popular "POW Freedom Bracelets" to Americans who made donations to them to support the POW/MIA cause. VIVA produced nickel-plated or copper bracelets and engraved them with the name of a POW or MIA, and the date he had been captured or been declared missing. They had bracelets packaged with a message printed on a piece of paper in the packing about the more than 1,500 POWs and MIAs in Southeast Asia. The message said:

> Aside from the inhumane treatment witnessed by those few who have returned, the most tragic aspect is that most of the families of these men do not know if their sons, husbands, or fathers are alive or dead. Hanoi won't tell them. This bracelet honors the man whose name is inscribed, and includes the date he was lost. It should be worn with the vow that it will not be removed until the day the Red Cross is allowed into Hanoi and can assure his family of his status and that he receives the humane treatment due all men.
>
> Distributed by VIVA (Voices in Vital America) a non-profit, non-political national student organization dedicated to the fact that progress and freedom can only be achieved and maintained by rational and responsible action.[5]

Also in the package were VIVA's address and phone number and a donation form to order more bracelets. VIVA and the League sold and distributed them. VIVA donated some of their proceeds to the League, but we had no way of knowing how much they collected, how they spent the rest of the donations they received, or how or if they really supported our cause. We had been burned by "Caring Americans," so I was initially erring on the side of caution about "fund-raising" efforts.

As a recognized nonprofit organization, the League was careful to account for all the expenses and receipts associated with the VIVA bracelets we sold and distributed from our national office. However, VIVA would not permit us to have any insight to their records of receipts, expenses, or what percentage of total receipts we were given. This made me and some of our Advisors and Board members very uncomfortable. We consulted our attorney, and he and the Board decided we'd continue allowing the bracelets, as they were a reasonably good source of unsolicited funds for us. Without a doubt, they also helped us to get the POW/MIA message out. I checked back into our financial records, and noted that VIVA had already given the League almost $9,000. The bracelets were a huge thing in America. Everyone seemed to be wearing them, so we continued to carry and sell them at the National office as did many of the state offices. However, in keeping with our charter and policy, the League did not officially endorse any organizations, including VIVA. That was a thorn in VIVA'S side. They were constantly nagging me to endorse them. We declined to do that, citing our policy, and the bracelet project continued unabated, with occasional donations from VIVA coming to our offices.

As National Coordinator, I also coped with a lot of speaking engagements, a huge amount of correspondence, and daily meetings that took me in all directions. I signed appreciation certificates to our many benefactors, gave interviews to the press, to radio and television stations, and ran the national office of the League. It did not take long for me to realize what a demanding responsibility I had accepted.

In early October 1971, the Viet Cong in South Vietnam released POW Army Sergeant John Sexton, who had been prisoner since August of 1969. According to newspaper accounts, his release was in exchange for our release of a North Vietnamese prisoner we had held in South Vietnam.[6] Every release brought a ray of hope that more might follow. On October 12, 1971, following my

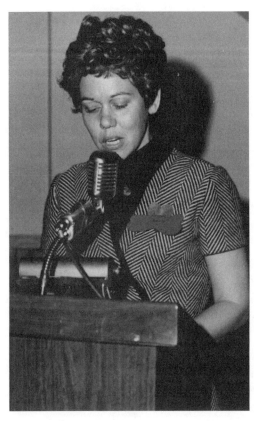

Evelyn Grubb accepts role of National Coordinator of the National League of Families of POW/MIA, Washington, D.C., October 1971.

first week as National Coordinator, I sent a telegram to the Provisionary Revolutionary Government of North Vietnam in Hanoi, which read:

> The National League of Families of Prisoners of War and Missing in Action in Southeast Asia welcomes the release of Sergeant John Sexton. We hope this release will lead to further prisoner releases for all parties involved. Information provided by you on the status of prisoners and MIA's would be appreciated.[7]

Of course there was no reply from the DRV, nor did I expect one. However, there was a lot of discussion in the news surrounding the selection of John Sexton for release.[8]

My daily meetings ranged from lobbying in Congress to meeting with representatives from the New York chapter of the Hell's

Angels; from talking to executives in the White House to luncheon at the Press Club. Two Hell's Angels from New York visited me after parking their "Iron Buffalos" on the American Legion's small porch. They offered their services to set up a POW/MIA Festival at Radio City Music Hall in New York City. They told me that lots of big names would be there, including a very successful musical group called "The Grateful Dead." I stopped them there. "The 'Grateful Dead' at a benefit for POW/MIAs? I hardly think that would be wise, or appropriate." They understood, apologized, and immediately said they would get someone else. They also assured me that they would do all the work, but needed formal sponsorship by us before Radio City officials would even consider it. I told them that was a legal issue, and I'd ask our legal counsel to join us if possible. I called Charlie Havens, and asked if he could possibly come to the League office right away.

"What's up, Evie?" he wanted to know. "Anything serious?"

I said cheerily, "Not really. Two members of Hell's Angels Motorcycle Club are here . . . I need your opinion on a benefit they want to hold for us."

"The Hell's Angels? Want to hold a benefit for us? I'll be right there."

Charlie came over, heard them out, and gave them the same straight answer he'd given VIVA:

"Sorry. The League of Families cannot sanction, sponsor, or endorse any activities but its own." So that idea for a benefit was shelved.

The American Legion representatives offered to clean and paint our offices. *That* we could accept with pleasure.

General Don Hughes called from the White House to inform me that the November 20 date for our Board meeting would be a good time for us to meet with Dr. Henry Kissinger. It would be in the Executive Meeting Room next to the Oval Office. I accepted with pleasure, hoping this session would go better than the last one. We were cleared in advance by White House Security, and on the day of the meeting, we entered through the West Gate and were escorted directly to the meeting room as we had been before. This time, the promised speaker, Dr. Henry Kissinger, Nixon's National Security Advisor, was able to join us.

It was a good and informative meeting. Dr. Kissinger was always kind and most courteous to us. He made us feel that he was very open to listening to us and answering our questions. He also was extremely well-informed and knowledgeable about our POW/MIA situation. He gave concise and specific answers to just about everything we asked him. Personally, I was amazed that he found the time to meet with us like that, and to hear our needs and concerns about our imprisoned or missing loved ones. It raised him pretty high in my esteem.

On most weekends, I joined the busy I-95 traffic heading southward to see my boys and participate in various activities with them, the Carlsons, Mother, and our Colonial Heights neighbors.

"I'm glad this National Coordinator job with your League is only for a year, Evie," my Mother remarked one weekend evening. "We all miss having you home. I hope by the end of the year this will be over and done with, and things can get back to normal. You and the children need to get on with your own lives."

What is "normal" any more, I wondered. Does she think we are not getting on with our own lives? Does she think that I don't wish that my life for the past five years, and for God knows how long into the future, could be for only one year, and then it would 'get back to normal?' Whatever that was? Loyal as always, even if she disapproved, I knew that Mother would be there to back me when I needed her, and I was truly grateful to her. I also realized then how different our lives, our families, and our country had become from what it was in my Mother's youth, or the way it was until the agony of the Vietnam War tore our country asunder. I couldn't help but wonder if we'd ever see "normal" again. I was different, too. My whole life and outlook were different. Seeing the children on weekends also brought home how independent and self-reliant the boys had become since I'd started working with the League. Jeff always asked me about my work, and seemed interested to hear about what I had done all week. Roland and Van had begun asking questions about the war, and the POW/MIA issue. They actually listened to my answers about those things, too. Roy was just thrilled to have Mommy home, for at least three minutes. Then he was ready to go outside and play.

Before I knew it, my first months as National Coordinator had passed, and I realized that I, too, was growing—in confidence, independence, and self-reliance. I was making broadcasts over Radio Free Europe and meeting with important Washington figures. I no longer spent idle hours daydreaming about where we'd go next, or what we'd do "when Newk comes home."

This was my life now, all I could really count on. I was firmly ensconced in the here and now, not the past. When tomorrow came, whatever it brought, I felt confident that I could face and handle that, too.

I was no longer the angry woman I'd been for so long. I could even handle Jack Anderson's one-sided perspective. He published a column in *The Washington Post* on October 27 1971, headlined, "Wives of POWs Create Problems." In it, he intimated that President Nixon was manipulating the POW wives and families for political gain. Andersen claimed that Nixon was trying to keep us quiet while he strategized the U.S. pullout from Vietnam so that he would look good when the POWs were released.[9]

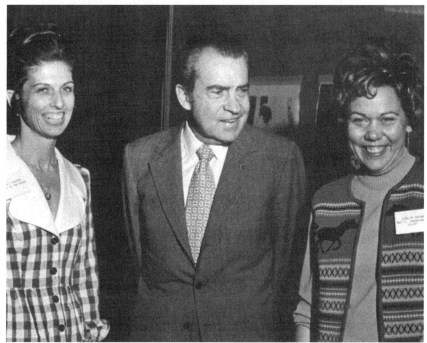

League Chairman Carole Hansen (left) and National Coordinator Evelyn Grubb (right) meet with U.S. President Richard M. Nixon.

Grubb family files

Anderson also sniped at the creation of the League of Families, saying, "A Defense Department lawyer, Charles Havens, who had worked on the POW issue at the Pentagon, stepped into the unpaid volunteer job as counsel for the league shortly after leaving the government . . . the league's advisory board was also selected with the active, if informal, advice of military officers. Most of the advisors are outspoken hawks on the war; some are retired military officers. No outspoken doves are active on the board."[10]

He accused President Nixon of being overly-solicitous toward the POW families and of stroking us by offering us briefings with his national security advisor, Dr. Henry Kissinger. Anderson also claimed that the Nixon administration had a hand in the proposals that were voted on at the National Convention of the League of Families, and that we were blocking the "militant minority" of POW families from making the League a more politically active organization.[11]

"Those who favored a more militant role would have had to vote to dissolve the league," wrote Anderson. "The Convention also swarmed with dashing officers, sent over from the Pentagon, who assisted the wives, and in some cases, berated wives who opposed President Nixon's Vietnam policies."[12] After reading that, I didn't know whether to laugh or scream. Mr. Anderson certainly went to great lengths to make us look like a bunch of airhead female ninnies who couldn't think for ourselves.

Mr. Anderson apparently couldn't fathom that we were activists *for our cause* and that we could do that without being party banner carriers or political activists. In point of fact, the League's Constitution required us to remain nonpartisan, and that's the way most of us preferred it. Our activism for the POWs and MIAs had nothing to do with our private political or religious beliefs, although of course we each had those. Nor did it depend upon President Nixon or the Pentagon and its "dashing officers." It was centered on what we were trying to accomplish, which was to get access to those who could help our POWs receive fair, decent, and humane treatment under the Geneva Conventions, and get them accounted for and returned home as soon as possible. We wanted North Vietnam to identify the prisoners, allow free correspondence, and most of all, release the sick and wounded, so they could come home.

Dr. Kissinger *always* listened intently and with great politeness to what our representatives of the League had to say. He gamely fielded our questions, which often were pointed and occasionally even rude. Except for one time, he never became visibly angry and never lost patience with us at those meetings. He always treated us with courtesy. We had the strong impression he really cared about us and our situation. Anderson's accusations made it look like he was patronizing us, and using us to further the Administration's agenda, and I deeply resented that.

Unfortunately, Jack Anderson's article was the opening salvo to what would soon become a major schism in the League of Families. Some of the wives and family members, like Valerie Kushner, Louise Mulligan and others, felt that political activism was the only way we would ever solve our problem. That was against the League's charter.

At the next board meeting, Joan Vinson announced that she would be the new Nonpartisan Political Activity Chairwoman at the League. The American Legion had given her rooms above our offices for her use. She requested that Betty move up there as her secretary, and that she get funding from the Board. I was pleased to learn that Joan had now found a suitable activity with which she could remain an active member at National level within the League, but wasn't required to commit to a term of office. Joe McCain also was still with us as a volunteer, still doing an admirable job with the Discrepancy Display and Report.

At about that same time, we received the first design of the POW/MIA banner, which would also become the official flag of the League of Families of POW/MIA. League member Mary Hoff, wife of MIA Michael Hoff, had contacted Norman Rivkees, Vice President of Annin & Company, the largest manufacturer of flags in the world, (including the Armed Services flags of the United States,) and commissioned them to design a special flag to be the standard of the POW/MIA for the League of Families. The design project devolved to graphic designer Newt Heisley, a former World War II pilot. This flag design was a challenge dear to Heisley's heart. His own son, Jeffrey, had become seriously ill during Marine training. When he returned home on leave to recuperate, he was gaunt and thin, and reminded his father of the condition of POWs returned from being prisoners of war since World War II, in photos he'd seen. He sketched his son's profile, and incorporated it into the starkly moving and very impressive flag design.

When the design was completed, it was in the normal black and white configuration of such designs, awaiting colors to be assigned to the various elements. Above the white circle containing the silhouette of a young man in the field of black that was the flag's background, the acronyms POW and MIA were reversed out in big white letters, with a white five-point star separating them. A curved string of linked chain underscored the silhouette circle, and below that, in simple block letters reversed out in white against the black background, was the League's new motto:

YOU ARE NOT FORGOTTEN.

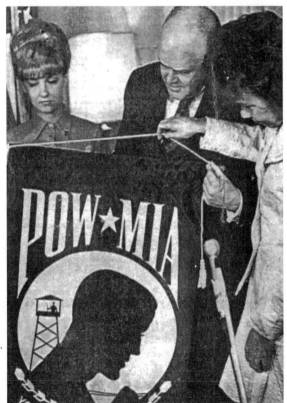

League of Families National Coordinator Evelyn Grubb presents first rendition of the POW-MIA flag in banner form to Secretary of Defense Melvin Laird, October 1971.

Grubb family files

It was a poignant, moving image of our situation. We immediately ordered the first rendition of it in black and white. In late October 1971, I had the great honor of presenting the first POW/MIA flag, in the form of a banner he could hang in his office, to Secretary of Defense Melvin Laird at the Pentagon. I was so proud of that design! It was a talisman for our cause, and amazingly it became symbolic of the POWs and MIA to all Americans.

That flag and its motto have remained an enduring emblem of the POW/MIA cause and the crusade of the League of Families. It flies in tandem with, and just below, our National Colors, the Stars and Stripes. Its design was never copyrighted and remains in the public domain. Annin & Company still manufactures and sells the flag.[13]

Early in November the League received a telegram from the Royal Swedish Embassy in response to our request that they help us bring pressure on the government of North Vietnam for humane treatment of our POWs. It said,

> Vietnamese officials in Hanoi informed [Prime Minister] Thorsten Nilsson that the captured military men in DRV [Democratic Republic of Vietnam] are given a lenient and humanitarian treatment. According to information further passed to Mr. Nilsson, arrangements will be made for forwarding mail and parcels to forthcoming Christmas in accordance with the regulations issued last year by the DRV government.[14]

I sighed. It was pretty much the same old line from the North Vietnamese, the one they had fed us for years without taking any action. I had thought, hoped, the situation might improve now that other governments were inquiring, but it was not so.

In late October, I had sent a telegram to Prime Minister Indira Ghandi of India about her earlier concern and interest in the POW and MIA family situation. Ms. Ghandi had met with some of the family members when they were in her country and had made inquiries to North Vietnam on our behalf. I requested a meeting with her when she visited Washington in November. Unfortunately, her schedule did not permit a personal meeting, So I sent her a note while she was in Washington, asking,

Will you, as Chairman of the ICRC [International
Committee of the Red Cross] pursue new initiatives to
assist with the repatriation of our prisoners as was done during the Indo-China War? Time drags on for all of us so
closely connected with this conflict, and very little seems to
be accomplished to relieve the anxiety of those involved.
The amount of mail from prisoners has never been adequate, and in recent months it has decreased alarmingly.[15]

I also enclosed a list of our MIA, and requested that she inquire
as to the status of the missing men if possible. In closing, I wished
her a pleasant and successful visit in our country. The following
week, I received a note from the First Secretary of the Embassy of
India that acknowledged receipt of my letter. The note said, "I have
been instructed to assure you that India will continue to do whatever she can in the matter."[16]

We heard that President Nixon would soon be making a statement about his plan to end the war in Vietnam. We were anxious
to learn whether that statement would include any strong language
about them handing over all our POWs and MIAs.

However, there were others who preferred more political activity on the home front. Val Kushner and Louise Mulligan broke
their ties with the League to campaign for a new American president and administration that they felt would be more receptive to
insisting on the immediate release of the POWs and accounting for
the MIA. In July, Mrs. Louis F. Jones and Mrs. James L. Hughes,
both MIA wives, had founded the activist POW/MIA Families for
Immediate Release. This group strongly advocated what its name
implied, and that was commendable. This is the group in which Val
and Louise became active. I was sorry to see them leave the League
of Familes.

I had a meeting scheduled on November 10 with Clark
Clifford, who had been Secretary of Defense during President
Johnson's last term. Bonnie Metzger and I met with him at his elegant suite of private offices in Washington. Mr. Clifford was very
receptive and cordial. He told us his opinions on the war, especially the POW aspect of it, and said he appreciated our position and
our concerns.[17] It was his opinion that President Nixon had no real
plan for the POW/MIA situation to put forward right now and

likely wouldn't address it in his upcoming talk. That distressed me. I asked what he thought we could do to rectify Nixon's possible omission of the return of the POWs in his speech. Mr. Clifford suggested that the League make a forceful statement *beforehand*, requesting that President Nixon set a specific date for the return of all POWs in Southeast Asia. As we stood to leave, Mr. Clifford took out his checkbook and personally contributed $1000 to the League. I was very grateful to him for that gesture of support to us.

Some of us privately agreed with Mr. Clifford's statement that the situation looked grim and that, if the President didn't make a strong statement, lobbying by the League for such a statement would be necessary. I took Mr. Clifford's sage advice, although I didn't ask for a specific date. Instead, on November 12, I sent a telegram to President Nixon on behalf of the League, and copied Dr. Henry Kissinger, General James "Don" Hughes, Defense Secretary Melvin Laird, and Secretary of State William Rogers:

> President Nixon: The National League of Families of American Prisoners and Missing in Southeast Asia anxiously awaits your November 15th message to the nation concerning Vietnam. Many families are desperate. We expect a positive POW/MIA solution as part of that message. The men must not be kept waiting indefinitely. We're depending on you Mr. President.[18]

President Nixon held a press conference on November 12, the same day I sent the telegram. Several questions regarding POW/MIA matters were put to him by members of the press. All POW/MIA families received a verbatim recap of that presidential press conference from General Hughes at the White House, attached to the Air Force Headquarters newsletter of December 22 1971. General Hughes added in his cover letter, "I would like to emphasize, however, that whenever the President uses the term prisoners of war he intends to include those who are missing in action, and he is genuinely dedicated to obtaining an early accounting for all the missing as well as for the release of those who are held prisoner."[19]

In his press conference ot November 12, when questioned if he had "any reason for encouragement about the release of prisoners of war from any source?" The President said several times, "No reason for encouragement that I can talk about publicly." That seemed to me to be a tongue in cheek confirmation of the rumors about Kissinger's secret peace talks. President Nixon went on to make statements about the status of peace negotiations in Paris and the prisoner of war issue that alarmed many of the POW/MIA families. When a press questioner asked,

> Mr. President, you said there was no movement on the prisoner of war issue. Is there anything at all to report on negotiations either through Paris or through some other means?"
> PRESIDENT NIXON: I would respond to that only by saying that we have not given up on the negotiating front. . . . I, however, would not like to leave the impression that we see the possibility of some striking breakthrough in negotiations in the near future. But we are pursuing negotiations in Paris and through whatever other channels we think are appropriate.
> QUESTIONER: There has been no progress, either publicly or privately, on getting the release of our prisoners?
> PRESIDENT NIXON: I do not want to give any false encouragement to those who are the next of kin or who are close relatives of our prisoners. I can only say that we, on our part, have taken initiatives on a number of fronts here. So the possibility of progress in the future is there. As far as the enemy's position is concerned, it is still intransigent.

What frightened us most was that the President intended to remove our armed forces from Vietnam without a negotiated settlement or any other definite agreement for release of our POWs and with only a small contingent (about 45,000) of troops remaining there as a negotiating tool. As President Nixon expressed it:

> . . . maintain a residual force for not only the reason—and this is, of course a very primary reason—of having something to negotiate with, with regard to our prisoners, but it is also essential to do so in order to continue our role of leaving South Vietnam in a position where it will be able to defend itself from a Communist takeover. Both objectives

can be fulfilled, we believe, through a negotiated settlement. We would prefer that. If they are not fulfilled through a negotiated settlement, then we will have to go another route and we are prepared to do so.[20]

In a nutshell, the President and Commander-in-Chief of the United States of America had just admitted publicly that he was still floundering for solutions. The enemy was not giving an inch on anything. Our morale sagged lower in the face of those pronouncements.

The League decided to address in writing the families' fears and concerns about the return of their servicemen. The Leagues "task force" drew up a list of constructive action items for the services to consider regarding the rehabilitation of both our men and their families when they came home. When finished, we had a sizeable list of actions to present to our advisors and White House liaison people:

- The government should make transportation arrangements to get the POW wives and families to wherever the men were taken upon their initial return, and as soon as possible following their arrival back to the United States.
- A "casualty assistance officer" should be assigned to each POW and his family immediately. That person should be tasked to contact the family (wives and parents) at least monthly to get to know them, their particular situation and needs, and what might be needed when their POW or MIA returned (or didn't), to perform the most efficient liaison possible under these unusual circumstances.
- For our men, any and all personnel who would be dealing with these men should be trained in a "code of conduct" toward them, to avoid any undue stress from feelings of guilt, inadequacy or any suicidal tendencies.
- Provide the returning men with routine physical and dental care for the rest or their lives and professional psychological counseling for at least 5 years following their return. The counseling program should be designed to help the men achieve educational, emotional and social adjustment to a world many of them haven't seen in 5 to 8 years—years during which major social and cultural changes have taken place

in the United States, the world, and their families.

- Provide each man with a personal packet of tapes of common new vocabulary and social phrases and customs, along with an update on how the services have changed during that period in respect to pay scales, protocol, uniforms, rules and regulations.
- Discuss the startling changes they will encounter in behavioral matters, like religion, morals, customs, sports, music, ethnic and racial issues, urban pollution, and the like.
- Include an "overview update" on major news events, as well as a list of prominent national and international figures that had died during the time they were incarcerated and isolated from such news.
- Gently advise them, especially those for whom correspondence had been minimal, that their wives will be, in most cases, dramatically changed women, not only from the standpoint of age, but as women who had assumed a much stronger head of household role while their husbands were away for so long.
- Have the psychologists inform them that some wives might have difficulty adjusting to a POW mate's return, just as the POW will have difficulty adjusting to all the major changes in lifestyle, activities, dress and discipline that have taken place during his years away.[21]

It wasn't until we made this list and read it over several times that we began to understand the true depth and width of the chasm that would have to be bridged when the men came home.

In my capacity as Coordinator, there were many diverse personalities with whom I had to meet, listen to their ideas, and embrace their problems. At times it seemed like I had a million different activities to oversee: fundraising, letter writing, the color of bumper stickers, seeking information from North Vietnam, and lobbying the U.N. and the White House for more action. I sensed it was going to be a long and difficult year, and I would need more skill and diplomacy than perhaps I possessed to weather it, but I was determined to persevere and learn.

"Political neutrality" for the League was one of the biggest tightrope issues for me to walk. On the one hand, I was happy to be working in an office that had important ties to the current administration, and to the movers and shakers who could make things happen. How else could we have approached the key people who would decide the fate of our men and this war? On the other hand, I had to keep both my personal position and the office of the National Coordinator of the League politically neutral. Unfortunately, I didn't always succeed at that on the personal side.

We enjoyed wonderful, and mostly willing, cooperation from our many influential contacts in Washington. Having our head-quarters located in the capital allowed us access. We could visit and speak on short notice with representatives from Congress, the White House, the State Department, the Red Cross, the Pentagon, and heads of all branches of the U.S. military. We stayed abreast of important matters, pending legislation, and decisions that strongly affected us as families of POWs and MIAs. Our mission to promote the return of our men and the well-being of their families was a difficult job. We didn't need to enter into political activism in our own country because we were involved in plenty of it abroad, walking a tightrope between monitoring the Paris Peace Talks, dealing with the stubborn North Vietnamese, and trying to invoke the Geneva Conventions.

Arriving home on weekends, I tried hard to leave the League problems behind in Washington and just enjoy being with the boys, Mother, and the Carlsons. On Mondays, I endured the stuck-in-traffic commute back up to Washington, D.C., and upon arrival, dove back into the office regimen all over again. As seriously as we took our work, there were always office incidents to get us laughing. A young woman called one day thinking that the "League of Families" was a family planning group. She asked if we could recommend the best contraceptive to use. Bonnie replied, "I'm not sure what the best is, but the women in our office practice total abstinence, and that works very well."

As the years dragged on, not every POW and MIA wife followed the path of abstinence or fidelity. Society seemed to expect that these young women would wait like prayerful nuns while watching their peak sexual and childbearing years slip away. We were given no ray of hope that we might ever see our husbands again, yet we were to expected to embrace the sacrifice of our best years to loneliness, anxiety and fear.

The upright men in Congress and the State Legislatures, many of whom were no saints themselves, blamed and condemned POW/MIA wives in the strongest terms for any lapses of fidelity. I received a telegram that November from Harrisburg, the capital of Pennsylvania (Newk's and my home state), which served to underscore the moral and legal mood of our nation's leaders:

> The State Legislature (of Pennsylvania) . . . called on the wives of servicemen missing in action in Vietnam to be faithful. The Legislature passed and sent to the Governor a bill providing that a wife be disinherited if she remarries before her husband is found or declared dead. The final vote in the Senate was 45-0. The bill also disinherits any child born more than nine months after the woman's husband is declared missing. In either case, the estate would be handed over to the soldier's relatives.[22]

The legal implications that prompted the bill were apparent in the accompanying transcript of the discussion in the legislature before the bill was passed. A Pennsylvania resident, who was the wife of an MIA helicopter pilot shot down in 1968, had gone ahead and remarried before her husband was declared dead by either Congress or his branch of the military. Representative William Wilt, who introduced the bill, was quoted as saying,

> The parents are concerned because if their son is declared dead at some later date, his wife could admit she perjured herself on the second marriage certificate. Then she could have that second marriage annulled and collect on the estate of her first husband. After she gets the money, she could go and remarry her second husband again. The parents were told [by attorneys] that "only an act of the Legislature could protect the estate." Rep. Wilt further declared, "The Defense Department feels a Missing-in-Action is not dead until he is officially declared dead. His salary is placed in escrow in Washington.[23]

The legal aspects of marrying before the determination of death interested me from both a personal and a League standpoint. As mentioned earlier, Iris Powers was one who had learned the risks inherent with remarriage without physical evidence of a body all too well. As noted earlier, her husband turned up alive following the end of World War II, after being MIA for years and ultimately declared dead. He came back, and there she was married to someone else. None of it was her fault, but there surely must have been extreme emotional trauma for all three people concerned.

There was no question that time took its toll on the wives, just as time and the rigors of incarceration were doubtless taking a toll on our men. The wives of POWs and MIAs were locked in invisible cells of silence and waiting. Many could not stand the loneliness and fear or the deprivation of emotion and being loved. So they embarked on affairs. Some even moved in with their lovers, caring little about what society or their families might think. Since they'd broken no laws, there was little the government could do to punish them. Others divorced their absent mates after finding someone else to establish a life with, or have children with, before their child-bearing years were gone.

Tangee Alvarez was one who gave up. Her husband, Navy Lieutenant Everett Alvarez, was the first POW captured in North Vietnam (August, 1964) and one of the examples the League used to demonstrate how long the men had been imprisoned. We were shocked to learn in December 1971 that Tangee had divorced her husband in absentia and remarried. Her marriage created an uproar in the national press, an outcry in Congress, and general denunciation of her character. Did she really deserve that? Who can sit in judgment on the length of human endurance? Who else had walked in her shoes for seven years to earn the right to condemn her? Everett Alvarez continued to endure his fate, suffering, marking time, hoping the government would someday make a move to free him, but Tangee had decided to move on with her life.

Other wives, like Evelyn Guarino, remained faithful and hopeful. Like most of us, Evelyn worried about how a gap in their married life and in the lives of their four sons could ever be overcome. At least she'd had occasional correspondence from her husband over the years. Evelyn Guarino was very active with the League's speaking and letter writing campaigns in Florida. Three of their sons had grown up, married and had children while their father

remained a POW in Hanoi. Their oldest son, Allan, was now
grown, and an Air Force pilot himself. Allan had served in Vietnam
while his Dad was still a POW there. When and if the POWs were
released, Col. Larry Guarino (shot down as a young Air Force
Major aged 44, in 1965, with four young sons) would return to his
family a grandfather, find his eldest son a young Air Force pilot, and
meet daughters-in-law and grandkids he'd never seen. How would
he react to this extended family, after so many years in solitary confinement?[24]

These were the things we thought about at the League, for we
all faced the somewhat scary, and at the same time exhilarating and
hoped-for, eventuality of our POW's return home. That, or else the
more sorrowful truth revealed. I believed that was my ordained
fate—accepting the finality of widowhood, with grieving families
to console, fatherless children to rear, and grandfatherless grandba-
bies to welcome into the world alone someday.

Meanwhile, there was the present, so I pushed my own circumstances aside for the time being. I had a preliminary meeting at the
United Nations on November 17, and the League Board met again
with Dr. Henry Kissinger at the White House on November 18. At
this critical juncture in the peace negotiations, we figured the more
pressure the families could bring to bear, the better.

I returned to the U.N. on November 29, this time accompanied
by astronaut Admiral Alan Shepard, League member Joe McCain,
and several others. Ambassador George H.W. Bush greeted the
League representatives at the U.S. Mission to the United Nations.
Then, Rita Hauser and Admiral Alan Shepard spoke to a U.N. delegation of nearly one hundred people. They talked about my petition and the POW/MIA situation in general. They specifically
addressed ways in which the failure of North Vietnam to adhere to
the Geneva Conventions in their treatment and accounting of
POWs affected not only the men's families, but the world at large.
Then Joe McCain did his usual excellent presentation of the
Discrepancies, and everyone seemed very impressed with that.
Afterward, Ambassador Bush asked to see my Petition, and asked
me some questions about it, and my thoughts on the violation of
the Geneva Conventions.

Then he asked Joe and me to explain the Discrepancy Board to him in more detail. We were very flattered and grateful that he showed such intense interest in the work we were doing on these two issues.

I felt that it was a very successful trip. I couldn't believe that soon it would be December again. The boys and I faced another holiday season without Newk, our sixth. I concentrated on League business so I wouldn't have to think about that. Gratefully, I turned my attention instead to the League's finances.

Thomas V. Jones, President and Chairman of Northrop Corporation, signed a letter to heads of major U.S. corporations. In it, he supported the League and requested they encourage their companies to have fundraisers or make donations to support the League and its cause. He reminded the corporate officials that "whatever our views on that [Vietnam War] issue, we can stand united on the POW/MIA question." He asked them to help the League of Families finance a national publicity campaign for 1972. "American industry has an obligation to help these families in their

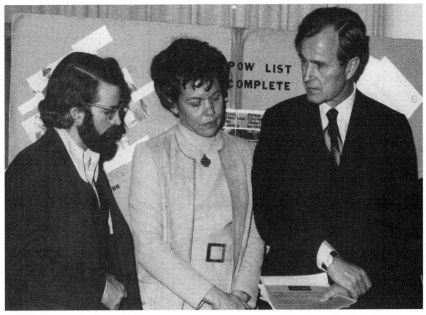

Joe McCain and Evelyn Grubb meet with United Nations Ambassador George H.W. Bush, to present her Human Rights Petition to the United Nations, Human rights violations by North Vietnam regarding U.S. POWs and MIAs. December 1971.

C. Zumwalt, Grubb family files

mission. I urge your generous support for this worthy organization."[25]

Ross Perot continued to support our efforts. He called me that December and suggested that the League send a delegation to Paris and that I contact the White House to see how they reacted to the idea. He said he'd find a sponsor for our trip, *if* we were willing to follow his advice on how to handle the trip, and *if* we'd take some of the kids, and some tapes, with us. That was typical Ross—he always wanted things done his way.

I arranged a meeting with Secretary of Defense Melvin Laird on the morning of December 15 to discuss several things. My first order of business was the suggestions we had made regarding the needs of our men and their families upon repatriation. Secretary Laird advised us that there was already a firm, adequate plan in place. He reminded us that most POWs would need to undergo debriefing and treatment in military hospitals, some only for a short time, others perhaps longer. I responded that families must be prepared for these delays and made aware of the reasons behind them. Secretary Laird offered to set up an appointment for us with Dr. Wilbur to discuss any problem areas. Dr. Wilbur was developing repatriation plans for the DOD. We then discussed how the military might handle promoters who wanted to latch onto the POWs for commercial purposes.

I brought up the idea of a trip to Paris to the Peace Talks from the League's, not Mr. Perot's, standpoint. Laird agreed that the families needed to do something positive. We suggested that some of the families fly to Paris with family tapes and extensive news coverage, pick up the mail that had been sent by Americans to the DRV representatives of the Paris Peace Talks, and deliver the mail to Hanoi.[26] Defense Secretary Laird was interested in the idea and suggested that we could time the trip to coincide with Ambassador Porter's stand on the failure of Hanoi to abide by the Geneva Conventions.[27] He said he'd check on it and get back to us.

Meanwhile we started planning the trip. We lined up contacts at AP, CBS, *Newsweek* and other media outlets that might cover the story. On December 20 we discussed ideas for the Paris trip with Dr. Roger Shields, and covered the actions we wanted to take.

• Bring family tapes to Paris to be sent to Hanoi as Christmas presents for our men being held there as POWs, presented in person by representative POW families to the DRV representatives in Hanoi.

- Hold a vigil of the families in front of the DRV Embassy in Paris.
- Tour the warehouse full of undelivered letters with reporters and show the American public how little the DRV cared about their effort.
- Make personal pleas to the DRV to show our goodwill and request humane treatment.
- Point out that although we were proceeding with "Vietnamization" of the war and withdrawing our troops, the DRV had shown no action of reciprocity as promised. Suggest they release all U.S. prisoners being held in South Vietnam as a gesture of their good will.
- Publicize that the mail flow from our men has not improved. It has gotten worse. In the period May-October 1970, the families had received a total of 130 letters from known POWs in Vietnam. This year, in the same period, a total of only 170 letters had been received from the Vietnam prisoners. During either period, there were no letters from POWs held in Laos and Cambodia. For just the prisoners *we knew about,* the minimum mail requirements under the Geneva Conventions were 4000 letters and 8000 cards in each of those six month periods.

As the war marched on toward another New Year, more American men joined the captured or missing list, and more families joined the League. For any other organization, an increase in membership is a positive statistic. But for the League of Families, our goal was to go out of business, after all the POWs and MIAs were either home or identified.

By December 20, 1971, Pan American Airways had committed twenty complimentary seats for the Paris trip and Ross Perot had offered to finance it. We had high hopes for what we might accomplish. It was holiday time again. The families had nothing to cling to, and from the looks of things, nothing to hope for. We had to do *something* to sustain hope.

The boys and I were invited to participate in the White House

Christmas Tree lighting ceremony, and we did. It was a beautiful, touching and very inspiring event. Two rows of magnificent Christmas trees were installed on the lawn in front of the White House. Each tree was decorated with ornaments upon which were written the names of Vietnam POWs and MIAs from every state and territory of the United States. The White House incorporation of our men into the national Christmas celebration helped the families face another lonely holiday season.

I drove back home to Colonial Heights from Washington on December 23, determined to create a happy, normal Christmas for my own family. The boys were waiting for me and could barely contain their excitement.

"Wait till you see our tree," Roy announced proudly.

"Yeah," Roke added, a mischievous glint in his eye. "We cut it down ourselves. It's a real Christmas tree."

They pulled me into the living room, and I burst out laughing. I couldn't help myself—it was the funniest tree I had ever seen!

"Isn't it a great tree, Mom?"

"Yes, it's a great tree," I gasped, still giggling, remembering the gorgeous indoor White House trees, and the others that stood outside it, equally magnificent, lining the White House lawn. The ornament with Newk's name on it hung on the Pennsylvania Christmas tree.

Our magnificent tree at home in Colonial Heights had a trunk that was turned and bent like a crooked old man, and had barely 15 branches on it. But it was the first tree the boys had ever found in the woods, cut down, and dragged home themselves. It was *their* Christmas tree. Bruce Carlson had taken Mother and the boys to the woods "to find and cut us a *real* Christmas tree" as Roy put it. We decorated the tree with abandon, and that scrawny, crooked tree brought outright laughter and joy to our Christmas that year, something we'd nearly forgotten existed.

We spent Christmas Day at Mother's. Bruce and Sharon Carlson were there with us, and Mother cooked her usual fantastic dinner. It was a cozy, warm-glow kind of family occasion. My gratitude to Bruce and Sharon was boundless. They brought such normalcy to the boys' lives! They were and are truly wonderful, caring people. We are still in touch.

Newk, of course, was very much in our thoughts and prayers that Christmas of 1971. I realized that my longing for him now was not the kind of deep, tearing pain of grief and anger I'd felt on each of the previous five Christmases. This longing was different. Our crooked and bent lives, like our Christmas tree, were different now, too.

Six years of silence from Newk had resulted in six years of unbelievable anxiety, pain and grieving, bewilderment and, for me, a lot of deep, unfathomable anger. This year, I made sure there was room and time for laughter, a lot of spiritual uplift, and unfettered joy in celebrating Christmas for our family, and our boys. It was the least I could do in memory of the man I loved, who loved the holidays like a kid himself.

President Nixon and his two chief negotiators, national security advisor Dr. Henry Kissinger and Philip Habib of the U.S. delegation to the Paris Peace Talks, worked during Christmas to try and broker a peace agreement that would extricate us from the Vietnam War with honor. Not surprisingly, the Democratic Republic of Vietnam remained as recalcitrant and uncooperative as ever. Habib, a career diplomat who had served as U.S. minister-counselor at the Saigon Embassy from 1965-1966, was a specialist in Vietnamese affairs. But even with his and all of Dr. Kissinger's expertise, the U.S. delegation could make no identifiable "public" progress toward peace. Nor were there any positive prospects for the release of our POWs.[28]

Given that, none of us were shocked or surprised when the League's December trip to Paris was not as successful as we'd hoped it might be. I was not with the group that went to Paris. Too much was going on at the office in Washington. One incident during that trip, though, really stood out. The families did not get the approval they sought to fly onward to Hanoi. They remained in Paris and tried to bring world attention to the plight of the POW/MIA families. They requested an appointment to meet with representatives of North Vietnam who were in Paris. The North Vietnamese delegates to the Paris Peace Talks, and the North Vietnamese Embassy, flatly refused. The League visitors were 0 for 2, with the jury still out on the world attention try, but our League group had one last idea up their collective sleeves, and elected to go for it full bore.

Before they departed for Paris, we'd learned that the boxes and bags of the thousands of letters sent by Americans to the Democratic Republic of Vietnam in care of their representatives in Paris had been shoved into a warehouse there, and totally ignored. After they arrived in Paris, our League group had somehow procured two big dump trucks and, with the help of a team of international volunteers, had somehow gained access to that warehouse. They filled both truck beds with the bags of neglected letters and drove them to the front gates of North Vietnam's Embassy. There, they tried to deliver the letters to the DRV Ambassador. When the guards refused to admit them, our group simply backed the trucks up to the closed front gates, and unceremoniously dumped all the letters there! Before they drove away, they had left sacks of letters piled to the very top of the gates. For awhile, no one could enter or leave the DRV Embassy by its front entrance.[29] Our little group pulled the "letter blockade" off nicely (with tacit help from the French). The POW/MIA families and the League got great press and television coverage in the United States and Europe. It also boosted our morale to have made even that small, silly triumph over the stonewall tactics of the North Vietnamese, who were "still intransigent," as President Nixon had put it.

Most importantly for our purpose, the people of the world had seen on television and in the newspapers and knew from the piled-high bags of letters that the American people had written, that we were indeed concerned about our missing and imprisoned men. We cared about them and wrote letters to Hanoi that said so. Lots of letters. Enough letters to obscure the front gates of the DRV Embassy from view. We had scored our point.

As the year waned, the Vietnam War continued, and more men became POWs. On the night of December 29, 1971, I wrote in my journal:

> The reality must come sooner or later to them that the men held in a prisoner of war/missing in action status are in a most precarious predicament—both in Southeast Asia and here at home. It is this reality that shatters the confidence of their families in our government, in our Administration, and in our fellow Americans. I am surrounded by a sea of suspicion. We families live day by day torn between faith

and fear—a dual existence that is unbearable, yet must be borne. Our men, who should be heroes, have become symbols of terrible futility, with no reasonable solution to their desperate situation. The families—compromised in political complicity, are floundering for solutions—any solutions—that will get their men out of that Hell called the 'Southeast Asia conflict.' I rarely cry any more, but tonight I weep for them all, and most of all for my four sons. I cannot counsel them any more to have faith, or to have hope—for at this point I have lost both myself.

After six years of limbo, I still had plenty of questions, and no answers. But I still had three powerful things to see me through the rest of this . . . 1) Family—Mother, the Grubbs, my brother Bill's family, Newk's sister Beverly, and our four sons; 2)My Faith in God. That gave me the determination to keep marching forward. 3) The League of Families. That kept me focused and saved my sanity during these longest years. Since I could still pray, I could add a fourth: 4) Hope for others, since for this family I believed all hope was gone.

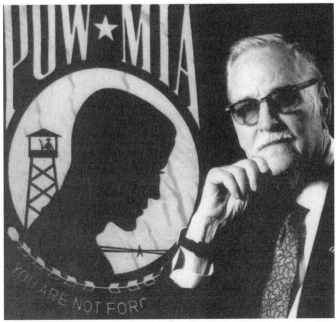

Newt Haisley, pilot and WWII veteran, designer of the POW/MIA flag.

9 Searching the World for Solutions

TIMELINE . . . 1972 . . . <u>WORLD</u> . . . ISRAELI ATHLETES AT MUNICH OLYMPICS KIDNAPPED, MASSACRED . . . NIXON VISITS CHINA . . . WWII JAPANESE SOLDIER FOUND ALIVE IN CAVE ON GUAM AFTER 27 YEARS . . . <u>VIETNAM</u> . . . NIXON REVEALS SECRET PEACE TALKS . . . NORTH VIETNAM INVADES SOUTH IN EASTER OFFENSIVE . . . U.S. MINES, BLOCK-ADES HAIPHONG HARBOR . . . THREATENS BOMBING RESUMPTION . . . <u>USA</u> . . . WATER-GATE BREAK-IN . . . FBI HEAD J. EDGAR HOOVER DIES . . . *THE GODFATHER* WINS BEST PICTURE OSCAR® . . .

To be the wife of a man who is MIA or a POW is to live in a suspended world where life must still go on.
—Lt. Clemmer L. Slayton, USAF

January 1972 opened a new fiscal year, and I was pleased to hear from Dr. Herb Ladley that the League of Families was in much better financial shape than it had been when I became Coordinator three months ago. We were solidly in the black at the moment, but our situation was fluid, and we'd need to raise more funds soon. One of our most dedicated advisors, Dr. Ladley kept tabs on our precarious finances. My daily routine was a continuous round of phone calls and meetings. I had a full schedule every day that often went into late at night.

Carole Hansen, Chairman of the Board, presided at our January Board meeting. Herb Ladley informed us then that "we are receiving about $2 now, for every $1 spent." This amount was not enough to accomplish our goals, but better than being in the red, I thought.[1]

Next, we learned that our campaign to get television network air time for our PSAs (public service announcements) being created by the Ad Council had been stopped in its tracks by a "strong complaint" to the FCC by someone. Our attorney, Charles Havens, informed us about this news. The League had put a substantial amount of money and effort into those ads. Charlie said that he had personally spoken with Dean Fritchen of the Ad Council, but did not know who had sent a "strong complaint."

"He wouldn't give me proof in writing about it," Charlie replied. "He just said, 'It's because they are controversial, with no explanation.'"

SSC&B Ad Agency had developed both 30-second and 60-second spots for us. I had seen them. They were very moving presentations and were completely nonpolitical. Therefore, the "controversial" complaint to the FCC had to be from some powerful antiwar individual or group. "Well, let's be sure to remind the Ad Council that the League still has a credit of $11,000 with them," said Dr. Ladley, clearly annoyed. "We'll want that money put to some good use in the near future."

I was more than annoyed. "I have an appointment with the Ad Council in New York on January 10," I said. "Shall I cancel it?" The consensus of the Board was that I should keep the appointment. I was anxious to find out just who had made that complaint to the FCC, and why.

"I could write letters to the presidents of the three major networks and ask for their ruling on our TV spots in writing," Charlie suggested. We approved that. After that blow, I was pleased to inform the Board and advisors that the League would receive $20,000 from a POW/MIA Christmas Seals campaign from our Colorado Springs chapter. That brought a smile back to a lot of faces, especially Dr. Ladley's.

1972 was also a Presidential election year. We discussed the feasibility of participating in the platform committee meetings prior to the Democratic and Republican National Conventions. Our appearance at both parties' platform committee hearings would help gain some national publicity for our cause. However, it might be construed by some members as overtly political. Given that our innocuous TV spots had been construed as "controversial," which was enough to block them, I was understandably concerned with protecting the League's nonpartisan position. The Board decided that addressing both major parties equally wouldn't be seen as overtly political, and the Board finally agreed that we'd send a representative to speak to both Platform Committee hearings.

On January 10, I met with our Ad Council team in New York and explained our position on the TV spots and the rationale behind them. The Ad Council representatives wanted to bring an "idea man" in to brief me. "No, thank you." I said. "I don't need to talk to an idea man, since our spots are already completed, and I've seen them. They are short, non-controversial, nonpolitical, and have been approved by our Board. We are ready for your *commitment* to air them, on the part of the Ad Council."

They countered that our agency, SSG&B, would be willing to go ahead with our publicity spots, but only as paid advertising by us, not as PSAs. SSG&B had estimated that the cost to the League for that would be about $20,000. I ended the meeting there. Something deeper was behind all this "controversial" stalling.

I took the suggestion that we have the spots aired as paid advertising to our next Board meeting. We decided it would be too costly for too little exposure. We tabled the project. Later, we learned from the FCC that the complaint had come from our own defectors: "The POW/MIA Families for Immediate Release," the splinter, politically active group started by Val Kushner and Louise Mulligan. I couldn't fathom that when our mutual goal certainly was to improve POW/MIA conditions and obtain prisoner identification and immediate release of the wounded! I guess they were putting all their backing on total, unconditional, immediate release of the prisoners. We all wanted that, but I didn't see it happening without a peace agreement. Whatever their reasoning, they had deliberately sabotaged us, and succeeded in derailing our effort to raise public awareness through PSAs. We'd just have to wait for the response from Charlie's letters to the network presidents to see what they had to say.

I was discouraged, but the great response we had to the full-page publicity piece we ran in *Reader's Digest* was a consolation. We received tremendous response from that piece, many with enclosed donations. It proved to us that ordinary people in America *were* interested in the POW/MIA cause, which was gratifying.

On January 15, 1972, I had a letter from Colonel Luther, informing me that Newk's promotion to Lieutenant Colonel was now official.[2] That was another feel good/feel bad moment for our family. We were of course proud that this had occurred. We were devastated at the thought that we couldn't share and celebrate this great milestone with Newk. The Air Force didn't congratulate us either, but stated only, "We have advised the Air Force Accounting and Finance Center of this promotion and they will make appropriate changes . . . "

January 25 was cold and raw in Washington. One year from now, the elections would be over, and whoever has won the Presidency will have been inaugurated. What would this year bring to our suffering families, I wondered? That evening, I settled in front of the television at the apartment in Foggy Bottom to watch President Nixon speak to America about our latest proposal to end the war. In a surprising turn, Nixon openly discussed the status of the war and POW situation in Vietnam. He described the war situation as it had been when he took office: We had 550,000 American fighting men in Vietnam and an average of 300 per week killed in action. He observed that "the only thing that had been settled in Paris at that time was the shape of the conference table." He certainly spoke the truth there. I had often commented that the Paris Peace Conference table should be shaped like a toilet, with a giant flusher that could be activated whenever the talks stalled, which seemed to occur almost daily.

President Nixon said that he believed he had only two options for peace: 1) the path of negotiation, which, though preferred, had not worked (and hearing that, my heart almost stopped at what might be coming), and 2) the path of Vietnamization, the option he had chosen. Well, neither was working all that well. Our troops in Vietnam had been withdrawn in substantial numbers, but the South Vietnamese government was still too weak to fend off the communists from the north. The President continued,

> Two weeks ago, you will recall, I announced that by May 1st, American forces in Vietnam would be down to 69,000. That means almost one half million Americans will have been brought home from Vietnam over the past three years. In terms of American lives, the losses of 300 a week have been reduced . . . to less than 10 a week.

He revealed then that Dr. Henry Kissinger had indeed been conducting secret peace negotiations in Paris since August of 1969, which confirmed the rumors that had circulated for the past three years. The President said that the French President Georges

Pompidou had arranged twelve secret peace meetings between Dr. Kissinger and North Vietnamese Minister Xuan Thuy. He said that General Alexander Haig was with Dr. Kissinger during those secret negotiations. President Nixon continued,

> Now, however, it is my judgment that the purposes of peace will best be served by bringing out publicly the proposals we have been making in private.

Then President Nixon listed the long series of proposals that Dr. Kissinger had made, all of which had been totally rejected by North Vietnam. He listed some proposals North Vietnam had made that the United States had rejected. Then came description of some that were partly accepted and partly rejected by both sides and one that the North Vietnamese presented in public and the United States negotiated in private. Whereby, the President said, the Vietnamese berated us publicly for not responding to their proposal when they knew full well we had responded to it privately.

> They induced many Americans in the press and in the Congress into echoing their propaganda—Americans who could not know they were being used by the enemy to stir up divisiveness in this country.

President Nixon also revealed that the United States and the DRV Government of North Vietnam had agreed in October to hold another meeting in late November of last year. It was now January, and Nixon still hadn't heard anything more from the North Vietnamese. Meanwhile, they continued to increase their troop infiltration into Laos and Cambodia.

The speech went on and on. I was nearly asleep by the time he finally addressed the POW/MIA situation. He said he'd instructed Ambassador Porter to present *our* peace plan next Thursday at the Paris Peace Talks, and the essence of the plan was (I held my breath):

> Within six months of an Agreement:
> • We shall withdraw all U.S. and allied forces from South Vietnam.
> • We shall exchange all prisoners of war.
> • There shall be a cease-fire throughout Indochina.

- There shall be a new Presidential election in South
Vietnam.

I let my breath out—whoosh! He included the exchange of
POWs in the proposal for peace! *But . . . he'd said nothing about
accounting for the MIAs or those who had died in captivity!* Perhaps the
accounting of MIAs was part of "exchange all prisoners of war." I
jumped up to get paper and pen so I could make some notes on
questions for our next meeting with Dr. Kissinger. I also quickly
wrote down two other statements by the President that caught my
attention, lest I forget them:

1. We will pursue any approach that will speed negotiations.
2. Because some parts of this agreement could prove more
   difficult to negotiate than others, we would be willing to
   begin implementing certain military aspects while negotiations continue on the implementing of other issues . . .

I didn't like that at all! "Any approach" sounded ominous and
left everything open-ended. "Other issues" *might* mean the return
of the POWs or the accounting of the MIAs and those who died
in captivity, or it might not. The Geneva Conventions called for
specific accounting of those known to have died in captivity. I definitely wanted a full accounting from the DRV for Newk, and for
any others who died while in the hands of the North Vietnamese.

The President spoke on, but my attention wandered. I worried
over the phrases that pertained to our POW/MIA cause. *Those
statements are going to be open to a lot of interpretation,* I realized.
Wrap-up statements like "We are ready to negotiate peace immediately . . ." and "We want to end the war not only for America but
for all the people of Indochina . . ." floated in my consciousness. It
was an election year, all right, and Nixon wanted to be re-elected.
When President Nixon looked like he was finishing his speech, I
shook myself, sat up straighter, and paid close attention.

This has been the longest, the most difficult war in
American history. Honest and patriotic Americans have
disagreed as to whether we should have become involved at
all nine years ago; and there has been disagreement on the
conduct of the war. The proposal I have made tonight is one
on which we all can agree. Let us unite now, unite in our

search for peace—a peace that is fair to both sides—a peace
that can last.[3]

The President thus far had failed to fulfill the promise of his
first campaign: to end the war, and bring the prisoners home. Four
more long years of war had passed. He was cornered now and fighting back. He was also caught in a vise. An end to the Vietnam War
would assuredly get him reelected. *But at what cost to our men and
their families? Would he leave some behind, dead or alive?*

Following that speech, one positive thing happened: The families of POWs were suddenly receiving more letters from Hanoi.
That was something to applaud.

Meanwhile, the League made no further progress with the Ad
Council and the public service project than Dr. Kissinger had made
with the Vietnamese at the Paris Peace Talks. We hadn't received
the check for the Christmas Seal donations from the Colorado
chapter yet, either. We were hurting financially. The good news was
that the Colorado check was expected to be considerably higher
than $20,000 and possibly closer to $30,000. I welcomed that, since
our working fund was down to $8,000, not enough to cover our
immediate overhead. But we were not operating in the red, and that
was a plus. Unfortunately, there was no quick solution in sight to
our financial dilemma, and no solution to our goal: Achieving
humane treatment and full accounting for our POWs, MIAs, and
KIA (in captivity).

Charlie informed us we had received the letters from the heads
of CBS, NBC, and ABC television networks, telling us they would
not run the League of Families' public service spot. Again, antiwar
politics reared its ugly head, as it often did lately. Despite the
President's urging that we unite as Americans in our quest for
peace, the antiwar protesters, many of them famous national figures, marched, cursed, demonstrated, and practiced civil disobedi-
ence. Some, like Jane Fonda, went to Hanoi and gave aid and comfort to the enemy.[4] All while North Vietnam, and some Americans,
refuted the League of Families' attempt to give aid and comfort to
our American men being held as POWs there. The protesters
spoke adamantly and raucously against the war, the U.S. government, and its policies. They vilified our American servicemen and
POW's for even participating in the war. They got plenty of free

TV exposure from CBS, NBC, and ABC, and reams of press coverage, all of it free. That frustrated and angered us because it played right into the hands of the North Vietnamese, whom we now knew from former POWs took every opportunity to capitalize on the dissent in the United States and use it against the helpless prisoners.[5]

Everyone rioting and marching seemed to be in favor of individual freedom without restriction. It was hardly surprising that in such a hostile cultural climate the war was a lightning rod for rebellion, a reason to shatter and toss out the old rules. Those of us who represented the U.S. military felt spurned, taunted, reviled and ignored by this new social wave, and we were bewildered and deeply hurt by it. This election year promised to be one of the most angry, volatile election years in history. It seemed to me that the world had become a theater for violence. The violence of Vietnam was an ongoing nightmare. There also were airplane hijackings, race riots, attempted assassinations, fighting in Ireland, fighting in the Middle East, and always more difficulties with Russia, as the "Cold War" continued.

I was aware of all that was going on and concerned about it. However, I realized I had to stay focused on our League's goals. We were going to get our fighting men out of those hellhole prisons of Southeast Asia! Politics aside, the fate of these men mattered to us and should matter to every American. So we struggled with changing attitudes and floundered for solutions ourselves. It was like being caught in a time warp, a psychedelic nightmare from which we couldn't awaken.

The League was preparing for another "Mayday!" meeting on May 5-7 at the Marriott. In the midst of advance preparations, Jan and Cathy Ray decided to resign from the League. Their resignations couldn't have come at a worse time. Fortunately, Lou Stockstill, author of the POW article in *Reader's Digest,* now our Press Advisor, had agreed to run this year's meeting. Lou, always resourceful, would surely find a couple of good volunteers to replace the Ray girls for the Mayday meeting, but I knew I'd really miss them on a day-to-day basis at the national office.

On March 10, 1972, I was invited to the White House for a signing ceremony where President Nixon declared March 26- April 1 a "National Week of Concern for the POW/MIAs." That

"Week of Concern" had become an annual event that included nationwide ceremonies, prayer meetings, and expressions of sympathy coordinated and executed by our fantastic State Coordinators of the National League of Families. It created national recognition of our cause during that week, and was a time we definitely paused to remember and pray for our men. I wished the Week of Concern could create some solutions, too. Our State Coordinators did an excellent job of organizing their State's communities in this endeavor and helped plan and execute events in their respective states.[6]

The League also had a soft spot in its heart for the children of POW/MIAs. These children suffered the same pain that my four sons were enduring. They needed to know that their dads were not forgotten, and were important to America. I was always pleased to learn about the great numbers of Americans, including some who had lived through World War II and Korea, and some of our great sports figures, who were showering our POW/MIA kids with the total generosity of heart and spirit for which Americans are known all over the world.

Football star Johnny Unitas and Carmella La Spada had formed a group called "No Greater Love" backed by sports greats Joe DiMaggio, Althea Gibson, Joe Louis, Jesse Owens, Arnold Palmer, and Ted Williams. The membership of No Greater Love consisted of stellar athletes from just about every American and Olympic sport. The group's mission was for a "nonprofit national volunteer organization to serve hospitalized veterans, servicemen overseas," and to be a "program of friendship and care for America's special children, like the 2050 children of Americans who are Prisoners of War or Missing in Action in Indochina."[7]

"No Greater Love" arranged for the children of POWs and MIAs to attend sporting events, meet sports figures and other dignitaries, and receive sports memorabilia and calendars. Major magazines like *Sports Illustrated* and sporting goods companies also participated. This group provided a great boost to the kids' morale and I will be forever grateful to them for what they did to cheer my family during those dark days.

Jeff was now 15, Roland (Roke) was 10, Stephen (Van) was 8, and Roy was 5. Although Jeff could seldom attend, due to high school activities and later his college schedule, they all enjoyed the

"No Greater Love" activities that they could participate in. They always received sports calendars at Christmas. In 1971, First Lady Patricia Nixon and her daughter Julie had attended "No Greater Love's" Christmas party for the POW/MIA children, a big thrill for all of the kids that were there. Jeff was still being very supportive of the League's cause by giving talks, and writing thank you letters for me to people who wrote Letters to Hanoi.[8]

Military organizations also helped the children of the POW/MIA families. The Red River Valley Association, a Vietnam-related military group, established a scholarship fund for children of men who were lost or flew missions over North Vietnam. In 1971, they awarded fifteen $1,000 scholarships. The chairman of their scholarship fund, Colonel Howard C. Johnson, told me they would do the same again in 1972. The midshipmen from the Naval Academy volunteered to be Pen Pals for the POW/MIA kids and the Air Force Academy looked into sponsoring a similar program. Another organization, called "Alaskans Care POW/MIA" offered a summer vacation in Alaska to any graduating high school senior who was the child of a POW or MIA. Their Alaskan Safari 1972 included deep sea fishing, canoe trips, gold panning, glacier explorations, and trips to the north slope oil fields. The organization provided airline travel, accommodations, expenses, and constant supervision for the kids.

The League also worked through its state chapters to get state-sponsored college scholarship programs for POW/MIA children. State-sponsored scholarships for the kids of their POW/MIA servicemen would be an immense help to the families. We were gratified when Congress passed a bill that required the service academies to offer automatic entrance to all academically qualified POW/MIA dependents. These kids had only to follow the established application process through their congressional representatives.

Now that we had our own official banner symbol of the League of Families to use on our media pieces, we continued to concentrate heavily on publicity to keep the POW/MIA issue before the public. In addition to the new POW/MIA flag and banner, we created bumper stickers, billboards, and bus and subway publicity cards for the state chapters to distribute. I was seeing POW/MIA related bumper stickers on more and more cars as I drove home to Virginia on Friday evenings and back into Washington on Monday mornings. And the VIVA bracelets also were in great evidence on peoples wrists. Some wore more than one bracelet.

Congressman and former professional football player, Jack Kemp (R-New York), helped Evie and the families coordinate with the National Football League for military flyovers in the Missing Man formation and announcements about the POW/MIA cause at major football games. Most of our missing husbands enjoyed sports, so we were delighted to keep our absent men in the hearts and minds of American football fans. Another 1972 project was the worldwide voyage of the *Star of Peace* flying our POW/MIA flag and carrying our banner. Businessman Conrad Mikulec owned the three-masted schooner and provided free board and bunks to the all volunteer crew.

On March 24, 1972, I traveled to New York with Charles Gentry, Charlie Havens, and Joe McCain to meet the newly elected Secretary General of the United Nations, Kurt Waldheim of Austria. Colonel Mel Adams, assigned to the U.S. delegation, met us and drove us to the U.N. Building. After coffee with the U.S. mission, Secretary General Waldheim received us in his suite of offices. He was charming and openly sympathetic.

"I had family members missing during the Second World War, and I can feel for what you are going through," he said. I found it gratifying that he identified personally with our pain and anguish.[9]

Joe McCain presented his Discrepancy Report again. That featured lists, files, and a large poster board display of men known to have been captured alive but never acknowledged by Hanoi or the Viet Cong. Joe had taken our haphazard collection of discrepancy information and organized it into individual files of personnel records, proofs of capture, and published photos of the men after capture, like Newk's and Charlie Shelton's.[10] He had also developed the powerful display board with lists, photos, news clippings, and ID cards of servicemen known to be captured, but not acknowledged by the North Vietnamese. We often used Joe's Discrepancy Report and his Discrepancy Board when giving POW/MIA talks.

Joe was extremely good at presenting the Discrepancies, and we availed ourselves of his time and willingness whenever possible. Joe

McCain was a very personable young man. Slightly built, with a dark beard and ready smile, he was intense, friendly, and participated actively in the League. He was always eager to be at the office. He brought youth, boundless energy, and enthusiasm to the task. He bonded with the POW/MIA kids when they visited the national office. He played the spoons to astonish his small fry audience, and even his adult colleagues, when things got too serious around the office. As I saw it, family members like Joe McCain were the lifeblood and heart of the League and its mission. He was a staunch and reliable volunteer. The families, and their impossible position and heartache, were why we had formed the League in the first place. We were amateur volunteers. And here we were at the United Nations that March, in the office of the new Secretary General, where Joe did his usual excellent job of presenting the Discrepancy Report. We wrapped our visit by holding a press conference on the second floor. Then we lunched in the Delegates' Dining Room.

When we returned to Washington, D.C., Charley Gentry critiqued our trip to the U.N. "We did all right, but we could have done better. We should have given heavier accent to the Geneva Conventions and emphasized the other signatory nations' *responsibility* to bring pressure on North Vietnam to adhere to those Conventions."[11] Charley volunteered to write to Secretary-General Waldheim and U.S. Ambassador Stillman and request that the applicable sections of the Third Geneva Convention be read before the General Assembly.

That March, a story came out in the *Penn State Alumni Association Magazine* about Newk and me. It featured my work with the League of Families. The magazine gave substantial space to my petition to the United Nations. I knew that my late father, and Newk's Uncle Roke, and Newk, all would have been proud to read it. I missed them all, so very much! That article also brought me back into touch with former classmates and friends of ours. Many of them wrote to express their sorrow and support and hoped Newk would return alive.

Meanwhile, at the League in Washington, I arrived one morning to find that a major crisis had developed. Someone was leaking information to the press about our meetings with Dr. Henry Kissinger! Kissinger was incensed about the information leaks, and he believed they came either from me, the League Board, or someone on my office staff. His staff member informed me that Dr. Kissinger was seriously considering canceling all future briefings with the League, if we were unable to determine the source of the leaks, and put an immediate stop to them. The thought that we might lose the candid and open dialogue we enjoyed with Dr. Kissinger or lose the access we had to privileged information on the progress of the peace talks, the war, or the POW/MIA situation, was simply unthinkable. I was horrified at the mere thought, and was almost certain the leaks couldn't have come from any of our League Board, or our staff members. I knew they certainly weren't coming from me. So it was a big shock to us all when one of our Board members admitted that he had actually concealed a tape recorder in his pocket at one meeting and taped Dr. Kissinger's remarks. Worse, he admitted he was the one who had later met with the press and leaked to them what Dr. Kissinger had said![12] I was appalled to learn that one of our Board members would do such a thing. The Board met and formally reprimanded the transgressor and the Board and I sent letters of apology to Dr. Kissinger. So did the guilty Board member, who knew he had jeopardized the League's credibility and had almost destroyed our future ability to meet with Dr. Kissinger. He was abjectly sorry and the rest of us were very angry at him, but the damage had been done and could not be undone. Fortunately, Dr. Kissinger accepted our apologies. Most important of all, he graciously continued to meet with us. However, after that incident, the format of the meetings changed. Attendance was more restricted and closely monitored. Also, the candidness and easy give and take that we formerly had enjoyed with Dr. Kissinger was more subdued. But he still answered our questions. To my eyes, he was looking more tired and overworked each time we saw him. I didn't comprehend how he stood the pressure of flying all over the globe constantly, always trying to put recalcitrant people together and create some kind of peace agreement. Yet, when he was with us in a meeting, he acted like we were the only people on his agenda at that time. I wished I could learn to do that.

The 1972 presidential campaign was heating up, and I'm sure that brought even more pressure for Kissinger to "do something" with the North Vietnamese. President Richard Nixon was the Republican Party's candidate for reelection, and George McGovern looked strong as the quintessential anti-war Democratic candidate. Many POW/MIA wives jumped into the political campaign arena, feeling it was finally their opportunity to express their personal views and their anger and frustration about U.S. war policy. Their participation did not please the military services. In April, the League received an Air Force communication, via Mary Crow, that criticized the information packets distributed by Joan Vinson's Political Action Committee.[13]

Early in April 1972, I learned that U.N. Ambassador Stillman had called Frank Sieverts, our liaison at the State Department, to say that the spokesman for the United States was going to present a statement on the violation of human rights of the POWs to the Human Rights Commission at the U.N. shortly. That was great news! I told Frank to let us know when he had the date, and we'd try to have someone there from the League. Our petition had gotten some response after all.

Elaine Hoffman, an MIA Mom, eased my correspondence backlog when she volunteered to be my personal secretary to replace Betty. She was the answer to my prayers. She soon knew my writing style and drafted letters for me. We thought alike and were compatible in every way. Her volunteer services were invaluable. My agenda continued to be packed with meetings, many now about the upcoming "Mayday!" meeting. I also needed to generate a nominating committee to select the next slate of League officers to run for election at the next National Convention in September. I had already decided that I would not be available as a candidate for a League office again. I felt that by the end of my term in October, I'd have accomplished all I could for the League of Families. The job of National Coordinator was time-consuming and filled with pressure, far more than I'd anticipated at the beginning of my term. I knew that a couple of members were interested in being the National Coordinator and that they would bring new ideas and fresh enthusiasm to the job. For me, it was time to leave. I needed some time to face my private realities and to reconnect with my sons and help them prepare for the difficult times we'd probably be facing soon. I had agreed to serve on the Board, though, which would keep me in touch with what was happening at the League.

Later that month, Bill Mitchell of the Committee to Re-Elect the President called me to say that there was a good possibility that Senator Bob Dole (R-Kansas) would again be attending our "Mayday!" meeting. We had invited all the members of Congress and the prospect that someone as prominent as Senator Dole might attend, and encourage others to attend, was very exciting news.

We also had initiated a project in tandem with the National Home Study Council to send foreign language text books to the POWs. My brother Bill already had the books committed, and they were delivered to our office pending free shipment to Hanoi. I first asked TWA for help shipping them to Southeast Asia. Dick Triby responded to my request, saying, "I'm sorry Evie, but only military flights are being cleared into Laos now, so TWA is out as far as carrying books is concerned." Maybe sending them via Bangkok, Thailand, would be easier, I thought. So, I called Pan Am next. Don Hittle called back to say he was sorry, but Pan Am could not help us unless our request was urgent to national interests. "Why don't you check with Air Vietnam or Royal Thai Airways?" he suggested. "Maybe they'll be able to help you."

I hung up and sighed. Then I wondered, "Why *can't* this project be urgent to national interests?" I picked up the phone again. Like waving a magic wand, everything came together. A couple of days later, I had approval to support our project as urgent to national interest. Don Hittle asked that the cases of books be delivered the next day to the Eastern Airlines Shuttle. Eastern had volunteered to fly the cases of books from D. C. to LaGuardia in New York. There, an American Courier volunteer would drive them to the Pan Am plane at Kennedy. The Pan Am plane would fly them to Russia, where the books would be transferred to a Russian Aeroflot and hopefully flown to Hanoi. Amazingly to me, all that did happen. However, given the previous behavior of the North Vietnamese regarding mail and packages, it was not really surprising to learn later that the POWs never received the books. Even so, the excitement and ingenuity of cooperation between multiple agencies was wonderful to witness, and again, generated some great publicity for our POW/MIA cause. It also made them feel like they had tried to do something good for our men, and it renewed my faith in American spirit and ingenuity and our "can do" ability to get things done. I needed that, because the optimism I'd felt early in the year, when President Nixon announced his peace overtures to the DRV, waned when the talks had brought no visible results months later. Here it was May, the 1972 election was looming, and the President became more aggressive about the War and resumed the bombing of North Vietnam.[14] A reporter from the *New York Times* called me to ask, "How does the League of Families feel about the bombing of Hanoi?" I referred them to our Board Chairman Carole Hansen for a response. She said, "If it will end the war and get the prisoners home, we are for it."

The Chairman of the American Communist Party, Gus Hall, returned from Hanoi and blamed the bombing for his inability to bring mail from the POWs. Cora Weiss announced that no POW mail would come via her group either, until the bombing stopped. I felt that these people were openly blackmailing the families. They were punishing us with needless anxiety and anguish. But then, we were like fish in trapped in a deep barrel, and they had the guns, so why not? Was Dr. Kissinger experiencing this kind of frustration at the peace talks, I wondered?

Lou Stockstill had once commented to me, "Evie, I'm continually amazed at the naiveté of the League in dealing with the media." Since Lou was in charge of the upcoming "Mayday!" meeting, I asked him to set up seminars that would instruct League members on how to prepare for press conferences and other media events, to stay out of trouble and still obtain optimal publicity for the League's mission. Everyone was much better at public relations after his seminars!

By the time Friday, May 5, arrived, I had worked nonstop as the National Coordinator for seven months. I still had to select a theme and write a speech to open the "Mayday!" meeting. I had finally decided what I would talk about.

First, I wanted to speak about the failure of the peace negotiations to address the return of U.S. POWs held in areas of Indochina *other than* Vietnam. I was concerned that the release of the American prisoners in Vietnam was being included in the negotiations, but there was little or no mention of the release of American POWs in South Vietnam, Laos, or Cambodia where prisoners were known to be held.

Second, I wanted to mention the sloppy coordination of official POW/MIA records in Washington. Since my initial discoveries while checking Newk's records, I had learned that there were multiple information dossiers on each POW/MIA. These were kept not only by his military service, but also by the Central Intelligence Agency, the Defense Intelligence Agency, and the Department of Defense. None of these records were being coordinated, matched, reviewed for correctness, checked for accuracy, or cross-checked and referenced. There didn't seem to be any single oversight authority for these important records. The left hand didn't know what the right hand held, and vice versa. As for the families . . . they didn't know which set of records to believe.

When the Mayday Meeting arrived, I opened my welcome speech with a strong question and answer.

> When wars end, don't ALL prisoners return, as a matter of course? The answer is a resounding NO! . . . In the Vietnam conflict, *five different Southeast Asian countries* are involved, and we have men either missing or held prisoner in each of them. Each country has a separate government from North Vietnam's, governments that will have to have a say in a settlement and in prisoner repatriation. Our military, or our government, will have to address that. In Cambodia and China, there are only a few men, but bargaining for a few may well be as complicated as bargaining for many. Most of us are already aware of the 'bargaining power' of the North Vietnamese. They discuss only what they want to, and only when they want to. Now, there is discussion going on with North Vietnam. With Laos, there has never been any dialogue, and the blind hope that settling the war with the North Vietnamese will lead to an automatic settlement in Laos seems to me to be fantasy of fantastic proportions. Too often the political talk about 'prisoners' means only those men held in North Vietnam. Do you realize that over half the men were captured in other countries? The words Laos, Cambodia, South Vietnam and China must become an automatic part of the negotiators' vocabulary when they talk of prisoner returns and accounting for the missing. It is up

to us to make sure that those other countries are included as part of the bargain of war settlement. It is something that we can—that we must do!

The United States must be prepared for all contingencies to deal with each country. The Department of Defense must be ready with information on *all* our men, and most importantly, our adversaries in Southeast Asia must be forced to a settlement that meets our requirements. When a man's life depends on facts recorded some four to six years ago, no excuses of 'lost records' should be allowed to jeopardize his destiny. Every known item that exists on every man must be placed on record in one location. Computers must be made available, and every fact, rumor, photo, or description from everywhere must be gathered and made available in one place for quick access. Perhaps it is time to be alarmists!

. . . This is the challenge for the coming year, and it is a challenge that requires many hours of work and effort. With your help, the League can do it . . . the challenge rests with us! The rousing ovation I received told me that I touched a nerve with the audience.[15]

Shortly afterward, Sergeant Everhart of the Association of the U.S. Army called our office and asked what they could do to help the League.[16] I replied, "Tell your organization we need money to keep going." On the following Wednesday he handed me a check, bless him.

Several of us had been working on a League trip in late May to Switzerland to meet with the International Committee of the Red Cross at their big meeting. We had also arranged to present our case to several other countries while we were in Europe. "Getting press coverage for this trip will be a good way to bring more international attention to our POWs in Southeast Asia, *vis-à-vis* the Geneva Conventions," Carole Hansen reported to the Board. "I mentioned the trip to President Nixon in a recent meeting and he assured me the White House would help." She turned to me, "Check with Brent Scowcroft for some good contacts in Europe, Evie. He'll be glad to help you." Brent was another of those wonderful folks who were always there when we needed them. He had struck up a friendship with my son Roke, who had sat at his table at a dinner function once, and Brent always asked about him, and wanted to know how he was doing. None of them knew just how important those small personal expressions of interest were to families and kids that were outcasts in America, derided by their friends as Jeff and Roke often were, because of the antiwar sentiment and our association with the military. Mean people never stopped to think that we were suffering the separation from, and possible loss of, our most loved one, too.

I planned to be along on this trip to test foreign waters and to see if I could scare up some information about Newk, or the other men on the list of Discrepancies, like Charlie Shelton. I would be accompanied by Lou Stockstill, as the League's official News and Information Director, Joe McCain as Chairman of the Discrepancy Committee, Carole Hansen our Board Chairman, and Nancy Perisho, Assistant Coordinator for Illinois. Nancy, who traveled with us at her own expense, was the designated representative for the MIA families. We arrived at the Geneva airport May 22, 1972, in the early morning. The air was crisp, and the sky a brilliant blue. Chestnut trees with fragrant blossoms were in full bloom. One sniff and I was transported back to our little trailer house of long ago in Chambley, France, where two large chestnut trees had stood in our front yard. I pictured Newk there, holding the hands of Jeff and Roke, two little tykes then, as they had walked toward our old black Citroen car parked between the trees to go shopping. I was overwhelmed by the sweet memory of that scene and, without warning, tears began to stream down my cheeks. When the others noticed and expressed concern, I pulled myself together, and explained,

"Sorry . . . I'm having one of those happy/sad memories of Newk that sometimes comes with a particular view or smell. This time, it was the blooming chestnut trees."

Our main goal in Geneva was to present the Discrepancy Report to the International Committee of the Red Cross and to show North Vietnam's crass refusal to adhere to the tenets of the Geneva Conventions. We met with Idar Rimstad, U.S. Ambassador to Switzerland; Kaj Falkman, a deputy in the Swedish Foreign Ministry, Secretary General of Red Cross Societies Heinrik Beer; Assistant to the ICRC President, Michel Barde; and

Jean Ott, delegate for Southeast Asia, along with staff members from their offices. Joe gave a compelling presentation of the Discrepancy Report. While the ICRC officials attending were cordial to us, they didn't offer much hope or specific help. They expressed reluctance to pursue the discrepancies by inquiring about any individuals by name, and when we asked about pressing the DRV for capture cards, Monsieur Barde assured us that had been tried before with no response. On the other hand, Heinrik Beer was very sympathetic and unequivocally supportive of our efforts. He agreed to study the problem further and gave us a list of other Red Cross officials to see. At a later meeting, we also learned from Mr. Rameseyer, Assistant for the Minister of Switzerland, that the Swiss had sent an Ambassador to Hanoi but his credentials had not yet been presented. He tentatively suggested that, when they had been presented, the Swiss might then be able to address this issue again.[17]

Carole Hansen and I ate breakfast on our lovely balcony in the mornings, enjoying the beauty of Geneva and its lake before setting out for our stressful all-day sessions of pleading and begging for help from the international allies we needed to come to our aid.

Tired after all the meetings, with little to show for it except exposure of the League and our cause, I returned to my hotel room that evening, to find a jarring Telex there from home. Jeff and his girlfriend had been in an automobile accident with our Volkswagen. "Thankfully, no one was hurt," it said. I grabbed up the phone receiver and placed an overseas call with the operator. Then I paced my room for hours, waiting for the call to go through an overseas connection. I was poised to take the next plane home. Finally, the operator rang me back with an open line through to the States. Jeff answered and assured me all was indeed well there, or at least it was in hand. "Whitey is taking care of everything legal, and Bruce helped me get the VW to the repair shop. It's really okay Mom, don't try to come home, we're just fine." So I calmed down, hung up, and went on with the business of the trip.

The next day Nancy, Carole, and Lou drove to Bern, the capital of Switzerland, to formally present our pleas to the Swiss government. They met with Paul Andre Rameseyer of the Ministry of Foreign Affairs. Joe McCain and I stayed behind in Geneva and

continued meeting with the International Red Cross and some of
the people on the list we'd been given. When it was time to leave, I
felt that in general, our meetings had been promising. Joe was less
enthusiastic, and not optimistic.

We went from there to Paris, site of the still-flagging peace
negotiations, where we had seven meetings scheduled. Carole
Hansen privately met with Mr. M.S. Petsanghane, the Pathet Lao
Representative in France, while the rest of us met with Mr.
Froment-Maurice, the French Director of Asian Affairs at the
French Foreign Ministry. Predictably, Mr. Petsanghane recited the
North Vietnamese party line to Carole. As she related later, it went
along the lines that American prisoners in Laos are victims of Mr.
Nixon's bad politics. They have a superior life and receive better
food than the Laotians themselves enjoy. He said that instead of
demanding a list of names from Vietnam, we should be demanding
a halt to our bombing over there. We also tried to arrange some
meetings with the Viet Cong and the North Vietnamese delega-
tions to the Paris Peace Talks, but they wanted no part of us. Our
meeting with the French Croix Rouge (Red Cross) was equally
frustrating. President Carraus and his staff refused to offer any help
in publicizing our Discrepancy lists. However, we were able to visit
and speak with representatives at several foreign embassies in Paris.
Joe pitched his Discrepancy Report to every one of them, and was
reasonably well received.

The next morning we were offered an eleventh hour hearing at
the French Foreign Relations Ministry. At the meeting, Joe gave his
Discrepancy Report and followed with a question and answer session. The French showed little empathy for our situation. That
meant that we left without receiving any promises from them for
specific action to help our cause. Froment-Maurice claimed we
were under a misimpression about the French POWs following
their departure from Vietnam in 1954 when they lost at Dien Bien
Phu. "Within 30 days of the signing of our agreement with Hanoi,
all French POWs were fully accounted for." Afterward, Joe grumbled that he was shocked at that statement and thought they were
rewriting history. "Can you believe he said they've done everything
they can and he trusts the Viet Cong? Their attitude was unbelievable, Evie!" After all we'd done as their World War II Allies, Joe was

clearly outraged at the French Foreign Ministry official's attitude towards us. I couldn't disagree on that. We'd seen how "eager" they were to help us. Not a bit. I was glad to leave.

Lou was waiting at the curb in a taxi with my luggage. I was wound up and frustrated with the meeting. "The French may have warned us not to get involved in Vietnam, but that doesn't mean they have to ignore this issue of it," I complained.[18] "They're supposed to be our Allies. They need to help us bring world attention to this cause!"

"Well, just relax now, Evie. You'll need all your energy for the next group," Lou reminded me, "We have learned we don't always get the response we hope for. But it will be a success, simply because we are here telling our story, using real people like you and Joe and Nancy, who are directly involved, and have suffered a lot." Lou was a true diplomat and a great public relations guy. As he'd promised if I'd just attend the meeting, Lou got me to my flight on time. Then he headed north to Stockholm and Oslo with Joe, Carole, and Nancy Perisho.

I flew on to Brussels alone, where I was met by Russ and Genevieve Davis whose son was MIA. Joe McCain had wanted to accompany me on this leg of the trip, but Chappie James had remained adamantly against it. Joe had to go on to the countries in Western Europe with the other group. Given that our next stop would be Bucharest, Romania, still a Communist ruled country, I could understand that. Joe's brother was already a POW of the Communists in Vietnam. His father, Admiral John McCain, was in command in the Pacific. Chappie was right to object. There was just no sense in tempting Fate. Russ and Gen Davis lived in Brussels, where Russ was European representative for American Aluminum Products. They were a lovely couple, very warm, welcoming and helpful. They also both spoke fluent French.

"We appreciate very much what you and the League accomplish for all the POW/MIAs, including our son, Evelyn," Russ greeted me. I liked both of them right away, and we were soon very comfortable together. We went straight to my hotel as I was scheduled to present Joe's Discrepancy Report to representatives of the Belgian Foreign Relations Office within the hour. At that meeting, the Davises heard the Discrepancy Report for the first time. As always, I ended with an appeal for assistance from the Belgian government. I asked them to appeal to North Vietnam and its allies to provide a full accounting of the prisoners and those Missing in Action. Gen and Russ had already briefed me on how to approach the dignitaries to get their best response and we did receive sincere sympathy and kindness from the Belgians, but they offered no specific commitment of help or action. That afternoon, Gen took me shopping. Lou had left my best outfits in my hotel room, when he packed for me while I was at that French Foreign Ministry meeting. He didn't think to look in the closet. When I got to Brussels, I discovered that two pantsuits were all I had to wear to all these meetings. Fortunately, I found two dresses there in Brussels that were perfect for my needs.

Early the next morning, the three of us flew to Vienna, Austria. There the Davises and I secured the first promises from a foreign government to help the POW/MIA cause. We met with Mr. Walter Wodak, Secretary-General of the Austrian Foreign Affairs Ministry. After seeing our Discrepancy Report, which I presented, he said he would have the Austrian Embassy in Moscow contact the North Vietnamese Embassy there and question them about these discrepancies. He agreed to request a complete list from the North Vietnamese of all American military held as POWs or known to be dead. He also assured us of Austria's willingness to function as a Protecting Power for the neutral internment of American POWs, as provided for in the Geneva Conventions,[19] until a final peace agreement was reached. What a satisfying moment it was for me when I heard a heartfelt, "Yes, we can do something to help your cause," for the first time during that trip. Toward the end of our meeting, the subject turned to more general conversation. Russ Davis and Walter Wodak discovered they had a mutual friend whom they both admired. After that, Mr. Wodak took a personal interest in Russ and Gen's missing son. Through that connection, he became interested in the overall POW/MIA dilemma. His personal attention helped immensely later when we met with Mr. Hans Polster, Secretary General of the Austrian Red Cross.

Mr. Polster was initially cool to us and disinterested. However, after we expressed our surprise at the difference between his attitude and the warm reception we'd received from Secretary-General Wodak, his attitude changed. He immediately warmed to the Discrepancy presentation and took careful notes. The next day, we met our own Ambassador to Austria, John Humes, and his assistant, Mr. Paul Bergman, at the U.S. Embassy. After briefing them, they promised to contact Mr. Polster and encourage him to pressure the ICRC on our behalf.[20]

On the following day, May 30, we were on a plane again, this time to Bucharest, Romania. Russ had business friends there who could escort us around the city and provide an interpreter when needed. Although Romania was ostensibly part of the Communist Bloc, Bucharest had a U.S. Embassy, as well as embassies for North Vietnam and the National Liberation Front (Viet Cong.)[21] We hoped to make our point with all three.

We'd already spoken with countless dignitaries in four European capitals: Geneva, Paris, Brussels, and Vienna. As I approached meetings with new dignitaries in a Communist country, my confidence was a measure of how much I had grown, personally, and in handling high-level meetings about serious issues since becoming active with the League. However, Russ and Gen cautioned me strongly on the pertinent security aspects of our visit to Romania.

"You must remember to speak only in generalities, especially in the hotel and in your room, Evie. If we need to speak privately about specifics, we will take a walk and mingle with pedestrians. Understand that we'll be followed, observed, and likely eavesdropped on at all times. Most Romanians would like to be friendly, but being friendly to us can be dangerous for them." Having to watch every word I spoke was a sobering introduction to the world of people who are not free and open and who fear speaking out.

When we landed in Bucharest, our pilot parked on the tarmac a fair distance away from the terminal. When I emerged from the aircraft into the bright sun, I was stunned to find armed Romanian soldiers surrounding our plane, their rifles pointed toward us.

"Don't be frightened, it's normal. It's the way they welcome all foreigners," Russ whispered. The greeting was a grim reminder that I was no longer in the free world. I couldn't imagine what Mother would think or say if she saw this airport scene, and me there. But the militant welcome aside, the Romanian officials actually treated us very well and processed our visas, entry papers, and luggage with great courtesy and efficiency.

The city of Bucharest appeared to be frozen in the past century. It was somewhat somber-looking, its buildings in dire need of upkeep and modernization. When I got onto the elevator, it gave a big jolt, and we all gasped aloud. Then it started chugging until, to my relief, it jerked to a shaky stop at the seventh floor. I tipped the bellboys, and they were very grateful, but my heart was still thumping as I walked to my room. I stood looking out of the window in my room, thinking. I wanted very much to tell my boys how lucky we were to be citizens of the United States where we can smile, laugh, and talk without fear. The Romanians didn't live that way, but they *had* signed the Geneva Conventions, so they were important to my mission.

We attended five meetings in Bucharest. The first was with Constantin Babeanu, Director of North American Affairs in the Ministry of Foreign Affairs. He was an especially valuable contact because he had recently returned from a posting in Hanoi. Mr. Babeanu was courteous and attentive to our requests. He said he

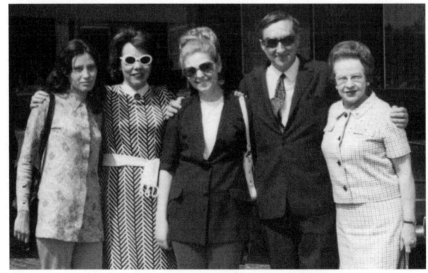

Grubb family files

League National Coordinator Evelyn Grubb and MIA parents Genevieve and Russ Davis (in sunglasses) in Bucharest, Romania, with Romanian escorts. May 1972.

recognized our concern about the Discrepancies and believed Hanoi had created a credibility problem with their lack of cooperation. The Romanian Red Cross representative, Andrei Dorobantu, Director of International Relations, was also very polite, but neither one gave us any promises to help our cause. Nevertheless, they had heard us out, and that was a plus.

The next morning, Gen, Russ, and I took a bold step and made an impromptu, unescorted visit to the North Vietnamese Embassy. We had no appointment, although we wouldn't have been given one if we'd asked for it through channels. Surprisingly, we were invited inside without question. There was no tirade, no ordering us out. We asked politely for a meeting with the Ambassador and were told that he was not available. Then we were ushered in to see Mr. Doan Hung Ke, a junior official, who courteously allowed me to go through our Discrepancy Report presentation. Our communication was in French. But because my command of French was inadequate for the Discrepancy Report, I presented it in English, with Russ translating for me. Mr. Ke even accepted the written materials without objection. Afterward, he made no comment. Then he presented us with a handful of pictures of bombed buildings, broken bodies, and weeping women. We took the pictures, looked at them, and nodded solemnly without comment. I requested that he pass our information on to the Ambassador and he said he would, but there was little he could do. I handed him a copy of my Petition and the League's Petition to the United Nations, and we left. I was feeling flushed with that success, so we decided to try the same surprise tactic at the embassy of the South Vietnamese Peoples Provisional Revolutionary Government (the Viet Cong).[22] We received a very different reception there. A Romanian clerk let us in the door. Once we were inside, the Vietnamese staff was horrified to discover we were Americans. We took a look around the reception room while a loud discussion about our presence went on in the next room. None of us spoke Vietnamese, so we couldn't understand what was being said. I noticed a tall, narrow, lighted cabinet with a shelf display of spoons, bowls, and ashtrays. Photos of American plane crashes lined the back of the shelf. The artifacts were probably made from planes they'd shot down, I figured. The shelf above held a display of Vietnamese postage stamps with images of American

POWs taken during various stages of capture. Thinking one might be Newk, I approached the cabinet to get a better look.[23]

A Viet Cong soldier, obviously a guard, jumped between me and the cabinet, completely blocking my view. He fixed me with a chilling glare and said sternly in halting but clear English, "We do not accept you here. I must request you leave—now!"

I stepped back and said nothing, even though I wanted to shout back at him. Russ came over and tried to hand him a copy of the Discrepancy Report, but he would neither accept our written materials nor allow us to leave them anywhere.

"May we please make an appointment to meet with your official Representative later today?" I requested.

"That will not be possible, Madame. I say again, leave now! You do not have appointments. We do not invite you here."

The loud discussion continued in the next room. No one had returned to speak with us. Seeing the angry color rising in my face, Russ discreetly took my arm. "We'd better go . . . *now* . . . he said quietly. We turned and left. I was relieved that no one followed us or tried to catch up with us. That evening we flew back to Brussels, and the next morning I said farewell to the Davises. I truly hoped their son would be found.

I then crossed the English Channel to rejoin the rest of our League group in London. Carole and Joe had already met with Lady Angela, Countess of Limerick, President of the British Red Cross and Chairman of the Permanent Commission of the ICRC. Joe had figured out that she was the highest-ranking Red Cross official in the world. They had presented the League's Discrepancy Report to her. Joe pointed out that some American POWs, like Newk (whose photos taken by the North Vietnamese were included in the display), "are now said to be dead, but as you can see here, Newk Grubb was in apparent good health in these photos, taken soon after his capture." Lady Angela had studied the Discrepancy display carefully. "I think you should disseminate more information like this worldwide. It is most interesting," she told them. Joe had concluded his presentation by saying, "These others, captured in the South of Vietnam, have been seen in prison camps by men who have escaped or been released, but, in violation of the Geneva Conventions, their names do not appear on any prisoner list provided by Hanoi. We ask, Lady Angela, that you use the influence of your government to help us pressure the governments of North Vietnam, the (Viet Cong) in South Vietnam, the Pathet Lao in Laos, and the Khmer Rouge in Cambodia to openly identify the men they hold captive. It is vital that they clarify these discrepancies, tell us who they are holding captive, and alleviate the agony of the families of the more than 1700 missing men."

Joe had also pointed out that each prisoner should be allowed to fill out and mail a capture card as prescribed by the Geneva Conventions. But none had ever been given one.[24]

Everyone who presented Joe's report made the same points. In all our meetings on that trip, each of us stressed that Protocol III of the Conventions, Article 12 relative to the Treatment of Prisoners of War, was not being upheld and that better methods needed to be devised for its enforcement. We were convinced that the majority of Americans would not be satisfied with any resolution of the conflict in Vietnam until all U.S. Prisoners of War, and any Missing in Action, were fully identified and accounted for, as required by the Geneva Conventions. We always noticed that, like Lady Angela, those who heard the Discrepancy Report and saw Joe's detailed charts were being made aware of the problem for the first time. Many asked pertinent questions and took careful notes. That pleased us. We had been well-received and attentively listened to in most of the countries we visited. Joe told me that Norway had been particularly promising. In Oslo, Per Kleppe, Minister of Trade, representing the Foreign Minister that day, was impressed by Joe's display and said that since Norway was in the process of opening diplomatic relations with Hanoi, he would recommend that Norway transmit the Discrepancy information to the North Vietnamese. Otherwise, this was a matter that he feared would affect the peace settlement. He would not, however, offer Norway's help in transmitting mail to, or receiving mail from, the POWs held in Hanoi. He considered the Discrepancies a more important matter. Our League delegates left there very satisfied. In Stockholm, the Swedish Ministry had not been as nice as they had been on previous contacts. Joe said that Rune Nystrom, who had written me with the confirmation of Newk's death, scoffed at the Discrepancies Report. Nystrom's assistant, named Berg, had been "blatantly rude," according to Joe. So we got no help there at all.

They had then called on a Mr. Pietrei, the Swedish Ambassador to Vienna, who had spent six years as Ambassador to China in Peking, among other important assignments. He said he found it not at all out of character that the Vietnamese would not disclose all the POWs . . . he said they'd do that to "keep the Americans guessing," and added that Hanoi is "fiercely independent" and doesn't like taking direction from Moscow or Peking. Joe, Carole, and Nancy agreed that was a very informative session for the League.

We left knowing that our trip had at least generated a lot of interest in our cause by our European allies and had opened their eyes to some of the serious issues we faced. Thanks to Russ and Gen Davis, we had even managed a personal visit with some North Vietnamese diplomats, definitely a first for the League and for me. I agreed with the Countess of Limerick, as did Joe and our Board, that we needed to continue to highlight Joe's Discrepancy Report in our attempts to turn world opinion in our favor. The Discrepancy Report and display Board appeared to be the key because it demonstratively proved that the North Vietnamese were not treating the POWs humanely as required by the Geneva Conventions. Also the signatories were doing nothing to stop what they were doing.

We flew back to the United States and briefed Ambassador Porter at the State Department in Washington the very next day. The trip was a publicity success. We were glad we went, but we were also very happy to be home again.

Summer vacation began for the boys, but the office requirements kept me in Washington more than at home. The Presidential campaign was in full swing, and proposed solutions for ending the Vietnam War were prominent in the rhetoric. Even though the League remained nonpartisan, we couldn't help being aware that the outcome of this campaign would directly affect everything we were working for. We were also aware that time was running out for the League. The American public wanted the United States out of Vietnam, period.

We could only hope that Dr. Kissinger had a firm grip on the peace negotiations and would provide us with a viable agreement to end the war before November's elections. We fervently hoped that the Administration would include *all* American prisoners and missing in Southeast Asia in the peace deal, not just those held in Vietnam, or worse, only North Vietnam.

I started the year riding a wave of optimism with the President's speech, but peace had not come, and now I could feel a sense of discouragement and bitterness rising in me again. I deeply despaired at the "out at any cost" attitude of the American public. Why should men like Newk fight and die for people who obviously don't give a damn about what happens to them? When did the people of our country become so selfish and uncaring? How can any country survive without a strong military force? Who'd want to serve in a military force and put their life on the line every day, for an uncaring public? Why can't a country as big and strong as ours get enforcement of the Geneva Conventions? Why can't we win this war and get *all* our prisoners freed, all our troops home with honor, after all they've suffered and endured? Who or what in the world are we afraid of?

I wrestled with these thoughts, fought my personal grief, and dealt with the daily business of the League. Would we, the POW/MIA families, ever have truthful answers to our questions? I sighed. Probably not.

Not long after I returned from Europe, I received a letter from Genevieve and Russell Davis, the friends I had met on my League visit to Belgium. They said, in part:

> We are no less concerned for our future than for the past, and we shudder at the opportunities that will be missed. We still believe that there is a key, a solution, to success . . . but who holds that key? Is it President Nixon or is it really Kissinger? I cannot help but wish that the answer was in Paris at the Peace Talks. What needs to be said that cannot, or should not, be said publicly? There is certainly enough being said publicly that does NOT favor the U.S. or help members of the League. 'Nuf said. I am just adding another viewpoint. Please be sure we receive information about the dates of the Convention (in October), etc.
>
> Best,
>
> Gen and Russ[25]

That concluding paragraph summed up my own thoughts exactly. I said a silent prayer, probably the thousandth one, for Dr. Kissinger's efforts in Paris to be successful.

10 We Are Many ... They Are Few

TIMELINE . . . 1972 . . . <u>WORLD</u> . . . IDI AMIN BEGINS REIGN OF TERROR IN UGANDA . . . BOBBY FISCHER (USA) BEATS BORIS SPASSKY (RUSSIA) IN CHESS . . . <u>VIETNAM</u> . . . JANE FONDA SITS ON ANTI-AIRCRAFT GUN IN NORTH VIETNAM . . . B-52 BOMBERS BEGIN POUNDING HANOI . . . <u>USA</u> . . . PRESIDENT NIXON REELECTED . . . DOW-JONES INDUS-TRIAL AVERAGE BREAKS 1,000 FOR THE FIRST TIME IN HISTORY . . . OAKLAND WINS WORLD SERIES . . .

There is always inequity in life. Some men are killed in a war and some men are wounded. Some men never leave the country. Life is unfair.
—John F. Kennedy, 1962

I was delighted whenever Sybil Stockdale was around and could visit me at the League's Washington office. On her most recent visit, she'd commented that it was in the best shape ever. She also complimented me on the latest treasurer's report, saying it was the best she had seen to date. That really cheered me up a lot and being Sybil she also gave the staff a big lift, too. "You are all doing a great job. I am both grateful and proud to be one of what has become an effective, efficient, hard-hitting team." She requested that all current Board members run for office again, and she proposed a slate of officers for the coming year that would name me again as National Coordinator. However, I had already made my decision not to run again. I was pleased and honored with Sybil's vote of confidence in my work as National Coordinator. The confirmation I'd gotten from the Swedish government on Newk's death in captivity had provided no additional details. The U.S. government and the Air Force still weren't prepared to accept it as fact. The North Vietnamese had lied about so many things, we simply could not trust that statement. Nevertheless, I was certain that the next year would bring many changes to my life. There would be personal and family decisions to make. It clearly was time for someone else to take the reins of the League office.

I informed Sybil of my decision and the reasons behind it. "I've loved my work here at the League's national office, Sybil. It made a huge difference in my life and my outlook. We've accomplished so much this past year! Someone else should have that chance now. I'll have enough to deal with in the near future regarding Newk's situation, as I'm sure you can imagine."

Sybil accepted that news graciously and asked me to stay on the League Board of Directors. I said I'd be happy to do that. Sybil said, "Good. Now, as for the National Coordinator, I agree with you that the war might end soon, leaving a large number of MIAs still unaccounted for. Therefore, if you're stepping down, the reins of the League of Families should rightfully pass to the families of the MIAs, don't you think?"

"Absolutely." I agreed wholeheartedly with that, as did the rest of the Board members. At our July 1972 Board meeting, Bob Brudno introduced a motion that provided for the orderly succession of any elected Board member or Officer who resigned after the return of their POW or MIA family member. We agreed with his proposal and passed the motion.[1]

Also that July, a newsletter from the Air Force acknowledged that the latest POW lists from Hanoi had the names of 24 more servicemen—16 Air Force and 8 Navy—who had been captured since November 1971. We learned also, that upon their return to the United States, the repatriated POWs would initially be assigned to a military hospital. That would be for medical evaluation and some mental and emotional decompression, I supposed. If the immediate family wanted to stay near to the hospital to be with their family member, they would be entitled to do so at government expense. That news was encouraging because it indicated that some specific planning was now underway for the repatriation of our POWs.[2]

The announcement of these plans, together with the resumption of bombing and the mining of Haiphong harbor instituted by President Nixon earlier in the year, gave credence to Sybil's belief and my fervent hope that we could anticipate release of the POWs in the very near future. Excitement and anticipation permeated the families of the League around the country. Unfortunately, there was a flip side to the positive electricity we felt. Some of our own citizens were working against us and our efforts.

That summer, a number of American civilians, who had publicly disagreed with the country's position on Vietnam, traveled openly to Hanoi. They were greeted by the North Vietnamese with open arms. They apparently had no qualms or fear of legal consequences that might result from blatantly meeting with and befriending the enemy.

The North Vietnamese had never allowed the families of POWs to go to Hanoi. These families, including mine, denied all access to their men, now suffered the additional pain of seeing the North Vietnamese welcome these arriving citizens: actress Jane Fonda, former U.S. Attorney General Ramsey Clark, Cora Weiss, and David Dellinger, to mention a few.[3] They reviled the sacrifice of our American POWs in Hanoi and elsewhere. They raucously denied the suffering and/or death of those men and their families.

In Fonda's case particularly, they flagrantly consorted with the enemy, and espoused the enemy's side against their own country. Jane Fonda made a second trip to Hanoi in July 1972. There at her own request, she taped radio broadcasts that denounced the U.S. bombing of North Vietnam. She also met a few Hanoi POWs, who were forced to meet with her, and she famously posed for pictures aboard a large enemy antiaircraft gun, wearing a DRV Communist military helmet. Jane Fonda was (and still is) an actress, and therefore was accustomed to seeking large audiences, posing, and getting major attention in the media. She certainly attracted plenty of that. However, like many families in the League and the military, I despised what she did and felt she should either be summarily stripped of her American citizenship, or tried for consorting with the enemy forces. As an American citizen, she certainly had a right to express her personal beliefs. But many U.S. citizens felt then, and still feel, that "Hanoi Jane" Fonda (as they nicknamed her) and the other U.S. citizens who went to Hanoi did not have the right to commit overt acts that directly aided and abetted the enemy's cause.

Her highly publicized actions and statements, and her behavior in Hanoi, dealt our country, the League of Families, our POWs and MIAs, and our dedicated military forces and their families some very serious and painful propaganda low blows, for which many of us may never forgive her.

The same goes for Ramsey Clark, who also traveled to Hanoi that summer. Following his return, he claimed that American

POWs "are receiving humane treatment."[4] His claim was based on staged meetings with only 10 U.S. prisoners. The League knew from returned prisoners that this was not true and wanted to publicly counter his statement. We decided to meet with him in person before taking any overt action, such as public censure. On August 16, 1972, Bonnie Metzger, Lou Stockstill, and I met with Ramsey Clark at his offices in Washington, D.C. Mr. Clark told us that he had taken about 400 family letters to Hanoi with him, including 102 letters to men missing or captive in South Vietnam. He informed us that he'd brought back 112 letters from POWs in North Vietnam and 17 letters from men captured by the Viet Cong in the south. Some of the letters were from three new writers who were classed as MIA. One had been carried as "missing" since 1969, he said. These same letters *proved* the North Vietnamese were lying and in egregious violation of the Geneva Conventions. Apparently, these facts didn't occur to Mr. Clark. As we spoke, Mr. Clark nodded toward some bags stashed in the corner of his office. They apparently contained the letters he was talking about. Bonnie had not heard from her injured POW husband in a long time. She became visibly excited.

"Mr. Clark," she said, "My last name is Metzger. Do you know by chance if one of those letters might be for me, from my husband?"[5]

He replied very coldly that he didn't know. His tone implied that he didn't care, either. I stepped in.

"Well, Mr. Clark, since those bags are sitting right there may we help Bonnie go through them to see if there is one for her?" I thought it was a reasonable request. I knew personally the pain Bonnie was experiencing at the silence from her young husband.

Clark's tone turned icy. "No, you can't. You'll have to wait until Cora Weiss' group distributes those letters. They are going directly to her first." With that, he turned away and refused to look at Bonnie, who sat quietly with tears running down her face.

I was seething. How was it possible that this man, that *anyone*, could be that cruel, that cold, that uncaring? He was an ice cube of a man. Obviously, Ramsey Clark had not carried those letters home in a gesture of human compassion. He intended to use them as blackmail, as ammunition to advance his and Cora Weiss' agendas!

I was appalled that any American, especially a former American *official*, could behave that way to an innocent, grieving young woman like Bonnie.

The meeting continued, but I for one was no longer feeling obliged to be civil or cater in any way to this man.

While in Hanoi, Clark informed us, he had asked to see 50 or more POWs and had asked to see several prisoners (military and civilian) by name. His request was denied. The North Vietnamese allowed him to see only 10 prisoners, all of their choosing.

"Are you sure those weren't showcase prisoners that you saw, Mr. Clark? They've done that before," I said.

"No, I don't feel that the ten men I saw were what you call showcase prisoners!" he responded angrily.

I then asked for the names of the prisoners he'd seen. He pulled out a sheet of paper and handed it to us without comment. We orally reviewed the list, pointing out to him that of the ten men he had seen, eight were among those taken prisoner this past December (1971) and were therefore recent captives of less than a year. The other two had repeatedly been exhibited by the DRV to visitors during the past two and a half years and paraded as examples of their "humane treatment" of our POWs.[6]

I was still seething over his callous treatment of Bonnie, but I tried to keep my voice calm.

"How could you possibly have assessed, from those 10, the reality of the condition of the hundreds of other POWs in Hanoi? Why not include some of the ones who have been prisoners for seven years or more? I bet it was because they wouldn't let you see those men, that's why! Our effort to get humane treatment for our American POWs is being seriously jeopardized because of the actions of a few people like you, Cora Weiss, and Miss Jane Fonda, Mr. Clark," I said, as angrily and coldly as he had spoken to us.

"On what do you base such an assumption, Mrs. Grubb?" Clark gave me a thin, arrogant smile.

"On the basis of your questionable information, limited exposure to a small number of prisoners, and your preconceived bias about your country, our men's patriotism, and the war, Mr. Clark," I replied. "Visitors to Hanoi like you and Miss Fonda see and hear only what the North Vietnamese government *wants* you to see and hear. Then you come back and make broadly generalized, widely disseminated public statements, based on your weak third hand assumptions about the men being held there and their circumstances. The few long-term prisoners who have returned tell a vastly different story of very *in*humane and brutal treatment, Sir."

Hearing that, Mr. Clark stopped smiling, and his attitude toward us became considerably more negative. We offered him some facts, including information from Joe's Discrepancy Report and details reported by the POWs who had been released. He was obviously not interested in facts, but he allowed us to speak our piece.

Even our diplomatic Lou Stockstill took a swipe at Clark, saying, "We sincerely hope, Mr. Clark, that your future public statements will be tempered to reflect some of these facts we've just given you."

"Well, here are a couple more facts for you, Mr. Stockstill," Clark rejoined, with barely concealed sarcasm.

Possibly in a brief attempt to placate us, or to show us up, Clark told us that during the course of the two hours he'd spent with the ten POWs he was allowed to see, each man had been allowed to take his tape recorder into a corner of the room and record a two minute message to his family. He said he had not heard the tapes himself (which we didn't believe for one second) but had furnished them directly to ABC-TV. He'd been told that the recordings would be reproduced on individual tapes and sent to each man's family. That news, at least, did placate me some, as it was something positive. But not much, considering his attitude and the damage he'd done just by going there. I made clear what I thought about him and the trip he'd made. I didn't comment further, and we were soon ushered out.

I was elated when some high-profile figures in the United States took Ramsey Clark to task publicly and reviled his Pro-Communist activities. Congressman Bob Sikes (D-Florida), movie actor Charlton Heston, and political columnists, Rowland Evans and Robert Novak, were just a few of those who castigated Clark. Congressman Sikes' press statement said, in part,

> I have been gravely concerned about the statements made by
> Mr. Ramsey Clark concerning the so-called 'humane' treat-

ment that he believes our Prisoners of War are receiving . . . he saw only 10 POWs, saw them in what not even he could deny may very well have been a 'staged production' and in the presence of their captors. The truth is that we do not know, that no one knows, that our men are being treated humanely . . . Every thinking American, every concerned American, every American with the milk of human compassion . . . knows full well that every time North Vietnam has briefly parted the curtain on the (U.S.) prisoners of war that we have seen only what they wanted us to see, and heard only what they want us to hear. How Ramsey Clark could believe otherwise is beyond my comprehension.[7]

Joe McCain went on the offense, too, bless him. He countered the effects of Clark and Fonda by using the Discrepancy Reports and statements made by returning POWs to prove them wrong at various group meetings all over Washington, D.C. He also met with Cooper Holt and Phelps Jones of the Veterans of Foreign Wars (VFW), who asked him to address the VFW convention in Atlanta in August.[8] He also did a radio show on WAMU-FM with

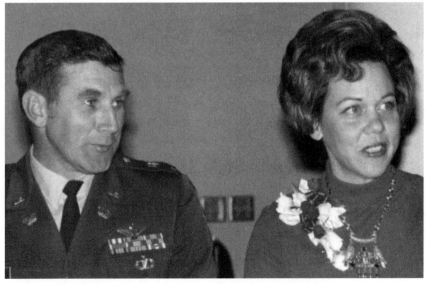

Army helicopter pilot WO Laird Osburn and Evelyn Grubb at a press conference in Wichita, Kansas,1972. POW Osburn was released by Cambodian authorities in March, 1969.

Lou Stockstill and Joan Vinson.

I went to Wichita, Kansas, to appear at a Press Conference with former POW Laird Osburn, an Army Warrant Officer helicopter pilot, who had been captured in Cambodia by the Viet Cong. He had been held as a POW of the South Vietnamese for a short time and was among 10 U.S. Army prisoners the Viet Cong turned over to Cambodian authorities. They in turn released Osburn along with three other Army POWs, John Fisher, Querin Herlik and Robert Pryor, in March 1969.[9]

The rumor mill was working overtime that summer and fall with various people guessing when the POWs would be released. We heard that Senator Barry Goldwater believed that the POWs would be home within 90 days. Family hopes soared, only to be dashed again when it didn't happen. Someone questioned the League about whether there was truth in the rumor that some POWs had been secretly transferred to China. We replied that we had no way to investigate or confirm that. There was a rumor that the Justice Department intended to sue the POWs for making anti-U.S. statements while imprisoned. General Chappie James assured us there was no way that would happen, and no truth to that rumor.

The national political scene churned up enormous waves that alternately lifted and then dashed down our hopes. The fate of our men hung somewhere between Henry Kissinger's well-honed negotiating skills and the outcome of the November 1972 Presidential election. The end to the Vietnam War and the status of the POW/MIAs were high priority issues with both the politicians and the American voters. The candidates, of course, were very aware of that. Aspiring office-holders cleaved to the POW and MIA cause to help them win elections in November.

The League was not spared waves of criticism during that fractious time either. Some claimed we were too political; others complained we weren't political enough. In early August, I traveled to Miami to present our issues to the Republican Platform Committee. My remarks at that meeting reflected the League's basic position:

> No cold recital of statistics about our prisoners and
> missing can do justice to their plight. We have talked about

their tragic situation since 1963, when the first man was listed as missing. Now, 9 1/2 years later, 1800 more men have been added to that 'missing' list, 500 of them during President Nixon's Administration alone. I come to you today as one voice speaking for 1800 men who are silenced behind the curtain of captivity. They request that your platform state explicitly that any resolution of United States participation in the war must provide strong safeguards for the release and full accounting for all Prisoners of War and Missing in Southeast Asia. I cannot stress too strongly the need for a full accounting of these men. Missing in action is not another word for 'dead' . . . MIA also means that our enemy has not identified all of the men they are holding captive. . . . our men have been held captive longer than any Americans in any war. Our men survive because of their persistence, because of their dedication, and mostly because of their faith, the faith that you will have the persistence and the dedication to bring them home safely to their families, and soon. Have we done enough? As President Nixon said to us when proclaiming the National Week of Concern for POWs and MIAs last March, 'Nothing will ever be enough until the men are home again.'[10]

A week later, I heard another pro-Vietnam, anti-American broadcast by Jane Fonda from Hanoi aired on the radio. I wanted to throw up. I was heartily sick of her antics against our country, and our valiant men.

Phyllis Galanti, Sybil Stockdale, and Joan Vinson attended the Republican Convention for the League, where President Nixon and Vice President Spiro Agnew were again nominated.

Joan Vinson also attended the Democratic National Convention in Florida on behalf of the League's Political Action Committee. There was great chaos outside the convention as antiwar activists rioted in the streets of Miami. The police had a difficult time controlling them and resorted to heavy riot control tactics. Joan reported to the office by phone, "Many people are being tear-gassed as they go into and come out of the Convention Hall. Others are suffering just from all the tear gas being used."

Val Kushner was also at the Democratic Convention and stated her support of the Democratic candidate, George McGovern. She then went on the campaign trail to promote him for President. A marker of attitudes about women activists at that time came in the September 29th issue of *Life* magazine, where in an article called "P.O.W. Wife" that POW wife Evelyn Guarino called "very unflattering to POW/MIA wives," a member of the Appleton, Wisconsin Kiwanis Club, where Val had just spoken on behalf of McGovern, was quoted as saying, "She has nice legs, but she's been brainwashed."[11] It was 1972, and women activists still "got no respect," as comedian Rodney Dangerfield would say. These preelection upheavals and comments mirrored the dramatic change American society had undergone in the last few years. The shocking shootings of student protestors by National Guard military at Kent State University in Ohio in 1970 had reawakened anti-military hostility and prejudices.[12] There had never been, not even during the Great Depression, such open and volatile demonstrations against our government. Never had rank and file Americans publicly denounced and vilified our democratic ideals, and how they were being administered, to the extent that was happening now.

I began to worry about my four sons and what kind of omen this was for their future. As a teenager, Jeff was aware of the demonstrations and upheavals, and occasionally he agreed with them. However, he did get involved with our League efforts on behalf of his Dad. I knew he'd soon have to register for the draft. I was concerned about that of course, but I didn't think he'd actually be called up because of Newk's as yet unresolved status.

I had changed drastically too. I looked at myself and my sons differently now. Instead of trying to see us through Newk's eyes as I had in the early years of his captivity, wondering if he'd approve, and worrying how we'd react to him after such a long absence, I now looked at myself and our sons with my own eyes, just their Mom's eyes, in the present. I began to enjoy them for who they were in relation to me, not to us, meaning Newk. With great help from Mother, the Grubbs, and the Carlsons, I was the one who had been responsible for them, who had raised them for nearly seven years now. I liked what I saw in our boys. I liked who they were, framed by our home and their activities today, not as things were six or eight years ago.

Newk and other long-time POWs or MIAs, if and when they returned, might still envision "home" as it had been when they were shot down. They were in for a big surprise. Home as it was now would be a huge adjustment for them when they saw their kids: teenage boys with long, flowing hair, teenage girls in short-short skirts, many of them running away from home, sleeping on roads and porches, freely experimenting with sex, carrying on at rock concerts, smoking marijuana, freely expressing themselves, sometimes in profanity laced language. How different things would be from what they recalled! How would they ever adjust?

Every time I looked at my sons now, I thought with deep emotion about Mother and Dad Grubb, and how they must feel. I was shattered enough about the thought of my lost husband. After the pain and grief I had experienced losing our only daughter, I coud not even begin to imagine how Newk's parents felt about losing their only son, nor could I imagine myself coping with losing any one of the four sons I loved so very much.

In early September, the League received the announcement that three POWs: Navy Lieutenant Mark Gartley, Air Force Major Edward Elias, and Navy lieutenant Norris Charles, would soon be released. Surprisingly, Gartley's mother and Charles' wife were being allowed to accompany Cora Weiss, David Dellinger, Richard Falk, and Reverend William Sloane Coffin to Hanoi to bring them home. We learned through news reports that the families had refused U.S. military assistance in bringing their men home, even though the three POWs were still on active military service.

At the League, we were of course very excited, and not in a position to be concerned about the political or military implications because no matter their families' political persuasions, the POWs would be home again, bringing current news with them about the prisoner situation in Hanoi. We immediately tapped all our contact lines for more information, but got precious little. What we did hear was that the three released POWs would go from Hanoi to Moscow on a Russian Aeroflot plane. Beyond that, there was no other information. Then we learned that David Dellinger was out of jail on bond and would have to get permission to leave the United States to accompany Weiss' group and escort the released

POWs home.[13]

Then the rumor mill produced something even more unbelievable. Word got out that Jimmy Hoffa, the former head of the Teamsters' Union, whose conviction and prison sentence had inexplicably been commuted by President Nixon in December of 1971, would be going to Hanoi under a special permit from the government on some kind of peacekeeping mission![14] That was a shocker. Initially, we discounted it as pure rumor but then Charlie Havens called to tell me he had talked with Frank Sieverts at the State Department and there was "lots more to this than we know . . . about Hoffa." So . . . it wasn't simply a rumor! Then around September 10, we heard that the United States had rescinded Hoffa's travel permit and cancelled his mission to Hanoi because of the press leaks about it. At the League, we continued to wonder what was going on.

I lunched with Frank Sieverts, Charlie Havens and Charles Gentry on September 12, and Frank told us that the Hoffa stories were true. Hoffa had been scheduled to go to Hanoi on a government mission. Now Frank Seivert had to explain to Jimmy Hoffa that the leaks about his upcoming trip did *not* come from the Government. That was all we learned.

What connection could there possibly be between President Nixon and a criminal like Jimmy Hoffa, I wondered? Then I had to dismiss the question from my mind. I think I'd reached the point where nothing would surprise me any more, no matter how ludicrous it appeared. A convicted-then-pardoned criminal being invited to act for our country in the area of foreign relations with the President's personal approval simply boggled the mind. What next?

I participated in a "Today" show interview from New York by remote hookup. Bill Monroe and Barbara Walters were in New York, and Bill Moyers was with me in Washington. The sound connection was poor. At one point, it broke down completely. I couldn't hear Barbara Walters' questions, so Moyers whispered, "just talk about POW issues." So that's what I did.[15]

Much later, when I was at the White House to attend a meeting with Dr. Kissinger, Barbara Walters happened to be seated in the same reception room. One of the White House aides introduced us. I commented that we'd already met on the "Today" show.

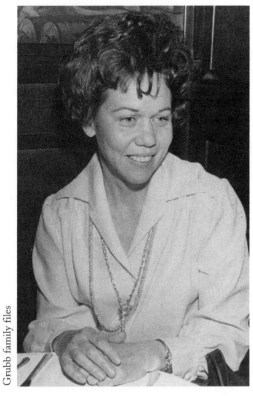

League of Families National Coordinator Evelyn Grubb at a business lunch with officials in Washington, D.C., September 1972.

She stared at me for several moments, as though trying to place me, and then said,

"Grubb? Oh . . . you waffled on answers to my questions."

That stunned me.

"I would never waffle on answers to questions about the POW/MIA situation, Ms.Walters," I replied. "My husband is a POW who is rumored to have died in captivity. I take that very seriously." At that she raised her eyebrows in a questioning way. So I said, "Actually, it was your sound connection between New York and Washington that 'waffled' . . . and then broke. We couldn't hear you at all. Bill Moyers told me to just talk about POW/MIA issues until the sound problem was fixed, so I did. Apparently no one informed you about that."

"Apparently not," she said. With that, she turned away and pointedly ignored me.

As the League's Annual Convention in October and the November Presidential elections drew closer, the League office was

busier than ever. Newspapers, television and radio stations bom-
barded us with requests for interviews. The impending release of
the three POWs was big news, and there was much speculation and
disagreement in the media about it. It seemed like everyone
referred people to the League for answers to their questions. We
had none to give. We didn't know any more than they did.

A few days later, I called Dr. Roger Shields. He was in charge
of POW liaison and was coordinating prisoner release details for
the Department of Defense. I asked him if it would be possible for
me and some of the other POW/MIA family members, or League
Board members, to be at the airport to represent the League of
Families when the three POWs being released by Hanoi arrived.
He said he didn't know when or where they'd be arriving, or even
how, but he thought that was a good idea.

"I'll try to get you set up with the necessary permissions for
attending," he said.

On Monday, September 25, Frank Sieverts called the office to
say that the three POWs and their escorts had left Hanoi for China
and would probably be in Moscow by Wednesday. Mary McGrory
from the *Washington Star* called for an interview with me. The
office phones rang constantly. We were inundated with requests for
speakers at various conventions and meetings, including our own
annual League of Families of POW/MIA Annual Convention slated to take place in Washington in three weeks.

On Tuesday, September 26, Dr. Roger Shields called me. "The
route for the released POWs might be Peking to Moscow to
Copenhagen, and they might arrive in the United States as soon as
Thursday evening."

By Wednesday, everyone was in a high state of expectancy. In
the midst of the maelstrom, Charlie called to tell me the Pentagon
was attempting to clean up their POW/MIA personnel files and
make them presentable for the media, starting with the files on
these three POWs now on their way home. I almost cheered—
finally! Larry McIntosh from *Newsweek* called, and wanted to do an
interview. I scheduled an appointment with him for that Friday
afternoon, which would be, from all indications, immediately after
the return of the three POWs.

Roger Shields called me again. "The released POWs informed

us that, to assist in future releases, they felt they should come back by commercial aircraft rather than military. We've heard they were two hours late landing in Moscow and Gartley is apparently very fatigued." I could tell from Dr. Shields' tone that he was concerned about the physical effect of such an arduous trip on the men. He felt they should have traveled by military medical evacuation plane with a doctor and nurse aboard to attend to them. "But I do have good news for you, Evie, you're cleared to go to New York to welcome them home. We estimate they'll be arriving at JFK airport around 7 p.m. tomorrow night."

I was excited to hear that, and was at JFK Airport the next evening when the plane transporting the ex-POWs and their families pulled up to the gate at 7:30 p.m. Greeting that flight was one of the most memorable events of my life. When I got near the plane, my heart constricted and just for a moment I thought, *why couldn't this be Newk?* Then I realized that every POW/MIA family, hundreds of them, were feeling and thinking the same thing. I should just be happy for these three and their relieved families. I was escorted aboard the plane and met everyone aboard. There was no celebrating onboard. Everyone looked exhausted from the long trip home. I expressed my happiness, and the great joy of the League of Families at having them home. Lt. Mark Gartley, who had been a prisoner for just over four years when he was released, was gaunt. Despite his obvious fatigue and physical frailty, he wanted to talk.

"The League of Families of POWs? Great. I have so much to tell the families, when can I talk to them? Soon, I hope. I don't want to forget a thing."

I immediately invited him to attend our Convention in three weeks, and he'd be a featured speaker. "That's where you'll get to meet and speak to the most families all at once, but only if you feel well and up to doing that. We'd be thrilled to have you there."

He accepted on the spot and swore he'd be there. I knew that he accepted in the excitement of the moment and that his appearance would have to be processed through the right channels. However, I didn't say that to him. I felt sure Frank Sieverts and Charlie and Dr. Shields would help make it happen, but only if Gartley's health and well-being were up to an appearance before the public then. I welcomed them back and left. They were whisked away to a military hospital. The ensuing days were a blur of work, calls, interviews and spotlights on the returned POWs.

The time for the October convention finally arrived. It would be my last hurrah, marking the finale of my year as National Coordinator, and time for the election of a new slate.

I'm happy to say that Lt. Mark Gartley did come to the Convention. He looked much healthier, more rested, and very snappy in his brand new Navy uniform. It was quite a change from POW garb. He was smiling broadly and appeared very glad to be there to speak to us. He was our opening banquet speaker, and I had the pleasure of introducing him. His appearance was a huge lift to the families because he was living proof that the rest of our POWs might actually get to come home one day soon.

Having been briefed on our concern over the enormous news and cultural gap that our men might experience after so many years of captivity, Gartley was able to reassure us that life within the prison camps was not a total blackout as far as news of world happenings was concerned. "News trickled in to us via North Vietnamese news broadcasts, and also from the newly captured prisoners," he reported. He didn't say exactly how that was done, but we were glad to hear they were at least getting news, any news. Gartley's speech was brief, emotional. He received a standing ovation at the end. I could tell it meant a lot to him to have been there.

Dr. Henry Kissinger was scheduled to be our celebrity speaker at the closing banquet, and we were all very much looking forward to what *he'd* have to tell us about the peace negotiations, too. The morning of the banquet, I received a phone call from the White House.

"I'm sorry, Mrs. Grubb, but Dr. Kissinger will not be able to attend tonight. He sends his sincere regrets."

"Oh Lord, don't tell me!" I exclaimed. My heart sank. Had there been another leak to the press?

"Now we don't want you to be worried or upset," the caller soothed. "We are sending you a substitute speaker. We think you'll be very pleased with him. The President has decided he will come to speak in Mr. Kissinger's stead."

"Oh! . . . oh, my." I was momentarily at a loss. Then I managed to say, "Well that's just wonderful. Thank you! We're very honored."

"I knew you'd appreciate that, Mrs. Grubb. We're counting on you to help expedite the special arrangements that need to be made for his appearance. Oh, and you and Mrs. Hanson will be on hand to greet the President on his arrival and escort him into the dining room, won't you?"

We will? Of course we would! I was nervous, and delighted. "Of course. We'll be very honored." I replied. I couldn't wait to share this news with Carole Hansen and the Board. We'd all met the President in person several times before, so this would not be my first experience seeing him. Also, we weren't naïve. Of course the President's visit smacked of political maneuvering, with the election only weeks away, and doubtless there were those out there who couldn't wait to point that out to us. But we were a relatively small part of the U.S. electorate, and having the President of the United States as our closing speaker was a distinct honor, no matter when, why, or how it had come about. We were thrilled to welcome him.

The hotel was soon swarming with technicians, security folks, and all the hoopla that accompanies the President of the United States when he makes a formal appearance. Sure enough, there had to be one wet blanket around. That same afternoon a POW/MIA father member came up to me, and without any preamble lit into me.

"I think this is all a farce! Why should you women be dining in a fancy room, wearing evening clothes, and we fathers have to put on dinner jackets, while our loved ones languish hungry in prison camps, wearing God only knows what?"

Sudden attacks like that on what we were doing never failed to stun me. At least I could understand his bitter attitude, he was one of us, and under the same kind of unbearable strain we'd endured for so long. So I answered as kindly and gently as I could,

"Believe me, I understand how this may make you feel, but, if you knew how lonely it is for so many family members, and how much they've suffered. This is the only chance we do get to dress up the way we once could. We gather with others who are in the same situation and present a united face to the nation. I think it is very important that we represent our sons and brothers, our fathers, and husbands by looking our very best and being at our very best, as they'd expect us to at a meeting like this, to make them proud of us. And they'll be proud to know some day that their Commander-in-Chief was here to talk to us."

"No, I don't agree with you at all! Frankly, I think it's just a big waste of time and money," he snapped and stalked away.

I'm not a schooled diplomat, but at that moment I think I understood how Dr. Henry Kissinger and others must feel when their long and tiring efforts to negotiate a truce, or to pour a little oil on troubled waters somewhere, are met with implacable resistance, or worse, harsh criticism and cold rejection. Yet diplomats have to swallow that and press on, and so following their example, I did, too. I squared my shoulders, pushed the encounter from my mind, and resumed preparations for the President's arrival. I knew that what we were doing was the right thing.

The evening of his speech, Carole Hanson and I were dressed in our finest, standing just inside the hotel entrance, ready to greet the President upon his arrival. I was a bundle of nervous tension. The motorcade arrived with sirens, police escort, and all that. After greeting us, we escorted the President and his entourage to the entrance to the ballroom. He stood for a few moments outside the ballroom with us and politely inquired about our husbands' situations. We told him, and added a few comments about Joe McCain's Discrepancy Reports. For some reason, Joe's report caught his interest, and the President began questioning us intensely about the Discrepancy issue. Someone nudged Carole that it was time for her to move toward the doors. Carole started to back away, and President Nixon looked up. Carole stopped immediately. He continued talking to both of us, deliberately directing his remarks at Carole. Then a senior aide stepped up to the President and said quietly, "It's time for your speech, Mr. President."

Nixon's face underwent a sharp change and he snapped, "I'll tell *you* when it's time for my speech! Right now, I'm interested in this conversation, right here, with these two ladies."

Carole immediately stepped forward again. I was frozen to the spot.

"Thank you, Mr. President." The aide murmured, and stepped back. President Nixon smiled at us as though nothing had happened and continued conversing with us for another minute or two.

Then he nodded at Carole that *he* was ready to go in. We took our places for the grand entrance.

The doors opened, the President of the United States was announced, the familiar Presidential "Ruffles and Flourishes" sounded, and I was all goose bumps as we marched into the room. I could feel the lump in my throat and the tears starting to sting my eyes.

It is difficult for me to describe what I saw there. The League of Families may have been a group torn in many directions by political issues, impossible grief, frustration, and years of ongoing stalemate; but when our President walked into that room, he was greeted with a wildly enthusiastic standing ovation. Tears streamed from many eyes as we stood united, the proud and loving families of all those imprisoned and missing American servicemen. The President was our men's Commander-in-Chief. That night, all our hopes were pinned squarely on his shoulders. He was the only person in the world who had the final power to do something for us, and we were thrilled to have him in our midst.

Predictably, in his speech he promised to bring the POWs home and account for the missing in the very near future. That message was the one everyone wanted and hoped to hear. President Nixon's surprise appearance that night electrified and capped our League convention beyond anyone's wildest dreams. It certainly thrilled me to be part of it, and it ended the Convention and my term as National Coordinator on a joyous and hopeful note. It had been quite a year! Afterward, I was sad but relieved that my term was over.

I was delighted when Phyllis Galanti was chosen to replace Carole Hansen as Chairman of the Board; Helene Knapp became the National Coordinator, replacing me; Sara Francis Shay stayed on as the Liaison with State Coordinators; Iris Powers would continue to oversee the Rest, Rehabilitation and Recovery Committee in charge of plans for the returning POWs and MIAs, whenever that might happen. I was elected to serve as a member of the Board of the League for the upcoming term.

The days following the 1972 League Convention were packed with activity. I enjoyed making Helene's transition as Coordinator a smooth and friendly one. However, I left the position of National Coordinator with mixed emotions. I had truly enjoyed being part of the Washington scene. It had been a difficult, challenging, demanding, and exhilarating position, and I had worked very hard for a year. It would be sad to leave, but I was glad to let go of the reins. Being on the Board would allow me to remain current and involved, but to a lesser degree, with League and POW/MIA issues. I looked forward to doing that without the minutiae and infighting of the day-to-day activities, and that was really all I wanted or needed.

It wasn't long after the Convention, October 26, 1972, when Henry Kissinger electrified the United States, and indeed the world, when he uttered the four magic words that we'd waited so long to hear: "peace is at hand." We didn't hear the words "We believe that . . ." preceding the magic four, nor did we hear much of what he said after that.[16] We were delirious that peace was *finally* within his, and our, grasp. In the League, we'd been disappointed so many times before, we could only hope fervently that this time it would actually come to pass.

I knew that I'd soon have to make some serious plans for our future, especially if in the final resolution it would be without Newk. We'd have to leave the military scene, and the life, that we'd been a part of for so long. Fortunately, I was a much stronger, more independent, self-assured woman who had come to accept her husband's probable fate. I had heard yet another secondhand report from Hanoi (albeit still not an official government acknowledgment from the DRV) that Newk was one of several POWs who had supposedly died of wounds associated with his bailout, although I didn't believe for a minute that was the cause of his death. Whatever the cause, more likely he died at the hands of interrogators, from what I'd been told of conditions there. I also had accepted that, like the loss of our baby daughter, however horribly it had happened, what had been done couldn't be undone. I was now convinced I was indeed a widow and not a POW wife. Only the details of time, place and actual cause are in dispute. Forty years later, they still are.

I knew I wasn't going to give up fighting for official acknowledgment of Newk's death in captivity. I wanted notification in the manner that complied with the Geneva Conventions. I wanted that compliance from North Vietnam, although I didn't expect to get any truthful information from them about Newk's death at that time. I also believed, and still believe, that since they knew he was dead, and probably where his remains were, they knew where and how he died and was disposed of afterward. We deserved to have that information, and to get his remains back.

In my final days in the transition of Coordinators, in late 1972, I received another call from Colifam (the Coalition of Families) who had been given information by Cora Weiss that 278 letters came out of Hanoi with her, several of which were "duplicates" (several letters from one POW). On the dearth of letters, given that there were many more prisoners than letters coming back, Cora Weiss had given Colifam two reasons why more letters were not coming out:

> 1. There was now a longer clearance process for letters at both ends because the DRV claimed that families and the men had devised secret codes over the years for communicating, used 'funny ink' and other things found in letters.
> 2. Some men were not writing letters home any more. The DRV claimed this was due to fatigue or because some men had elected to break their ties with home by not writing. Letters brought too many memories, and too much pain and longing, and made surviving in the camps that much harder.[17]

That information, although some of it about the codes was true, brought an incomprehensible sadness to the families. We could imagine the despair and desperation our men must have experienced after so many years of being virtually abandoned by their countrymen. Now we learned that it drove many of them to withdrawal, isolation, and depression of the worst kind. We feared for their mental health as well as their physical health. This latest news added urgency to our appeals for their release.[18]

Newk had been gone from us for seven years. He'd left for Saigon in the fall of 1965. The League of Families, after all the years of hard work, had done much, but still had not succeeded in arriving at that elusive destination of resolution we'd all sought. The prisoners were not home, and the missing were still missing. Worse, more were being killed in action, more prisoners were being taken, and more men went missing in action every week. Would it never end? I was not at all surprised when, in November 1972, President Nixon was reelected. I hoped his election was a sign that Dr. Kissinger's "peace is at hand" might actually come to pass.

Not long after I completed my year as Coordinator and the transition was done, Mother surprised me with a cruise to the idyllic Mediterranean island of Majorca—just the two of us. The Carlsons had agreed to continue to stay with the boys until we returned. When we were on the beach one afternoon in Majorca, Mother told me that, although initially she had strongly objected to my job in Washington as National Coordinator of the League. "Over the year, I saw what a positive thing it was for you, Evie, how it strengthened you for going on, and I want you to know I am very, very proud of you and the wonderful job you did there for the League."

No praise could have touched me more, or been better for my heart and soul, than accolades from Mother, who had objected so strongly to it all, but nevertheless had stood staunchly by me and her grandsons. She was a true champion.

As we sunbathed by the Mediterranean, rekindling our mother/daughter bond, regaining enough strength and energy to face the months ahead, the words of poet Percy Bysshe Shelley played over and over in my mind, like a mantra.

> Rise like Lions after slumber
> In unvanquishable number—
> Shake your chains to earth like dew
> Which in sleep had fallen on you—
> Ye are many—they are few.

Shelley's command must have been an omen. The North Vietnamese were being recalcitrant again about the peace agreement. So, in that bleak December of 1972, on President Nixon's order, we Americans rose "like Lions after slumber." Weary after more than a decade of stalemate and war, disheartened by the endless peace talk hassles in Paris with no results, threatened at home with mutiny and revolt from our own citizens, the chains of patient acceptance that had bound us to the Vietnam War finally snapped. President Nixon stepped up to the plate and ordered our enormous

Air Force B-52s into the air to bomb Hanoi.[19] He meant business. The United States shook off its chains, and the noise they made falling to the earth was fierce.

11 Home with Honor and Tears

TIMELINE . . . 1973 . . . WORLD . . . ARAB & ISRAELI YOM KIPPUR WAR . . . OPEC DOU-
BLES OIL PRICES . . . SYDNEY AUSTRALIA OPERA HOUSE OPENS . . . VIETNAM . . . PEACE
AGREEMENT SIGNED . . . USA . . . VIETNAM WAR ENDS AFTER 14 YEARS . . . POWs COME
HOME . . . WORLD TRADE CENTER OPENS . . . HENRY KISSINGER IS NAMED SECRETARY
OF STATE . . . NIXON RESIGNS . . . GERALD FORD SWORN IN AS U.S. PRESIDENT . . . AVER-
AGE ANNUAL WAGE IN U.S. $12,900 . . . AVERAGE HOME COST $32,500 . . . *THE STING*
WINS BEST PICTURE OSCAR® . . .

> *Today unbind the captive,*
> *So only are ye unbound;*
> *Lift up a people from the dust*
> *Trump of their rescue, sound!*
> —Ralph Waldo Emerson

The relentless bombing of Hanoi by our B-52 bombers had begun on December 18, 1972. It stopped for Christmas Day and resumed the day after Christmas. The POW/MIA families worried and prayed, aware of both the destruction being visited on recalcitrant Hanoi and the danger to their men being held in or near Hanoi. Rumors were rampant. One that didn't bear thinking about was that the North Vietnamese might retaliate by publicly executing many or all of our POWs. The United States was risking all now, including the lives of the existing POWs and creating new POWs from the bomber crews. In one night alone, five B-52 bombers were shot down over North Vietnam.[1] I ached for the families of the newly captured, or missing, or killed in action crew members. I prayed that some would be rescued and that we were not going to be in a situation again where they would have to spend five years or more in the kind of anguish and despair that so many of us already had endured. It seemed I held my breath so much during that time, I barely breathed. Eleven days later, on December 29, 1972, the newscasters on all stations announced that the President had ordered the bombing of Hanoi to cease. I could only hope that meant that *serious* peace negotiations would soon be in progress again. That night I prayed for Dr. Henry Kissinger and his team to hit a home run. It all must have worked because, three weeks later, President Nixon appeared on television and spoke the words the nation had waited nearly 14 years to hear:

> We have today concluded an agreement to end the war and bring peace, with honor, to Vietnam and Southeast Asia.[2]

He then gave the details of the cease-fire. He said that all Americans held as prisoners in Indochina would be released within 60 days with the fullest possible accounting given for those still listed as missing in action. Oh, dear, I thought . . . did prisoners in Indochina mean only those in North and South Vietnam? Did it include U.S. POWs held elsewhere, like those reportedly in or moved to Cambodia, Laos, and China? Why didn't he say *all* U.S. prisoners and missing in Southeast Asia? Mother startled me out of my thoughts.[3]

"How are you feeling through all this, Evie?"

I was feeling weary and very sad. "Peace with honor," the President had said. What honor was there in this whole, tragic mess? What positive objectives had our country achieved for the South Vietnamese, for the Cambodians and Laotians, or ourselves, with this 14-year war? What objectives had we gained from this bloodbath that we would point to with pride in years to come? What did we have now, that we didn't have before, that would justify the more than 55,000 lives lost, the countless wounded, or the ordeal of separation and human suffering that the POW/MIA families had to survive? What of all those lost years that could never be recovered? What is there about this war that can ever justify our loss of Newk?

I didn't want to get Mother upset again, so I kept my tone neutral when I replied, "I truly don't know how I feel, Mother. I know it's way past time to end this war. I also know that the end will bring official confirmation of Newk's death. That will be a terrible moment for all of us, but we must know for sure. I worry a lot about Mother and Dad Grubb. I'm prepared for whatever comes, but I know in my heart they are praying for a miracle."

"What about the boys? Do you really think they believe as you do, Evie, that their Dad is truly gone and not coming home?"

"Yes, I believe they do, Mother. We've moved beyond expecting miracles. But I should warn you now that I intend to continue fighting for official Geneva Conventions notification from the government of North Vietnam, and for Newk to come home to rest."

Mother looked out the window and sighed. I think she, like the Grubbs, still believed she might see Newk walk through our front door. The faith in miracles I'd held for seven years of silence from Newk had dissipated with Cora Weiss' announcement. Now, for me, even faint hope was gone. The North Vietnamese had reported Newk's death to at least three different sources, but to my knowledge, none of those reports had been addressed to our government. They certainly hadn't reported it directly to me in any acceptable way. Of course, they had waited five years before even admitting Newk was "dead." That wait, so callously brutal to us, his family, had afforded them adequate time to cover their tracks and expunge any evidence of how he, and perhaps some other POWs, had actually perished.

The holidays had ended. It was mid-January 1973, and the boys and I prepared to attend President Nixon's inauguration. As his triumphal second term began, Nixon was riding high on his success in bringing an end to the war. He had gotten to announce it before the official end of his first term in office, so technically he had kept part of his campaign promise.

He didn't get the POWs home by then though. Our price as a family had been the highest . . . Newk suffering and dying as a prisoner of war, gone forever from our lives. Jeff, and maybe Roland, would remember Newk a little. Van and Roy wouldn't. None of them would ever have a chance to really know their wonderful father, be able to learn from him, confide in him, or share their accomplishments with him, as they grew to manhood. They would miss sharing with him their life's achievements and milestones, and seeing his pride in them shining from his eyes as they graduated and became men. The impact on each of us of our loss of Newk was beyond comprehending.

On January 16, I attended the League Board meeting in Washington, then remained in the city for a CBS phone interview with John Cochran and another appearance on the Fulton Lewis radio show. It was freezing that January and my apartment was a warm place to hang out and recover between inaugural events, so the boys joined me up there on Saturday. The inauguration of the U.S. President was as exciting as we knew it would be.

The boys had the pleasure of meeting and speaking with so many people, memorably Colonel Sanders, the Kentucky Fried Chicken icon, who sat near us in the bleachers. He looked just like the drawings of him; he was cordial and a true southern gentleman. The boys were very excited and impressed by him.

It was at the January Board meeting of the League that I learned that the United States had finally received two official lists of POWs from North Vietnam: the first was a list of those who would be returning, and the second was of those who had "died in captivity." Finally, I saw the truth I'd sought for so long. There, in black and white, in an official government document, among the list of men who had died in captivity, was Newk's name. It was a stark and painful moment. No reason for his death and no details were given, just his name. Everyone at the Board meeting expressed

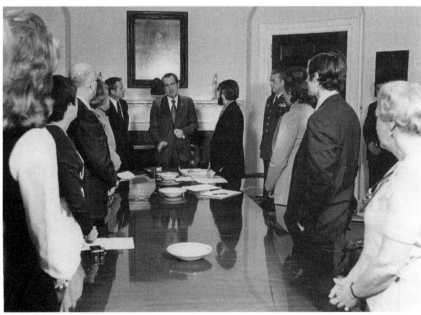

President Richard M. Nixon addresses the League Board January 26, 1973. To the President's left are: Joe McCain, Scott Albright, Evelyn Grubb, Bob Brudno, Iris Powers. To the President's right are George Brooks, Nancy Perisho, John Coker, Judy Irsch, Darleen Sadler, and (not seen) Phyllis Galanti, Board Chairman.

Grubb family files

their sincere condolences. After my initial and understandable reaction to seeing Newk's name in official print as being dead, I was able to continue with the meeting.

That night, Joe McCain tendered his resignation from the League. His brother, Navy Lt. Commander John McCain III, would soon return with the liberated POWs. Although the Discrepancies remained an important issue, Joe's work with the League was essentially completed. I was sad to hear he was leaving. Joe was a dear, kind friend and I knew I'd miss him a lot. We were honored when President Nixon stepped into our Board meeting unexpectedly, to commend us on our work for the POWs and MIAs.

Although Newk was now officially listed as deceased, our government did not rush to change Newk's or my official status.[4] I remained in "official limbo" and guessed it would be that way for awhile longer. I'd been in this "neither wife...nor widow" phase for so long, it didn't really make a difference now. My life continued as it had for the past seven years, except that now there were additional things to manage and people to console. When the two lists were published in the papers, more condolences followed.

I decided it was time for me to start looking for a real job—as much for my mental health as anything else. I constructed my resume and began sending it out. With all the boys in school, I truly believed I'd do better if I had a daily schedule of work to go to. Several weeks later, I accepted Conrad Mikulec's kind offer of a short-term position as the Washington, D.C., area representative for his fire extinguisher company. I enjoyed my new job at Mikulec's company. It was both interesting and challenging for me.

As the date neared for the return of the POWs, I experienced a series of emotional highs and lows and couldn't seem to move forward with my life. I told Sybil Stockdale about it, and she suggested I see a psychiatrist and get some counseling.

"That will help you find direction for the next part of your life, Evie. It really helped me when I went through a rocky period in my life a year or so ago." Sybil was happily anticipating being reunited with her Jim, who would be in the first group of POWs released, but she still cared enough to be concerned for me.

I acted on her advice, but my experience wasn't a positive one.

At 42 years old, I was hardly naïve, but I never expected to encounter a sexual predator in sheep's clothing in a mental health practitioner's office. If I'd wanted seduction, I could have found it anywhere in Washington, D.C. Sadly, experiencing that when I was fragile and at my most vulnerable fractured my trust in the mental health profession. I know now that I should have called the police. Instead, I went home, took a long, hot bath, cried for the first time in a long while, and then went on with my life.

It was mid-February 1973, around Valentine's Day when the first Vietnam POWs came home to enormous excitement, extensive press coverage, and a heroes' welcome. The country united to greet them in a way that was as poignant as it was unexpected. The country wanted—needed—heroes to heal the national wounds, and the returning POWs were available to be knighted. Their homecoming was the magic pill that eased the frustration and despair over leaving a war in which so many had died. It had been a very long war, one that our young people like Jeff had watched on the evening news for all of their formative years.[5]

As I watched the POWs' joyous return on television, I also felt deep regret that we couldn't be one of the happy families waiting to welcome our husband and father with open arms and tears of joy. I couldn't keep my tears from welling up and spilling over. But as each former POW, one after another, descended the stairway of the U.S. Air Force plane and took his first step back onto home soil, I felt true delight in my heart for them and their families. There were so many familiar names to which I could now put a face, and so many friends I deeply cared about who would celebrate today and return to their homes as a family again. Al Brunstrom was among them, and he, Helen, and daughter Kathy had a joyous reunion that was seen in newspapers around the world. [A painting was made of the photo of that moment, entitled *Homecoming* which is part of the Air Force Art Collection. Col. (Retired) Al Brunstrom was kind enough to provide us a copy of it for publication here.]

The returning POWs also had much ahead of them, both good and bad. Would the returning husband and/or father like the changes in his wife or in the attitude and behavior of his kids? Could a POW family ever put together a normal life again? A huge price might be exacted for all the years spent apart without any

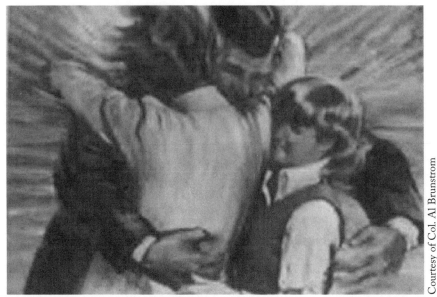

Hanoi POWs Return: February 1973: USAF Col. Al Brunstrom, reconnais-
sance pilot, (Newk Grubb's wingman) is reunited with his wife Helen and
daughter Kathy, 13, after 7 years apart. Brunstrom was shot down and cap-
tured in April 1966, 3 months after Newk Grubb. A rendering of "Joy at
Travis," painted by artist Amado Gonzalez, is in the U.S. Air Force Art
Collection.

meaningful communication, but that wouldn't be known for some
time yet.

Without a doubt, the men had also changed. They'd lived so
long in captivity, and had suffered and seen so much horror. They
had lost close friends while in there and many had lost family members, too. Their knowledge of past events was sparse, and their
mental status might be fragile or damaged. Physical or mental damage resulting from the rigors of long incarceration or torture might
not be manageable for the family, and necessary adjustments might
be extremely difficult. Only time could resolve the problems associated with assimilation of these men back into their changed families and country. No one could hazard a guess how long that might
take, or even if it would ever happen.

Americans didn't give the rigors of assimilation for these
returning POWs much thought. They wanted to celebrate, to exult
in the "feel good" moment of now. They wanted to parade their

returning heroes, see them on television, interview them, and bombard them with love, welcome, adulation, and parties. It was so American! Whether this was good for the men or their families, mentally or physically, was immaterial.

James S. Copley, Chairman of the Copley newspapers, helped the returning men catch up on world events by producing a booklet called *In Brief. . . for the P.O.W.: A Catch-up on News from Missing Years*. It was a handy booklet containing a digest of news, about the Vietnam War, the world, the United States, arts, music, and our accomplishments in space, plus a list of the deaths of well-known figures, year by year, from 1965 to 1972. The Department of Defense gave the booklet to each returning POW upon his arrival in the United States. I received one, too, as a Board Member of the League of Families. Each MIA family got one too, to tuck away in hope.[6]

I could sympathize and empathize with the MIA families. As I remarked in a subsequent interview, watching the return of the first POWs was the "happiest sad day" of my life.[7] There were still questions about the possibility of men left alive in Cambodia, Laos, maybe even China. The men listed to be repatriated were, according to the March 1973 issue of the *Air Force Magazine,* "555 American prisoners of war, far fewer than had been hoped for." In another segment of the article, "POW/MIA Action Report," the League "deplored the fact that there was no information at all about fourteen of the men expected to be included." Also, "Even more shocking was that the list . . . received from Laos named only seven military...three civilians, far below expectations."[8]

Well, where were all the others? The League had openly expressed our hopes that supplemental lists would be coming. Meanwhile, the MIA families remained condemned to continue the same worrying, wondering, and endless quest for information that I had endured for so long. In Laos alone, 294 Americans remained unaccounted for, some of whom were known to have been captured. Many of us hoped that the returning POWs could provide information about many of these missing American comrades.[9]

For me, a constant round of high and low points followed. There were condolences about Newk and letters of congratulations on my term as National Coordinator that came in the same mail delivery. The Hell's Angels sent me a telegram of congratulation on the return of the POWs. I received a letter from Leona Angell of Michigan, a divorced, single mother of three kids aged 13, 10, and 7, who had worn Newk's POW bracelet. She wrote:

> I have never taken it off since I put it on. I pray your man gets home. I hear you have 4 children, you sure have your hands full being alone, maybe it won't be long and you won't be alone. Hope so. I'm the type of woman that has a hard time with kids alone, as you well know how that goes. Have you heard anything about your husband? Please let me know . . . I have worn your husband's bracelet for so long, it's part of me. The black in the letters wore off because I even wash dishes with it on. God, I hope he comes home! I don't know why a person has to go through so much . . . will send you a picture later on, and do send one to me. Am thinking of you all. Take care always, Leona Angell.

I thought a lot about Leona and wished with all my heart that I could write her back with happier news. I knew exactly how she felt. I didn't know why a person had to go through so much either. Another letter was from Ed Prina of Copley News Service (a dear friend with a big heart) which said in part,

> I want to tell you how distressed I am that things did not turn out better. Although you were as well prepared mentally as anyone could be, it must have been terribly wrenching when the official word came. Hopefully, one or more of the returning POWs will have some information on what happened.[10]

As the furor over the POWs' return abated, I decided to accept a more permanent job offer from Leadership Systems, Inc., a management assessment firm in Silver Spring, Maryland. It was past time for me to begin a new life for myself and our family, one that wasn't continually grounded in false hope. I was still on the Board of the League and would remain deeply involved in MIA issues for awhile. I was still determined to secure official notification of the circumstances of Newk's death and to see that his remains were returned home. Mother had cried and grieved for Newk for several days after the news was confirmed, and the Grubbs had retreated to grieve for their son as well.

Then, here came Hanoi Jane Fonda again! Incredibly, given the national glowing mood of happiness about the return of the POWs, irrepressible actress Jane Fonda continued her diatribe by defaming our returned POWs. Those poor guys had been back barely two months before Jane publicly responded to their reports of torture inflicted by the North Vietnamese:

"We have no reason to believe that U.S. Air Force officers tell the truth. They are professional killers."[11]

She who had sacrificed nothing dared to speak that way about men who *had* sacrificed years of their lives so she would be free to spit out her lies. I brushed her silly antics aside. Those of us who had sacrificed and knew what it meant had to get on with our lives.

During those first couple of months, I had begun to make some serious decisions. I had decided we'd move to Silver Spring, Maryland, where I would be working. I would sell the Colonial Heights house and buy a new one there. It meant we'd be closer to Washington, D.C., with its many museums and activities that the boys and I could easily get to and enjoy. Also, it made access easier for me to handle the legal affairs that would be required regarding Newk's death, and also for my efforts with the League and the military command to have Newk's body or remains returned. Another, and the most important reason, was that I wanted our family to begin again in a completely new environment, away from the house and area where we'd spent too much time in sadness and anxiety, waiting and hoping for good news from or about Newk.

Meanwhile, all hell was breaking loose in Washington. Accusations were levied against President Nixon and his staff regarding the Republican-engineered break-in at the Watergate Hotel the previous June during the presidential campaign to illegally wiretap the offices of the Democratic Party. The investigation of illegal actions by the Republican Committee to Re-Elect the President (often pegged by the acronym CREEP in the newspapers) had been all but forgotten in the euphoria over the end of the Vietnam War. Five men proven to be directly or indirectly employed by CREEP had been convicted, and now it was rumored that people much higher up in the government, with much closer ties to the Nixon Administration, had been involved in the break-in or its aftermath. President Nixon and his Administration tried to distance themselves from the Watergate investigations, but that only served to widen the sphere of investigation. Rumors blew like a winter blizzard through Washington, the pinnacle city of rumor-mongering.[12]

The MIA families feared that the Pentagon was going to take advantage of the public's fixation on Watergate to quickly declare all servicemen still missing as PFD—Presumptive Finding of Death. Many firmly believed that the Pentagon's attempt to close these still-open files was a ploy by President Nixon and his Administration to get the whole POW/MIA issue buried once and for all. And no wonder! With Watergate, the Nixon people had all the problems they could handle. They didn't need to field questions about missing men in Southeast Asia.

"We're being Watergated right under the table," some MIA families declared angrily. "We're not going to cave that easily."[13]

With at least 1300 American men still listed as missing, the Virginia Chapter of the League of Families vowed to begin a new letter-writing campaign, this one to Congress and the President, to demand that no foreign aid be given to Vietnam until *all* remaining POWs in Southeast Asia had been repatriated and the MIAs accounted for.[14] The initial letters sent to Congressmen said, quite simply and clearly:

> As American citizens, we urge you not to contribute one cent to the rebuilding of North Vietnam until all of our men are home or accounted for. We have peace with honor. That is the American way. But, to honor America with peace, you must first honor those who kept that peace. As the Congress for the people of the United States, it is up to you to see that Vietnam does not become another Korea! BRING THEM ALL HOME.

In April, the State Coordinators for the League reported that they were distressed and discouraged. Angry words erupted at the Board meeting after reading their complaining letters. Attorney Dermot G. Foley of the New York League chapter wrote about the anger of the MIA families over the "wording of Article 8(b) of the

Cease-Fire Agreement with North Vietnam . . ." Foley wrote in part,

> . . . the League should become considerably more aggressive on the MIA question . . . the position of the M.I.A. question in the spectrum of priorities utilized by our government in negotiating the Vietnamese cease-fire, was totally inadequate . . . if the League finds that it cannot do so now, then would it not be fair and proper to so inform the membership so that those who wish to become more active can do so through other channels . . . ?[15]

At the same time, a document sent to the Foreign Claims Settlement Commission[16] on behalf of the MIA families said, in part,

> We now know from information provided by former prisoners who have been repatriated that many men were allowed to die in captivity and that others were killed. But inasmuch as many prisoners were held in solitary confinement or isolation for long years during the early stages of their imprisonment, it is highly likely that other captives may have died or been killed during this period without even being known to prisoners who have now been set free.
>
> . . . We believe that these circumstances, when considered in all of their combined implications, should encourage the Commissioners to exercise the widest possible latitude in deciding the validity of all claims. In absence of proof that the man was NOT captured, we think the benefit of all doubts should be resolved in favor of his eligible survivors. If such judgments cannot be made under current law, we would hope that the responsible Congressional Committees would take such action as may be necessary to provide the commission with essential authority. For that reason we are sending copies of this letter to the Chairmen of the House Interstate and Foreign Commerce Committee, and the Senate Commerce Committee.[17]

I knew that nothing could be done in the near term. Americans wanted the whole Vietnam War to disappear from the national consciousness, even though it wasn't yet settled in many areas. The

United States would probably be funneling money overseas to rebuild Vietnam before the glue was dry on the envelopes that contained the letters sent to Congress and the Commerce Committee!

The League chapters in Virginia and Maryland wanted to send a delegation to Southeast Asia, particularly Laos, to seek information about missing men. I was a living, breathing supporter of their determination. I hadn't, and wouldn't, give up on getting official notification and Newk's remains returned from North Vietnam.

People made wonderful tributes to Newk. In May, the boys and I were present for the dedication of the first Freedom Tree, which was planted at Roy's school, Lakeview Elementary School in Colonial Heights, Virginia. The tree was dedicated to Newk under the sponsorship of the Beta Sigma Phi Sorority. Over 150 parents, children, and dignitaries attended. Our dear friend Whitey Lemmond spoke briefly about Newk. As I stared at that little tree, struggling to survive, I thought that it was a fitting tribute to Newk, who loved the outdoors above all, and liked nothing better than to tramp through the woods and hunt and fish in the shade of tall trees.[18]

When asked to say something, I spoke from my heart when I said, "My sons and I are deeply honored at having Newk remembered in this way. This Freedom Tree symbolizes the hope and growth for America's future."

VIVA also made and donated the plaque that was placed under the tree. Their representative announced that VIVA would furnish a similar plaque to any city in America that planted and dedicated a Freedom Tree to POWs or MIAs.

I was also happy that something positive had come from this tragic year because it was Mom and Dad Grubb's 50th anniversary that year, and there was precious little joy in their hearts to mark that great occasion.

That July, most of the POW families whose loved one had been repatriated withdrew from the League of Families. The rest of us remained active members. Charlie Havens, our legal advisor, stayed on too. From then on, the League concentrated its efforts on the identification and recovery of the prisoners who died in captivity and the remaining 1300 or more MIAs.[19]

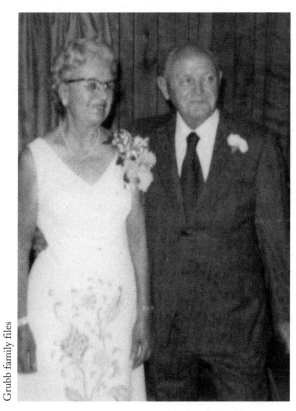

Grubb family files

Newk's parents, Mr. and Mrs. Newlin W. Grubb, celebrate their Golden (50th) Wedding Anniversary, July 1973. The senior Mr. Grubb was a Class of 1920 graduate of Penn State University.

Iris Powers' son, Lowell, missing since April of 1969, was still MIA. Iris remained active with the League and continued as head of the RRR (Repatriation, Rehabilitation, and Readjustment) Committee. She was a very strong influence in redirecting the League's focus as was Joan Vinson, whose husband, Bobby, missing since April of 1968, also remained MIA.

I had a happy yet poignant reunion with Al Brunstrom, Newk's wing man, who was present when Newk was shot down. Later, Al was also shot down and taken prisoner by the North Vietnamese. In answer to my question about any information he'd ever heard regarding Newk in Hanoi, he replied, "I heard as much as anybody, Evie, and it's pretty darn little."

> Newk could always find a hole in the weather, and one glance told him where we were. We had several targets that day, most were socked in weather. Suddenly, he flew up into the cloud cover, saying "I'm hit."

Then I heard his beeper that meant his chute had opened.
The A-1's went in within an hour, taking heavy fire, but
found nothing. Unfortunately there was a DRV military
installation nearby. He was likely captured immediately, no
chance to evade. When I was shot down three months later,
I got to Heartbreak prison in Hanoi at about 2 a.m. and was
thrown into a cell. I heard the name "Risner."[20]

He paused, remembering.
"I know who Risner is," I said.[21]
Al returned to the present and continued his story:

Right after I heard Risner's name, I was taken to a quiz
(interrogation) room. I was kept sitting on a little low stool,
for many hours, being interrogated by various Vietnamese.
They asked questions on military tactics, especially target
information. One of the interrogators pointed to map of
Hanoi and the area around the city, with decreasing size circles on it. He said "until x date you bombed to this, then to
this." Then he pointed to circles in Hanoi and said "when
here?" I was still giving them only name, rank, serial number and date of birth. The interrogator left and returned
some time later with a tape recorder. He turned on the
recorder and an American voice said, "Lt. Colonel
Robinson Risner," That got my attention. I listened carefully to a so-called confession. When it ended, there was a
click, a brief silence, and then another click and another
American voice came on and said, "This is Captain Wilmer
Newlin Grubb," At that point he immediately turned off
the recorder. Evie, it sure sounded to me like Newk's voice.
(We in the squadron called him "Newt.") I asked him to
turn it back on he said "no" and unplugged it. He asked why
I wanted to hear it. I said, "I know Capt. Grubb. I know he
is a POW. I want to hear what he had to say." He left the
quiz room with the recorder. About half an hour later the
door opened and Robbie Risner entered, with a guard.
Robbie had a watch in his hand and said they told him he
had thirty minutes to talk to me. Robbie asked what was
going on? He had no idea why he was there...they hadn't

told him anything. I said, "they played a tape that you made and when your part ended, there was a click, a silence, a click again, then another voice.'This is Captain Wilmer Newlin Grubb.' They turned the tape off there, and wouldn't play any more of it."

I told Robbie I knew Newt Grubb, I was his wingman when he was shot down, and had seen newspaper pictures of him on the ground and that he looked to be in good condition. I asked Robbie if he knew or had heard of Newt, and he said no, he had not heard the name. He said he heard them bring me in that morning, and as soon as the guards left he had called out to me. I'd heard him, but thought it might be a trap, so I didn't reply. He said he figured they played his tape when I didn't start answering their questions. They brought him in to talk to me, assuming he'd tell me they made him talk, and could make me talk, too. He described what they had done to him to make him make that tape. They had taken a rope and wrapped both arms tightly from wrist to elbow which completely cut off circulation. In a short time both arms went numb, started to turn black and blood started oozing out between the strands of rope. He reached a point where he knew he'd better do something, or lose both arms, so he taped the phony confession. He said, "I can't tell you to talk, and I can't tell you not to talk, that has to be your own decision. If you have to talk, give them as innocuous a story as you can come up with. Keep it simple, so you can remember it. You'll probably have to repeat it many times." He briefed me on prison camp conditions, and locations, described the tap code and how it worked, and said it was scratched into the wall in every room in Heartbreak. "Memorize it, learn to use it. When you get back to your cell, I'll contact you." His time was up and they took him away. The quizzing began again, and went on for two weeks, without any use of force. That started later—at the Zoo.

I'm so very sorry, Evie—for you and for the boys. You know how I felt about Newk. I wish I had more to tell you. They must have wanted to know from Newk when and where the bombing of North Vietnam would resume. Of course, he didn't know. I think the goon squad started out as amateurs (later they became professionals at it) and probably just went too far, and killed him trying to force him to tell them about targets, his missions, or to make that tape I heard the first words of that day at Heartbreak.[22]

Another returned longtime POW told me that he heard screams and yells of pain coming from the newcomer area about the same time Newk was reported to have died. Newk was the only newcomer captured that month to anyone's knowledge. It broke my heart to think that my Newk had died alone, tortured, bleeding from a ruptured spleen, in hideous pain, without ever having a chance to contact his family or see another American.[23] The thought devastated me and I was grief-stricken again. Nothing could or would be done, except to somehow force the North Vietnamese to own up to what they did. Too many other captives had died, too, with no explanation. The blankness of it, the not knowing, was the most upsetting. I was deeply grateful to Al for having told me all that he knew.[24]

Plenty of shocking things were coming out of Washington, too. On April 30, 1973, U.S. Attorney General Richard Kleindienst resigned, and so did President Nixon's two closest aides, John Erlichmann and H.R. Haldeman. That was a huge shock to the country. Then White House Counsel, John Dean, who had begun cooperating with federal Watergate prosecutors, was fired. We wondered what could possibly have blown up such a political storm, and how high would it go? It couldn't get much farther, we reasoned.

I turned my mind back to Newk and the sad and touching talk I'd had with Al Brunstrom. I desperately wanted to get Newk's remains back. I wanted him home, under his native soil, placed there with our loving care.

Not long after the POWs returned, Army Major Nick Rowe made a powerful and moving speech to the Military Chaplains' Association about the experience of being a POW. Major Rowe had escaped his captors in 1968 after five years of enduring the torment of captivity and the psychological experiments to which he was subjected. He accepted the association's National Citizenship

Award on behalf of all POWs and MIAs.

Rowe had spent 62 months under extremely brutal conditions as a prisoner of the Viet Cong in South Vietnam. He was carried as MIA while his family waited and clung to hope without a word of news, year after year, just as I had waited and clung to hope for some news of Newk. Only when three POWs from his camp were released in 1967, four years after his capture, did word of his status as a live prisoner come out. Rowe told the chaplains,

> The system under which we existed in the prison camps was not a 'haphazard' example of man's inhumanity to man. We underwent a sophisticated exploitation, a manipulation of human behavior in the classic sense, in that we were virtually in a laboratory situation . . . employing basic Pavlovian conditioning . . . the levels of manipulation began with the lowering of an individual to the level of an animal, struggling for simple physical survival. Degradation, dehumanization, humiliation, loss of identity, were their initial goals. Malnutrition, disease, physical mistreatment (torture) and isolation were their weapons. They sought to force us into abject compliance . . . they felt certain their system would crush our spirits and destroy our will to resist.

Rowe said that upon reflection about the horrors he survived, he felt that three faiths were the key to his survival: The first was his faith in God, the second his faith in his country, and the third his faith in his fellow Americans.

> With these faiths as a rock, as an anchor, I developed a resiliency which allowed me to continue . . . it was a test of values and faiths, and the captors were the losers.[25]

After reading that speech, I wondered how his fellow Americans, especially Jane Fonda and former Attorney General Ramsey Clark, would feel hearing Rowe's words? I wondered if they realized that, as fellow Americans, they had broken faith with him and his fellow captives during their darkest hours of torment?

On May 18, 1973, General Ogan, head of the POW/MIA Task Force, the Four-Power military team searching for additional missing and dead in Southeast Asia, spoke at a meeting of the League Board:

Negotiations have been slow. The first trip to Hanoi was
not very productive. Three grave sites were seen, two of
which were for men in the died-in-captivity category; the
names were written in North Vietnamese, dates of death
and initials of the deceased were in English; the third site
remains unidentified. On the second inspection trip to
Hanoi, 23 recently constructed grave sites were located. The
names were in North Vietnamese, initials and dates of
death in English. Members of the team are satisfied that the
gravestones, dates, and initials did match up with the names
of the 23 listed in the died-in-captivity category. 21 are in
an old French cemetery, 2 are in the first cemetery visited.[26]

The Board told him that we had been led to believe that
progress would be made toward the return of remains of those who
died in captivity. I wondered if one of those graves was Newk's.
General Ogan said that the State Department had agreed that they
should bring the lack of progress to the Kissinger-Le Duc Tho
talks that continued in Paris. This had been done, but the degree of
success was not yet known. He further advised us that "the U.S.
representatives probably will never be allowed to go to the cemeteries and exhume the bodies, but perhaps we'll be allowed to
observe [the Vietnamese do it, for positive ID.]" I didn't think that
sounded like good news.

Someone asked, "How long do you think it will take to get the
bodies in the American graves back to the United States for more
positive identification?"

His reply was, "Each one is an individual case." He said it was
his personal feeling that, "there will be a relatively short period of
time for the died-in-captivity cases as far as identification is concerned, but how or when they might be returned to this country is
a matter still being negotiated in Paris."[27]

The returned POWs had been home for three months. My status remained unresolved because Newk's remains had not yet been
retrieved, identified. or returned home.

One of the Board members asked Ogan about the MIAs, "Why
is our government willing to say our men are dead before the enemy
says they are dead? What about Dr. Shields' statement?"

Dr. Shields had recently made a public comment that some families thought blanket Presumptive Findings of Death (PFDs) would soon be forthcoming for many missing men, thus changing their status from MIA to KIA. His statement had raised a furor among the families that was still reverberating months later.

Ogan replied, "Dr. Shields has not said the men are dead. He has said that we have no information from any sources that indicate there are any other POWs, but this does not discount the possibility."

General Ogan had stated at one of our earlier regional meetings that he felt there were American men in Cambodia, and that Cambodia was one of the most likely places for us to look for some of the men who had earlier been identified as POWs but they had not been included on the North Vietnamese lists of those who died in captivity. At this meeting, we asked him for an update about Cambodia.

General Ogan replied that many things figured into the Cambodian situation, primarily the upcoming House and Senate votes on issues regarding Cambodia and the status of the Kissinger-Le Duc Tho talks. All this was very discouraging to the Board.

However, after hearing General Ogan's report, I felt certain that one of the bodies in those cemeteries he had mentioned was Newk's, and I was determined to verify it. I was equally certain that the investigation team had photographed or obtained photos of those gravesites. When I got home, I called the Air Force Casualty Office at Randolph AFB in Texas.

"Are there photographs of these gravesites General Ogan told us about? If so, I would like to see copies of them." I also requested updates on any news about the list of those who had died in captivity, and the location of my husband's remains. I was given the usual trite response, "You'll be kept informed, Mrs. Grubb."

By mid-May, I hadn't heard anything more about the gravesites, so I made more inquiries. Shortly thereafter, I received a letter from Colonel Luther from the Air Force Casualty Office with two enlarged black and white photographs. The letter said in part,

> Attached is a photograph of a marker which the North Vietnamese claim to be on the grave of your husband, Lieutenant Colonel Wilmer N. Grubb, and a photograph of

the graveyard. We will continue to advise you of information we receive pertaining to your husband. Please contact
us any time you feel we can be of assistance.[28]

Those photographs . . . the graves were so desolate! The graves
were mounded with what looked like sandy soil topped with a
slight growth of weeds. I thought that if they'd been in those graves
for seven years, they wouldn't look so much like new mounds; there
surely would be more growth covering them. Then I remembered
that General Ogan had said, "recent gravesites." So the remains had
been brought from elsewhere and hastily buried. A small grave
marker stuck up from each, very primitive. I got out my big magni-
fying glass. Newk might be buried under one of those mounds.

The second photo was a close-up. The grave marker was more
evident than in the other picture. Using the magnifier, I could make
out Newk's initials: "W. N." If there was a "G" for Grubb following
those two letters, it didn't show in the photo. Above the initials was
the inscription, "NG VAN GU CHET 4-2-1966." I put my face

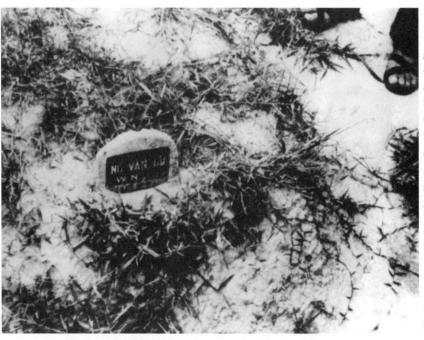

Official photo provided to Mrs. Evelyn Grubb, Grubb family files

*The North Vietnamese claim this is Newk Grubb's grave and grave marker
on one of 23 graves shown to U.S. inspectors in Hanoi, North Vietnam.*

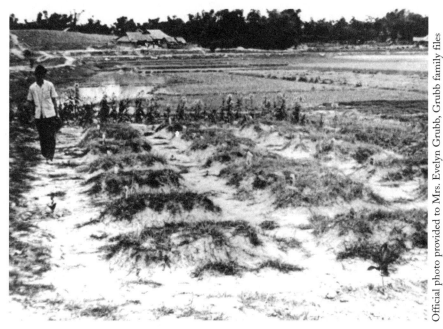

Official photo provided to Mrs. Evelyn Grubb, Grubb family files

Graveyard in Hanoi, North Vietnam, where North Vietnamese officials claim the remains of LTC Newlin W. "Newk" Grubb and 22 other POWs who died in captivity are currently interred. An American inspection team describes these graves as "recently constructed."

down next to the marker image on the cool surface of the photo. Tears came and slid slowly down my cheeks. These photos were all I'd received from where Newk drew his last breath. As time passed and I stared at those photos, the ugly desolation of the graves hardened my resolve to somehow bring my husband's remains back home. The photos were a sign for me to get busy.

I immediately wrote a note to Dr. Kissinger, asking him to please beef up his demands on the return of the remains of these men now that their graves had been identified.

I knew I also had to push for resolution and understanding of my financial situation when I became a legal widow. I volunteered to be a sample case study for other women, learning the many changes that would come with widowhood. These included insurance settlements and resolution and payment of government benefits. After it was done, I'd have one less concern when my status change became official. This was easier for me than for some other women because, in the fall of 1965, Newk had enacted a full Power of Attorney to me before he left for Southeast Asia. There were many types of Power of Attorney, but mine turned out to be the most beneficial for two reasons. First, it was an unlimited power of attorney, which meant I had full control of our assets and finances. Second, it would not expire until the day Newk was legally and officially declared dead by the U.S. government.

That hadn't happened yet because Newk's remains had not been exhumed and positively identified. In the meantime, I had enough time to consult with an attorney and gradually change things over into my name, using that Power of Attorney, so they wouldn't be held up in probate or litigation. The Power of Attorney had been very useful earlier when I dealt with the Air Force Finance Center in Denver. I had received Newk's full pay and allowances ever since.

Settling these issues was only the tip of the giant financial and bureaucratic iceberg I'd been required to grapple with all along the bumpy road of being a POW wife. Fortunately, I'd learned a lot in those seven years! I met with the Defense Finance Accounting Service, the IRS, and the Air Force Casualty Office. Each helped me review the various scenarios that a change in Newk's status from POW to KIA (Killed in Action) might bring. They calculated and listed various probabilities, and discussed with me the pros and cons of each for the boys and for me. They were especially helpful and kind in helping me plan for the day I received official notice of Newk's change in status. It was rewarding for me to see that our relentless activism had actually changed the military's bureaucratic attitude and behavior toward the wives, widows, and family members of the POWs and MIAs.

In Washington, the Watergate scandal just kept growing like a mushroom. In Paris, the North Vietnamese were failing to follow the peace agreements and did not return our men's bodies.[29] Despite his problems, President Nixon took the time to honor the returned POWs and their wives with a glittering reception at the White House.

On Watergate, the testimony of White House Counsel John Dean stunned the nation and implicated the White House, possibly even the President. This latest twist in the scandal overpowered everything else. We POW/MIA/KIA families were very dejected about the loss of momentum in pursuing the problems we had, but we were determined to continue pressing for closure, so that we could get on with our lives. We were gratified when the national commander of the American Legion said that the United States should apply military pressure to North Vietnam again, if necessary, to get information on the 1300 or more Americans still MIA.[30]

That summer of 1973, major dissension arose within the League over who had the power to accept or reject status changes for the missing men. In some instances, the wife wanted the status of the missing man changed to PFD to release her from bondage, but the parents or siblings didn't; in other cases, it was vice-versa. Some felt the military services should make the determination, but most families resisted that "solution."

Dermot Foley, League attorney in New York, filed a Class Action suit against the service secretaries that contested the legal validity of PFDs and enjoined the services against making status changes on missing men. On July 20, 1973, the U.S. District Court for the Southern District of New York granted the MIA families a temporary restraining order that prevented the service Secretaries from making any findings of death prior to July 30, 1973, while the courts researched the matter further.[31] The League refrained from taking a position on the lawsuit, as the Board agreed that status changes were a personal issue for each individual's family.

Helene Knapp, as National Coordinator, wrote President Nixon a letter with copies to Dr. Kissinger and Secretary of State William Rogers. The letter expressed the Board's disappointment that no statement from any of them concerning the Missing-in-Action issue had been made since Dr. Kissinger's return from Paris talks with Le Duc Tho. With the Board's backing, she had earlier invited Dr. Kissinger in writing to be the keynote speaker at our upcoming annual Convention in October, but still had not gotten a response. She had expressed our concern earlier about why he had not yet responded.[32]

Not long after that, Dr. Kissinger met with the League Board again. Our discussion with him centered on solving the POW remains and the MIA problem. He described how some teams were set up to find sites where the missing were buried and others were established to identify remains. He promised to accelerate progress in recovering the POW remains.

I asked him about Newk's remains. I was cheered when he replied, "I can assure you, Mrs. Grubb, that your husband's remains, along with the others, will be returned and soon."

"Thank you Dr. Kissinger," I replied.[33]

Afterward, we passed a motion to recommend that the next elected Board of the League continue to "push in the direction of promoting Congressional efforts and press coverage of all types on the MIA issue."[34] We were determined not to let the MIAs and the POWs who died in captivity become lost in the Watergate shuffle. The big Watergate news came at the end of July. The Senate Watergate Committee had learned of the existence of a tape recording system in President Nixon's office, and demanded the tapes for the time period under investigation. The president refused and the Committee threatened to subpoena the tapes.

While that dispute played out, the League remained focused on the issues that were now the League's top priorities: settling the process for status changes on MIAs, getting full accounting from Southeast Asia for the missing, and expediting the process to bring our men's bodies home.

We wanted countries like China and Russia denied most favored nation status and all financial aid withheld from Southeast Asian countries that participated in the war against us until our priorities were met, even if we had to mount another international letter writing campaign to accomplish our objectives.[35]

On October 20, 1973, in what the press dubbed the "Saturday Night Massacre," President Nixon fired special Watergate prosecutor, Archibald Cox. Deputy Attorney General William Ruckelshaus and Attorney General Elliot Richardson resigned. A short time afterward, Nixon appointed Leon Jaworski as the new special prosecutor. With all that was going on in Washington and despite Dr. Kissinger's good intentions and determination, it was no wonder that little or no progress was made on the MIA issue or the recovery of the bodies of the POWs who had died in captivity.

Nine months had passed since the signing of the Peace Agreements. We still had American troops in country, and North Vietnam was being as intractable as ever. Like many others, I felt our government had caved and was not pressing the North Vietnamese hard enough.

1973 was drawing to a close, and the status of MIAs and POWs who died in captivity, and their families, remained stagnant, controversial, and unresolved. Unfortunately, President Nixon's Administration was pretty much falling into the same sad state, but Watergate was being resolved, and fast.

It would soon be eight years since Newk had been captured. I was very much alive, but still shackled to an impenetrable wall, a prisoner of bureaucratic distraction and inertia. As 1974 dawned, I couldn't help wondering if and when I'd ever be released from my prison of being legally wife but actually widow. I asked myself the question, *Why can't they do something to get this over with?* The answer came back like a deep, hollow echo: *WATERGATE.*

We had major troubles in Washington. The Nixon Administration appeared to be on the verge of collapse. The country was absorbed in that. The Vietnamese gloated. Who would bother enforcing or policing the great Vietnam Peace Agreement?

In reply came another deep, hollow echo: *NOBODY.*

12 Journey's End: The Hero's Gate

TIMELINE . . . 1974 . . . <u>WORLD</u> . . . ASTROPHYSICIST STEPHEN HAWKING PROPOSES NEW BLACK HOLE THEORY . . . BALLET STAR MIKHAIL BARISHNIKOV DEFECTS FROM SOVIET UNION . . . <u>USA</u> . . . PRESIDENT FORD PARDONS EX-PRESIDENT NIXON . . . PATTY HEARST ABDUCTED BY SYMBIONESE LIBERATION ARMY TERRORIST GROUP . . . GIRLS ALLOWED TO PLAY LITTLE LEAGUE BASEBALL . . . HANK AARON BEATS BABE RUTH'S RECORD . . .

Show me a hero and I will write you a tragedy.
—F. Scott Fitzgerald

On Saturday, February 9, 1974, the League of Families Board met with Dr. Kissinger at the White House in one of our regular update sessions. He presented what he called "a wrap-up of the war." It was nearly a full year to the day since the surviving POWs had returned home. He was in good spirits, and I was emboldened to engage him and say, "Mr. Secretary, I am disappointed with what you just presented as the 'wrap-up of the war.'"

When Secretary Kissinger looked at me in surprise, I elaborated. "The known died-in-captivity POWs are still in their graves in Vietnam, sir. Although a year has passed since the live prisoners were returned and the graves of those who died in captivity have been identified, our 23 known dead have not been released by the enemy, nor returned for positive identification and burial. You promised me you would bring my husband Newk Grubb's body home, along with the other Americans who died in captivity, Secretary Kissinger. Where are they? When will we get them back?"

Our eyes met and held. The moment was so intense, it was as if we were alone in the room. No one made a sound. Finally, Secretary Kissinger said to me, very softly and kindly, "Mrs. Grubb, I'm deeply sorry it has taken so long. You will get your husband's body home soon. I do promise you."

Dr. Henry Kissinger was a man of his word, and I trusted him. He was focused, intent, confident. I had no idea what politics would conspire to get it accomplished, or what Herculean effort on his part would be required right in the midst of the turmoil still boiling in Southeast Asia, the Watergate scandal in Washington, D.C., threatening the stability of our government, and the controversy over the North Vietnamese failure to act to implement the Peace Agreement in Vietnam.[1] However, at that moment on that day, I knew that this man, Henry Kissinger, our Secretary of State, would somehow get Newk's remains home, and the other men's too. "Thank you, Mr. Secretary," I said, and smiled.

That was something to smile about. There wasn't much that brought a smile to my face these days and even less to make Dr. Kissinger smile. Nothing seemed to be going according to plan in Indochina.[2]

In mid-February 1974, less than a year after I was hired, I was laid off from my job. Economic times with inflation were tough in the United States and getting worse. The Vietnam War had taken a toll on the country in many ways. Perhaps it was for the best because only a week or so later Frank Sieverts from the State Department called to inform me that some of the died-in-captivity bodies from the North Vietnamese graves, including Newk's, might be returned "any day now."

"Oh, thank you Frank, and please thank Secretary Kissinger for me."

I immediately contacted Dr. Roger Shields' office at the Department of Defense. "Is my husband Newk's name on a list of returning bodies, and if so, could I see it?"

"Yes, his name is on it. I'm sorry, Evie, you can't see the list, but your husband's body likely will be returning very soon. You'll be notified as soon as we are."

I thanked him and called to alert Mother, who was visiting in Pittsburgh, and then Newk's parents, so they could prepare themselves to be ready to travel for the funeral. They were all relieved and excited about the news. That we'd have Newk home again, to bury him in Arlington was a major milestone in all our lives. The next week or so was full of tension and planning and anxiety. I did not want to leave the house and miss the call that Newk's body was due to arrive.

On March 8, I received another call, this one from a military official. I never registered his name because I was totally focused on the information he was giving me. He said that Newk's remains had been "provisionally" identified at the preliminary examination in Thailand and would be sent to the military forensics identification lab in Hawaii the following Wednesday. The lab would then make whatever further tests and identification measures needed for final, positive identification of the remains.

"Why is the identification process so time-consuming?" I wanted to know. I could almost feel my heart pounding. *What if the remains aren't Newk's?*

Although at first reluctant, the caller replied that because of the time that had elapsed, there could be no quick visual determination that it was Newk's remains that were in the grave marked as his. The remains had to be extensively tested for positive matches to Newk's blood type, height, physical features, and his medical and dental records. That helped me to understand but it didn't relieve the gnawing anxiety I was experiencing.

Two more weeks of tense waiting ensued. Then on March 21, 1974, I received calls from both the League of Families and the Air Force to inform me that Newk's body had been positively identified and was being flown to Travis Air Force Base in California. I breathed a great sigh of relief. "Closure is at hand," to paraphrase Henry Kissinger. I owed him a great debt. Thanks to him, Newk was coming home to us.

"Was identification of my husband's remains a difficult process?" I asked the Air Force representative who called me. He had seen the report from the lab in Hawaii.

"No Ma'am, his remains were matched to his records without great difficulty. Your husband had very few filled teeth, the blood type could still be matched, and all his bones were there, with the exception of one rib bone."

"Was there any information about the missing rib bone? I'm curious only for what it might contribute to determining the real cause of my husband's death in captivity."

"The North Vietnamese official death certificate, which as you requested is in the Geneva Convention format, accompanied the remains, ma'am. They claim the missing rib caused a ruptured spleen. They claim he suffered 'grievous wounds' on bailout."[3]

"That's not possible!" I blurted. Then I pulled myself back together, and thanked him for the identification work that had been done.

After looking at the photos of Newk very carefully again, I believed that the rib likely was missing because it had been broken by a rifle butt or other blunt object forcibly smashed into his midsection, either following capture, or in torture sessions aimed at eliciting information about his missions. It didn't happen on bailout as he was up and walking in those photos with no sign whatsoever of severe pain from any "grievous wounds on bailout." He had likely reached Hanoi in good shape. It was just more North Vietnamese propaganda.[4]

I also knew that, unless the United States demanded further medical evidence, such as a written report made by a physician at the date and time of death, we would never know whether Newk was fatally injured before or after making the tape that Al Brunstrom was convinced he had been forced to make. It was possibly the voice I'd heard on that tape all those years ago but couldn't conclusively identify it as Newk's. Most of the men in the camps had heard his name, so we knew he had reached the Hanoi prison camp alive. As the widely circulated North Vietnamese photos showed him, he was alert, stood upright, and appeared uninjured, except for some knee scrapes. So I was absolutely certain that whatever had caused Newk's death happened after he was taken prisoner by the North Vietnamese. The savage brutality of his captors, the merciless beatings and rope tortures, had been detailed and well-documented by the returned POWs in the year since their return from Vietnam.[5]

However, nothing was going to change this final reality. I couldn't allow myself to dwell on those thoughts or permit my anger to overwhelm me at this point. My final wish had been granted. What remained of Newk was out of that place and en route home for burial. I finally had been given proof that he had died in captivity. Now I could arrange a proper farewell for him. We all desperately wanted and needed to rejoice that Newk was back on home soil again and in the loving, caring custody of his family.

Dad Grubb chose to review the photos of his son's remains. I was grateful to him for doing that. It must have been a terrible blow to see what was left of his son that way. I went with Dad to review the autopsy report, but I could not go farther. I needed to remember Newk whole and smiling, not as a box of bones. Little was left now for us to do, except to mourn him, console one another, and lay him to rest in Arlington National Cemetery. Those arrangements needed to be made as soon as possible.

I had two weeks to plan his funeral and notify everyone. I had requested a plot close to where my father is buried and was assigned Section 8, Grave 658-E, only 30 feet away from Dad's gravesite. It is in a beautiful, peaceful spot at the base of the hill where General John J. Pershing rests. It overlooks the Washington Monument, the Pentagon, and the Potomac River.

One of Newk's best friends, Mike Nicolas, had done us the honor of escorting his remains from Travis Air Force Base in California to Washington, D.C. The funeral was scheduled for April 4, 1974. I prayed for a sunny day. President Nixon sent me a very nice letter the day before Newk's funeral:

> The White House
> Washington
> April 3, 1974
>
> Dear Mrs. Grubb:
>   Thank you very much for your deeply moving letter. Mrs. Nixon and I extend our heartfelt sympathy to you and your family at the end of your long and painful vigil.
>   Thanks to Wilmer Grubb and others like him, the American flag still flies proudly and unstained. Your husband rests in an America at peace—an honorable peace that his patriotism and your devotion helped to achieve.
>   That is something for which this generation and future generations owe you both an eternal debt. On behalf of all Americans, I thank you for your husband's dedication to the cause of freedom, and for your own unfailing courage as a wife, a mother, and a citizen. Our prayers and our thanks will always be with you.
>
> Sincerely,
> (Signed) Richard Nixon[6]

The day was cloudy on April 4, but no rain fell. I was astounded at how many people came to help us honor and say our farewells to Newk. The boys were tense and nervous about the ceremonials of the funeral, but we discussed it all ahead of time. I instructed Roke and Van to look to Jeff and our military escorts for what to do when necessary. Van and Roy would stay close to me, and I'd hold their hand when possible.

The brief Lutheran memorial service in the Arlington Cemetery Chapel, conducted by our own Pastor Cline, was impressive and lovely. After that, we lined up in cars for the procession to the gravesite. Roy clutched my hand. He was bewildered by it all, as any seven-year-old would be. Even so, he knew this was something important to do with Daddy—the Daddy he had never seen. All four boys behaved like young gentlemen, and I was extremely proud of them that day. I know Newk would have been, too.

Mother and the Grubbs also held up better than I expected considering their ages and all they'd endured over the past eight years. And I? Well, I thought I was emotionally prepared to handle the rituals that attend a hero's burial at Arlington, but I was wrong. The procession to Newk's gravesite was overwhelming. All those rows of headstones—nearly two centuries of national heroes—thousands upon thousands of them—blurred my vision and were forever seared into my memory of that day. I faced the reality of committing Newk forever to that hallowed earth with deep grief and enormous sorrow. Eight long, painful years had not diminished the love that had blossomed for us more than 22 years earlier, nor healed the profound pain and regret that I felt, and would continue to feel.

Outside Arlington Chapel, with great and precise ceremony, the military pallbearers lifted and loaded Newk's flag-covered casket onto a horse-drawn caisson. We were then taken in limousines over the hill near the Chapel, through the rarely opened Hero's Gate, and on toward the gravesite. Not far from the site, we got out of the limousines and stood, Roy on one side, clutching my hand, and Van on the other, equally close, as we waited for the caisson bearing Newk's body to arrive. Then we all walked behind the horse-drawn caisson bearing Newk's casket for the last 50 or so yards to his gravesite.

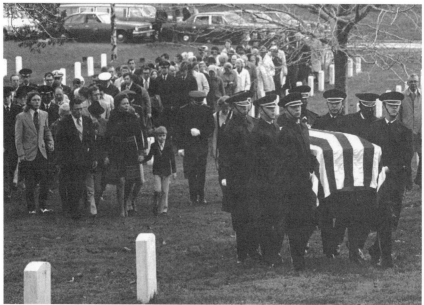

April 4, 1974: Lt. Col. Wilmer Newlin "Newk" Grubb's flag-draped coffin is transferred to his gravesite in Arlington National Cemetery. His widow, Evelyn Grubb, walks behind, with sons Roy, 7, and Stephen, 11, Following are Newk's parents, Mr. and Mrs. Newlin Grubb, Evelyn's mother, Mrs. Sally Fowler, and the couple's older sons Jeffrey, 18, and Roland, 13.

Jeff and Roke were immediately behind me throughout the graveside service. There were so many others there, and I could sense their comforting presence, as well as my brother's and Mother's, even though I couldn't see them. Newk's parents, too, were stalwart throughout it all. My body and mind had retreated into an emotional cocoon that somehow buffered and shielded me, yet I was keenly conscious of sounds and smells around me: the damp earth smell, the rustling of leaves, the horse harnesses jingling, the small scrape of Newk's casket being unloaded, the scent of the horses' sweat and the sound of their heavy breathing.

Much later, I learned that scores of attending military and former POWs, all in uniform, had escorted Newk's casket on foot from the Chapel all the way to the gravesite in a final, comradely gesture of respect.

Pastor Cline presided at the graveside service. I honestly did not remember much of what he said, except that I briefly came out of my mental fog when he intoned, "This is a man who was buried at least three times in Vietnam. Finally, he has come home to rest. And so we commit the body of our friend, Wilmer Newlin Grubb, to this earth and his everlasting spirit to the Lord."

It was almost over. Newk might be gone from us, never to return, but his earthly remains were at last home—in the earth of his country where he belonged. I had nothing more to fight for or to dread. It was done. All was still and quiet. We could hear birds. I shuddered when the first volley of the gun salute shattered the silence. I could feel Roy trembling, too, as he edged closer to my side. I patted his shoulder to comfort him. I held Van closer, too. They winced as each volley rang out. We clung together while Air Force jets roared overhead in the missing man formation—the final salute.[7]

The honor guard smartly lifted and folded the flag that covered Newk's coffin and presented it to me. Then another flag was produced and draped over Newk's coffin for a brief time. In the same precisely performed ceremony, it was removed, folded, and presented to Newk's parents. I loved that gesture of also honoring them.

"On behalf of a grateful nation," said Chaplain Boggs, the presiding military chaplain as he handed the tricorn-folded flag to me, "this flag is presented to you. It is a symbol of freedom and liberty, and of a country your husband served so very well." He repeated it appropriately to Newk's parents. As we stood, clutching our flags, all that we had left of Newk now, the final, mournful bugler notes of "Taps" began. Tears flowed freely from hundreds of eyes.

I had asked a friend to put a small container into Newk's grave before it was sealed. The container held some of the many POW bracelets that were engraved with his name and date of capture. So many family members, friends, and wonderful, caring Americans had worn his bracelet for so many years, and had sent them to me when they learned Newk had been officially classified as Died in Captivity.

And so ended our final good-bye to him. After that, we were escorted to Air Force sedans for the drive to the Arlington Annex, where I'd arranged a reception and refreshments for everyone who attended the funeral. There I learned that Newk's service was the fifth largest military funeral ever held in Arlington to date. It was

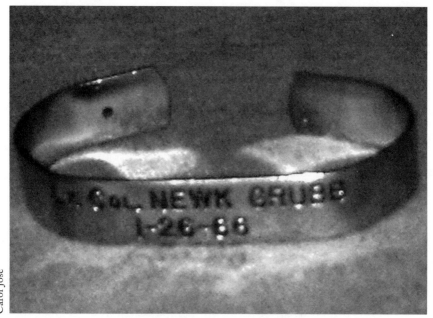

Carol Jose

One of the many POW/MIA bracelets engraved with Newk's name and date of captivity, January 26, 1966, worn in hope by hundreds of Americans. Evelyn buried some with Newk in his grave, Section 8, grave 658-E-1, Arlington National Cemetery.

not just family and friends who shook my hand to extend their condolences at the reception, but many ex-POWs, military and government officials, and members of the League of Families. Military friends whom Newk and I had come to know over the years made the trip to attend, including Jim (Col. James F.) Young, who had been one of Newk's roommates at the house in Saigon. Jim had also been shot down and held a POW in Hanoi. Fortunately, like Al Brunstrom, he had survived to return.

"Newk was one fine man, Evie," he said to me. "And one of the best reconnaissance pilots in the Air Force. Your sons had a father to be proud of. I'm just so sorry Newk didn't make it back with the rest of us."

"So am I," was all I could say. "But now at least we have him home. "

Former POW Fred Cherry was there, as was General Brent Scowcroft. I know there was a guest book at the reception for people to sign. I know that there were news photographers and other photographers there. Someone did a television video film of the ceremony. Unfortunately, the guest book disappeared, and I never received any copies of the films or photographs taken that day. I truly regret the lack of those. They would have been important mementos for our sons and grandchildren. There were articles and photographs in most major newspapers the following day, and many friends clipped and sent them to me.

The next few days passed in a blur of activities, condolence calls and farewells. Mother and Dad Grubb left to mourn their son in quiet at their Pennsylvania home.

On Sunday, I returned to Arlington with the boys and my family to say our private farewells to Newk. After a few moments by his gravesite, everyone walked away and left me alone with Newk. I had my senses about me by then, and I was able to say, just between us, the intimate and very personal farewell to Newk that I needed to make to have closure. Afterward, we all left Arlington. I felt a great sense of peace. My life could now come back into balance. We had done our utmost, and as I knew he would, Dr. Kissinger had kept his promise to bring Newk home again.

On April 17, I was surprised to receive another, more personal letter of condolence from President and Mrs. Nixon.

> The White House
> Washington
> April 16, 1974
>
> It is with great sadness that I have learned of the official confirmation of the death of your husband, Lieutenant Colonel Wilmer N. Grubb. The hope you held out for so long, and the immense ordeal you have suffered makes the news of his loss especially tragic.
>
> I know there is little I can say to ease your sorrow. But I do want to assure you that he has left a legacy that cannot die so long as men are willing to make the highest sacrifice for freedom so that others may live in a world at peace.
>
> Mrs. Nixon joins me in extending our deepest sympathy and our hope that the profound respect your husband has earned will sustain and comfort you in this time of

mourning. You and your family are in our thoughts and prayers.

Sincerely,

(Signed) Richard Nixon[8]

Actually, there was little time after that day to mourn Newk's death. I spent the next month coping with the blizzard of paperwork that widowhood required of me—legal, banking, financial, and insurance. I also needed to get back into the home front with the boys.

On April 20, 1974, I attended Kathy Plowman's memorial service for her husband Jim Plowman, who was missing in action.[9] Joe McCain also attended, and I was very glad to see him again. He expressed his condolences to me and went with me to visit Newk's grave. It was a special moment, a small victory over Hanoi that we both understood without saying anything. Newk was home at last. We had wrested official notification of his death from the DRV in the format provided for in the Geneva Conventions. We had won that one small concession in this. I was not only pleased to see Joe again, but also I was glad to share with him this one tiny victory in formally closing out one of Joe's Discrepancy Report files. I was glad to hear his happiness over the safe return of his brother, Lt. Commander John McCain III, from captivity, too, and to know that Bonnie Metzger's husband, Bill, who had been dreadfully wounded, had also made it back home alive.

Then suddenly it was June, and I realized with a jolt that Jeff's high school graduation was only two weeks away! The families were coming for it. It was time to plan something happy and joyous— Jeff's first big life milestone achieved, his high school graduation! A couple of days later, the phone rang. It was Air Force Headquarters.

"Mrs. Grubb, there will be a ceremony in Washington, at the Pentagon, on June 13 to award Lt. Colonel Grubb's service medals. We hope you and your sons can be present to accept these awards on your late husband's, and their late father's, behalf."

I thanked the caller and said we would be there. June 13 was the day before Jeff's graduation. The families would be here, so that was a good thing. I called Mother and Dad Grubb. "Can you arrange to come down a couple of days earlier so you can also attend the awards ceremony for Newk on June 13 at the Pentagon with us?"

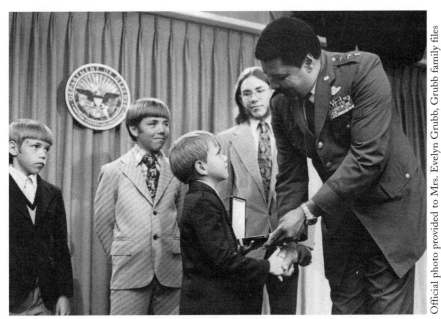

Official photo provided to Mrs. Evelyn Grubb, Grubb family files

June 13, 1974: Lt. General Daniel "Chappie" James presents one of Lt. Col. Wilmer N. Grubb's many citations and medals awarded posthumously to Grubb's youngest son Roy Fowler Grubb, 7, in honor of his father's service to his country. Roy, born 6 months after his father's capture, never saw his father.

"Of course, Evie. We'll be honored to be there with you and the boys."

I requested that Air Force Major General "Chappie" James conduct the ceremony. It was simple but impressive. Each of the boys accepted medals earned by their father.

Some of the awards honored Newk for feats I hadn't known about. For example, he was awarded the Distinguished Flying Cross for a mission he flew on December 21, 1965, just a few weeks before he was shot down. The citation read, "For 16 photographic passes over hostile territory at 1000 feet. On the seventeenth pass he received a direct hit, but continued to expose himself to enemy fire for two more passes, then brought his badly disabled aircraft back to his home base."

Besides the Distinguished Flying Cross, Newk was awarded the Air Medal with three oak leaf clusters, the Silver Star, two Purple Hearts, the Republic of Vietnam Service Medal, the National

Defense Service Medal, a Well Done Award for an outstanding feat of airmanship, the Armed Forces Reserve medal (Air Force), and several ribbons—the Outstanding Unit Award, Air Force Longevity Service with an oak leaf cluster, Small Arms Expert Marksmanship, and the Armed Forces Expeditionary Service with two oak leaf clusters. All of us, including Roy, left the ceremony with a new appreciation for, and great pride in, what Newk had accomplished in his Air Force career.

Jeff's graduation ceremonies broke us out of the somber mood that had descended again at Newk's award ceremony. Although I shed tears of emotion when our son walked across the stage to receive his diploma, wishing of course that Newk could have been there with me to share his important achievement, I was truly overjoyed for Jeff and happy for all of us. Through all the hard years, Jeff had remained level-headed and diligent in his schoolwork, and had earned his high school diploma. He did not fail, he did not quit, he overcame. Now he was proud, smiling, holding his diploma, and prepared to take the next step into his future. I felt certain that his three younger brothers would follow his and their father's lead. On June 29, I wrote this note to Chappie James[10] to thank him—he had always been a stalwart champion of my kids.

> Dear Chappie,
>
> Thank you very much for making Newk's posthumous Awards Ceremony so meaningful for all of us . . . most especially the children. Only Jeff remembers his father well, and it has been difficult to pass along to the three younger boys a mental picture of the good man Newk was. You helped do that. I think it is a tragedy that most Americans are unaware of the honor it can be to be known as a 'solid citizen,' with a genuine love of home, family, God and country. I think your words inspired that patriotic spirit in our small group. For myself, it has been an honor knowing you, Chappie. Too often, words of appreciation seem trite, but please know that my personal respect and admiration for you never wavered. Those long years of desperate waiting were bearable only because strong people like you were constantly working to solve the POW/MIA dilemma. For that reason, you being there to present Newk's

posthumous awards was especially significant. Although the ceremony concluded the book of life for a man we both hoped would survive captivity, you passed along to his sons, to the next generation, ideals that will never be forgotten.

Most sincerely,

Evie Grubb

On July 27, 1974, the Senate approved Articles of Impeachment against the President of the United States. President Richard Nixon resigned his office on August 8, 1974. The new President, Gerald Ford, was immediately sworn in. I knew very little about President Ford, and was relieved to learn that Dr. Henry Kissinger would remain as his Secretary of State, as many Vietnam issues were still pending.

Despite the provisions of the signed Paris Peace Agreement and our subsequent withdrawal of combat troops, the North Vietnamese moved boldly and rapidly into South Vietnam, and as they had with the Geneva Conventions, they pretty much ignored the important provisions of the Peace Agreement. Secretary Kissinger seemed the only slim hope we had for keeping Cambodia, Laos, and South Vietnam out of the hands of the Communists.[11]

Sadly, not many Americans cared one way or another at that point about what happened in faraway Southeast Asia. The threat of a Communist takeover there in the near future lent a special urgency to the League's desire to recover as many MIAs as we could, as soon as possible. I remained active with the League Board, and we worked on the many complex scenarios associated with the rapidly changing scene in Southeast Asia, not the least of which was getting Congress to allow money for the job.

Although not generally known then, in a report dated August 16, 1974, the DIA (Defense Intelligence Agency) reported that 294 Americans remained unaccounted for in Laos, of whom 5 were known to have been captured. According to the report, Special Intelligence (SI) indicated that:

- Navy pilot Barton S. Creed may have been captured but was probably dead;
- Air Force pilot David Hrdlicka, a known captive, was believed to have died in mid-1966;

• Eugene Debruin, acknowledged as captive by the Pathet Lao, had probably not survived;
• Air Force pilot Charles Shelton, a known captive, had probably died in mid-1966;

Civilian pilot Emmet Kay, downed in May, 1973, remained in captivity. (Kay was released in September, 1974).[12]

In late 1974, Iris Powers, Joan Vinson and I appeared before the Congressional Committee for Oversight of the Status of Missing Servicemen in Southeast Asia on behalf of the League of Families. We agreed that Iris, who had experience as both a wife and mother of an MIA in two different wars, would be our spokesperson.[13] We'd back her up if she needed help with any questions. After our introductions and background information were presented to the members of the Congressional Committee, Iris began with this statement:

> Your Committee has been charged with bringing to a conclusion one of the most frustrating problems ever faced by our country: an accounting of our missing men, both servicemen and civilians, in Southeast Asia. We do not envy you your job. Your willingness to expose yourselves to the baffling and emotionally charged issues, as they will unfold to you during your hearings, deserves the highest commendation. No one is more aware of the problems you will face than those of us sitting before you. We have traveled down the same road for many, many years.

She then gave a brief sketch of how the League of Families came into existence.

> In the beginning, it was simply a group of wives who banded together to bring public attention to the plight of their POW/MIA husbands. The first mass [national] meeting to bring our problem to the public was held at Constitution Hall on May 1, 1970, sponsored by this group. Families came from all over the United States, and even from Europe. Our first public event [as a national organization] was to invite Members of Congress, the military, and other government officials to an open house at our new space, generously donated by the Reserve Officers Association. So

many of you came we needed 'wall stretchers' to accommodate everyone. Our next project was a memorable one, too. At a joint meeting of Congress, we heard Colonel Frank Borman relate his travels around the world, seeking support for our cause from foreign governments.

As I listened to Iris speak to these eminent members of Congress, I noted with pride her confidence, professionalism, and determination as she delineated our views on the POW/MIA issue. She addressed the unresolved issue that remained after the POWs returned, the thorny problem of the missing. She asked these Congressmen to deal kindly with the MIA families and determine how to handle the fate of the missing and unaccounted for of that long war in Southeast Asia. Iris urged,

> Try with every means at your disposal to open up new avenues of communication with the North Vietnamese, and if you can arrive at new understandings with them; if you can find methods of reinstating the agreements in the Paris Peace Agreement that have been so flagrantly ignored; if you can develop procedures that will assure a proper accounting of even a portion of our missing men—that will allow U.S. search teams to comb the areas in which the men disappeared—you will have more than fulfilled your mission, and hundreds of MIA families will be forever in your debt. If these hearings can develop realistic policies to be followed in future conflicts, that too will serve a very useful purpose. May we also suggest that this Committee urge the convening of a new international assembly to study and revise the present Geneva Conventions pertaining to prisoners of war? These international rules need enforcement provisions that will assure their effectiveness. As they now stand—and as they were ignored during the Vietnam conflict—they are largely meaningless.[14]

Despite all she'd been through, Iris' voice rang with strength and sincerity at the end of our presentation. I realized then how much we had all grown as women and how much we had been able to get done for the POW-MIA families in the four years since Louise Mulligan had shouted that initial "Mayday!" at our first national meeting on the first of May, 1970.[15]

Today, many years later, I can still remember the sound of Louise's first cry of "Mayday!" I remember feeling like a huge door was opening in front of me, a door that had been blocked for years and that had kept me suffering—alone and in silence with my fear and grief.

The League of Families had pushed that door wide, and in the four years since then, had coalesced and evolved into a formidable international support group of families, heads of state, diplomats, devoted supporters—like Alan Shepard and Colonel Frank Borman, Anna Chennault, Johnny Unitas, Ross Perot — and a host of government officials at the United Nations, from various European countries, and in our own United States. We'd brought the plight of the unseen American POWs and MIAs to the attention of the world, and our own government, and we'd been a catalyst to ensure government support to their families.

I wondered, as I listened to the hearing, whether the Congressmen sitting before us could ever grasp or comprehend the excruciating pain that the three women before them had endured for more than eight years and were still enduring? What Iris Powers, Joan Vinson, and I, our families, and the thousands of MIA and KIA families, still had to endure? I doubted it. That kind of pain has to be felt deeply, lived with day in and day out, to ever be understood. No, they could not even imagine such pain, much less understand. It was there with us always, we were living it then as we fielded questions, explained thorny issues, and advised these Congressmen of the United States how to deal with the families of the MIAs.

As Iris went on speaking about the MIAs, I realized that my own mission with this group had at last come to an end. I had spent eight years living in limbo—neither wife nor widow—and had held tightly onto hope, until all hope was gone.

When official word finally arrived that I was indeed a widow I had fought to bring Newk home as fiercely as I knew Iris and Joan would fight to get an accounting of their loved ones and all the other missing warriors of the Southeast Asia conflict. I looked up from my thoughts to hear Iris saying,

> I've been condemned and vilified for seeming to care more

about the families than about the men themselves. But I believe that's the way our men would have wanted it, if there had been a choice. I resent having 'concerned citizens' tell me that they care more about my son than I do—and that has been done to me. Good God, I mourn my son Lowell today as much as I did 6 years ago. The need now to get on with the future of POW widows, MIA wives, children, and parents is more—far more—important than anything else.[16]

That reminded me that much of the work begun by us in the League was still unfinished. Truth be told, it might never be finished, but I hoped the League would continue on and not give up. It was now time for me to say my final good-byes—to the Vietnam War, to Newk, and to the League of Families. I knew then that I was truly ready to turn my full energies toward creating a new life with, and for, my children.

For this family, the Vietnam War had finally ended.

EPITAPH FOR A HERO
by Harry Dee

If I should perish overseas
In service to my Land
I shall have died a noble death—
Let none misunderstand.

I hope my body will be found,
Returned back to my home,
Where it was nourished and inspired—
No more to yearn, or roam.

Home is the soldier then from the war
Back to his family;
Home is the patriot at last,
Buried in majesty.

Pause, visitor, and cast a glance,
Upon a hero's grave;
Be thankful to breathe Freedom's air,
For which his life he gave.

In memory of Lt. Colonel Wilmer Newlin Grubb, POW/KIA
Section 8, Grave 658-E-1
Arlington National Cemetery
April 4, 1974
Vietnam Wall: panel O4E, Line 97

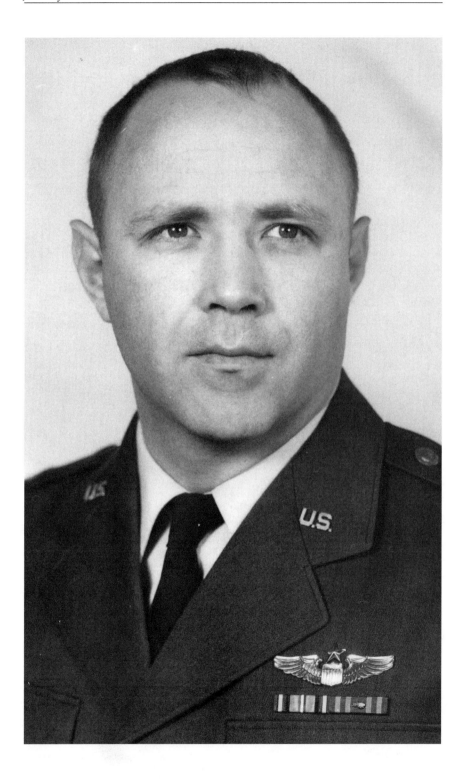

Appendix A
Military POWs Who Died in Captivity

NAME, RANK, SERVICE	CAPTURED	HELD IN	STATUS
Abbott, John, O5, USN	04-20-66	VN	KR
Adams, Samuel, E5, USAF	10-31-65	VS	KK
Arroyo-Baez, Gerasimo, E6, USA	03-24-69	VS	KR
Atterberry, Edwin L., O3, USAF	08-12-67	VN	KR
Bennett, Harold G., E4, USA	12-29-64	VS	KK
Burdett, Edward B., O6, USAF	11-18-67	VN	KR
Burns, Frederick J., E3, USMC	12-25-67	VS	KK
Cameron, Kenneth R., O5, USN	05-18-67	VN	KR
Cannon, frances E., E2, USA	01-08-68	VS	KR
Cobeil, Earl G., O3, USAF	11-05-67	VN	KR
Connell, James J., O3, USN	07-15-66	VN	KK
Cook, Donald G., O3, USMC	12-31-64	VS	KK
Delong, Joe L., E3, USA	05-18-67	VS	KK
Dennison, Terry A., O3, USN	07-19-66	VN	KR
Dexter, Bennie L., E3, USAF	05-09-66	VS	KK
Dexter, Ronald J., E8, USA	06-03-67	LA	KK
Diehl, William C., O3, USAF	11-07-67	VN	KR
Dodge, Ward K., O4, USAF	07-05-67	VN	KR
Dusing, Charles G., E5, USAF	10-31-65	VS	KK
Eisenbraun, William F, O3, USA	07-05-65	VS	KK
Ferguson, Walter, E6, USA	08-23-68	VS	KK
Frederick, John W., W4, USMC	12-07-65	VN	KR
George, James E., E4, USA	02-08-68	VS	KK
Godwin, Solomon H., W1, USMC	02-05-68	VS	KK
Gregory, Robert R., O3, USAF	02-12-66	VN	KR
Griffin, James L., O4, USN	05-19-67	VN	KR
Grissett, Edwin R., E4, USMC	01-22-66	VS	KR
Grubb, Wilmer N., O3, USAF	01-26-66	VN	KR
Hammond, Dennis W., E4. USMC	02-08-68	VS	KK
Hartman, Richard D., O4, USN	07-18-67	VN	KR
Heggen, Keith R., O5, USAF	12-21-72	VN	KR
Lyon, James M., O3. USA	02-05-70	VS	KK
Martin, Duane W., O2. USAF	09-20-65	VN	KK
Moon, Walter H., O4, USA	04-22-61	LA	KK
Moore, Thomas. E6, USAF	10-31-65	VS	KK
Newsom, Benjamin B., O4. USAF	07-23-66	VN	KR
Parks, Joe, E7. USA	12-22-64	VS	KK
Pemberton, Gene T., O4. USAF	07-23-66	VN	KR

NAME, RANK, SERVICE	CAPTURED	HELD IN	STATUS
Port, William D., E3, USA	01-12-68	VS	KR
Ray, James M., E3, USA	03-18-68	VS	KK
Rehe, Richard R., E3, USA	01-09-68	VS	KK
Reilly, Edward D., E4, USA	04-26-66	VS	KR
Roraback, Kenneth M., E8, USA	11-24-63	VS	KK
Salley, James, E7, USA	03-31-71	VS	KK
Schmidt, Norman, O5, USAF	09-01-66	VN	KR
Schumann, John R., O4, USA	06-16-65	VS	KK
Shark, Earl E., E5, USA	09-12-68	VS	KK
Sherman, Robert C., E4, USMC	06-24-67	VS	KR
Sijan, Lance P., O2, USAF	11-09-67	LA	KR
Smith, Homer L., O4, USN	05-20-67	VN	KR
Smith, William M., E3, USA	03-03-69	VS	KK
Stamm, Ernest A., O5, USN	11-25-68	VN	KR
Storz, Ronald E., O3, USAF	04-28-65	VN	KR
Sykes, Derri, E3, USA	01-09-68	VS	KK
Tadios, Leonard M., E5, USA	12-11-64	VS	KK
Terrilll, Philip B., E4, USA	03-31-71	VS	KK
Vanbendegom, James L., E4, USA	07-12-67	VS	KK
Varnado, Michael S., W1, USA	05-02-70	CB	KR
Versace, Humberto R., O3, USA	10-29-63	VS	KK
Walker, Orien J., O3, USA	05-23-65	VS	KK
Walters, Jack, O3, USN	05-19-67	VN	KR
Weskamp, Robert L., O2, USAF	04-25-67	VN	KR
Williams, Richard F., E8, USA	01-08-68	VS	KR
Young, Robert M., O3, USA	05-02-70	CB	KK
Zawtocki, Joseph S., E5, USMC	02-08-68	VS	KR

EXPLANATORY KEY:

RANK: Rank at date of capture; promotions continued until individual was officially declared deceased

CAPTURED: Date the POW went missing, or was captured

HELD IN: VN = North Vietnam; VS = South Vietnam; LA = Laos; CB = Cambodia

STATUS: KK = Captive, Died in Captivity, Remains Not Returned to U.S. Control; KR = Died in Captivity, Remains Returned to U.S. Control

Appendix B
Vietnam War Statistics

General Statistics:
- 3.4 million Americans served in Southeast Asia during the Vietnam War, including 514,300 offshore in Vietnam, Laos, Cambodia, and flight crews based in Thailand.
- Peak American troop strength in the Vietnam Theater was 543,400 in April of 1969.
- More than 55,000 U.S. Service Members were killed, or died.
- More than 150,000 were seriously wounded.
- 795 total Americans are known to have been captured during the Vietnam Conflict. This includes escapees, repatriated, and died in captivity for both U.S. military (725) and American civilians (70).
- PMSEA (Prisoners and Missing in Southeast Asia) lists 3,797 total Missing in the Vietnam War.

As of January 30, 2008, The National League of Families of POW/MIA lists these statistics:
- 1,763 Americans are still missing and unaccounted for from the Vietnam War, in these locations: Vietnam - 1,353 (North Vietnam-480; South Vietnam-873); Laos – 348; Cambodia - 55; Peoples Republic of China territorial waters -7 .
- 450 of these missing personnel were losses over water or at sea.

According to its website www.pow-miafamilies.org the National League of Families of POW/MIA seeks the return of all US prisoners, the fullest possible accounting for those still missing, and repatriation of all recoverable remains. The effort to accomplish this is ongoing.

PMSEA and POW "Mac's facts" are courtesy of Ex-Vietnam POW and U.S. Navy Captain (Retired) Mike McGrath, and NAM-POWs Corporation, a 501 (c) (19) veterans organization for the Vietnam era POWs. Go to: www.nampows.org

Tally of missing (MIA) is courtesy of the National League of Families of POW/MIA at 1005 North Glebe Road, Suite 170, Arlington, VA 22201. Go to: www.pow-miafamilies.org

Other statistics are from: http://vietnamresearch.com/history/stats.html

Bibliography

Books:

Alvarez, Everett, Jr. with Anthony S. Pitch. *Chained Eagle*. New York: Donald I. Fine, 1989.

Bigler, Philip. *In Honored Glory: Arlington National Cemetery, the Final Post*, 4th Ed. St. Petersburg, Florida: Vandamere Press, 2005. First published 1986.

Butwell, Richard. *Southeast ASIA Today And Tomorrow: A Political Analysis*. New York: Praeger, 1961;1964.

Corum, Robert: *American Patriot: The Life and Wars of Colonel Bud Day*. New York: Little Brown and Company, 2007.

Day, George E. "Bud." *Return with Honor*. Mesa, Arizona: Champlin Museum Press, 1989.

Guarino, Col. Larry. *A P.O.W.'s Story: 2801 Days in Hanoi*. New York: Ballantine/Ivy Books, 1st Ed. Mass Market 1990, Trade Ed.,1997.

Guarino, Evelyn and Jose, Carol. *Saved by Love*. Cocoa Beach, Florida: Blue Note Books, 2000.

Haney, Eric. *Inside Delta Force*. New York: Delacorte Press, 2002.

Howren, Jamie and Kiland, Taylor Baldwin. *Open Doors: Vietnam POWs Thirty Years Later*. Washington D.C: Potomac Books, Inc. 2005.

Hubbell, John G. *P.O.W.: A Definitive History of the American Prisoner-of-War Experience in Vietnam 1964-1973*. New York: Readers Digest Press, 1976.

Kissinger, Henry. *Ending the Vietnam War*. New York: Simon & Schuster, 2003

Korman, Stanley. *Vietnam: A History*. New York: The Viking Press, 1983

McGrath, John Michael. *Prisoner of War: Six Years in Hanoi*. Annapolis: Naval Institute Press, 1975.

Newman, Rick and Shepperd, Don. Foreword by Senator John McCain. *Bury Us Upside Down: The Misty Pilots and the Secret Battle for the Ho Chi Minh Trail*. New York: Presidio Press, Ballantine Books Trade, 2006.

Powell, Colin, with Joseph E. Persico. *My American Journey*. New York: Random House, 1995.

Risner, Robinson, Gen. *The Passing of the Night*. Connecticut: Konecky & Konecky, 1973.

Rowe, James N. *Five Years to Freedom*. New York: Ballantine, 2005. (Originally published 1971: Little, Brown & Company.)

Rochester, Stuart I. and Kiley, Frederick. *Honor Bound: The History of Prisoners of War in Southeast Asia 1961-1973*. Washington, D.C: Historical Office, Office of the Secretary of Defense,1988.

Shepperd, Donald W. (USAF Maj. Gen., Ret.) Editor. *Misty: First Person Stories of the F-100 Fast FACs in the Vietnam War.* 1st Books Library, 2002.

Stockdale, Jim and Sybil. *In Love and War: The Story of a Family's Ordeal and Sacrifice During the Vietnam Years.* New York: Harper & Rowe, 1984: Softcover: Bantam Books, 1985.

The Concise Columbia Encyclopedia, 2nd Ed. New York: Columbia University Press, 1989.

Magazines, Periodicals, Correspondence, Government Publications, and other Sources Consulted:

Air Force Magazine, 1501 Lee Highway, Arlington, Virginia 22209. Published monthly by the Air Force Association.

Air Force and Space Digest. Merged with AIR FORCE Magazine. See above.

Air Force Times. 6883 Commercial Dr. Springfield, Virginia 22159-0500.

Congressional Record, 1970-1971.

Journal of the Armed Forces. 6883 Commercial Dr. Springfield, VA. 22159-0500

News Release, Department of Defense, Office of Assistant Secretary of Defense (*Public Affairs*). No. 408-69.

POW Political Timeline Up to Son Tay, Appendix A. Military Thesis by Major John Mitchell, U.S. Marine Corps, 1997. Accessible online at www.globalsecurity.org/military/library/report/1997/Mitchell.htm

Reader's Digest. Pleasantville, New York.

Report of the Senate Select Committee No. 29 on POW/MIA Affairs. Chapter 7.

The American Legion Magazine. Go to: www.legion.org.

Third Geneva Convention of 1949 for the Treatment of Prisoners of War.

Time Magazine. Accessible online at www.time.com

Vietnam Information Notes. Office of Media Services, Bureau of Public Affairs, U.S. Department of State Publication, Washington, D.C. No. 9, August, 1967.

NOTE: Minutes of Board Meetings of the National League of Families; Evelyn Grubb's personal notes and correspondence, Official correspondence from military sources and organizations; Correspondence to and from The White House, to and from U.S. State and U.S. Government officials, United Nations Representatives, foreign government officials, and some articles cited in the chapter Endnotes, are extant in the Grubb family files.

Endnotes

Chapter 1

[1]Newk's tape to his family is in the Grubb family files, as are all family photos, tapes, letters and most documents quoted and/or reprinted herein.

[2]Grubb family files.

[3]USAF notification telegram, Jan. 26, 1966 (Grubb family files).

Chapter 2

[1]U.S. Secretary of State John Foster Dulles, speaking at the Geneva Conference, 1954: ". . . Indochina where the question of possible United States participation has to be considered . . . Communist conquest of this area would seriously imperil the free world position in the Western Pacific. President Eisenhower on April 16, 1953, said that "Aggression in Korea and in Southeast Asia are threats to the whole free community, to be met by united action." On Feb 12, 1955, he sent the first U.S. "military advisors" to South Vietnam . . . (*American Foreign Policy, 1950-1955*, Dept. of State Publication 6446, Washington, D.C., U.S. Govt. Printing Ofc., 1957).

[2]For full details on the two Taiwan Straits crises in the 1950's, go to: http://www.globalsecurity.org/military/ops/quemoy_matsu-2.htm.

[3]For information on the preparation and issuance of this Directive, see *Foreign Relations*, 1958-1960; Vol. IV, pp. 135-140.

[4]Secretary of State Dulles believed in nuclear deterrence through "brinksmanship" diplomacy to persuade an adversary to back down. (IV, "Kennedy and Cold War Brinksmanship" in *The Kennedy Mystique* by Russel D. Renka, March 3, 2006).

[5]The "Gulf of Tonkin incident" was an alleged pair of attacks by forces of Ho Chih Minh's Democratic Republic of Vietnam against two American destroyers on August 2 and August 4, 1964. (A report released in 2005 by the National Security Agency, indicated that the second attack did not occur.) This resulted in the Gulf of Tonkin Resolution, which granted President Johnson (and later Nixon) authority to assist any Southeast Asian country whose governments were jeopardized by Communist aggression. (*The Concise Columbia Encyclopedia*, 2nd Edition, New York: Columbia University Press, 1989, p.382).

[6]The domino theory—that if we allowed one small Southeast Asian nation like Vietnam to fall into the clutches of Communism, then neighboring SEATO nations like Thailand, the Philippines, and Pakistan would fall the same way—was the broad policy that goaded deeper involvement in the Vietnam civil war.

[7]Alvarez, a Navy pilot, launched from the aircraft carrier USS Constellation in an A4 Skyhawk over the Gulf of Tonkin on August 5, 1964. Headed toward Hon Gay, northeast of Haiphong, his aircraft was hit. Shortly afterward, he radioed: "I'm getting out. I'll see you guys later." He became the first American shot down, and first American POW in Hanoi, North Vietnam. (Hubbell, John G. *P.O.W.: A Definitive History of the American Prisoner-of-War Experience in Vietnam 1964-1973*. New York: Readers Digest Press, 1976, p.4).

Chapter 3

[1]USAF Telegram. (Grubb family files).

[2]President Johnson had offered Hanoi unconditional negotiations and, as a measure of goodwill, ordered a ceasefire on December 25, 1965. Captain Grubb was shot down in an unarmed reconnaissance mission on Jan. 26, 1966.

[3]Some military personnel functions had been moved from Washington, D.C., to the Headquarters, Air Force Military Personnel Center at Randolph Air Force Base, Texas.

[4]USAF telegram. (Grubb family files).

[4]Photos of Newk Grubb in captivity are from Grubb family files.

[6]Col. Lowery letter of Feb.5 1966. (Grubb family files).

[7]Al Brunstrom tape regarding Newk's last day. (Grubb family files).

[8]This photo of Newk Grubb was also published in Rochester, Stuart I. and Kiley, Frederick. *Honor Bound: The History of Prisoners of War in Southeast Asia 1961-1973.* Washington, D.C.: Historical Office, Office of the Secretary of Defense, 1998, p. 154).

[9]Al Brunstrom, Newk's wingman, would be shot down over North Vietnam three months later, and be a POW for nearly 7 years.

[10]The North Vietnamese were torturing POWs to get military information and propaganda statements when Captain Grubb was shot down. Wilmer Grubb was particularly vulnerable to being tortured, as he was the first prisoner captured since the cease fire 30 days earlier, and might be expected have current targeting information. When forced under extreme duress to make statements, many POWs disguised their statements in some way to let their family and nation know that their statements were not freely given. (Honor Bound, op.cit. p. 619 top; note 26 p. 631).

[11]USAF Telegram. (Grubb family files).

[12]The Casualty Officer assists the next of kin with receiving casualty services. In the case of a missing casualty, these services amount to keeping the next of kin notified of any changes in the airman's status and helping him or her resolve any military-related issues that come up.

[13]Col. Lowery letter to Personal Affairs Office, Randolph AFB. (Grubb family files).

[14]*Third Geneva Convention of 1949,* Section V, Article 71.

[15]See photo of this march of prisoners on cover of Guarino, Col. Larry. *A P.O.W.'s Story: 2801 Days in Hanoi.* New York: Ballantine/Ivy Books, 1st Ed. Mass Market 1990, Trade Ed., 1997, and also on the cover of *Honor Bound,* op. cit.

[16]Noted in Grubb family files.

[17]North Vietnam, a signatory, blatantly ignored Geneva Conventions on the Treatment of Prisoners of War. Various military sources, including OSD, confirm that besides not allowing POWs to send mail, an Information Bureau to keep the US advised of POW names and status wasn't created, and inhumane prisoner abuse, such as unsanitary conditions, solitary confinement, brutal torture, threats, exploitation, brainwashing, medical neglect and mental cruelty persisted for years. (*P.O.W.* op. cit.; *Honor Bound,* op. cit., debriefing and memoir accounts of returned POWs).

Chapter 4

[1]The torture sessions had shocked and subdued American POWs being held in "the Zoo". "All were appalled . . . Duffy Hutton's face was a mass of blue-red blotches: After he had been roped, his ankles and neck had been tied together across his back. He had lost consciousness . . . most of the blood vessels in his face had ruptured . . ." (*P.O.W.*, op. cit., pp. 202-203).

[2]"Both North Viet-Nam and the NLF (National Liberation Front) refused to observe the Geneva Convention provisions . . . their claims of humanitarian treatment of prisoners cannot be verified . . . majority of American prisoners have been isolated from every contact with the outside world. In the past 2 years there have been several incidents of abuse of American POWs, including the reprisal murder of three captured U.S. servicemen by the Viet Cong in 1965 . . . parading American pilots through the streets of Hanoi in 1966 ....The U.S. Government has formally protested the atrocities committed against U.S. personnel detained by the enemy . . . it is impossible to confirm the conditions under which prisoners are held by the enemy . . ." (*Viet-Nam Information Notes,* Bureau of Public Affairs, Dept. of State, August, 1967: Dept. of State Publication 8275 USGPO 1967 0-272-109).

[3]USAF letter, February 1967. (Grubb family files).

[4]USAF letter, April 1987. (Grubb family files).

[5]USAF letter, June 1967. (Grubb family files).

[6]*Life,* April 7, 1967.

[7]The United States government had been taking, similar actions since early 1966. (*Honor Bound,* op. cit., pp. 47, 99 et al).

[8]President Eisenhower wrote in 1954, "No one could be more bitterly opposed to ever getting the U.S. involved in a hot war in that region [Indochina] than I am; consequently, every move that I authorize is calculated, so far . . . to make certain that does not happen . . . any nation that intervenes in a civil war can scarcely expect to win unless the side in whose favor it intervenes possesses a high morale based on a war purpose or cause in which it absolutely believes." (Dwight D. Eisenhower papers, 1954, in John F. Kennedy Library).

[9]Letter from Lt. Col. J.G. Luther, Chief of Casualty Division, Randolph AFB Texas, 31 Aug, 1967. (Grubb family files).

[10]Air Force official letter on packages. (Grubb family files).

[11]USAF Captain Richard D.Vogel became a POW May, 22, 1967.

[12]Evelyn did not get the name of the Congressman who questioned her motives and worth, nor did she ask. But she never forgot that experience.

[13]American officials were quick to pronounce the Tet offensive "a military and psychological failure." In fact, militarily, the Communist forces won no new ground. The Administration's conduct of the war came in for heavy criticism. (*P.O.W.,* op. cit., p. 397). "The Tet offensive tripled their numbers. Within a four week span . . . the Communists in the South acquired more than 50 new U.S. prisoners, almost half of them civilians." (*Honor Bound,* op. cit., p. 446).

[14]The North Vietnamese had released three POWs, Black, Matheny, and Overly ,on February 16, 1968, as a "humane" gesture for Tet. The three men had been kept

in a camp designed for propaganda purposes, filled with recent captives who had limited exposure to the whole POW experience. The released men provided the U.S. military with their first intelligence on the POW camps and treatment, and also many POW names collected, memorized and passed from man to man, camp to camp. (*Honor Bound*, op. cit., p.366-369).

[15]U.S. Navy letter to Navy POW wives, 1968. (Grubb family files).

[16]*Third Geneva Convention of 1949*, Section V, Article 70.

[17]USAF letter March 1968. (Grubb family files).

[18]In early 1966, a State Department Committee on Prisoner Matters was established to solicit international support against the North Vietnamese charge of war crimes against the POWs. In July 1967, the Department of Defense created a PW Policy Committee headed by Paul Warnke, Assistant Secretary of Defense for International Affairs, to address the POW issue. By 1968, the committee's staff exceeded 100 persons. Responsibility for casualty status and assistance to the families, however, remained in the hands of the individual services. (*Honor Bound*, op. cit.) Author's Note: In 1966, the year Captain Grubb was captured, eight POWs died in captivity. For years, the United States refrained from direct charges of POW mistreatment for lack of documented evidence and concern about retribution against the prisoners. In May 1966, Navy POW CDR Jerry Denton, captured in July of 1965, blinked the word TORTURE in Morse code during a filmed interview. This raised public awareness, and ire, in the United States. (*Honor Bound*, op. cit., pp. 157; 183).

[19]USAF letter, March 1968. (Grubb family files).

[20]Col. Larry Guarino was in those Christmas 1965 propaganda photos. He says, "They blindfolded us, gave us a few pieces of candy to munch on while we waited, then Rabbit (one of the guards/torturers) demanded we 'confess to the priest how many times you have come up here, how many missions you have flown.' We knew we were in for a quiz-spiked (interrogation-recorded) church service . . . Our blindfolds were removed, Father Ho pressed on with the Mass, the photographers took their shots and filmed and we were given holy communion and taken back to the zoo." The POWs got no food except the candy. (*A P.O.W.'s Story: 2801 Days in Hanoi*, op. cit., pp. 76-77).

Chapter 5

[1]See Section 23 of the *Report of the Senate Select Committee of POW-MIA Affairs*, 1993. This issue is also addressed in a letter from Vice-Admiral J. Semmes Jr., Chief of Naval Personnel, dated 29 Jan 1968, wherein Adm. Semmes notes: "We have suggested to each of you that you avoid publicity concerning your husband's or son's status . . . this has been construed by some to be a concern for the safety of the husband or son. Our major purpose has been to avoid exposing you to harassment by "Anti-Vietnam-policy" agitators and to avoid invasions of privacy by well-meaning news media correspondents." (Grubb family files).

[2]Dr. Henry Kissinger, U.S. negotiator at both public and private Paris peace talks, reflected later in his memoirs, "The cause of frustration with Vietnam was not the

way in which America entered the war, but that it did so without a more careful assessment of the likely costs and potential outcomes." Kissinger also notes, "All this has come clearer to me with hindsight. My own views evolved only gradually . . ." (Kissinger, Henry, *Ending the Vietnam War.* New York: Simon & Schuster, 2003 pp. 38, 40).

[3]Peace talks, begun in Paris in 1968, stagnated during the latter part of President Johnson's regime, and remained so even after President Johnson ordered a bombing halt in October 1968. "No agreement was imminent in 1968. Hanoi was not prepared . . . to settle for anything other than total victory. . . . The stalemate was a dilemma that Nixon would inherit with his inauguration as President in January 1969. (*Ending the Vietnam War,* op. cit, p. 54)

[4]Evelyn Grubb's recollection of those events.

[5]*Pittsburg Progress Index* clipping, Feb. 9, 1969. (Grubb family files).

[6]White House Telegram, January 1969. (Grubb family files).

[7]Four-page letter dated Feb. 6, 1969, from Frank Sieverts, Special Assistant to the Under secretary of State, to Brigadier General Leo E. Benade, Military Personnel Policy, DOD, forwarded to "Navy Wives and Parents" of POW/MIA by Vice Admiral Charles K. Duncan, Chief of Naval Personnel, on Feb. 24, 1969. (Grubb family files).

[8]Grubb family files.

[9]Reprint of this article from the *Air Force and Space Digest,* October 1969 issue was given to Evelyn Grubb. (Grubb family files).

[10]U.S.Navy Captain Roger N. Netherland's remains were returned unilaterally by the government of Vietnam in September 1989. He is buried in Arlington National Cemetery , Section 5-E, Row 15, Site 5. Vietnam Wall, panel 19E, Row 84.

[11]On October 23, 1969, Kenneth O. Gilmore, Washington Editor of Reader's Digest, sent Evelyn Grubb an offprint of Stockstill's article in advance of publication. (Grubb family files).

[12]In his Thesis on the POW Political Timeline up to Son Tay, Major John Mitchell, USMC, states: "November 1969: President proclaims Nov. 9, 1969, a National Day of Prayer and Concern. U.S. makes major statement of concern in United Nations (UN) Human Rights Committee." For Mitchell's 1997 military thesis go to: www.globalsecurity.org/military/library/report/1997/Mitchell.htm.

[13]Dr. Joseph Elder's letter and notes. (Grubb family files).

[14]Ibid.

[15]Ibid.

[16]Ibid.

[17]Ibid.

[18] *Detroit Free Press,* Nov. 22, 1969. (Grubb family files).

[19](Henry) Ross Perot, Texas businessman and graduate of the U.S. Naval Academy, served four years as a naval officer. His failed attempts to deliver food and supplies to the POWs in North Vietnam were instrumental in bringing the plight of the POWs to the world's attention. *Wikipedia.*

[20]North Vietnam released three American POWs: USAF Major Norris Overly,

USAF Captain Jon Black and Navy Ensign David Matheny to Father Berrigan and Boston U. history professor Zinn, emissaries of David Dellinger's National Mobilization Committee in Feb. 1968, and another three prisoners, Navy Seaman Doug Hegdahl, Navy LTJG Robert Frishman and USAF Capt. Wesley Rumble in July of that year. (*Honor Bound,* op. cit., p.373;letter from Vice-Admiral B.J. Semmes, Jr., Chief of Naval Personnel. Grubb family files).

[21]Grubb family files.

[22]Air Force Col. Arthur Mearns, shot down over North Vietnam on Nov. 11, 1966, was listed as MIA until his remains were returned Sept. 30, 1977. He was buried in Arlington National Cemetery on Veterans' Day, Nov. 11, 1977.

[23]Weiss letter. (Grubb family files).

[24]*Congressional Record,* Jan. 26, 1970.

[25]USAF letter, March 1970. (Grubb family files). President Nixon brought POW issues into the open ("Go Public" campaign) in May of 1969 after receiving mounting indications of POW torture and pressure from the POW families.(*Honor Bound,* op. cit. p. 12.; Grubb family files.)

[26]"Mayday!" as a call for help in English is from the French *M'aidez!* (pronounced mayday) which translates to "Help me!"

[27]Perot worked on ways to help the POWs until their release in 1973. Although most people believe "United We Stand" originated with Perot's 1992 political campaign, it was used by Mr. Perot in 1970. Perot founded United We Stand as a POW/MIA awareness group with chapters in most states, which coordinated the League letter-writing campaign to the Vietnamese peace talks representatives in Paris. (*Time,* "The Odyssey of Ross Perot" Jan 12, 1970).

[28]The Military Services and the League of Families tracked these statistics.

[29]Unfortunately, there were conflicting year-by-year statistics on the POW situation. Artist and Vietnam Ex-POW John Michael "Mike" McGrath, Capt. USN (Ret.), author of *Prisoner of War: Six Years in Hanoi,* is the historian and current expert on POW statistics.

[30]Fact Sheet, National League of Families. (Grubb family files).

[31]*Third Geneva Convention for the Treatment of Prisoners of War.* Article 71.

[32]"The Air Force Association is a non-profit educational organization that promotes public understanding of aerospace power in the defense of our nation and supports the Air Force Family." From the AFA Mission Statement.

[33]"[Le Duc Tho, Hanoi's Special Adviser at the Paris Peace Talks] knew what he was about and served his cause with dedication and skill. That cause was to break the will of the United States . . . Any proposed settlement that deprived Hanoi of total victory was in his eyes a ruse by definition. He was there to wear me down. . . . In his view, the sole way to end the fighting was American acceptance of Hanoi's terms . . ." (*Ending the Vietnam War,* op. cit., pp. 113-114.

[34]League Bulletin, 1970. (Grubb family files).

[35]MIA Navy LTJG James Plowman: Plowman's wife Kathy identified him from a North Vietnamese photo just prior to December 1970; his parents identified him from a 1967 North Vietnamese photo. Even though there seems to be some doubt

that the two (Buzz Ellison) died, and that they may have been prisoners, their status remained MIA. By 1980, Plowman had been declared dead (PFD). Go to: http://www.pownetwork.org/bios/p/p043.htm.

[36]The DRV, Russia and China had published the photos of Newk through 1969. Cora Weiss was the first to claim in November 1970 that she had "an official list" from the North Vietnamese listing Col. Wilmer N. Grubb as one of six POWs who were "dead." See note 2, Chapter 6.

[37]Col. Larry Guarino, a senior officer and the tenth man captured and taken prisoner in Hanoi in 1965, adds substance to Evie Grubb's firm belief that the North Vietnamese jailers killed her husband, that he perished from mistreatment or torture. It was a belief she held until her own death 39 years later in December 2005. "In early 1966," Guarino notes, "we heard that the new shoot-downs were getting immediate torture for information vital to their [North Vietnam's] cause. The Vietnamese were questioning in four categories.…Military information of a timely nature had first priority. The V had learned from POW admissions under torture that a list of targets to be struck was published thirty days in advance. They probed to find out if the prisoner under interrogation knew the target list, or any part of it. "This would give them the opportunity to evacuate . . . personnel or . . . move out essential supplies or technical equipment. . . . The quest for information about our aircraft and new management capabilities was continual. Weapons delivery techniques and flight tactics were also important to the V[ietnamese] . . . [to] help them to devise defensive methods . . . Intelligence about newly installed electronics, and electronic countermeasures, was also of great military value . . ." (*A P.O.W.'s Story: 2801 Days in Hanoi*, op. cit., pp. 183-184) quoted with permission from the Author). Also: "On January 31, 1966 after a suspension of 37 days, the U.S. air attacks resumed, and with their renewal, the persecution of the American prisoners of war recommenced . Eight of the 1966 group would die in captivity . . ." (*Honor Bound*, op. cit., pp. 156, 157).

Chapter 6

[1]Evie's mother's fears were not idle ones. In 1971 alone, 90,000 people gathered outside Washington, D.C., to stage an anti-war march and demonstration in the capital. A bomb exploded in May 1971 in the Senate wing of the Capitol, which "has been the scene of bombings, shootings and other forms of mayhem since the early days . . . (David Stout, *New York Times*, July 25, 1998).

[2]*Third Geneva Convention for the Treatment of Prisoners of War.* Section 3, Articles 121, 122.

[3]In Evelyn Grubb's files, the document Cora Weiss brought back, with a list of names of 17 missing Americans is attached to a handwritten letter by Barbara Webster of the Committee of Liaison (COLIAFAM), dated November 16, 1970. Webster's letter says, " We are enclosing a copy of the written confirmation from the North Vietnamese, which is all the information we have. We are sorry to have to send this news to you, and extend our deepest sympathy." The fifth name on the list reads #5/ Grubb, Wilmer Newlin FV2211784 "dead." Also listed simply as "dead"

are: #1/ Atterberry, Edwin Lee; #3/ Burdett, Edward Burke; #9/Walter, Jack; #10/Griffin, James L.; #13/ Hartman, Richard D; of the 11 other men on the list only one, James J. Connell, was listed as "present in DRV detention camp." Connell may already have been dead at that time from the effects of severe beatings in 1969. Col. Larry Guarino reports in *A P.O.W.'s Story* (op. cit, p. 274): "Another person from there was my main man at the Zoo, J.J. Connell. JJ had been severely beaten . . . during the purge in 1969. He (Connell) and two other POWs were taken to the hospital in October of 1970 and neither was ever seen alive again." Connell's tragic story, one of torture so severe it drove him to insanity and death, is recounted in a number of POW books, notably *Chained Eagle,* (op. cit.) by Alvarez and in *Honor Bound* (op. cit.). The circumstances surrounding the deaths of known POWs, and the real cause of these deaths remains a mystery. Our government has failed to question or demand evidence of how or why they perished. Newk Grubb, J.J. Connell, and others who were reported "dead" were captured in reasonably healthy condition.

[4]*Congressional Record,* December 1, 1970.

[5]*Richmond News Leader,* Editorial, November 1970.

[6]The full text of Secretary Laird's report to the Senate Foreign Relations Committee is in the Grubb family files.

[7]*New York Times,* Dec. 12, 1970.

[8]David Bruce, Opening remarks, Paris meetings on peace in Vietnam, Dec. 1 1970. (Grubb family files).

[9]*The Review of the News,* (pp. 23-40) Belmont, Mass., (weekly) Vol. 6 No. 51, Dec. 23, 1970. (Grubb family files). No further information about this publication is contained in the file.

[10]Valerie's husband, Army doctor Capt. Floyd H. Kushner, a captive in South Vietnam, endured hideous conditions in a makeshift "camp." Captured November 30, 1967, he survived and was repatriated March 16, 1973. Kuschner testified later that six of the 22 men in his group of captives perished, "most of them in my arms . . . our ration was very low . . . we were horribly malnourished. People had malaria and dysentery . . . I don't know words that can describe how bad those times were." (*Honor Bound,* op. cit., pp. 463-467).

[11]*Air Force and Space Digest,* October, 1969.

[12]Major Arthur Stewart Mearns, USAF, MIA/KIA, was buried in Arlington Cemetery, November 11, 1977, in Section 11, grave #404-2. Lt. Col. Mearns' name is on the Vietnam Wall Panel 12 E, Row 55.

[13]The letter from President Nixon quoted here, dated Dec. 26, 1970, is more than three single-spaced pages in length. (Grubb family files).

[14]John Moore letter 15 Jan. 1971. (Grubb family files).

[15]Ibid.

[16]*Congressional Record* (E10958) of Jan. 2, 1971.

[17]BGen. Daniel James, Jr. letter Jan. 21, 1971. (Grubb family files).

Chapter 7

[1]Col. Bobby Vinson was declared dead (PFD) in 1977. Pieces of his F4D Phantom were located in 1996, and the family held a service and placed a headstone in Arlington Cemetery. Copilot Woodrow Parker's remains were identified. Col. Vinson's remains have not been retrieved, or ID'd per his widow, Joan Vinson, (March 2008). Bobby Vinson's name is on the Vietnam Wall, Panel 52E, Row 1.

[2]The White House Fellowship program gives outstanding young graduates an opportunity to work for a year in government assignments from the White House to the Justice Dept., the FBI, etc. (www.whitehouse.gov/fellows/home.html).

[3]In January 1970, Sullivan, Stauffer, Colwell & Bayles shortened its corporate title formally to SSC&B, Inc. A month later, SSC&B, Inc. purchased an interest in Lintas, creating SSC&B-Lintas, which made it the seventh-largest advertising agency in the world. Excerpted from the company history.

[4]Letter from Swedish Foreign Minister Rune Nystrom. (Grubb family files).

[5]The Third Geneva Convention allows for neutral powers (called Protecting Powers) to monitor the implementation of the conventions. North Vietnam did not do this. (*Diplomatic Conference of Geneva of 1949, Convention (III) relative to the Treatment of Prisoners of War,* 12 August 1949, Article 8.)

[6]Evelyn Grubb testimony, House Foreign Affairs Committee. (Grubb family files).

[7]Ibid.

[8]"Top of the News" Newsletter, no. 12, Volume 13 (Friday March 19 through Thursday March 25, 1971).

[9]Yale graduate and later United States President George Herbert Walker Bush received the Distinguished Flying Cross for Bravery during World War II and was an Ambassador to the United Nations (1971-1974). Evelyn Grubb admired him very much for the kind way he treated her and other members of the League when they called upon him at the United Nations.

[10]Ambassador George H.W. Bush in welcoming remarks to League members March 24, 1971. (Grubb family files).

[11]Ibid.

[12]Basic text of letters presented to the UN, March 1971. (Grubb family files).

[13]Enclosure to Sen. Bob Dole letter. (Grubb family files).

[14]This quote from her meeting with Dr. Shields is noted in Evelyn Grubb's writing in her personal engagement calendar, week of May 9-15, 1971.

[15]Ibid.

[16]U.N. Ambassador Stillman served concurrently with U.N. Ambassador George H.W. Bush. There were at that time several U.S. Ambassadors to the United Nations, who performed different ambassadorial functions for the U.S. Mission.

[17]Taken from a copy of Evelyn Grubb's Petition to the United Nations in the Grubb family files.

[18]Ibid.

[19]"The United Nations on Dec. 9 passed a strongly worded resolution calling for compliance with the Geneva Convention. . . ." Excerpt from President Nixon's open

letter to Evie Grubb and all POW/MIA families in Dec. 1970. (Grubb family files).
[20]Draft paper by John Moore. (Grubb family files).
[21]Ibid.
[22]Later, Perot learned from returned prisoners that their treatment did improve in direct correlation with his efforts. (Senate Select Committee no. 29 on POW/MIA Affairs Report, Chapt.7).
[23]For more about Everett Alvarez, who was repatriated alive in 1973, see the book he wrote later with Anthony S. Pitch about his POW experience. (Alvarez, Everett, Jr. with Anthony S. Pitch. *Chained Eagle.* New York: Donald I. Fine, 1989).

Chapter 8
[1]Col. Nick Rowe was assassinated by Communist insurgents April 21, 1989, while on assignment in the Philippines. (Rowe, James N., *Five Years to Freedom: The True Story of a Vietnam POW,* New York: Random House/Presidio Press Ed., 2005, About the Author).
[2]*Apollo 15* went to the moon, where the crew placed a memorial plaque, next to a small figure representing a fallen astronaut as a memorial to those who perished in space exploration.
[3]USAF letter (Grubb family files).
[4]The President signed the bill into law Nov. 24, 1971 as Public law 92-169. The families were notified of its passage in a newsletter from Air Force HQ dated Dec. 22, 1971. (Grubb family files).
[5]Copy included with packaging of POW/MIA bracelet. (Grubb family files).
[6]*Honor Bound,* op. cit., note 42, pp. 660- 661.
[7]National League of Families Telegram to North Vietnamese government, Oct. 12, 1971. (Grubb family files).
[8]Newspaper stories on Sexton's release (*Washington Post,* Oct. 13, 1971; *New York Times,* Oct. 12, 1971, *Philadelphia Inquirer,* Jan. 25, 1972; (*Honor Bound,* op. cit., note 42, p. 661).
[9]*Washington Post,* Oct. 27, 1971.
[10]Ibid.
[11]Ibid.
[12]Ibid.
[13]On March 9, 1989, the League's POW/MIA flag was installed in the Rotunda of the United States Capitol Building, the only flag to be honored in that way. On November 18, 1997, President Clinton signed into law the 1998 Defense Authorization Act. Part of that Act requires that the POW/MIA flag be flown from Military Installations, National Cemeteries, VA Medical Centers, and many other Federal Buildings. Since it is a declared national flag, when flown the POW/MIA flag flies in tandem with, and just below, the U.S. National Colors—the Stars and Stripes. It is the only other flag besides the Stars and Stripes that has ever been flown over the White House. Since POWs and MIAs come from every state, it flies on the same flagpole as the Stars and Stripes, and higher than state or other organizational flags. The POW/MIA flag is still manufactured and sold by Annin &

Company. Go to www.annin.com.

[14]Telegram, Swedish Embassy. (Grubb family files).

[15]League note to Indira Ghandi, Oct. 1971. (Grubb family files).

[16]First Secretary, Indian Embassy, note to League. (Grubb family files).

[17]Bonnie's husband, Navy LTJG Bill Metzger, captured 5/19/67, was "gravely injured" and looked after by injured and tortured "Red" McDaniel and other comrades in the "Vegas" prison camp. His wife Bonnie had heard nothing from her husband. Metzger's condition was described as "convinced of his imminent death, they (the North Vietnamese) bothered neither to treat nor to clothe him. . . . Lt. Metzger was left to lie naked, with gaping shrapnel wounds, broken leg bones and suppurating wounds in his arms, pus leaking onto the concrete floor, in stench so horrific the Vietnamese burned incense to counter it . . ." Saved only by the care of his fellow POWs, Lt. Metzger somehow survived until his repatriation on March 4, 1973. (*Honor Bound*, op. cit., pp. 302; 414-418).

[18]League telegram to President Nixon, Nov. 12, 1971. (Grubb family files).

[19]USAF letter, Dec. 22, 1971. (Grubb family files).

[20]The League received hard copies of press conferences like this. (Grubb family files). Rumors had been circulating that there were secret negotiations going on in Paris between Dr. Kissinger and chief North Vietnamese negotiator Le Duc Tho. These replies were an apparent reference to those rumors, later confirmed by Nixon, and by Kissinger in his memoirs. (*Ending the Vietnam War*, op. cit., p. 112).

[21]League action items. (Grubb family files).

[22]Telegram from Pennsylvania to League. (Grubb family files).

[23]Pennsylvania Legislative Transcript to League (Grubb family files).

[24]Evelyn Guarino describes her experiences during her husband's more than 7 years of captivity, and how things went when he returned home in 1973, in her book. (Guarino, Evelyn and Jose, Carol. *Saved by Love*. Cocoa Beach, FL: Blue Note Books, 2000 www.caroljose.com)

[25]Thomas Jones letter to heads of major U.S. corporations. (Grubb family files).

[26]This mail had never been delivered to Hanoi, but was stored in Paris.

[27]Ambassador William J. Porter was Chief Delegate to the Paris Peace Talks in 1971-1972. Ambassador to five countries, including South Korea, Amb. Porter died in 1973.

[28]As Kissinger later remarked in his memoirs, "Troop cuts poulticed public anguish at home, but they were destroying Hanoi's need to bargain about our disengagement." (*Ending the Vietnam War*, op. cit., p. 141).

[29]Evelyn Grubb's recollections of those events.

Chapter 9

[1]League Board meeting minutes, Jan. 1972. (Grubb family files).

[2]USAF letter, Jan. 13, 1972. (Grubb family files).

[3]Nixon's speech was televised January 25, 1972. Copies of President Nixon's speeches that addressed POW/MIA matters were provided to the League by the White House. (Grubb family files).

[4]Although she has since apologized for her shocking behavior in giving aid and comfort to the enemy during the Vietnam War, film actress Jane Fonda began speaking out against the Vietnam War in the early 1970s.

[5]The North Vietnamese used the divisive public attitude in the United States against not only the American POWs but also as a tool in refusing to negotiate peace on any terms except their demands that the U.S. capitulate. Examples: Kissinger's exchanges with Xuan Thuy, North Vietnam's plenipotentiary to the plenary peace talks. (Ending the Vietnam War, op. cit., pp. 87,89 210-211.)

[6]A letter confirming this "Week of Concern" went out on March 24, 1972 from the Department of the Air Force. "We stand ready to provide you every possible assistance in coping with the problems of waiting and the uncertainty of not knowing the status of your loved ones. Please be assured that we share your burden . . ." signed Robert C. Seamans, Jr, Secretary of the Air Force and John D.Ryan, General, USAF, Chief of Staff. Attached to that letter was a packet of information on items very important to the families, like the application forms for the 15 Red River Valley Association scholarships for children of POW/MIA men, and that Texas was exempting children of Texas Military personnel MIA or POW from state university tuition and fees. They also attached a list of medicines the Air Force Surgeon General's office would provide to families to include in packages to the POWs. They also cautioned that packages mailed to men that Hanoi had not acknowledged as POWs would be returned.(Grubb family files).

[7]Information and photos of childrens' activities sponsored by "No Greater Love" are in Grubb family files.

[8]In his talks to various civic and student groups, Jeff Grubb recapped the details of his Dad's capture and the aftermath, up to the notice of his Dad being dead, and said, "And so my mother, 3 brothers and I are left not knowing what to believe." Jeff and Roland Grubb, now grown men, have expressed that they still feel that way today. They have never received any evidence to prove, or give them closure, on how their Dad Newk Grubb actually died in captivity. All photos taken by the Vietnamese after his capture, or released after they claimed he was dead, showed him to be "in great shape," as Jeff expressed it in his 1972 talking points. (Grubb family files).

[9]Records and Photos of U.N. Visits and Joe McCain's Discrepancy Report presentations are in League Board Meeting Minutes, and in Grubb family files.

[10]Newk's friend, Charlie Shelton, was shot down in an RF-101 *Voodoo* over Laos in April 1965. He survived the crash, made radio contact, and was believed captured by the Pathet Lao. Officially listed as a POW by the U.S. government for years following the repatriation of U.S. prisoners in 1973, Shelton was declared dead (PFD) in 1994, but his ultimate fate is unknown. (*Honor Bound*, op. cit., pp. 281 & 614.) Shelton's widow, Marian, had committed suicide four years earlier, after searching for clues to her husband's fate for 25 years, per *The New York Times*, "The status change by the Air Force was requested by the Sheltons' children, who said it might help give them a sense of finality." ("Vietnam Era's Last P.O.W. Is Declared Dead by U.S.", *The New York Times*, Sept. 25, 1994.) According to Mike McGrath,

POW/MIA historian and statistician: because Col. Shelton's status as a POW of the Pathet Lao has not been officially confirmed by a sighting or other official notice, Shelton's status is not (at this point) confirmed as "POW/died in captivity." (Telephone conversation between author Carol Jose and Mike McGrath, November 2007).

[11]The first article of each of the four Geneva Conventions reads "The High Contracting Parties undertake to respect and to ensure respect for the present Convention in all circumstances." This is interpreted to include the endeavors by all Contracting Powers to bring a Power that fails to fulfill its obligations back to doing so. (Geneva Convention Commentaries provided by the ICRC, considered Guardians of international humanitarian law).

[12] "Kissinger Links Aid Bill to Talks" "His audience included the leaders of the major organizations of prisoners' families, including the Board of the National League of Families of Prisoners and Missing . . ." (*The New York Times,* Feb 3, 1972.)

[13]Grubb family files.

[14]On April 2, 1972, Nixon authorized the U.S. bombing of military and supply infrastructure all across North Vietnam. Operation Linebacker I continued until October 23, 1972, when Nixon halted the bombing after receiving indications that North Vietnam was ready to resume peace discussions. (www.militaryhistoryonline.com/Vietnam/airpower).

[15]Evelyn Grubb's Mayday speech is in Grubb family files.

[16]The Association of the United States Army is a nonprofit educational organization that supports the interests of America's Army and the men and women who serve in it. (AUSA website).

[17]Trip Notes on meetings with Government, ICRC, and other foreign dignitaries on this trip by League representatives are contained in the League minutes, along with Evelyn Grubb and Joe McCain's post-trip reports to the League, (Grubb family files and Evelyn Grubb's personal recollections of that trip, as told to co-author Carol Jose).

[18]President De Gaulle of France famously recommended that the United States not step into the Vietnam conflict between north and south, as Eisenhower earlier had warned him not to get France involved, and they had ignored him, too. In 1961,de Gaulle again strongly urged President Kennedy not to get more involved there, and predicted that the U.S. would find itself in a "bottomless quagmire"..if they did. (The French lost 55,000 troops there, almost as many as the Americans would.) Thus it is not surprising that the French would be adverse to helping us get out of that quagmire later, when Joe McCain approached them on his Europe trip for help regarding the conditions of our POWs. (http://www.spartacus.schoolnet.co.uk/2WWvietnam.htm).

[19]*Protocol III of the Geneva Convention for the Treatment of POWs,* Article 12.

[20]"Reaction to Discrepancy Presentation Report." May 21-June 4, 1972, pp. 4-5; and detailed "Special Report by Evelyn Grubb and Carole Hansen." (League of Families Board Meeting Minutes, July, 1972; Grubb Family Files).

[21]Pressured by the Communist Party of North Vietnam, the Communists in

South Vietnam organized as the National Liberation Front, called "Viet Cong," in 1961. (www.psywarrior.com/VCleafletsProp.htm).

[22]The communists in South Vietnam were known alternatively as the Viet Cong (by South Vietnamese), the National Liberation Front (by Communist party members) and the PPRG. (www.psywarrior.com/VCleafletsProp.htm).

[23]Former POW USAF General Robinson Risner also mentioned seeing North Vietnamese postage stamps made from photos of captured POWs. (Risner, Robinson, Gen. *The Passing of the Night.* Connecticut: Konecky & Konecky, 1973, p. 76) Author Carol Jose has obtained a rendering of such a stamp, depicting a downed American USAF F4H, with an injured American pilot being captured by three armed North Vietnamese female militia. Such postage stamps being displayed or used, like those seen by Risner and Grubb in different countries at different times, were clear violations of the Geneva Conventions, which prohibits such exploitation of POW captives for propaganda purposes.

[24]*Geneva Convention for the Treatment of POWs,* op.cit.

[25]Letter from MIA parents Genevieve and Russell Davis. (Grubb family files).

Chapter 10

[1]League Board Meeting Minutes, July 1972 (Grubb family files).

[2]Ibid.

[3]Actress Jane Fonda traveled to Paris in March 1971, where she met with the National Liberation Front (Viet Cong) and went to Hanoi in July, 1972, where she made radio broadcasts in which she accused her country of bombing civilians, and posed for photographs sitting on a North Vietnamese anti-aircraft battery used to shoot down U.S. planes. In 1973, when returned POWs claimed torture by the Vietnamese, she called them liars. (*Time,* Jan 3, 1972; U.S. House Committee on Internal Security, HR 16472 19-25 Sept. 1972; *Honor Bound,* op. cit., pp.180-81, 411, 566).

[4]The League of Families Special Report on meetings with Ramsey Clark. (Grubb family files).

[5]Bonnie Metzger's husband was still alive but severely injured and unable to write. He survived to return with the other POWs in 1973. (*Honor Bound,* op. cit. p 302).

[6]The Democratic Republic of Vietnam (DRV) refers to Communist North Vietnam.

[7]Congressman Sike's press statement. (Grubb family files).

[8]The mission of the Veterans of Foreign Wars (VFW) is to "honor the dead by helping the living through veterans, community, and national service and a strong national defense." (VFW website: www.vfw.org).

[9]*Honor Bound,* op. cit., p. 477.

[10]League presentation to Republican Platform Committee, August 1972. (Grubb family files).

[11]*Saved by Love,* op. cit., p. 179.

[12]On May 4, 1970, four students were killed by National Guardsmen at Kent State University in Kent, Ohio, following three days of anti-war protests and riots.

It was the cover story in Life magazine on May 15, 1970. The incident inspired the first nationwide student strike in U.S. history. Four million students protested and more than 900 American colleges and universities closed briefly. (*Life*, May 15 1970, *Wikipedia*).

[13]David Dellinger was one of the "Chicago Seven" group of protesters. He was tried and convicted in 1970 on charges of conspiracy and inciting a riot in the disruption of the 1968 Democratic National Convention in Chicago. The case was later overturned due to judicial errors. A lifelong pacifist, Dellinger worked with many anti-war groups during the Vietnam War. (*Wikipedia*).

[14]Jimmy Hoffa, the President of the Teamsters Union, was convicted in 1966 of jury tampering and fraud. President Nixon clearly mentions his personal participation in the "Hoffa pardon" on his White House tapes. (listened to by Carol Jose.) Hoffa was briefly slated to go to Vietnam in 1972, on a "peace-keeping mission" reportedly related to the POWs, which is how Evelyn Grubb, then National Coordinator of the League, became aware of this. Secretary of State Rogers cancelled Hoffa's plans, when word of the trip leaked to the press after prominent anti-war activists made statements from Hanoi, and the public found out. (*Time*, Sep 18, 1972).

[15]From notes in Grubb family files and Evie Grubb's personal recollections, as told to Carol Jose.

[16]Kissinger has said, "In my opening remarks, I uttered the phrase ('peace is at hand') that was to haunt me from then on" and, ". . . The press conference is now remembered, if at all, for the phrase. . . . In fact, the essence of the press conference was a detailed description of the terms of the agreement . . ." (*Ending the Vietnam War*, op. cit., Ch. 9, p. 375).

[17]Evie Grubb's personal notes, Grubb family files.

[18]The families learned later that the POWs had gone on a seven month "moratorium" on writing letters home. [The guards] "were so relieved when our seven month letter writing moratorium of 1971 was over. We could only hope that it was of some use against the Vietnamese in Paris," Guarino recalled. (*A P.O.W.'s Story: 2801 Days in Hanoi*, op. cit., p. 316).

[19]President Nixon halted the bombing of North Vietnam above the 20th parallel on October 23, 1972, after the DRV and U.S. agreed on a proposed settlement, and it held during the election. Reelected, Nixon began to consider the nonstop bombing of transportation, supply, and military infrastructure in Hanoi and Haiphong harbor around December 18, after Henry Kissinger reported that the North Vietnamese negotiators were creating problems and issues at the peace talks in France. Kissinger says, "Le Duc Tho..siezed the floor for a violent denunciation of our tactics . . . then rejected all proposals . . . he was willing to risk a breakoff in the talks . . . the immediate task was to save our national honor and position.." After several rounds of exhausting negotiations failed, "Nixon . . . agreed that we would have to step up military pressure." This concerted "Christmas bombing" for 12 days and nights by the B-52s finally brought the recalcitrant North Vietnamese back to the peace table for a final peace Agreement. (*Ending the Vietnam War*, op. cit., pp. 395-425).

Chapter 11

[1]*Honor Bound,* op. cit., pp. 552, 559.

[2]The White House provided the League with official transcriptions of President Nixon's speeches regarding the Vietnam War, POWs or MIAs. (TV address in Grubb family files).

[3]In 1972 and early 1973, American POWs were frequently shuffled around. They were scattered geographically throughout Southeast Asia, including Communist China. China released Vietnam captives AF Capt. Philip Smith and Navy CDR Robert Flynn (Vietnam War), and civilian John Downey, (Korean War) in March,1973. (*Honor Bound,* op. cit., Chapter 25 "Detours: Dissension and Dispersion" pp. 548, 554, 555, 563 (notes), 576, 577 ref. locations of different POW camps; p. 585, ref. China releases).

[4]The military services currently require that commanders obtain conclusive evidence before reporting the death of an individual. If the remains cannot be recovered, commanders may determine that conclusive evidence exists only if survival is deemed, beyond any reasonable doubt, to be impossible. (Current AFI 36-3002).

[5]*Time,* Feb 19, 1973 "A Celebration of Men Redeemed."

[6]The Copley booklet is in the Grubb family files.

[7]Evie's notes, Grubb Family Files.

[8]*Air Force Magazine,* March 1973; pp. 28-29. (Grubb family files). Also see reference 13 below re the Laos list, and further testimony before Congress in 1991 on these MIA issues when the POWs returned home.

[9]Later,POW/MIA Senate Select Committee report XXI addressed the Laos issue on MIA, also possible POWs left in Laos. As Ambassador Winston Lord, (Kissinger's executive assistant and team member at the secret Peace negotiations in Paris) testified: "The President in the end decided not to scuttle the agreement and resume the war over the MIA question. It was a very difficult decision. I believed then it was a correct one. I believe that still. Although we had strongly suggestive intelligence that the lists [were] incomplete, the American society would have blown apart if the President overturned the [Paris Peace] agreement and resumed the fighting. It is doubtful that Congress would have supported such a policy. Indeed, it would probably have prevented it. Remaining prisoners who were on the lists would not have returned. More Americans and Vietnamese allies would have been killed and captured." (http://www.aiipowmia.com/ssc/ssc21.html).

[10]Leona Angell letter. (Grubb family files).

[11]*Washington Star,* April 19, 1973.

[12]Watergate effectively distracted President Nixon's attention from monitoring the Vietnam Peace Agreement. Kissinger wrote, "By mid-April [1973] some 35,000 North Vietnamese troops had entered South Vietnam or nearby sanctuaries . . . In the past, this would have been the precursor to strong decisions. Not now. When Haig reported on April 15, Nixon procrastinated again. . . ." (*Ending the Vietnam War,* op. cit. pp. 467-468). Failure to act on the part of the United States assured the North Vietnamese that they could violate the treaty without fear of military retribution from the U.S.

[13]The families were right. Watergate was their Waterloo.

[14]The difficulty here is regarding the terms of the secret agreements to the Peace Accords. Congressional testimony gives additional insights into the "hot button" issues of: correct count of MIA; Controversy over PDF (Presumptive Finding of Death); POWs known alive but families not notified immediately; and science and methods employed for body identification accuracy in Hawaii in this report: (www.aiipowmia.com/testimony/handrws.html). That there was a "Laos List" is supported by many reports. A handful of POWs from Laos were sent to Hanoi and released there with other POWs. (League Board Minutes, Attachments, April, 1973, Grubb Family files).

[15]Attorney Dermot G. Foley's correspondence, Feb. 22, 1973. (League Board Minutes, Attachments, March 8,1973.) A "South Texas' concern: that Watergate will hinder getting all our men back. Will Nixon be too concerned with Watergate to work for our men . . . ?" (League Board Minutes, Attachments, May 1973).

[16]The Foreign Claims Settlement Commission is an independent agency within the Department of Justice that adjudicates claims of U.S. nationals against foreign governments. (www.usdoj.gov).

[17]Ibid.

[18]Clipping of Newspaper article, publication unidentified, clipping contains photo credit, "Staff Photo by Hank Bilyeu," (Grubb family files).

[19]The term "recovery" as used by the Defense Department, includes the recovery of captured, detained, evading, isolated, or missing personnel from hostile areas. The term "accounting" is usually limited to the recovery of persons in missing status. Accounting includes the return of the person, the person's identifiable remains, or credible evidence for another status, such as the Presumptive Finding of Death. (DoDD 2310.2 and 2310.7).

[20]"Heartbreak Hotel" prison camp became the in-screening and initial interrogation of most new POWS. New Guy Village nearby was also used for in-processing. Both were in Hoa Loa, the infamous "Hanoi Hilton." It has not been agreed who named Hoa Loa prison the "Hanoi Hilton," but Bob Shumaker scratched the message, "Welcome to the Hanoi Hilton" on a pail to greet Air Force Lt. Robert Peel in 1965. The nickname stuck. (*Honor Bound*, op. cit, pp. 90-96).

[21]Air Force Lt. Col. Robinson Risner was a Korean War ace pilot. A squadron commander in Vietnam featured on the cover of *Time* (April 23, 1965) as exemplifying the dedicated military professional of the Vietnam War. Reisner was shot down and captured over North Vietnam Sept. 16, 1965, September of 1965. Reports from early returning prisoners, and his own account in his 1973 memoir, revealed that he had been brutally tortured, many times. (*The Passing of the Night*, op. cit.).

[22]A note on an Arlington Cemetery website indicated that two other Ex-POWs, William "Bill" Tschudy (USN) and Herschel "Scotty" Morgan (USAF) had heard Newk Grubb's full prison camp tape recording played over the camp loudspeaker system (the irreverent POWs named it "CBS, Camp Bullshit System") in Briarpatch when Tschudy and Morgan were in cell C-3 there in Sept.1966. At author C. Jose's request, Col Al Brunstrom, who personally knows both men, con-

firmed this in a telecon with "Scotty" Morgan on April 19, 2008. Morgan recalled one statement Newk made on the tape was, "they made me fly, they paid me to fly . . ." Brunstrom also consulted Bill Tschudy, who recalled hearing the tape. Brunstrom/Jose conferred by email/telecom on March 5&6 and April 18&19, 2008, re the Tschudy/Morgan recollections and his own experience in Hearbreak. (www.arlingtoncemetery.net/wngrubb.htm).

[23] The speculation by fellow POWs that Newk most likely had been tortured to death for information, was painful but not surprising for Evie. She believed it. The League Board had already been briefed by the returning POWs about the extreme torture conditions in Hanoi. (Grubb family files).

. [24] Photo, p. 157, and End Note #26 p. 631, in *Honor Bound*, op. cit.

[25] The League Board received a copy of Maj. James "Nick" Rowe's acceptance speech on behalf of all POW/MIA. He is buried in Arlington Cemetery, Section 48.

[26] The Paris Peace Accords established a 60-day, Four-Party Military Commission to execute the tasks set forth in the Accords. The Accords also provided for a Four-Party Military Team to continue the search and accounting for missing personnel after the termination of the Four-Party Military Commission. This political team operated until the fall of the Saigon government in April 1975. (www.miafacts.org).

[27] Special Report with a recap of General Ogan's remarks to the League is in the League Minutes (Grubb family files).

[28] USAF letter, May 1973. (Grubb family files).

[29] The peace agreement Kissinger negotiated with Vietnam is variously referred to as the Vietnam peace agreement, the Vietnam Accords, the Paris Agreement or the Paris Accords, even by Dr. Kissinger in his book. Therefore, you may see it referred to differently in various quotations which are excerpted as they are written. Kissinger remarks that "after the events of the summer of 1973 Vietnam disappeared as a policy issue." In August 1973, Kissinger was appointed Secretary of State by Nixon, and Kissinger and Le Duc Tho were awarded the Nobel Peace Prize "for negotiating the Vietnam agreement."

[30] Notes in Grubb family files.

[31] League Board Minutes, July 1973. (Grubb family files).

[32] Helene Knapp, League letter to President Nixon. (Grubb family files).

[33] Kissinger's frustration with the failure of North Vietnam to abide by the Peace Agreement, the lack of progress of return of the bodies of POWs who had died in captivity, and the status of accounting for the Missing In Action was underscored in an article entitled, "Dr. Kissinger 'Extremely Dissatisfied' with MIA Accountability" in *DOD Commanders Digest*, Vol. 14, no. 23, Dec. 6, 1973, an edition that focused on MIAs. "The only cooperation we have received is the visit to gravesites of some 23 Americans who died in captivity in North Vietnam," said Kissinger.

[34] League Minutes, 1973. (Grubb family files).

[35] Asked why the United States completed the withdrawal of its troops without insisting that the Pathet Lao first identify and release U.S. POWs whom they were believed to be holding, Admiral Moorer stated: "Don't forget, [the President] was

getting tremendous pressure from the Congress, the public, and the *New York Times,* and the *Washington Post,* everyone you could think of. They had had a belly-full of this whole war. I think we almost would have had a rebellion if we had turned around and started fighting like hell in Laos again. That's my explanation of it." (POW/MIA Senate Select Committee Hearing XXI: www.aiipowmia.com/ssc/ssc21.html).

Chapter 12

[1]" 'We are extremely dissatisfied' with the results of the implementation to date of those provisions of the agreement that provide for an accounting for all persons held prisoner or missing in action, Dr. Kissinger reemphasized." (*DOD Commanders Digest,* Dec. 6, 1973, op. cit., p.16).

[2]Kissinger notes that in 1973 "Nixon was simply unable to concentrate his energies and mind on Vietnam. The record shows that he was engaged in incessant meetings and telephone calls on Watergate.... By the end of April 1973, therefore, both carrots and sticks for enforcing the Vietnam agreement were in tatters. When in June of 1973 Congress prohibited the use of military force 'in or over Indochina' the United States was effectively forbidden to enforce an Agreement for which over 55,000 Americans and hundreds of thousands of Vietnamese had given their lives . . ." (*Ending the Vietnam War,* op. cit., pp. 468- 469).

[3]The Geneva Convention death certificate from the North Vietnamese, claiming Newk died of "grievous wounds on bailout" gave his date of death as Feb. 4, 1966 and it accompanied the return of Newk's identified remains in March 1974. Official notification of "termination of the captured status" of her husband was sent 2 April 1974 in a detailed chronology letter from USAF Maj. Gen T. R. McNeil, Headquarters, USAF. President Nixon confirmed his death in a letter.

[4]Returning POWs in 1973 charged that the North Vietnamese captors deliberately broke the ribs of their prisoners and left them unset. "At Last the Story Can Be Told," (*Time.* According to *Time* internet archives, the publication date was Monday, April 9, 1973, but the article was probably published in the April 19, 1973, issue.)

[5]Ibid.

[6]Nixon letter, April 3, 1974. (Grubb family files).

[7]The missing man formation is an aerial salute that is flown by the military services to honor a dead comrade in arms. Four aircraft approach the site flying in formation and low. When directly overhead, one of the aircraft abruptly pulls up into a steep climb while the rest of the formation continues level flight until they are out of sight. (*Wikipedia*) For more information on Grubb's Arlington funeral see: www.arlingtoncemetary/wngrubb.

[8]Nixon letter, April 16, 1974, Condolence letter confirming Newk's death. (Grubb family files).

[9]In 1996, an MIA search team was sent to Ha Bac province in North Vietnam to investigate a 1967 report of a downed U.S. plane there. The team recovered pieces of a plane similar to an Intruder, and four bone fragments. DNA testing linked the

fragments to Navy LCDR. James Plowman, 23, and concluded that the crash was nonsurvivable. His remains were interred at Arlington National Cemetery on Sept. 20, 2006. (www.pownetwork.org/bios/p/p043.htm).

[10]Tuskegee Airman and Air Force General Daniel ("Chappie") James: In March 1970 Chappie became Deputy Assistant Secretary of Defense for Public Affairs and advanced to the rank of Major General. In September 1974, with the rank of Lieutenant General, he became Vice Commander of the Military Airlift Command at Scott Air Force Base, Illinois. In September 1975 he became the first black officer in the history of the United States military to attain four-star full General rank. Chappie retired from the Air Force in early February 1978, and passed away of a heart attack several weeks later. He is buried in Section 2 of Arlington National Cemetery.(www.arlingtoncemetery.net/djames.htm).

[11]In June of 1973, the U.S. Congress blocked the use of appropriated funds for any military activity in Indochina, including Vietnam, Laos, and Cambodia, beyond August 15, 1973. (Karnow, Stanley. *Vietnam: A History*, New York: The Viking Press, 1983, p. 656).

[12]During his debrief, Emmet Kay stated that he had no knowledge of any other Americans being held in Laos. He also said that he had been told by the Pathet Lao that he was the only American being held there and that all U.S. POWs were released in 1973 during Operation Homecoming. (www.aiipowmia.com/ssc/ssc21.html)

[13]Iris Powers' MIA son: On April 2, 1969, WO1 Lowell S. Powers, pilot; Major Butler, plus an unidentified crew chief and gunner comprised the crew of a CH47 helicopter (serial #67-18523) conducting a mission for Allied troops. Shortly after takeoff, the Chinook dropped back to earth, rolling down a ravine onto its left side. Maj. Butler radioed for help, giving location and evaluation. He asked pilot Lowell Powers if he was all right. Powers replied he was OK. Butler saw Powers release his harness and crawl back to the passenger compartment. Maj. Butler exited the aircraft through the left window, and never saw Lowell Powers again. No trace of Powers was found. The aircraft later caught fire and burned. (http://taskforceomegainc.org/p085.html).

[14]Iris Powers Congressional testimony, 1974. (Grubb family files).

[15]Louise's husband, Navy Commander James A. Mulligan, was captured in March 1966 and repatriated in February 1973. In prison camp in Hanoi, he became a "walking memory bank . . . and could recite 450 names of POWs from memory when released." (*Honor Bound*, op. cit., p. 105).

[16]Iris Powers Congressional testimony, 1974. (Grubb family files).

Index